PEDIATRIC SPINE SURGERY

SECOND EDITION

PEDIATRIC SPINE SURGERY

SECOND EDITION

Editor
STUART L. WEINSTEIN, MD

Ignacio V. Ponseti Chair of Orthopaedic Surgery
Department of Orthopaedic Surgery
University of Iowa Hospitals
Iowa City, Iowa

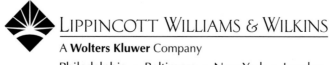

LIPPINCOTT WILLIAMS & WILKINS
A **Wolters Kluwer** Company

Philadelphia · Baltimore · New York · London
Buenos Aires · Hong Kong · Sydney · Tokyo

Acquisitions Editor: Robert Hurley
Developmental Editor: Anne Snyder
Production Editor: Steven P. Martin
Manufacturing Manager: Colin J. Warnock
Cover Designer: Mark Lerner
Compositor: Maryland Composition
Printer: Edwards Brothers

© 2001 by LIPPINCOTT WILLIAMS & WILKINS
530 Walnut Street
Philadelphia, PA 19106 USA
LWW.com

Printed in the USA

Library of Congress Cataloging-in-Publication Data

Pediatric spine surgery / editor, Stuart L. Weinstein.—2nd ed.
        p. ; cm.
    Includes bibliographical references and index.
    ISBN 0-7817-3151-8 (casebound)
    1. Spine—Surgery. 2. Spinal cord—Surgery. 3. Pediatric orthopedics. I. Weinstein, Stuart L.
    [DNLM: 1. Spinal Diseases—surgery—Child. 2. Orthopaedic Procedures—Child. WE 725
P3713 2000]
    RD768 P365 2000
    617.5′6059′083—dc21
                                                                00-061642

10 9 8 7 6 5 4 3 2 1

To L.K.W. and W.S.W.
for their love, encouragement,
understanding, and continued support

CONTENTS

Section V: Complications of Surgery 559

CONTRIBUTING AUTHORS

William A. Abdu, MD Associate Professor of Orthopaedic Surgery, Department of Orthopaedic Surgery, Dartmouth-Hitchcock Medical Center, One Medical Center Drive, Lebanon, New Hampshire 03756

Max Aebi, MD Orthopaedic Surgeon In Chief, Division of Orthopaedic Surgery, Royal Victoria Hospital; McGill University, Department of Orthopaedic Surgery, 681 Pine Avenue West, Montreal, Quebec H3A 1A1 Canada

Vincent Arlet, MD Associate Professor, Department of Surgery, McGill University, Division of Orthopaedics; Montreal Children's Hospital, 2300 rue Tupper, Suite C-1112, Montreal, Quebec, H3H 1P3 Canada

Marc A. Asher, MD Professor of Orthopaedic Surgery, The University of Kansas Medical Center, 3901 Rainbow Boulevard, Kansas City, Kansas 66160-7387

Thomas E. Bailey, Jr., MD Clinical Professor of Surgery, Orthopaedic, Medical College of Georgia, Chief of Orthopaedic Surgery, University Hospital, 820 St. Sebastian Way, Suite 8A, Augusta, Georgia 30901-2668

Randal R. Betz, MD Professor, Department of Orthopaedic Surgery, Temple University School of Medicine, 3401 N. Broad Street, Philadelphia, Pennsylvania 19140; Chief of Staff, Shriners Hospitals for Children, 3551 North Broad Street, Philadelphia, Pennsylvania 19140

Norbert Boos, MD Chief of Spine Surgery, Orthopaedic University Hospital Balgrist, Forchstrasse 340, CH-8008 Zurich, Switzerland,

David S. Bradford, MD Professor and Chairman, Department of Orthopaedic Surgery, University of California, San Francisco, 500 West Parnassus Avenue, MU 320 West, San Francisco, California 94143-0728

Jack C. Y. Cheng, MD Professor and Chairman, Department of Orthopaedics and Traumatology, Chinese University of Hong Kong, 5th Floor, Clinical Sciences Building, Prince of Wales Hospital, Shatin, New Territories, Hong Kong SAR

Samuel J. Chewning Jr., MD Miller Orthopaedic Clinic, Inc, Medical Center Plaza, 1001 Blythe Boulevard, Suite 200, Charlotte, North Carolina 28203

Haemish Crawford, MD Consultant Orthopaedic Surgeon, Starship Children's Hospital, Auckland, New Zealand

Bryan W. Cunningham, MSC Director of Spinal Research, Department of Orthopaedic Surgery, Union Memorial Hospital, 201 East University Parkway, Baltimore, Maryland 21218

Andrei A. Czitrom, MD, PhD Clinical Associate Professor of Surgery, University of Texas Southwestern Medical Center, Dallas, Texas 75230; Orthopaedic Center of Dallas, Suite C707, 7777 Forest Lane, Dallas, Texas 75230

Jesse H. Dickson, MD Clinical Professor, Department of Orthopaedic Surgery, Baylor College of Medicine, 6550 Fanning Street, # 1900, Houston, Texas 77030

Ron L. Ferguson, MD Shriners Hospital for Children 911 W. 5th, PO Box 2472, Spokane, Washington 99210-2472

Robert B. Forbes, MD Professor, Department of Anesthesia, University of Iowa College of Medicine, Iowa City, Iowa 52242-1079; Staff Anesthesiologist, Department of Anesthesia, Children's Hospital, 200 Hawkins Drive, Iowa City, Iowa 52242

K.Y. Fung Adjunct Associate Professor, Department of Orthopaedics and Traumatology, Chinese University, Shatin, New Territories, Hong Kong, SAR; Consultant Orthopaedic Surgeon, Department of Orthopaedics and Traumatology, 5th Floor, Clinical Science Building, Prince of Wales Hospital, Shatin, New Territories, Hong Kong SAR

Neil E. Green, MD Department of Orthopaedic Surgery, Room D4207, Vanderbilt University Medical Center North, Nashville, Tennessee 37232-2550

Michael Grevitt, FRCS Consultant Spinal Surgeon, Centre for Spinal Studies and Surgery, University Hospital, Queen's Medical Centre, Nottingham, NG7 2UH, United Kingdom

Charles F. Heinig, MD *(Retired)* Spinal Surgeon, Department of Orthopaedics, The Miller Orthopaedic Clinic, 1001 Blythe Boulevard, Charlotte, North Carolina 28203

John A. Herring, MD   Professor, Department of Orthopaedic Surgery, University of Texas SouthWestern Medical School, 5323 Harry Hines Boulevard, Dallas, Texas 75225; Chief of Staff, Texas Scottish Rite Hospital for Children, 2222 Welborn Street, Dallas, Texas 75219

Kamal Ibrahim, MD   Department of Orthopaedics and Rehabilitation, Loyola University, Maywood, Illinois 60153; M & M Orthopaedics, Downers Grove, Illinois 60515.

Kiyoshi Kaneda, MD   Department of Orthopaedic Surgery, Hokkaido University School of Medicine, Kita-15, Nishi-7, Kita-ku, Sapporo 060, Japan

Lee A. Kelley, MD   Peachtree Orthopaedic Clinic, 2001 Peachtree Road NE, #705, Atlanta, Georgia 30309

J. Ivan Krajbich, MD   Department of Orthopaedic Surgery, Shriners Hospital for Children, 3101 S.W. Sam Jackson Park Road, Portland, Oregon 97201-3095

Guy A. Lee, MD   Spine Surgeon, Orthopaedic Specialty Care, 2400 Maryland Avenue, Willow Grove, Pennsylvania 19090

Lawrence G. Lenke, MD   Associate Professor, Department of Orthopaedic Surgery, Washington University School of Medicine, #1 Barnes Hospital Plaza, 11300 West Pavilion, St. Louis, Missouri 63110

Thomas G. Lowe, MD   Woodridge Orthopaedic and Spine Center, P.C., 3550 Lutheran Parkway West, Suite 201, Wheat Ridge, Colorado 80033

Masafumi Machida, MD   Department of Orthopaedic Surgery, Nihon University School of Medicine, 30-1 Oyaguchi, Itabashi-ku, Tokyo 173, Japan

Paul C. McAfee, MD   Chief of Spinal Surgery, Department of Orthopaedic Surgery, St. Joseph's Hospital 7505 Osler Drive, Baltimore, Maryland 21204

John McClellan, MD   Department of Orthopaedic Surgery, University of Nebraska Medical Center, 600 S. 42nd Street, Omaha, Nebraska 68198; Nebraska Spine Center, 11819 Miracle Hill Drive, Suite 102, Omaha, Nebraska 68514

Robert F. McLain, MD   Section of Spine Surgery, Department of Orthopaedic Surgery, A41, The Cleveland Clinic Foundation, 9500 Euclid Avenue, A41, Cleveland, Ohio 44195

Arnold H. Menezes, MD   Professor and Vice Chairman, Division of Neurosurgery, University of Iowa Hospitals and Clinics, 200 Hawkins Drive, Iowa City, Iowa 52242-1061

Kan Min, MD   Orthopaedic Spine Surgeon, Orthopaedic University Hospital Balgrist, Forchstrasse 340, CH-8008 Zurich, Switzerland

Antonello Montanaro, MD   Second Division of Orthopaedic Surgery, Children's Hospital, Ospedale Bambino Gesu, Via Torre di Palidoro, 00050 Passoscuro, Rome, Italy

David J. Murray, MD   Department of Anesthesiology, Washington University School of Medicine, 3rd Floor, BUC South Campus, 880 S Luclid Street, St. Louis, Missouri 63110; Associate Director, Department of Anesthesia, St. Louis Children's Hospital, 5531 One Children's Place, St. Louis, Missouri 63110

Peter O. Newton, MD   Assistant Clinical Professor, Department of Orthopaedic Surgery, University of California, San Diego, 200 W. Harbor Drive, San Diego, California 92103; Chief of Scoliosis Programs, Department of Orthopaedic Surgery, Children's Hospital and Health Center, 3030 Children's Way, Suite 410, San Diego, California 92123

Christopher W. Reilly, MD, FRCSC   Department of Paediatric Orthopaedic Surgery, British Columbia's Children's Hospital, 4480 Oak Street, Vancouver, British Columbia V6H 3V4, Canada

Vittorio Salsano, MD (Deceased)   Second Division of Orthopaedic Surgery, Ospedale Pediatrico Bambino Gesu IRCCS, Via Torre Di Palinoro, Rome, Italy 00050

Mark A. Ross, MD   Department of Neurology, University of Kentucky Medical Center, KY Clinic (Wing D) - L445, Lexington, Kentucky 40536-0284

Harry L. Shufflebarger, MD   Chief, Department of Orthopaedic Surgery, Division of Spinal Surgery, Miami Children's Hospital, 3100 SW 62nd Avenue, Miami, Florida 33155-3009

Jason A. Smith, MD   Assistant Professor, Spinal Disorders Service, Department of Orthopaedics, University of California, San Francisco, 500 West Parnassus Avenue, MU320W, San Francisco, California 94143-0728

J. Andrew Sullivan, MD   Department of Orthopaedic Surgery, University of Oklahoma College of Medicine, 940 NE 13th Street, CHO 2MR2000, Oklahoma City, Oklahoma 73104

Stephen J. Tredwell, MD, FRCSC   Professor, Department of Paediatric Orthopaedic Surgery, British Columbia's Children's Hospital, 480 Oak Street, Vancouver, British Columbia V6H 3V4, Canada

Francesco Turturro, MD   Pediatric Orthopaedic Surgery, Second Division of Orthopaedic Surgery, Ospedale Pediatrico Bambino Gesu IRCCS, Via Torre di Palidoro, Rome, Italy 00050

John Webb, FRCS   Director, Centre for Spinal Studies and Surgery, University Hospital, Queen's Medical Centre, Nottingham NG7 2UH, United Kingdom

James N. Weinstein, DO, MS Professor, Department of Community and Family Medicine, Dartmouth Medical School, 7251 Strasenburgh Hall, Hanover, New Hampshire 03755; Director, The Spine Center, Dartmouth-Hitchcock Medical Center, One Medical Center Drive, Lebanon, New Hampshire 03756,

Stuart L. Weinstein, MD Ignacio V. Ponseti Chair of Orthopaedic Surgery, Department of Orthopaedic Surgery, University of Iowa, Iowa City, Iowa 52242

Thomas S. Whitecloud III, MD Professor and Chairman, Chief Spine Surgeon, Department of Orthopaedics, Tulane Medical Center, 1430 Tulane Avenue, New Orleans, Louisiana 70112

Thoru Yamada, MD Division of Clinical Electrophysiology, Department of Neurology, University of Iowa College of Medicine, Carver Pavilion, Iowa City, Iowa 52242

Michael R. Zindrick, MD Department of Orthopaedics, Loyola University, 550 West Ogden Avenue, Hinsdale, Illinois 60521

PREFACE

Pediatric Spine Surgery is devoted primarily to surgical approaches and techniques. The challenges of choosing the right operative approach and the right technique are among the most difficult a spine surgeon faces. These choices may profoundly affect outcomes.

This book thoroughly covers intraoperative considerations, including anesthetic considerations, neurophysiology and spinal cord monitoring. With their considerable experience and expertise, the authors of each chapter provide complete and in-depth coverage of each subject. The presentation of surgical approaches and techniques is well detailed and illustrated, but this volume is more than an atlas. Operative approach chapters describe variations in technique, and specific advantages, disadvantages, and complications. Technique chapters emphasize indications, contraindications, pitfalls, and the etiology, prevention, and treatment of complications. Chapters on implants place strong emphasis on basic science, particularly on biomechanics, in addition to detailed explanation of surgical techniques.

Pediatric Spine Surgery is aimed at the senior resident and practicing pediatric spine specialist. It should also be of interest to orthopaedic surgeons and neurosurgeons.

Stuart L. Weinstein, MD

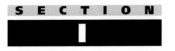

SECTION

I

INTRAOPERATIVE CONSIDERATIONS

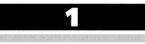

ANESTHETIC CONSIDERATIONS

DAVID J. MURRAY
ROBERT B. FORBES

Before the introduction of ether anesthesia into clinical medicine in 1846, attempts at surgery, including amputations and repair of congenital deformities, were performed on pediatric patients without any effective form of anesthesia or analgesia. Children were simply physically restrained while the surgical procedures were completed with lightening speed and predictably dismal outcomes (118). As the advantages of general anesthesia and its ability to abolish pain were recognized, an impression grew that ether anesthesia could be safely and effectively administered by anyone, including orderlies, nurses, and occasionally even the patient's parents (18). This led to numerous complications and catastrophes, and for much of the next century, anesthesiology, as a specialty, rarely received the respect it deserved. Consequently, there was great difficulty attracting dedicated physicians with the special interest and expertise necessary to anesthetize young children safely for complex surgical procedures.

Despite this initially slow progress, the specialty of pediatric anesthesia did ultimately emerge as the unique requirements of pediatric patients were recognized and as new drugs, technology, and clinical expertise were developed to address these demands. Today, pediatric anesthesiologists caring for children undergoing spinal surgery have a sophisticated array of pharmacologic agents and monitoring equipment at their disposal. Both the emotional and physical well-being of each child are of paramount concern and are incorporated into the anesthetic care the child receives as he or she is guided through the perioperative period.

PREANESTHETIC EVALUATION

The purpose of the preanesthetic visit is to establish rapport with the child and family, assess the patient's medical condition, identify potential anesthetic problems, and develop an anesthetic plan. Although the preoperative evaluation must be adapted to the clinical situation, it usually begins with a thorough review of the hospital chart. The child's state of health, medications, and the presence of other coexisting diseases should be evaluated, with particular attention paid to problems encountered during

D. J. Murray: Washington University Clinical Stimulation Center, Department of Anesthesiology, St. Louis, Missouri 63110.
R. B. Forbes: Department of Anesthesia, University of Iowa College of Medicine, Iowa City, Iowa 52242.

previous anesthetics and to any family history of anesthetic complications. Results of laboratory evaluations, radiographs, and medical consultations should be reviewed. After reviewing the child's hospital chart, the anesthesiologist interviews the patient and parents to obtain a more complete medical history with attention directed toward factors that are pertinent to the child's anesthetic management. The emotional state of the child and parents must also be evaluated and their fears or concerns addressed. Finally, a careful physical examination is performed in a gentle, nonthreatening manner.

The Respiratory System

The airway and respiratory system of an infant or young child differ anatomically and physiologically from the respiratory system of an adult (Fig. 1). These differences predispose the infant to airway obstruction and can make endotracheal intubation more difficult (56). Differences in pulmonary physiology make children more prone to atelectasis and hypoxia than adults and contribute to a higher incidence of perioperative respiratory complications. Their airways are small, and resistance to airflow is high. The ribs are horizontally oriented and cannot provide substantial lung expansion from the "bucket-handle" effect seen in adults. Also, the cartilaginous ribs of an infant may retract inward when the child generates negative intrathoracic pressure on inspiration. Alveoli in the pediatric lung are small, have a relatively high surface tension, and are prone to atelectasis. The muscles of respiration are more susceptible to fatigue. In addition, children also have high oxygen consumption, and their rapid respiratory rate provides the higher minute ventilation required to meet their additional oxygen requirements. All these factors combine to leave children with little pulmonary reserve to call on if airway obstruction or respiratory failure occurs. Therefore, careful preanesthetic examination of the pulmonary system is essential if complications are to be avoided.

Signs or symptoms of acute airway disease, such as fever, cough, wheezing, or abnormal breath sounds, should prompt further evaluation and perhaps consultation with a pediatrician. A careful history and physical examination should reveal whether the disease is adequately controlled or whether additional treatment is needed before surgery (67).

The Cardiovascular System

The cardiovascular system, like the respiratory system, develops and matures rapidly during early childhood. Immediately after

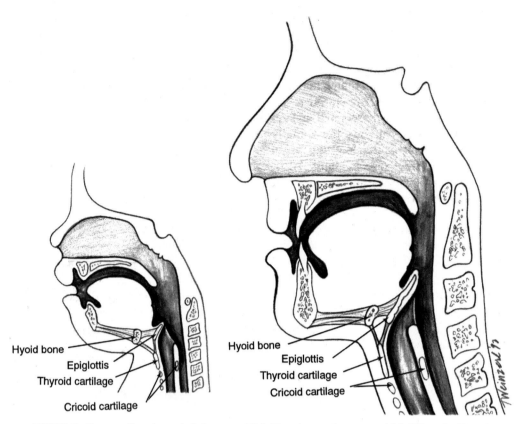

FIGURE 1. Comparative airway (adult versus child). The airway of a young child differs significantly from that of an adult. The tongue is large, the mandible is small, and the epiglottis and larynx are positioned higher in the neck, making exposure of the vocal cords during laryngoscopy more difficult.

birth, there is a change from fetal to neonatal circulation, with functional closure of the foramen ovale and ductus arteriosus. Anatomic closure of these shunts may not occur for days or weeks, and 20% to 30% of the adult population may have a patent foramen ovale. In children, particularly premature infants, an increase in right atrial pressure can open the foramen ovale or ductus arteriosus, producing a right-to-left shunt and cyanosis. A newborn's myocardium contains a larger proportion of connective tissue and is relatively noncompliant. Compared with an adult, a newborn must maintain a higher cardiac output and, because the left ventricle is relatively noncompliant, has limited ability to augment cardiac output by increasing stroke volume. Therefore, children are highly dependent on heart rate to maintain an adequate cardiac output.

Autonomic control of the cardiovascular system is immature at birth. The myocardium and peripheral vasculature have fewer sympathetic receptors than occur in adults. Consequently, sympathetic stimulation and peripheral vasoconstriction may not maintain blood pressure in a hypovolemic or hypotensive neonate. In contrast, parasympathetic innervation of the heart is active, and vagal stimulation can cause severe bradycardia in children. By about 5 to 6 years of age, a child's cardiovascular system functions much like that of an adult. If a heart defect is known or suspected, the preoperative evaluation should include an electrocardiogram, chest radiograph, hemoglobin, and hemo-

globin saturation. For accurate diagnosis of specific lesions, evaluation of their physiologic effects, and institution of appropriate treatment, consultation with a cardiologist may be necessary. When a child with congenital heart disease comes for surgery, it is particularly important that the patient receive appropriate prophylaxis against subacute bacterial endocarditis.

Fluid and Electrolyte Balance

Intravenous administration of water and electrolytes is an integral part of anesthesia care, and an assessment of fluid balance is essential during the immediate preoperative period. Young children have a high total-body water content (40% of body weight) that decreases during the first year of life to 20%. Dehydration can occur rapidly during periods of fasting. Neonates manifest hypovolemia by decreased peripheral perfusion, hypoxia, metabolic acidosis, hypothermia, and hemoconcentration. In older children, changes in weight, along with a history of fluid loss such as emesis, diarrhea, or gastric suction, are evidence of developing dehydration. Signs of dehydration include dry mucosa, tachycardia, tachypnea, oliguria, sunken fontanelles, and decreased skin turgor. Blood pressure and mental status are well preserved until a patient is 15% dehydrated. Urine specific gravity and urine sodium may also be useful when assessing a child's fluid requirements. If the child appears dehydrated, serum electrolytes should be measured to distinguish hypernatremia and hyponatremia and to help guide perioperative fluid therapy. Any abnormalities must be corrected before elective surgery.

The Nervous System

A careful history and physical examination should identify disorders of the neuromuscular system and provide an assessment of the severity of the abnormality and its effect on the child's anesthetic management. Children admitted to the hospital with traumatic injuries must be evaluated for signs of intracranial pathology, including bleeding or cerebral edema. An altered level of consciousness, nausea, vomiting, and papilledema all suggest the presence of increased intracranial pressure. This can have a profound effect on anesthetic management because the volatile anesthetics, hypoxia, and hypercarbia may all adversely affect a patient with a serious head injury by increasing cerebral blood flow and exacerbating intracranial hypertension.

In children with seizure disorders, the serum levels of anticonvulsants should be determined before surgery and drug doses adjusted to ensure that serum levels are in the therapeutic range.

Muscular dystrophy and congenital myotonias may be associated with impaired respiratory function, cardiac dysrhythmias, and an altered response to succinylcholine that can produce a sustained muscular contracture, interfere with ventilation, and produce severe hyperkalemia precipitating cardiac arrest. Finally, with the increasing use of regional anesthesia for postoperative analgesia, it is important that existing sensory or motor deficits be documented during the preanesthetic evaluation.

The Hematologic System

The two primary reasons for hematologic evaluation before anesthesia and surgery are to ensure that the child's blood volume and oxygen-carrying capacity are sufficient to meet oxygen demands throughout the perioperative period (108) and to identify the presence of any situation, either a preexisting disease or medications, that may interfere with normal coagulation and contribute to excessive intraoperative bleeding (103).

A minimal acceptable hemoglobin concentration necessary for elective surgery is difficult to define in children patients because their hematocrit changes with age. A newborn infant has a high concentration of fetal hemoglobin. After birth, the hemoglobin concentration begins to fall, and by 3 months of age, it may be as low as 10 g/dL (95). After a nadir in red cell production at 3 months of age, hemoglobin production increases, so that by 1 year of age, a normal hematocrit is observed. Although childhood anemia is often a result of nutritional deficiencies, the presence of other important diseases, such as thalassemia, sickle cell anemia, or leukemia, must be evaluated before elective surgery.

Coagulation disorders are rarely asymptomatic. Only if the child has a history of easy bruising or excessive bleeding after minor injuries or surgery or if drugs such as antiinflammatory medications are used should coagulation studies, such as prothrombin time, partial thromboplastin time, fibrinogen level, platelet count, or bleeding time, be obtained.

TABLE 1. AMERICAN SOCIETY OF ANESTHESIOLOGISTS CLASSIFICATION OF PHYSICAL STATUS

Class	Description
I	A normal, healthy patient
II	A patient with a mild systemic disease
III	A patient with a severe systemic disease that limits activity but is not incapacitating
IV	A patient with an incapacitating disease that is a constant threat to life
V	A moribund patient who is not expected to survive 24 hours with or without surgery
E	A patient undergoing an emergency procedure

Laboratory Studies

The laboratory tests ordered before anesthesia and surgery should be selected only after completing a history and physical examination (76,96). The general medical condition of the patient and the nature of the surgical procedure determine the appropriate laboratory tests (75). A battery of screening tests is costly, and even the minimum requirement of a hematocrit and urinalysis in healthy children older than 1 year of age does not detect asymptomatic disease in otherwise healthy patients.

A healthy child having a minor elective procedure in which blood loss is expected to be minimal may not need any laboratory or radiologic examinations. Studies evaluating the usefulness of chest radiographs (135), hemoglobin or hematocrit determinations, urinalysis, coagulation studies (103), electrocardiography, and biochemical panels to assess hepatic and renal function in symptom-free patients found that unexpected disease was rarely identified (128). The ideal method for selecting laboratory tests before anesthesia is to take a careful medical history, complete an appropriate physical examination, and order only those tests that are indicated from signs and symptoms elicited by the history and physical examination. From the information obtained during the preanesthetic assessment, each child can be assigned an American Society of Anesthesiologists (ASA) physical classification (5), which is useful for estimating anesthetic risk and anticipating outcome (Table 1).

PREOPERATIVE PREPARATION

Physiologic Preparation

Anesthesiologists can play an important role in alleviating the psychological stress that children and their families experience in the perioperative period. Sources of anxiety for children change as they mature. The preoperative preparation required depends on the child's age, previous experience with anesthesia and surgery, and support received from family (120). An important goal for an anesthesiologist is to establish rapport with the patient and the family and gain their trust and confidence. This can best be accomplished during the preanesthetic visit by providing simple, straightforward explanations of the events that will occur. Questions from the child or the parents must be answered honestly, and it is important to reassure the patient that his or her concerns or anxieties will be taken seriously and that the child will be treated with empathy while in the operating room. Many hospitals have special tours or slide shows that introduce children to the hospital and the operating room and that demonstrate many of the situations they will encounter when they come for their surgery. With careful preoperative preparation, many children come to the operating room with their parents in a calm and cooperative state of mind, making pharmacologic sedation unnecessary.

Preanesthetic Medication

Newer anesthetic agents permit anesthesia to be induced quickly and pleasantly. Liberal visitation policies allow parents to stay with the child during induction, which eliminates a major cause of preoperative anxiety and reduces the need for heavy sedation. However, many anesthesiologists continue to premedicate children before surgery. The most common reasons for administering premedication are to lessen anxiety, provide sedation and analgesia, produce amnesia, and block unwanted autonomic reflexes.

There has been a long search for the ideal drug to sedate children before surgery. What is required is a medication that is easily and painlessly administered; results in all children being calm, yet arousable; and is eliminated quickly so that postoperative recovery is not delayed. To date, this ideal premedication for children does not exist, and it probably never will. Consequently, combinations of drugs are frequently used in an effort to create an effective but safe sedation regimen. No combination of drugs, nor route of administration, has been found that is consistently effective in all children, and as the number of drugs in the combination increases, so does the incidence of complications.

The types of drugs most commonly used to produce preoperative sedation include sedative-anxiolytics, narcotics, and anticholinergics (62,72). The timing and route of administration of the premedication are also extremely important. Fear of intramuscular injections is widespread among children, and intramuscular injections should be avoided whenever possible. In addition, there is increasing interest in administering a variety of premedicant drugs in new ways, such as nasal instillation (65,134), transdermal patches, or oral transmucosal fentanyl citrate (45). The onset and duration of action of preoperative medications should also be kept in mind to ensure that they will be effective when they are needed most. In a large, busy operating room, last-minute changes in the operating schedule and delays in communicating instructions can make the appropriate timing of sedation difficult. After the medication has been given, the child should be disturbed as little as possible if the drugs are to be maximally effective.

Sedative Anxiolytics

Benzodiazepines are the medications most widely used for perioperative sedation because they are effective anxiolytics and amnestics and are well tolerated by patients. In years past, diazepam was the most commonly used benzodiazepine for preanesthetic sedation. It is well absorbed orally, producing peak plasma levels in 30 to 90 minutes. It has little effect on postanesthesia recovery. However, response to diazepam is highly variable, and enterohepatic recirculation can result in increased drowsiness and increased plasma concentrations 6 to 8 hours after administration.

Midazolam is a newer benzodiazepine that has largely replaced diazepam for sedation before surgery. It can be given intramuscularly, orally, nasally, or rectally and has a more rapid onset and shorter duration of action than diazepam (134). In addition to producing sedation and anxiolysis, it provides excellent amnesia. It is infrequently associated with nausea, vomiting, or excitement. Because its duration of action is less than an hour, the administration of midazolam must be carefully timed so that the maximal effect occurs when the child arrives in the operating room.

Lorazepam is also an effective anxiolytic, amnestic, and sedative that can be used for preanesthesia sedation. Its onset is slow and its duration of action prolonged; hence, it is not widely used for preoperative sedation in children.

Narcotics

Morphine and meperidine are excellent analgesics, but, when used alone in a child without pain, they can cause dysphoria. For this reason, opiate premedication is often combined with a barbiturate or benzodiazepine. Additional disadvantages of narcotics as premedicants are the nausea and vomiting associated with their use and the respiratory depression that occurs, particularly in infants. The cardiovascular effects of morphine and meperidine are minor, but unless a child has pain, there is little need to give narcotic premedication.

Anticholinergics

Anticholinergics are commonly administered to children before surgery to prevent vagal bradycardia during manipulation of the airway or associated with the use of halothane or succinylcholine. Atropine is the anticholinergic most commonly used in children, and it not only blocks the vagal effects on the heart but also is an effective drying agent. Numerous side effects are associated with the use of atropine and the other anticholinergics, however. They inhibit sweat gland activity, producing an increase in body temperature and a flushed appearance and, in large doses, can cause confusion and agitation.

Glycopyrrolate can also be used as a preanesthesia medication. It is a more potent drying agent than atropine but causes less tachycardia. Because of its quaternary ammonium structure, glycopyrrolate does not cross the blood-brain barrier and does not cause the central nervous system effects that can be seen with atropine. In addition, it decreases the volume and acidity of gastric secretions.

In summary, there is no one premedication that is significantly better than another. Much more important is establishing in the child and the parents a sense of trust and confidence in the anesthesiologist and in the anesthesia care that will be provided.

Fasting

Prolonged fasting is believed to decrease the potential for vomiting or regurgitation during induction and, therefore, reduce the risk for pulmonary aspiration of gastric contents. In early studies of morbidity and mortality associated with pediatric anesthesia, pulmonary aspiration of gastric contents was a common cause of anesthetic mortality (7). Recent studies suggest that the risk for pulmonary aspiration is small in healthy children having elective surgery, although there are factors that do increase the risk (130). These factors are usually easily identifiable and include conditions that slow gastric emptying, such as trauma, pain, administration of narcotics, diabetes mellitus, or ASA physical status III, IV or V.

Although solid food may take several hours to pass through the pylorus, clear liquids are emptied from the stomach soon after being ingested. Several studies have shown that clear fluids consumed until 2 hours before the induction of anesthesia do not adversely affect the volume or acidity of gastric contents when compared with patients who have fasted for 6 hours or more (32,34). Therefore, more liberal fasting guidelines can be recommended that include oral intake of clear fluids up until 2 hours before surgery (7).

In patients who are at risk for an increased volume of acidic gastric contents, even prolonged periods of fasting cannot ensure that the stomach will be empty. For these patients, the preoperative administration of a histamine-2 receptor blocker and antacids may decrease gastric volume and increase pH. In addition, specific steps should be taken during the induction of anesthesia to reduce the risk for regurgitation and aspiration.

ANESTHETIC PRINCIPLES AND PHARMACOLOGY

Theories of anesthesia have attempted to define a single mechanism by which a variety of dissimilar anesthetic agents produce anesthesia. Although the mechanisms of anesthesia remain poorly understood, general anesthesia can be described as the presence of four interrelated, but separate, conditions:

1. Amnesia
2. Analgesia
3. Hypnosis
4. Muscular relaxation

Suppression of reflex responses (e.g., glottic closure, vagal reflexes, baroreceptors) is considered by many to be an additional requirement for general anesthesia. An increasing inventory of inhalation and intravenous drugs makes the above division of anesthesia into a number of interrelated conditions useful, particularly in understanding how combinations of drugs can be used to produce general anesthesia.

Inhalation Anesthetics

In the mid-1800s, inhalation anesthetic techniques using ether and later nitrous oxide and chloroform were introduced. Among the agents in use today, isoflurane, desflurane, and sevoflurane are compounds derived from the first inhalation anesthetic, diethyl ether. Halothane, a halogenated alkane, is slightly different from the ether compounds and was the most commonly used volatile agent in pediatric anesthesia until sevoflurane was introduced into clinical practice in the early 1990s.

Uptake and Distribution

Anesthetic uptake and distribution are similar for all the inhalation anesthetics. The pharmacology of the inhaled drugs is best understood by considering their similarity to oxygen uptake (110). Inspired gases are distributed to alveoli, cross the alveolar-capillary membrane, and dissolve in blood. Arterial blood transports the anesthetic agent to the brain. Anesthetic agents have a high lipid solubility compared with air and oxygen and rapidly enter the central nervous system. A number of variables alter the speed of onset of inhalation anesthesia: inspired anesthetic concentrations, alveolar ventilation, solubility of the anesthetic in blood and brain, magnitude and distribution of cardiac output, and alveolar to pulmonary artery anesthetic partial pressure gradient.

Volatile anesthetics are liquids at room temperature and have low boiling points. Therefore, the drugs can be vaporized by passing a known volume of carrier gas, usually oxygen and nitrous oxide, through the liquid. The precise delivery of a uniform inspired anesthetic concentration requires an agent-specific vaporizer that provides a constant percentage of volatile agent regardless of total gas flow, room temperature, and atmospheric pressure. The anesthetic delivery system includes a breathing circuit with one-way valves and a carbon dioxide (CO_2) absorption system to prevent rebreathing of CO_2.

Minimum Alveolar Concentration

Minimum alveolar concentration (MAC) is a measure of anesthetic potency. It is defined as the alveolar partial pressure associated with no movement in response to a skin incision in 50% of patients (57). MAC is similar to a drug's effective dose in 50% of patients (ED_{50}) and is helpful in determining an inhaled anesthetic's potency, in comparing side effects of different anesthetics, and in defining a therapeutic index. Alveolar anesthetic partial pressures reflect central nervous system partial pressures when an equilibrium exists between the central nervous system and the alveoli. For this reason, end-tidal gas measurements can be used to estimate anesthetic partial pressures in the central nervous system. Nitrous oxide, a relatively weak anesthetic, has a MAC in children of more than 100% and is used primarily to reduce the concentration of volatile anesthetic required or as an adjunct to intravenous anesthetics (90). Halothane, the most potent inhalation anesthetic, has a MAC in healthy adults of less than 1 vol%; isoflurane and sevoflurane have MAC values of 1.2 and 1.8 vol%, respectively (22,46,57) (Table 2).

Nitrous Oxide

Nitrous oxide (N_2O) was one of the first inhaled anesthetics used, and it remains an integral part of anesthetic practice 150 years after its introduction. N_2O is used in more than 90% of general anesthetics in children because of its low toxicity and minimal cardiovascular and respiratory side effects (87,89). N_2O

TABLE 2. COMPARATIVE PROPERTIES OF INHALATION ANESTHETICS

Property	Nitrous Oxide	Halothane	Enflurane	Isoflurane	Sevoflurane	Desflurane
Approximate duration of use in anesthesia	150 years (1846)	40 years (1954)	30 years (1964)	20 years (1971)	9 years (1990)	6 years (1993)
Boiling point	Gas at room temperature	50°C	56°C	48°C	48°C	18°C
Minimum alveolar concentration in infants	100 vol%	1.1 vol%	1.9 vol%	1.6 vol%	2.7 vol%	9.0 vol%
Cardiac depression	Minimal	Yes	Yes	Yes	Yes	Yes
Respiratory depression	Minimal	Yes	Yes	Yes	Yes	Yes

is a weak anesthetic when used alone, but when added to volatile anesthetics or narcotics, N_2O reduces the dose of narcotics or other agents required for anesthesia (90). This also reduces the cardiovascular and respiratory side effects of more potent volatile anesthetics in children (89). The low solubility of N_2O enables a high partial pressure to be achieved rapidly in the alveoli and the central nervous system, and analgesic and amnestic effects can be achieved with N_2O concentrations of 50% to 70%. The major disadvantage of N_2O is the high partial pressures required in the inspired gas, which necessarily reduce the inspired oxygen concentration. Also, nitrous oxide crosses membranes more readily than air or oxygen, significantly increasing the volume or pressure in gas-containing body spaces (44).

Side Effects in Children

All volatile anesthetics depress cardiovascular performance in a dose-related manner in children and adults (86,88,92,136). The major hemodynamic effect of these anesthetic agents is depression of myocardial contractility, but additional effects on heart rate and rhythm, venous return, and arteriolar dilation contribute to the cardiovascular changes associated with these agents (48,86,88).

The volatile agents also depress respiratory function. Minute ventilation decreases as a result of a fall in tidal volume. Volatile anesthetics alter muscle tone, and intercostal muscle weakness results in a fall in resting lung volume. The decrease in functional residual capacity not only alters lung volumes but also contributes to small airway closure. Control of ventilation is also altered by inhalation anesthetics. An increase in ventilation that normally occurs in response to hypoxia or hypercarbia is severely impaired in patients who receive even subanesthetic concentrations of inhalation anesthetics (70).

Hemodynamic depression leading to cardiac arrest is cited as a major contributing cause of increased anesthetic morbidity and mortality in children. The increased anesthetic requirements in children result in a smaller margin of safety between anesthesia and cardiovascular toxicity (68,88,111). In the presence of cardiovascular disease, hypovolemia, or anemia, an even smaller margin of safety exists between anesthesia and lethal cardiac depression. Improved noninvasive monitoring devices have enhanced anesthesiologists' ability to recognize cardiovascular depression, but the need for safer anesthetic drugs for children remains a priority.

Although increased hemodynamic sensitivity is believed to be the most important factor responsible for the higher incidence of anesthetic-related morbidity and mortality in children (68,90), respiratory effects of inhalation anesthetics are also more profound in infants than in adults. A more compliant chest wall in infants leads to a greater fall in lung volume during anesthesia. A higher basal metabolic rate, increased oxygen requirements, and an upper airway more prone to obstruction also contribute to the increased risk for hypoxia during anesthesia in children (25,126).

Intravenous Anesthetics

At present, no one intravenous drug can produce all the elements of anesthesia—amnesia, analgesia, muscle relaxation, and hypnosis. Consequently, inhalation and intravenous drugs are often combined to produce anesthesia. The principal advantage of drug combinations is that lower doses of multiple drugs, each titrated to achieve a specific anesthetic goal, can be used, reducing side effects. The disadvantages of such combinations are the increased frequency of drug interactions and the additive respiratory and cardiovascular side effects.

Most intravenous anesthetic drugs have high lipid solubility and rapidly enter the central nervous system. The initially high concentration of drug in the central nervous system decreases over a period of minutes as drug redistribution to other body tissues occurs. Drug redistribution after an intravenous bolus is the primary factor in termination of central nervous system anesthetic effect. Metabolic and excretory mechanisms then eliminate the drug from the body.

Ultra-short-acting barbiturates (thiopental, methohexital) provide rapid induction of anesthesia and are frequently used intravenous induction agents. Respiratory and myocardial depression occurs, but in healthy patients, the cardiovascular side effects from an induction dose of barbiturate are minimal. Other intravenous drugs, such as midazolam, diazepam, etomidate, and propofol, can also rapidly induce anesthesia. Although these compounds are structurally different from barbiturates, all have high lipid solubility and rapidly penetrate the central nervous system.

Ketamine also rapidly enters the central nervous system but has a different central nervous system effect (132). Nystagmus, amnesia, profound analgesia, and a dissociative dreamlike state occur with ketamine. Ketamine was purported to maintain airway reflexes and spontaneous ventilation better than other intravenous drugs. However, airway reflexes are depressed by ketamine, and aspiration of gastric contents can occur during dissociative anesthesia with ketamine. The disadvantages of ketamine are the increased airway secretions, prolonged recovery, and unpleasant postoperative dreams and persistent nightmares that may follow its use. In addition, ketamine is associated with a high incidence of nausea and vomiting. An advantage of ketamine is its sympathomimetic effects, which may be particularly valuable during induction of anesthesia in hypovolemic, hypotensive patients. Ketamine is also useful in patients with severe asthma who benefit from the bronchodilation caused by sympathetic stimulation.

Narcotics

For many years, anesthesiologists depended on intravenous hypnotic agents and inhaled anesthetics, and spontaneous ventilation was maintained with almost all anesthetics. Until tracheal intubation and positive-pressure ventilation became routinely available, narcotics were used primarily to treat postoperative pain. In patients with severe cardiovascular disease who often tolerated inhalation anesthesia poorly, large doses of morphine were found to provide anesthesia with excellent cardiovascular stability even though a prolonged period of respiratory support was required. The long duration of action of the two most commonly administered postoperative narcotic analgesics, meperidine (Demerol) and morphine, still limits their use during the intraoperative period, particularly for brief operations (74).

New synthetic narcotics (sufentanil, alfentanil, remifentanil) helped decrease some of the side effects of opiates (38,71,84). The greater lipid solubility and minimal vasodilation of new opiates produce rapid and profound analgesia with minimal circulatory effects. Like intravenous anesthetics, rapid redistribution of narcotics from the central nervous system limits the duration of analgesia and respiratory depression. Anesthesia with remifentanil, sufentanil, or alfentanil is characterized by a stable cardiovascular system; with careful titration, postoperative respiratory depression is less of a problem, but only skilled personnel who are familiar with airway management should administer these potent opiates.

Neuromuscular Blocking Drugs

Neuromuscular blocking drugs are classified according to their action at the neuromuscular junction. Succinylcholine and D-tubocurarine, introduced into clinical practice 50 years ago, are prototypes of the two main classes of paralyzing drugs. The depolarizing drugs are represented by succinylcholine and the nondepolarizing drugs by D-tubocurarine.

Succinylcholine is the only depolarizing neuromuscular blocking agent currently available. Succinylcholine binds to the acetylcholine receptor site at the postjunctional neuromuscular end plate, causing depolarization and paralysis of short duration as a result of its rapid hydrolysis by pseudocholinesterase. A small proportion of patients have a genetic abnormality that results in a pseudocholinesterase enzyme that does not metabolize succinylcholine and produces profound, prolonged paralysis (more than 8 hours) after a single intravenous dose. Patients with pseudocholinesterase deficiency have no signs or symptoms of under-

lying disease but may give a family history of prolonged paralysis after anesthesia.

Many of the side effects caused by succinylcholine relate to its depolarizing action at the neuromuscular junction. With the generalized tetanic muscle contraction that occurs when succinylcholine depolarizes the neuromuscular junction, an increase in intragastric, intraabdominal, intraocular, and intracranial pressure may result (29). Muscle fasciculations caused by succinylcholine are also believed to be responsible for the postoperative myalgia experienced by some patients. In healthy patients, a transient rise in serum potassium of 0.4 to 1 mEq/L occurs after succinylcholine administration. Case reports describing cardiac arrest due to potassium efflux in children with undiagnosed muscle disease has led to debate about the appropriate use of succinylcholine in children (106). If new, rapidly acting nondepolarizing neuromuscular blocking drugs become available, succinylcholine will undoubtedly be replaced in clinical practice. Similar potassium efflux also occurs in patients with lower motor neuron disease or burns as a result of changes in the muscle membrane and neuromuscular junction. Severe hyperkalemia (more than 10 mEq/L) leading to cardiac arrest has been reported in children with muscle disease (58).

Succinylcholine's structural similarity to acetylcholine can also produce autonomic side effects, including bradycardia, salivation, and flushing. Finally, succinylcholine can trigger masseter spasm and malignant hyperthermia and is contraindicated in susceptible patients (104). Despite succinylcholine's multiple side effects, the rapid, profound neuromuscular blockade of short duration makes it a valuable drug in the anesthetic management of selected children and adults (37).

The curarelike neuromuscular blocking drugs produce muscle paralysis by competitively antagonizing acetylcholine's action at the presynaptic and postsynaptic receptors of the neuromuscular junction (29). Two different pharmacologic classes of drugs produce competitive neuromuscular blockade: the steroid group, represented by pancuronium (pipercuronium, vecuronium, rocuronium); and the benzylisoquinoline group, derived from D-tubocurarine (atracurium, doxacurium, mivacurium). The groups differ slightly in their cardiovascular effects, metabolism, excretion, and duration of action.

The effect of competitive neuromuscular blockers can be reversed by the use of anticholinesterase drugs (neostigmine, edrophonium, pyridostigmine), which prevent acetylcholine metabolism. This increases the concentration of acetylcholine at the receptor site and displaces the competitive neuromuscular drug, thereby reversing neuromuscular blockade. Neuromuscular blocking drugs do not produce hypnosis, amnesia, or sedation. Almost all patients who describe awareness during anesthesia and surgery have received a neuromuscular blocking drug as part of their anesthesia management.

INDUCTION OF ANESTHESIA

Although there are many ways to induce anesthesia in young children, the chosen technique should be safe, quick, and uncomplicated. Both the child and the family should be made to feel as comfortable and relaxed as possible, and the induction should be carried out in a controlled and gentle manner. Dramatic changes in the child's emotions or physiologic status can occur quickly and contribute to a higher incidence of critical events during induction of anesthesia in this group of patients.

Preanesthetic Preparation

Before the induction of anesthesia is begun, all the anesthetic equipment and drugs that will be required must be available and checked for proper functioning. Appropriately sized laryngoscopes, endotracheal tubes, stylets, face masks, oral or nasal airways, and suction must be close at hand. Pulse oximeter and temperature probes, electrocardiogram electrodes, a correctly sized blood pressure cuff, an intravenous administration set, and a selection of intravenous catheters must be available before beginning the induction. The room should be comfortably warmed. When the child is in the operating room, a quiet, tranquil atmosphere must be maintained to minimize the risk for a forceful, stormy induction.

Parental Presence

Awareness of the importance of parental participation in the medical care of children has increased in recent years, and parental presence during the induction of anesthesia is becoming increasingly common. Parents who have received a careful explanation of what to expect as their child is anesthetized can provide reassurance and support to a frightened or anxious child, greatly diminishing the need for preanesthetic sedation (64,113).

Not every child needs a parent present during the induction of anesthesia. Infants younger than about 6 to 8 months of age are rarely distressed when taken away from their parents. Older children with a strong sense of independence may prefer to go to the operating room without their parents. Children who are critically ill undergoing emergency surgery or who present potential anesthetic problems are perhaps best induced without their parents. Parents must understand that their participation is invited, not required. Whether parents choose to remain with their child or not, they must be given a careful explanation of what is to be done. The risks and complications of anesthesia should be briefly described and any questions answered. Finally, they should be assured that their child will always be treated with gentleness and extreme care.

Monitoring

The American Society of Anesthesiologists has established standards of monitoring that must be met when providing anesthetic care. A precordial stethoscope, electrocardiograph, blood pressure cuff, inspired oxygen analyzer, pulse oximeter, end-tidal CO_2 analyzer, temperature probe, disconnect alarms, and monitors should all be placed before inducing anesthesia and disconnected only at the end of surgery when the patient is being transferred to the postanesthesia care unit.

Techniques

Anesthesia can be induced by the inhalation of nitrous oxide and a volatile anesthetic agent, such as halothane or sevoflurane, or by the intravenous, intramuscular, rectal, or transmucosal administration of a wide variety of anesthetic drugs, including barbiturates, benzodiazepines, narcotics, ketamine, or propofol.

The choice of a specific induction agent and the method of administration depend on the age and emotional state of the child, his or her medical condition, the nature of the surgical procedure to be performed, and the familiarity of the anesthesiologist with the chosen technique. Each of the following induction techniques can be used safely and effectively in a variety of clinical situations. It is the responsibility of the pediatric anesthesiologist to assess each child carefully and to choose the best technique for that child.

Inhalation Induction

Anesthesia in children is most commonly induced by having them breath a potent volatile anesthetic agent. This provides a safe, rapid onset of anesthesia that is well accepted by most children. Although the smell of the anesthetic is unpleasant, an inhalation induction avoids the need for an injection until after the child is asleep. In addition, it can be done with the child lying down or sitting on the operating table or in the parent's lap.

The anesthetic is delivered by placing a face mask gently over the child's face, then gradually increasing the concentration of the volatile agent until the child loses consciousness. Nitrous oxide alone will not produce anesthesia, but it is often combined with the more potent agents, such as halothane or sevoflurane, to speed anesthesia induction because it is odorless, equilibrates rapidly in the brain, provides excellent analgesia, and reduces the concentration of volatile agent needed to produce anesthesia (87,90).

Halothane, isoflurane, and sevoflurane cause significant dose-dependent myocardial depression (88,89,92,136). Stroke volume, cardiac output, and blood pressure are all decreased by the concentrations of halothane, isoflurane, or sevoflurane required for anesthesia (86,88,89). Isoflurane frequently causes tachycardia that helps maintain cardiac output (88). In contrast, high concentrations of halothane can result in bradycardia (92). In addition, cardiac dysrhythmias are more common during halothane anesthesia, particularly if endogenous catecholamines are administered by the surgeon to produce vasoconstriction and reduce bleeding.

Halothane, isoflurane, and sevoflurane also cause respiratory depression as the concentration is increased (70), and isoflurane's pungent odor often results in coughing, breath holding, and laryngospasm during induction (69). Similar airway irritability occurs at the end of surgery as the patient emerges from isoflurane anesthesia (47). Because of the increased incidence of hypoxia associated with these respiratory complications, many pediatric anesthesiologists prefer halothane or sevoflurane to isoflurane, despite the theoretical hemodynamic advantages offered by isoflurane.

Intravenous Induction

Intravenous induction of anesthesia in children offers a rapid, relatively pleasant onset of anesthesia if intravenous access can be quickly and easily achieved. Intravenous techniques are less common because many children are fearful of needles and will not cooperate while the intravenous catheter is placed. For an intravenous induction, the most easily cannulated veins must be identified ahead of time, and a knowledgeable assistant who can distract and gently, but effectively, restrain the child while the intravenous line is being placed is required. In older, more cooperative children, the use of a topical (119) or local anesthetic using a 32-gauge needle usually permits a relatively painless insertion of an intravenous catheter.

Thiopental, an ultra-short-acting barbiturate, is one of the most common intravenous agents used to induce anesthesia in both children and adults. It has a short duration of action because of its rapid redistribution in the body. Ultra-short-acting barbiturates cause myocardial depression and peripheral venous dilation, but hypotension is uncommon in healthy, well-hydrated children (31). Respiratory depression, airway obstruction, and apnea can all occur after administration of an induction dose of thiopental; hence, the anesthesiologist must be prepared to control the airway, maintain ventilation, and provide supplemental oxygen as the child loses consciousness.

Propofol is a newer intravenous agent with high plasma clearance and short elimination half-life that allows rapid induction of anesthesia and prompt postoperative recovery (114). Propofol has cardiorespiratory effects similar to those produced by thiopental (15) and is painful on injection, which can be distressing for children (63). Pain may be minimized by injecting the drug into a rapidly running intravenous line in a large vein or by injecting a small dose of lidocaine with the propofol. As well as being an effective induction agent, propofol can be administered as a continuous infusion to maintain anesthesia throughout the surgical procedure (114).

Ketamine can also be used intravenously to induce anesthesia. By stimulating the release of endogenous catecholamines, ketamine helps maintain cardiac output and blood pressure in patients with cardiovascular instability (132). It also causes bronchodilation. Smaller doses of the drug produce intense analgesia and a dreamlike state that allows painful procedures to be done in a conscious, but dissociated, patient. Postoperative nightmares and disturbing flashbacks make ketamine an unsuitable intravenous agent for routine use in healthy children.

Rectal Induction

Induction of anesthesia by the rectal administration of methohexital or thiopental is a safe, pleasant technique for anesthetizing young children younger than 4 or 5 years of age (49–51). It can be administered quickly and painlessly by inserting a soft plastic catheter several inches into the rectum while the child is being held by a parent. Although rectal methohexital provides a pleasant induction, variation in the rectal absorption and systemic availability of the drug makes rectal administration more unpredictable than intravenous or inhalation induction. Depending on the dose and concentration of the methohexital solution used, more than 90% of children are asleep within 10 minutes (49). Complications associated with the use of rectal methohexital include hiccoughs, apnea, defecation, and damage to the rectal mucosa and delayed recovery (51). In healthy chil-

dren, there is no change in blood pressure or cardiac output associated with the rectal administration of methohexital, although a slight increase in heart rate may occur (50). Oxygenation and ventilation are usually well maintained, but appropriate monitoring, particularly pulse oximetry, should be used during the induction and while the child is being transported into the operating room.

Other Techniques

In children who become extremely agitated before the induction of anesthesia or who have behavior problems that make it impossible for them to cooperate, rapid and reliable anesthesia can be achieved with intramuscular ketamine. In recent years, there has been increasing interest in the use of oral transmucosal fentanyl (45) and nasally administered agents, including fentanyl, sufentanil (65), and midazolam (134). Although transmucosal induction is useful in some children, the sedation or level of anesthesia achieved is less reliable than that after intravenous, inhalation, or rectal anesthetic inductions. It is unlikely that transmucosal induction of anesthesia with the presently available drugs will replace more common inhalation or intravenous techniques.

Airway Control and Endotracheal Intubation

After anesthesia induction, maintaining a patient's airway is of paramount importance. Placing the patient in the "sniffing position" with the neck flexed on the thorax and the head extended at the occipitocervical junction is often all that is required to open the airway. If necessary, the jaw and tongue can be displaced anteriorly to open the airway and permit unobstructed ventilation. In this position, most patients can be effectively oxygenated and ventilated using a face mask and bag. If soft tissues in the upper airway continue to obstruct the airway, an oral or nasal airway can be inserted to maintain a clear airway. During many surgical procedures, anesthesia can be maintained with a face mask and spontaneous or assisted ventilation. During spinal surgery, the prone position mandates endotracheal intubation, which in most children is accomplished safely and easily during direct laryngoscopy.

Compared with adults, children have a large tongue and relatively small mouth owing to a slightly receding mandible. In addition, the larynx is located more cephalad than it is in an adult, and the epiglottis is longer, is stiffer, and tends to obscure the glottic opening. The narrowest part of a child's airway is the cricoid cartilage. For this reason, an endotracheal tube may pass easily through the vocal cords but fit too tightly at the level of the cricoid cartilage, compressing tracheal mucosa and leading to submucosal edema. After extubation, obstruction and stridor may result from submucosal edema. Most of the complications of endotracheal intubation, including postintubation croup, can be avoided by performing a gentle intubation with an appropriately sized endotracheal tube (123).

After induction of anesthesia, intubation can be performed with or without the use of a neuromuscular blocking agent. Neuromuscular blocking drugs provide profound muscle relaxation so that intubation can be achieved with a lower concentration of volatile agent. This reduces the incidence of hypotension and other cardiovascular side effects that occur during administration of high concentrations of volatile anesthetics. The disadvantage of a neuromuscular blocker is that it removes the patient's ability to ventilate spontaneously. Therefore, before administering these drugs, it is critical that the anesthesiologist be able to ventilate the patient with a bag and mask.

A variety of formulas have been derived to choose an appropriately sized endotracheal tube. The most common is as follows: tube size (mm ID) = 16 + [age in years ÷ 4]. Another easy method is the use of an endotracheal tube with the same diameter as the child's little finger. These are only guides for choosing the correct tube size, and both larger and smaller endotracheal tubes should be available. Pediatric endotracheal tubes are uncuffed to minimize airway trauma; thus, it is important that the correct size be used. Large tubes can cause postintubation croup or subglottic stenosis if intubation is prolonged. If the tube is too small, a large leak around the tube could prevent effective ventilation. Tube size can be confirmed by checking the size of the leak around the tube. Ideally, it should be possible to ventilate the lungs and hear a small leak at 20 to 25 cm H_2O airway pressure. It is important to remember that the pediatric trachea is short; the distance between the vocal cords and carina in a newborn may be as little as 4 cm, making accurate placement of the tube critical. Correct placement of the endotracheal tube can be confirmed by auscultating equal bilateral breath sounds and observing the chest wall for any asymmetric movement that may indicate endobronchial intubation. In addition, the anesthesiologist should auscultate over the stomach, check the tube for mist during expiration, and carefully monitor the patient's hemoglobin saturation and end-tidal CO_2 concentration. If there is any doubt about correct endotracheal tube placement, the tube should be removed and ventilation established with a bag and mask. When the patient is stable and well oxygenated, intubation can be repeated.

Complications that can occur during direct laryngoscopy include minor trauma to the lips, tongue, or other soft tissues; dental trauma; sore throat; hoarseness; subglottic edema; and stridor. Serious complications are rare but include vocal cord injuries, tracheal or bronchial perforation, and unrecognized esophageal intubation. These types of injuries can usually be avoided by ensuring that the patient is adequately anesthetized and relaxed before attempting intubation, maintaining flawless technique during laryngoscopy, and monitoring carefully to confirm that the endotracheal tube is correctly placed.

MONITORING DURING ANESTHESIA

The goal of monitoring during anesthesia is to obtain information about drug effects, assess anesthesia machine and breathing circuit integrity, and measure the patient's physiologic function so that as conditions change, action can be taken to avoid catastrophic complications. With better techniques for acquiring physiologic information and the adoption of standards of patient monitoring, anesthetic morbidity and mortality have been reduced. Although standards for intraoperative monitoring of oxygenation, ventilation, and circulation have been adopted by the

ASA, training and vigilance are required to integrate and interpret clinical signs and physiologic monitoring (6).

These monitoring recommendations recognize that the most serious anesthetic-related complications are hypoxia due to respiratory problems and cardiovascular collapse due to hemodynamic depression or inadequate volume replacement. General anesthesia causes hypoventilation due to central nervous system depression. Central and peripheral ventilatory control mechanisms are depressed, and the normal responses to hypoxia and hypercarbia are markedly impaired during anesthesia (70). A hypoxic patient fails to increase ventilation during anesthesia, and the early cardiovascular signs of hypoxia (tachycardia or hypertension) observed in conscious hypoxic patients are absent. Because observation is not a reliable method of detecting cyanosis, early recognition of arterial hypoxia requires sensitive monitoring techniques, of which pulse oximetry is the most reliable.

In addition to the impaired control of ventilation and the absence of the usual signs of hypoxia, anesthesia and surgery have a variety of deleterious effects on the relationship between pulmonary ventilation and perfusion. Higher inspired oxygen concentrations are required to maintain a normal PaO_2 during the perioperative period.

Respiratory Monitoring

During anesthesia, a number of different devices are used to monitor the adequacy of ventilation and oxygenation. All anesthesia machines have an inspired oxygen concentration monitor to ensure that an adequate concentration of oxygen is being delivered to the breathing circuit. In addition, if the central supply of oxygen is interrupted, a fail-safe device automatically stops the flow of N_2O, so that a hypoxic gas mixture cannot be delivered to the patient.

Tidal volume, respiratory rate, and minute ventilation are

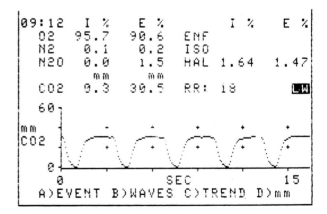

FIGURE 2. Capnography provides breath-by-breath analysis of inspired and expired gas concentrations. Gases are continuously aspirated and analyzed from the connector attached to the endotracheal tube. The waveform provides information about inspired and alveolar O_2, N_2, N_2O, CO_2, and halothane concentrations, which predict arterial concentrations. This normal capnogram indicates the CO_2 concentration of alveolar gas (30.5 mm). A simultaneous arterial CO_2 concentration is 32 mm.

measured using a spirometer, and carbon dioxide, oxygen, and anesthetic gas concentrations are analyzed throughout the respiratory cycle. Carbon dioxide measurements in inspired and expired gas (capnography) are useful to assess the adequacy of ventilation (Fig. 2), and the changing pattern of carbon dioxide concentration within the breathing circuit can provide diagnostic information that helps detect improper functioning of the anesthesia circuit, rebreathing of anesthetic gases, and hypoventilation, bronchospasm, or pulmonary embolus.

Pulse oximetry uses the color difference between oxygenated and deoxygenated hemoglobin to quantify hemoglobin saturation (12) (Fig. 3). normally, saturation is maintained at greater than or equal to 95% until the Po_2 falls below 65 mm. In low tissue flow states, such as with vasoconstriction due to hypothermia, an arterial waveform may not be detected, and arterial saturation cannot be determined. The presence of carbon monoxide, methemoglobin, sulfhemoglobin, or other substances alters light absorption and may cause erroneous oxygen saturation values. Fortunately, few clinical conditions significantly alter pulse oximetry, and the correlation between measured arterial oxygen saturation and functional oxygen saturation derived by pulse oximetry is greater than 0.95 when oxygen saturation is between 70% ($po_2 = 40$ mm) and 95% ($Po_2O2 = 65$ mm), making pulse oximetry an essential monitor (Fig. 4).

Cardiovascular Monitoring

Cardiac rate and rhythm changes, as well as st-t wave abnormalities, can be detected using the electrocardiogram. In children, most intraoperative changes in the electrocardiogram are related to respiratory complications, anesthetic overdose, or inadequate vascular volume and manifest as tachycardia that can rapidly progress to bradycardia (68). In studies of cardiac arrest during anesthesia, bradycardia occurs just before cardiac arrest in more than 95% of children (25,68). For this reason, bradycardia in infants and children is an ominous sign of significant hypoxemia unless proved otherwise.

Heart rate must be interpreted relative to a child's age. A heart rate of 90 beats/min is normal in an anesthetized 2-year-old, but a neonate who has a heart rate of 90 beats/min has serious bradycardia that requires immediate action.

Blood pressure measurements must also be interpreted based on normal values in relation to age. For example, in newborns, systolic blood pressure is 60 to 70 mm hg. When blood pressure is normal, it suggests that cardiac output and tissue blood flow are adequate. A fall in blood pressure is a nonspecific sign and can be related to decreased blood volume, depressed myocardial contractility secondary to drugs or disease, venous pooling, or arterial dilation (Fig. 5). several factors often exist simultaneously during surgery (115).

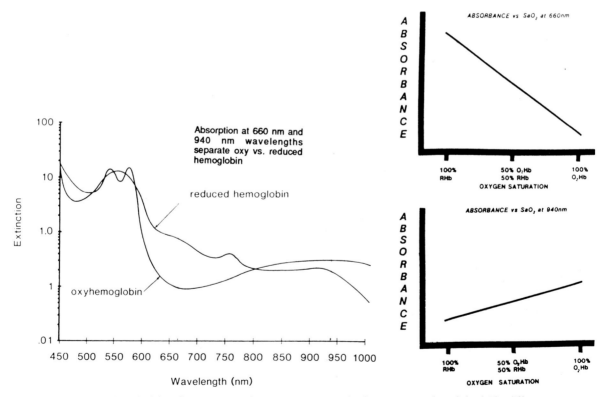

FIGURE 3. Principles of oxygen saturation measurement: extinction versus wavelength (nm). The differential absorption spectrum of oxyhemoglobin and deoxyhemoglobin at 660 and 940 nm is used to determine the proportion of oxyhemoglobin and deoxyhemoglobin present in arterial blood. Changes in absorption of two wavelengths of light are used to quantitate oxygen saturation. The presence of carbon monoxide, methemoglobin, and sulfhemoglobin interferes with the interpretation of saturation.

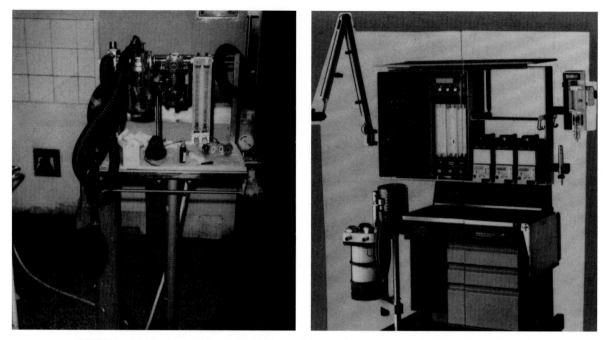

FIGURE 4. Anesthetic machines. *Left:* Simple anesthetic machines with oxygen and nitrous oxide tanks and two anesthesia vaporizers (ether and halothane); there is no special monitoring equipment. This machine dates from the 1950s. *Right:* A modern (1992) anesthetic machine with anesthetic capabilities similar to those of the machine on the left. The N_2O and O_2 flowmeters are similar, but there are three vaporizers instead of two. N_2O and O_2 tanks are replaced by central hospital supplies of O_2 and N_2O. The primary difference between the machines is the addition of monitors, safety devices, and a ventilator. Respiratory and cardiovascular monitoring equipment includes a pulse oximeter, spirometer, gas analyzer, ventilator alarms, oxygen analyzer, and automated blood pressure device. A backup battery system is required to power the monitors and alarms.

Central venous pressure measurements alone rarely provide sufficient data upon which to base clinical therapy, but when combined with other hemodynamic measurements, such as heart rate and direct arterial pressure (83), central venous pressure is often valuable. Intraoperative central venous pressure monitoring should be considered when (1) estimated blood loss is expected to exceed 50% of blood volume, (2) major fluid shifts are anticipated, (3) preoperative abnormalities suggest that traditional signs of fluid management will be difficult to assess, and (4) special intraoperative management is being considered, such as hemodilution, induced hypotension, or deliberate hypothermia. Repeated measurement of central venous pressure over a prolonged period of time is more useful than a single measurement.

Temperature Measurement

During anesthesia, peripheral and central thermoregulatory mechanisms are depressed, and compensatory mechanisms to maintain thermal homeostasis are absent (55). Unless steps are taken to prevent heat loss, hypothermia occurs during surgery. In addition, malignant hyperthermia, a rare genetic disease leading to sustained muscle contraction with associated metabolic acidosis, hyperkalemia, and hyperthermia, can develop at any time during the perioperative period in susceptible patients. Therefore, temperature monitoring is an important standard of anesthetic care.

Neurologic Monitoring

Assessment of spinal and lower brain stem function during general anesthesia requires complicated electrophysiologic monitoring. Electroencephalogram (EEG) monitoring is helpful in detecting significant cerebral cortical ischemic events during operation, but separating changes in spinal cord and lower brain stem function from baseline eeg activity and anesthetic drug effect using cortical sensory evoked responses is more difficult. Sophisticated equipment for sensory stimulation and processing the EEG are required to differentiate the evoked responses from baseline EEG activity (60). High concentrations of volatile anesthetics, hypothermia, and hypotension can all decrease the amplitude of, prolong the latency of, or eliminate evoked responses. Other anesthetics, including narcotics, benzodiazepines, and nitrous oxide, may also alter somatosensory evoked potentials.

Intraoperative Wake Up

Electrophysiologic sensory monitoring does not assess motor function during spinal surgery. Therefore, intraoperative awakening is often used in addition to sensory evoked potentials to assess gross motor function. When anesthetic management includes a wake-up test, patient preparation begins in the preoperative period. The patient must be able to cooperate with instructions and have adequate motor function to accomplish the movements. With newer, highly soluble synthetic opiates (remi-

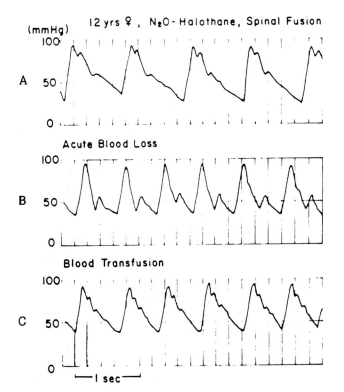

FIGURE 5. Direct blood pressure measurement. Changes in the contour of the arterial waveform often provide clues to the status of intravascular volume. **A:** Before blood loss, the full systolic arterial wave in this healthy child suggests adequate intravascular volume. **B:** The narrow systolic wave suggests less aortic filling, probably as a result of inadequate vascular volume secondary to blood loss. **C:** After transfusion, the character of the arterial waveform is restored, suggesting adequate restoration of vascular volume. (From Shimosato S [1983]: Blood pressure pulse. In: Shimosato S, ed. *Anesthesia and cardiac performance in health and disease*. Springfield, IL: Charles C. Thomas, pp. 80–99, with permission.)

fentanil, sufentanil, alfentanil), in combination with nitrous oxide and neuromuscular blocking agents, the anesthetic can be tailored to provide a brief period of response to verbal command. Inhalation or intravenous anesthetics are discontinued before the wake up, and if residual neuromuscular blockade is present, an anticholinesterase can be used to antagonize the block. As soon as purposeful movement occurs, an intravenous induction agent, such as thiopental, is administered to reestablish anesthesia. Excessive movement during the wake-up test can exacerbate blood loss, lead to extubation and loss of intravenous access, or dislodge the surgical hardware with potentially catastrophic consequences. Vigorous diaphragmatic activity can decrease intrathoracic pressure, leading to air embolus if there are open epidural veins above the level of the heart. For this reason, the surgical field is often flooded with saline immediately before wake up.

Neuromuscular Monitoring

The effect of neuromuscular blocking drugs on synaptic transmission can be measured by observing the magnitude of the muscle response to stimulation of a motor nerve. As paralysis develops after administration of a neuromuscular blocking drug, the motor response of the adductor pollicis to ulnar nerve stimulation shows a gradual decrement. With larger doses of a relaxant, the twitch response may disappear completely. Neuromuscular recovery can be confirmed by clinical signs as well as by the neuromuscular twitch response using train-of-four ulnar nerve stimulation. Four supramaximal stimuli, separated by 0.2 msec, are applied, and the difference in motor response between the first and fourth response correlates with the degree of neuromuscular blockade.

INTRAOPERATIVE FLUID MANAGEMENT

Maintenance Fluids

General principles of pediatric fluid therapy can be difficult to describe because fluid requirements and electrolyte regulation continually change as a result of growth and development (14,53). In addition, fluid requirements change rapidly during the perioperative period, and replacement solutions must reflect differences in the proportion of losses attributed to fluid sequestration, blood loss, and maintenance fluid requirements (53,54,85). Maintenance fluid replacement in children must include water required for increased caloric expenditure resulting from growth and development and greater insensible water losses.

When fluid management is based on weight alone, adjustments need to be made to replace the additional fluid required in a child. The advantage of fluid replacement regimens based on body weight is the ease with which rapid and precise repetitive weight determinations can be made on a daily basis. A useful maintenance fluid replacement formula that relates fluid requirements to body weight is:

0 to 10 kg: 4 ml × weight in kilograms for initial 10 kg
11 to 20 kg: add 2 ml for each kilogram over 10 kg (up to 20 kg)
21 kg: add 1 ml for each kilograms over 20 kg

The composition of a maintenance fluid must be based on energy requirements and electrolyte losses. If no energy substrate is provided, catabolism of glycogen and protein provides basal caloric needs. Catabolism of body proteins and glycogen is to be expected when pediatric or adult patients are not allowed enteral intake. When enteral nutrition is not possible, intravenous caloric intake must be substituted. Hypertonic intravenous dextrose solutions (25%) would be required to meet even basal caloric requirements in this setting, but intravenous hypertonic dextrose solutions are irritating to peripheral veins and would also result in hyperglycemia. Five percent dextrose solutions provide only 20% maintenance caloric requirements, but because these solutions are isotonic when compared with body fluid, 5% dextrose is a convenient way of limiting protein and glycogen catabolism (116). Electrolytes lost in urine, sweat, and feces can be added in the form of sodium, chloride, and potassium.

Intraoperative Fluid Losses

When compared with maintenance fluid requirements, intraoperative translocation fluid losses (third-space losses) are often more difficult to determine. Thirty years ago, the concept of fluid replacement during surgery was radically altered by studies defining the magnitude of fluid translocation during surgery, which showed that intravascular fluid loss to the interstitial fluid space during abdominal surgery was profound, exceeding 10 ml/kg per hour^{-1}. An ultrafiltrate of plasma is lost to the third space; therefore, replacement fluids must be isotonic to maintain normal electrolytes. In the postoperative period, fluid sequestration, an increased metabolic rate, and continued third-space fluid accumulations contribute to additional fluid requirements. Fluid lost to tissue edema and interstitial spaces during surgery is reabsorbed 48 to 72 hours after surgery as vascular integrity is restored and tissue healing occurs.

Inappropriate Antidiuretic Hormone Secretion

Major surgery leads to profound neuroendocrine stress responses. Endogenous cortisol, epinephrine, renin, aldosterone, and antidiuretic hormone are released during surgical stress. Cortisol and epinephrine inhibit gluconeogenesis, glycogen breakdown is enhanced, and blood glucose levels become elevated during the perioperative period, even when maintenance glucose solutions are withheld. Aldosterone, renin, and antidiuretic hormone are also released during stress, leading to water retention and a decrease in urine output. In most operative settings, the stress response and hormonal release are short-lived, but inappropriate release of antidiuretic hormone may continue for an extended period and cause continued reabsorption of H_2O without Na^+. Hyponatremia, increased vascular volume, and continued urinary loss of sodium are characteristic of the syndrome of inappropriate antidiuretic hormone release. Manifestations of the syndrome in the perioperative period are most frequently seen 48 to 72 hours after surgery, when continued inappropriate antidiuretic hormone release and liberal hypotonic fluid intake can lead to hyponatremia. Fluid restriction and diuretics usually resolve moderate hyponatremia (Na^+ less than 120 mEq/L), but with severe hyponatremia (Na^+ less than 110 mEq/L) associated with cerebral irritability or seizures, a small volume of 3% nacl (about 60 mEq Na^+ per 100 ml) may be required to increase sodium concentrations. Inappropriate antidiuretic hormone release may occur in any setting associated with profound stress, but healthy adolescents having major spinal surgery seem particularly susceptible to hyponatremia and water retention associated with the syndrome of inappropriate antidiuretic hormone release [13]. Careful attention to fluid management, urine output, and serum and urine electrolyte determinations helps diagnose this perioperative problem.

Intraoperative Blood Loss

In the near past, surgical blood loss in the pediatric patient was often managed by replacing 1 ml of blood for each milliliter of blood lost. The risks of transfusion have now led to a reassessment of this approach to blood transfusion. In acute blood loss, initial fluid resuscitation and volume expansion can be readily accomplished with crystalloid solutions. Fortunately, operative blood loss is rarely both massive and acute, and initial intraopera-

TABLE 3. AGE AND ESTIMATED BLOOD VOLUME

Age	Body Weight (kg)	Estimated Blood Volume per Donor Units^a
1 wk	3	240 mL/0.5 donor units
1 y	10	700 mL/1.5 donor units
4 y	20	1,500 mL/3 donor units
Adult	70	5,000 mL/10 donor units

^{a} Adult donor units of whole blood.

tive blood replacement is usually managed with crystalloid solutions until blood component therapy is indicated [59]. Indications for the use of blood components in the perioperative setting usually include at least one of the following:

- A deficit in oxygen-carrying capacity (red cells or whole blood transfusion)
- Decreased platelets or other formed elements of blood (platelet transfusion)
- Inadequate clotting factors to maintain surgical hemostasis (fresh-frozen plasma)

With the availability of crystalloid and colloid solutions, intravascular volume replacement is no longer considered an indication for blood transfusion. Because red blood cells constitute up to 40% of the intravascular volume, however, red cell and intravascular volume deficits often occur concomitantly. Even though vascular volume on a milliliter per kilogram basis is greater in children than in adults (a neonate's blood volume is 80 ml/kg, compared with 70 ml/kg in an adult), the entire blood volume of a 3-kg normal newborn is less than half a unit of whole blood [53]. Blood volume declines with growth, and by 1 year of age (10 kg), relative blood volume is similar to that of an adult (Table 3).

In neonates, extracellular fluid space is 40% of total-body weight, with 8% intravascular (80 ml/kg) and the remainder interstitial (32%) [53]. In adults, the extracellular fluid space is 20% of body weight, with 7% (70 ml/kg) intravascular and 13% interstitial (Fig. 6). interstitial fluid space declines rapidly after

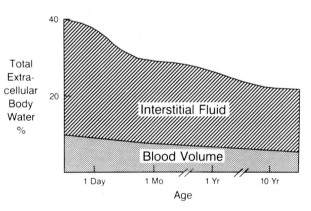

FIGURE 6. The changing relationship between blood volume and interstitial fluid in different pediatric age groups. The newborn has a large extracellular fluid space (40% of body weight) in comparison to the adult (20% of body weight). In neonates, blood volume represents only one fifth of the extracellular space; by 1 year of age, blood volume is one third of the extracellular fluid space.

birth, but interstitial and intravascular fluid relationships do not become adultlike until children are 4 or 5 years old. A large interstitial fluid space relative to intravascular volume in children results in a larger volume of distribution of crystalloid replacement solutions. Achieving the same intravascular volume replacement for blood loss in children as that recommended in adults requires more than 3 ml of crystalloid for each milliliter of blood loss.

Blood loss in an adult triggers a variety of cardiovascular compensatory mechanisms that can sustain adequate blood pressure, cardiac output, and blood flow to vital organs. Initially, blood loss is well tolerated in adults because only a small proportion of the entire blood volume is in arterial and capillary beds. Blood pooled in venous capacitance vessels is rapidly recruited by venoconstriction. An increase in heart rate and cardiac contractility can maintain blood pressure, cardiac output, and tissue blood flow in an adult until blood loss in excess of 20% of the entire blood volume has occurred (1 l of blood loss). In a child, particularly a neonate or infant, blood pressure and tissue blood flow may be compromised when intravascular volume decreases by even 10%. Vasoconstriction of splanchnic, skin, and muscle venous capacitance vessels in neonates and infants is less effective in maintaining blood pressure and tissue blood flow during hypovolemia. In an infant, more than half of the entire cardiac output is directed to high oxygen demand tissues, such as the brain, myocardium, and kidneys, which can autoregulate blood flow (53). Increases in heart rate and myocardial contractility in response to volume deficits are not as effective in increasing cardiac output and maintaining tissue blood flow in a child. For these reasons, hypovolemia is well tolerated by a young child, and inadequate tissue perfusion may occur in a child who sustains a 10% loss of blood volume.

Red Cell Replacement

Even though the hematocrit is high (45% to 50%) in the neonatal period, erythropoiesis does not keep pace with red cell losses. By 2 to 3 months of age, the normal hematocrit is 30%. As iron stores are replenished and erythropoiesis increases, the hematocrit reaches adult values by about 1 year of age.

Little information is available to define the red cell mass required in neonates and infants to maintain adequate tissue delivery of oxygen, but a high oxygen consumption and limited ability to augment cardiac output suggests that anemia may not be as well tolerated in neonates as it is in older children and adults. A hematocrit of 21%, suggested as a lower limit in healthy adults (27), is probably too low for neonates and infants.

An appreciation of the difference between a normal preoperative hematocrit and a hematocrit that merits transfusion is important in limiting unnecessary transfusion (16). If adequate vascular volume is maintained during the acute blood loss, red cell transfusion can be withheld until the red cell mass approaches the point at which oxygen-carrying capacity may be compromised. For example, a healthy 12-year-old patient weighing 60 kg with an initial hematocrit of 40% would have a red cell mass of 1,680 ml (based on a blood volume of 70 ml/kg or 4,200 ml), but this patient could sustain adequate oxygen delivery with only 900 ml of red cells (hematocrit of 21%). If gradual

blood loss of 2,000 ml occurred during surgery and was replaced with crystalloid preparations, the postoperative hematocrit would be 21%. Despite a large volume loss, homologous red cells are not required. The appropriate timing of blood transfusion can also decrease the need for red cell transfusion. This is particularly important if only a small volume of autologous blood is available (Fig. 7).

Blood transfusion risks include the parenteral transmission of infection as well as a number of acute problems related primarily to blood preservatives and changes that occur during blood storage. Citrate in the blood preservative chelates calcium to prevent clot formation. During blood storage, gradual metabolic and respiratory acidosis develops, potassium concentrations increase, and physical changes occur, including agglutination of red cells, platelets, and leukocytes. Blood storage also decreases 2,3-diphosphoglycerate (dpg) levels in plasma and shifts the oxygen dissociation of hemoglobin to the left. Few, if any, of these changes lead to major clinical symptoms or signs even in patients who require large volume transfusion.

Platelet And Coagulation Factor Replacement

The decision to replace platelets or coagulation factors is not as easily made as the decision to replace red cells because the simplest clinical monitor—increased surgical blood loss—can occur in patients who have no coagulation abnormalities (26–28,35).

Similar to red cells, platelets and coagulation factors are lost during hemorrhage. In addition, these coagulation elements are activated and incorporated into hemostatic plugs to seal vascular defects. In contrast to red cells, coagulation factors and platelets have an extravascular distribution and can be released into the circulation during periods of stress (91). For these reasons, a variety of coagulation tests may be required to define whether a hemostatic abnormality exists and determine whether blood components may be needed to correct the problem.

The severe bleeding reported in unprepared hemophiliac patients during minor surgery attests to the importance of the coagulation mechanism during surgery. When hemostatic abnormalities are the cause of hemorrhage, bleeding from wound edges will be unresponsive to electrocautery, or suture ligature and clot formation will be absent (24). Considerable reserve of hemostatic function exists, and increased bleeding during surgery does not occur until coagulation factor levels fall to less than 30% of normal (24,91).

A normal hemostatic mechanism does not prevent blood loss that results from either large vessel disruption or a large pressure gradient between the disrupted vasculature and the interstitium. In these situations, bleeding continues until intravascular pressure equals extravascular pressure. Frequently, increased bleeding during surgery is attributed to hemostatic disorders without considering the contribution of pressure gradients and major vessel disruption. A patient in the prone position who has increased intraabdominal pressure and elevated epidural venous pressure from improper positioning will experience increased blood loss during spinal surgery.

In situations in which significant blood loss is anticipated, preoperative assessment of coagulation provides an initial guide

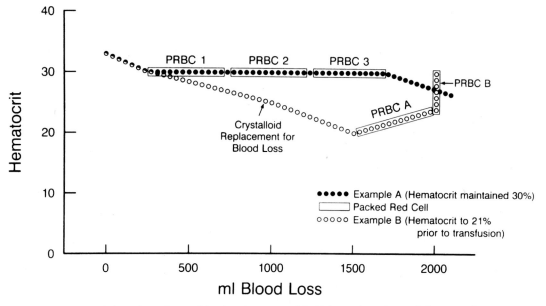

FIGURE 7. Timing of autologous blood replacement. This 60-kg patient donated three autologous units before surgery and has a preoperative hematocrit of 33%. **A:** The goal of intraoperative blood replacement is to maintain a hematocrit of 30% throughout the procedure. All three autologous units are administered during the intraoperative period of a 2,000-mL blood loss. No additional autologous blood is available in the postoperative period, and the final hematocrit is 27%. **B:** The goal of blood replacement is to maintain vascular volume with crystalloid until an intraoperative hematocrit of 21% is observed. Autologous blood will not be administered until 1,500 mL of blood is lost. One unit of blood administered at the conclusion of the procedure results in a postoperative hematocrit of 26%. A second unit administered in the recovery room increases the patient's hematocrit to a level greater than that observed when the approach has been to maintain a hematocrit of 30% throughout the operation. One additional autologous unit is available for continued losses in the 48 hours after surgery. Larger volumes of crystalloid or colloid solutions are required to maintain vascular volume during the intraoperative period in part **B**.

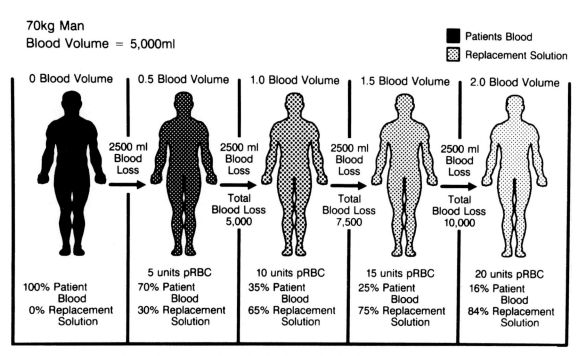

FIGURE 8. Dilutional changes in the patient's original blood volume occur as solutions are used to replace blood lost. The proportion of clotting factors and platelets left correlates with the original blood volume because clotting factors and platelets are not restored with red cell preparations.

to hemostatic factors. In patients with a preoperative coagulopathy related to disease or drugs, coagulation factor replacement may be needed early in the operative course. Dilutional changes associated with massive blood replacements can often be predicted, but the diagnosis is difficult when disseminated coagulopathy complicates massive hemorrhage. Evaluation of all coagulation factors and administration of multiple coagulation components may be required to correct the coagulopathy (91) (Fig. 8).

Packed red cells contain only a small amount of plasma, with minimal coagulation factor activity and no platelets; therefore, replacement therapy using packed red cells and crystalloid leads to a dilutional coagulopathy. Estimates of platelet and coagulation factor levels based on dilution, however, are frequently too low because coagulation factors and platelets, distributed outside the vascular space, are released during the stress of anesthesia and surgery (33,91). In a disseminated coagulopathy, coagulation factor activation may occur as a result of release of tissue thromboplastin into the circulation. Severe tissue trauma and shock can also result in coagulation factor activation and consumption, and platelet and coagulation factor decreases can be much greater than those expected from dilution alone. Coagulation factor activation and consumption are the primary reasons that prophylactic platelet or clotting component transfusion based on anticipated declines has no clinical merit in massive blood loss (24,25,91).

Thrombocytopenia and coagulation factor deficits that contribute to surgical bleeding occur concomitantly, but usually not until more than one blood volume has been replaced with packed red cells. In disseminated coagulopathy as a result of shock, sepsis, or thromboplastin release into the circulation, dramatic declines in platelet counts and fibrinogen levels may occur, and multiple blood components may be needed to achieve surgical hemostasis. Even though red cell scavenging techniques are effective in preserving red cells, these washed red cell solutions are devoid of coagulation proteins and must be considered when assessing whether a coagulopathy is caused by dilution or consumption.

HEMODILUTION

Hemodilution is a useful technique for reducing the allogeneic blood transfusion requirements of patients who are unable to participate in preoperative autologous blood donation (30). Children or adolescents who are excluded from autologous donation because of low body weight can participate in hemodilution, including patients who have severe cerebral palsy, myelomeningocele, or spinal muscular atrophy. Hemodilution can frequently be used to supplement other techniques used to reduce allogeneic blood product usage, such as autologous donation and cell-scavenging techniques.

Hemodilution may be acceptable to many Jehovah's Witness patients, provided the autologous blood removed remains connected to the phlebotomy site by means of the intravenous tubing.

The principles of hemodilution include the following:

1. Removal of a large volume of autologous blood immediately before the operative procedure
2. Replacement of autologous blood removed with crystalloid or colloid solutions
3. Loss of fewer red cells from the surgical field because of the low hematocrit
4. Replacement of autologous whole blood at the end of the operation to restore an acceptable postoperative hematocrit.

During the operation, a relatively profound anemia is expected to achieve a higher hematocrit in the postoperative period.

The limits of hemodilution are determined by assessing factors in tissue oxygen delivery, including hematocrit, blood viscosity and volume, oxygen saturation, oxygen content, and tissue blood flow (80,93). As the hematocrit falls, oxygen content is decreased, but lower blood viscosity decreases flow resistance and enhances microvascular capillary blood flow. Therefore, oxygen delivery can be maintained at a lower hematocrit (80). This produces a situation in which similar oxygen delivery can be achieved without a change in cardiovascular work at hematocrits between 30% and 45%. At hematocrits of less than 25%, even with improved microvascular tissue blood flow due to the lower blood viscosity, cardiovascular work must increase to sustain oxygen delivery.

The critical red cell mass is the lowest hematocrit that allows oxygen delivery to be maintained by cardiorespiratory mechanisms without acidosis secondary to anaerobic metabolism. The myocardium and central nervous system are at greatest risk for hypoxia because these tissues maximally extract available oxygen delivered by the coronary or cerebral arteries under normal circumstances. At hematocrits of less than 20%, myocardial metabolism becomes compromised. Subendocardial ischemia and myocardial infarction can occur even in healthy patients when the hematocrit is less than 15%. In the liver and kidneys, an increase in oxygen extraction usually sustains organ function at hematocrits of less than 20% (23), but centrilobular hepatic necrosis and acute renal failure may occur when hematocrits fall below 15%. Despite the tissue hypoxia that may occur when the hematocrit is less than 15%, case reports indicate that sustained hematocrit decreases to 15% are possible without adverse sequelae (16,27,43,59). The presence of underlying medical disease, the increased metabolic requirements associated with the perioperative period, and anesthetic and surgical effects on perioperative pulmonary function make defining the lowest safe hematocrit more difficulty for individual patients.

During intentional normovolemic hemovolemic hemodilution, the hematocrit is decreased by replacing the patient's blood with crystalloid until a lower hematocrit is achieved (30). Autologous whole blood, removed and stored in citrate solution, must be replaced with a larger volume of crystalloid or colloid solutions to maintain a normal intravascular volume (16,30,59). If vascular volume is not maintained during hemodilution, the hemodilution will be less effective in preserving red cell mass during surgery, and inadequate tissue blood flow and anaerobic tissue metabolism may occur because of the combination of anemia and inadequate vascular volume. The more blood removed before surgery, the fewer red cells will be lost during the operation (e.g., A patient with a hematocrit of 40% will lose twice as many red cells as a patient with a hematocrit of 20%) (30). Of note, large volumes of crystalloid or colloid are required to sustain vascular volume. Extracellular fluid accumulation and peripheral edema are to be expected in the postoperative period. Postoperative diuretics may help to reduce edema but can create an additional source of electrolyte disturbances.

In summary, the basic principles and requirements for intentional normovolemic hemodilution are as follows:

1. The lower the hematocrit is after hemodilution, the more effective hemodilution will be in preventing red cell loss during surgery.
2. Preoperative and intraoperative blood loss should be replaced with crystalloid or colloid solution.
3. Blood volume must be monitored and maintained during hemodilution and throughout the operative procedure.
4. Cardiovascular monitoring is used to assess vascular volume continuously. Persistent tachycardia and electrocardiogram changes suggestive of myocardial ischemia are usually the first signs of inadequate oxygen delivery as a result of anemia. Frequent blood gas assessments are recommended to ensure adequate tissue perfusion. Serial hematocrits help confirm blood loss estimates and evaluate fluid replacement.
5. Autologous red cells should be withheld until most operative blood loss has occurred.
6. Profound hemodilution should not be combined with other techniques that impair tissue oxygen delivery (induced hypotension).
7. Intraoperative hematocrits of less than 20% are to be expected with hemodilution.
8. Normovolemic hemodilution will not provide an acceptable postoperative hematocrit if blood loss exceeds a patient's blood volume. In these settings, hemodilution should be combined with additional blood conversation techniques (e.g., autologous preoperative donation or scavenging red cells).

Hemodilution is particularly useful in patients who cannot participate in an autologous red cell deposit program or if autologous deposit has not provided enough red cells for the anticipated operative procedure.

HYPOTENSIVE ANESTHESIA

Multiple factors influence blood loss during surgery, including the surgical procedure, surgeon, duration of operation, venous blood pressure, arterial blood pressure, tissue blood flow, and hemostatic mechanism. For this reason, studies attempting to define the efficacy of induced hypotension in decreasing blood loss often do not provide a convincing correlation between lowered blood pressure and decreased blood loss. Blood pressure reduced by deliberate hemorrhage was reported to be an effective technique for creating a bloodless operative field by Cushing (36), who recognized both the hazards and the benefits of induced hypotension. Improved monitoring techniques, more rapidly acting and controllable hypotensive agents, and a more complete understanding of the physiology of induced hypotension have helped to reduce complications associated with the technique (112,124).

The relationship between perfusion pressure, tissue blood flow, and tissue oxygen demands is important in defining the limits of hypotension. Setting a limit for induced hypotension is more difficult than setting a limit for a decline in red cell mass, primarily because oxygen delivery to tissues is not as closely related to blood pressure as it is to hematocrit. When blood pressure is reduced by arteriolar vasodilation, tissue blood flow and tissue oxygen delivery may increase even at extremely low perfusion pressures. At the other extreme in situations of hemorrhage or decreased myocardial contractility, tissue blood flow may become inadequate because of vasoconstriction, and tissue ischemia may occur although blood pressure is maintained in the normal range.

Indications

In most settings, induced hypotension is used to decrease intraoperative blood loss, improve operative conditions, and shorten surgical time. In procedures in which blood loss is expected to approach 50% of blood volume, induced hypotension can reduce blood loss by 50% (60,78). In the presence of underlying medical conditions that might be further compromised by the use of deliberate hypotension, a careful assessment of risks and benefits must be made. Some of these conditions commonly observed in posterior spinal surgery include cardiovascular disease, such as the cardiomyopathy of duchenne muscular dystrophy and cyanotic congenital heart disease, renal insufficiency, cerebral trauma, and hepatitis.

Intraoperative Considerations

Adequate anesthesia depth should be established before inducing hypotension, and vascular volume must be assessed throughout the period of hypotension. Additional invasive monitoring is required to determine urine output, direct arterial pressure, and acid-base status. Central venous or pulmonary artery pressure monitoring may also be indicated. The surgical procedure and anticipated operative findings should be well defined. Induced hypotension should not be used if acute massive blood loss is a major concern. If a complication of anesthesia or surgery occurs, induced hypotension should be discontinued.

Methods Of Inducing Hypotension

After a stable anesthetic depth has been achieved, deliberate hypotension can be induced by a variety of methods. When hypotension is induced to decrease operative blood loss, it should be maintained at a constant level throughout the period of surgical dissection. A constant decrease in blood pressure is usually more effective in reducing blood loss than fluctuating periods of profound hypotension throughout the procedure.

The most common method of producing short-term blood pressure reduction is the use of direct-acting vascular smooth muscle dilators. Although the level of blood pressure has been emphasized as important in reducing blood loss, many experts believe that to reduce blood loss, tissue blood flow to the operative site must also be decreased for hypotension to be effective. Controlled studies have not defined the best method of inducing hypotension to decrease blood loss. For this reason, multiple approaches exist.

Vasodilators

Nitroprusside, the most potent agent used to produce deliberate hypotension, is a direct arterial vasodilator. The major risks of nitroprusside relate to lethal cyanide toxicity when high doses (more than 8 μg/kg per min) are used or when the drug is used for prolonged periods (1 mg/kg per 24 hours) (2). Nitroprusside has five cyanide groups that are rapidly metabolized in the body, primarily to nontoxic metabolites. Usually, an insignificant proportion of nitroprusside is metabolized to free cyanide, but when high concentrations of cyanide overcome the usual metabolic pathway, cyanide (CN$^-$) is produced. When cyanide accumulates, cytochrome oxidase inhibition prevents oxidative metabolism, and anaerobic cellular metabolism results in a metabolic acidosis. Cardiac arrest occurs when high CN$^-$ levels disrupt cellular metabolism. Cyanide toxicity should be suspected when tachyphylaxis develops to nitroprusside or if acidosis and hypotension occur and are unresponsive to discontinuation of nitroprusside and intravascular volume expansion. The elevated cyanide levels can be reduced by providing alternative binding sites for CN$^-$, either methemoglobin or thiosulfate. An infusion of sodium nitrate converts hemoglobin into methemoglobin and binds CN$^-$ in an emergency setting.

Nitroglycerin and trimethaphan are also direct arterial vasodilators used to induced hypotension. Nitroglycerin, although less toxic than nitroprusside, is a less potent vasodilator (137). Methemoglobin formation can occur with prolonged infusions of nitroglycerin. Trimethaphan, a ganglionic blocking drug, is not as fast acting or as reversible as nitroglycerin or nitroprusside, and patients often develop tachyphylaxis to the hypotensive actions of trimethaphan. Adenosine, the end product of adenosine triphosphate metabolism, also produces vasodilation by direct effects on vascular smooth muscle and appears to be useful for inducing hypotension (98).

Adrenergic-Blocking Drugs

Sympathetic nervous system modulation of blood pressure can be divided into α- and β-adrenergic effects. β-Receptors primarily affect myocardial contractility and heart rate and have additional effects that produce arterial vasodilation. Propranolol, esmolol, and other β-blocking drugs decrease myocardial contractility and heart rate and are often used in addition to direct arterial vasodilators. Labetalol, a drug combining both α- and β-blocking qualities, decreases contractility, heart rate, and vascular tone; it has a longer half-life than esmolol. In addition to these fast-acting intravenous agents, a variety of other antihypertensive agents have been used to decrease blood pressure preoperatively.

Volatile Anesthetics

Volatile anesthetics at high concentrations are effective in decreasing blood pressure, primarily by depressing myocardial contractility. If complications of hypotension develop, inhalation anesthetics cannot be reversed as quickly or as reliably as short-acting vasodilators. Isoflurane, the most commonly used inhalation anesthetic, produces hypotension by increasing skin and muscle blood flow as well as by depressing myocardial contractility. Anesthetic concentrations required to produce hypotension often eliminate somatosensory evoked responses. If a wake-up test is indicated, volatile anesthetic concentrations must be decreased long before the intraoperative wake up. For these reasons, short-acting vasodilators and β-blocking drugs are more often used to decrease blood pressure in children during spinal operations.

Uncontrolled hypotension leading to cardiac arrest and postoperative neurologic deficits, either temporary or permanent, are the chief complications of induced hypotension. Many of these complications relate to intraoperative management problems, such as a too rapid decrease sustained for a prolonged period, underestimation of blood loss, improper monitoring, or poor patient selection.

PHARMACOLOGIC METHODS TO DECREASE SURGICAL BLEEDING

Drugs that increase coagulation factors and platelet levels potentially reduce surgical bleeding and provide another approach to limiting blood and reducing transfusion during spinal surgery. The pharmacologic agents that have been used to prevent blood loss include desmopressin (DDAVP), epsilon aminocaproic acid (Amicar), tranexamic acid, and aprotinin (Trasylol). All of these drugs have been studied during cardiopulmonary bypass or liver transplantation (109) in patients with multiple abnormalities in hemostasis and major intraoperative blood loss. Even though these agents may be efficacious during major operations in these types of patients, their application in children who require major spinal surgery may not offer similar benefits. At present, there is no evidence to indicate that a preexisting or acquired bleeding disorder is the major factor in blood loss in patients with idiopathic scoliosis. In patients with a preexisting or acquired coagulation abnormality, these drugs can potentially play an important role in reducing blood loss.

Desmopressin

Desmopressin is deamino-8-D-arginine-vasopressin (DDAVP), an analogue of vasopressin. Desmopressin can be extremely beneficial in limiting surgical blood loss in patients with mild or moderate hemophilia and in patients with von Willebrand disease. The stimulation of factor VIII and von Willebrand factor release from endothelial stores is often the only treatment necessary in patients with von Willebrand's disease or hemophilia who require minor surgery. Desmopressin (DDAVP), by increasing von Willebrand factor, also improves platelet aggregation and reduces bleeding time. This additional benefit of desmopressin indicates that this drug may be of benefit in a variety of surgical settings, including scoliosis surgery (61). These preliminary results in surgical patients given desmopressin did show reduced bleeding, but randomized double-blinded controlled trials suggest that the only subgroup of patients who benefited from this therapy are patients on long-term aspirin therapy. More recent studies in placebo-controlled clinical trials suggest that even in a carefully selected groups of patients who have a minor or moderate platelet abnormality, DDAVP may not result in reduced bleeding. A recent study in patients with idiopathic scoliosis has found no reduction in blood loss in DDAVP-treated patients and suggests that the therapy should be reserved for patients with underlying coagulation disorder (1).

Antifibrinolytics

Aprotinin, tranexamic acid, and aminocaproic acid prevent fibrin breakdown and clot lysis. These drugs are often beneficial in situations associated with fibrinolysis and platelet dysfunction, such as cardiopulmonary bypass and liver transplantation. There are considerable pharmacologic differences among the antifibrinolytic drugs.

Epsilon Aminocaproic Acid and Tranexamic Acid

Amicar and tranexamic acid are synthetic antifibrinolytic agents that, when given prophylactically, can reduce blood loss and transfusion requirements during liver transplantation and cardiopulmonary bypass (18,109). These synthetic inhibitors of fibrinolysis adhere to the lysine-binding sites of plasminogen and plasmin and inhibit the conversion of plasminogen to plasmin and interfere with plasmin's ability to cleave fibrinogen and fibrin. Because these agents inhibit clotting, one of the concerns with these drugs is their prothrombolic potential, which may lead to vascular thrombosis. These agents may be useful in patients expected to be at increased risk for blood loss.

Aprotinin

Aprotinin is a broad-spectrum serine protease inhibitor with antiinflammatory and antikallikinin properties, but at concentrations exceeding 50 KIU/mL, it has potent antifibrinolytic properties (76). Aprotinin's antiinflammatory properties reduce elastase release and inhibit complement- and kallikrein-mediated activation of neutrophils and platelets. Aprotinin may also preserve platelet integrity and function by inhibiting proteolytic alterations in von Willebrand factor and platelet glycoprotein Ib and IIb/IIIa receptors. Aprotinin's dual mechanism of action as both an antifibrinolytic and an agent that augments platelet activity may explain why blood loss–complicated cardiopulmonary bypass and liver transplantation is reduced by 40% to 50% (76). Aprotinin is considered helpful in reducing blood loss in patients who have recently received potent platelet inhibitors based on their ability to minimize platelet dysfunction or reverse platelet inhibition. This drug is associated with a higher incidence of allergic reactions than the synthetic antifibrinolytic and is also an expensive prophylactic therapy.

ANESTHESIA FOR SPECIAL PROBLEMS
Traumatic Spinal Cord Injury

One of the chief anesthetic concerns when managing a patient with an acute traumatic spinal injury is preventing progression of the neurologic injury. Securing an airway in a patient with a cervical spine injury must be accomplished with minimal neck movement. A team approach is particularly helpful, with the anesthesiologist attending to the airway and the surgeon maintaining head and neck position with axial traction throughout airway management, tracheal intubation, and patient position. Awake fiberoptic intubation techniques are frequently the best method of securing an airway, but topical anesthesia in a well-sedated patient is imperative to prevent excessive coughing and movement when the tracheal tube is placed in the sensitive glottis and trachea. The presence of a full stomach with the attendant risk for aspiration frequently complicates airway management in cervical spine injury and underscores the importance of preoperative discussion between surgeon and anesthesiologist about intraoperative airway management.

In acute spinal cord injury above T6, the abrupt disruption of sympathetic innervation to the vascular produces vasodilation and hypotension. When cord dysfunction extends higher than T1, sympathetic control of heart rate is also interrupted, leading to bradycardia (127). Venous capacitance vessels dilate, and compensatory baroreceptor responses to decreased vascular volume are lost. Position changes and positive-pressure ventilation frequently aggravate hypotension in patients with "spinal shock." Cardiac responses to increased ventricular volume are also altered in spinal cord injury patients, and small changes in intravascular volume can lead to pulmonary edema, even in patients with normal cardiac contractility. As spinal shock resolves 24 to 72 hours after injury, a return of sympathetic tone may result in a shift in blood volume from the dilated venous capacitance vessels to the central circulation.

In patients with chronic high spinal cord injury, severe hypertension due to autonomic hyperreflexia may occur. Autonomic hyperreflexia results when visceral or somatic stimulation below the level of spinal cord transection produces a generalized sympathetic response. In patients with cord transection higher than T7, this produces hypertension, headaches, sweating, vasodilation above the level of the transection, and intense vasoconstriction in denervated areas below the transection. Severe hypertension in susceptible patients can result in cerebral hemorrhage. General or regional anesthesia is often required to control this autonomic response in susceptible patients who require surgery.

An additional anesthetic concern in paraplegia is the hyperkalemic response to succinylcholine. In denervated muscle, the entire muscle membrane, rather than just the neuromuscular junction, may respond to succinylcholine by depolarization. Potassium efflux after succinylcholine can increase serum K^+ to more than 10 mEq/L, leading to cardiac arrest.

Upper Respiratory Infection

A difficult preoperative problem is dealing with a child who has symptoms suggestive of an upper respiratory infection. In the past, a runny nose often resulted in cancellation of the surgical procedure until the symptoms resolved, but this is not always appropriate. The first step in evaluating a child with a runny nose is to determine the etiology of the problem. Allergies are common and cause symptoms that mimic an upper respiratory tract infection but cause few perioperative problems. Parents can often help differentiate allergic symptoms from an acute infectious illness because a child with allergic disease tends to have a chronic runny nose and shows little change in day-to-day activities, such as eating, sleeping, or playing. In contrast, a child with an upper respiratory tract viral infection has increased airway secretions, airway reactivity, malaise, rhinorrhea, sneezing, congestion, cough, and sore throat as well as temperature higher than 38°C. The risk of anesthetizing a child during an upper respiratory infection is not clearly defined, but perioperative complications are more common in these children (39,121,122). The airway changes associated with upper respiratory infection often persist for several weeks; therefore, an ideal approach would be to postpone elective surgery for at least 3 to 6 weeks. This may not be a practical solution because upper respiratory tract infections are frequent (five to eight infections per year) in young children, and it may be impossible to find a time when a young child does not have, or is not just recovering from, a respiratory infection.

No single course of action is correct for all children with a runny nose, but it is important to establish a consistent approach to the management of children with this constellation of symptoms. In many cases, the operation can proceed, but elective surgery should be delayed in the following circumstances:

1. There is evidence of lower respiratory tract involvement (e.g., wheezing, bronchi, or coarse rales) by auscultation or abnormal chest radiograph.
2. The child has a temperature of more than 38°C associated with symptoms of an upper respiratory infection.
3. A stridorous cough or severe sore throat is present.
4. Any systemic symptoms (e.g., fatigue, malaise) or a change in daily activities is noted by parents.

Laboratory and radiologic examinations usually add little useful information, but a marked leukocytosis or changes on a chest radiograph would support a diagnosis of acute respiratory infection and indicate that elective surgery should be postponed.

Down Syndrome

Trisomy 21 is the most common chromosomal abnormality, and the constellation of morphologic, physiologic, and neurologic changes associated with Down syndrome affects anesthetic management. Operative intervention for neuraxial problems in some patients with Down's syndrome may be required for atlantoaxial instability (133). Anesthetic concerns in these children relate to morphologic changes in the upper airway. A large head, macroglossia, and small airway caliber relative to size create problems with perioperative airway management. Airway obstruction during anesthesia induction is a particular concern in patients with Down syndrome. Symptoms of chronic obstructive upper airway disease can often be ascertained by a history of snoring, apnea, or cyanosis while asleep. Postoperative upper airway obstruction

and edema due to their relatively small airway size may result in postintubation croup in patients with Down syndrome.

Atlantoaxial subluxation is a serious manifestation of the generalized ligamentous laxity that occurs in Down syndrome, and care must be taken if extension or flexion of the neck occurs during tracheal intubation (133). Fiberoptic endoscopy and intubation with the child's cervical spine maintained in a neutral position to prevent extensive neck flexion or extension is possibly the safest way to secure the airway in a child with Down syndrome.

An additional concern is congenital heart disease, which occurs in more than 40% of patients with Down syndrome (99). The two most common abnormalities, arterioventricular canal defect and ventricular septal defect, result in high pulmonary blood flow leading to pulmonary vascular changes and, if uncorrected, pulmonary hypertension. Operative repair of congenital heart disease often does not correct the pulmonary hypertension. Persistent pulmonary hypertension may lead to other pulmonary problems and right ventricular failure. Decreased immune surveillance and poor leukocyte function in patients with Down syndrome can result in pulmonary infection in the perioperative period.

Congenital Heart Disease

Congenital heart disease is most often described according to the anatomic or morphologic cardiac defect that exists. Atrial septal defects, ventricular septal defects, and patient ductus arteriosus, the most common congenital heart defects, are anatomic abnormalities that result in shunting of blood flow. The pressure difference between the lower-pressure pulmonary and higher-pressure systemic circulation usually results in a left to right shunt across the defect. Before operative closure, the increased pulmonary blood flow due to a left to right systemic to pulmonary shunt may require diuretic and digoxin therapy to decrease symptoms of congestive heart failure. Transposition of the great arteries or tetralogy of Fallot often creates more complicated pathophysiologic changes. When prior palliative or corrective cardiac surgery has been performed, an assessment of the special perioperative management required often becomes even more difficult. The most important initial step in assessing patients with congenital heart disease is to determine the physiologic impact of the underlying congenital heart disease on the day-to-day functional activities of the child and to define the current medical therapy required to control symptoms and signs of heart disease.

Muscular Dystrophy

Spinal stabilization procedures are often required in patients who are already severely compromised from a respiratory standpoint by progressive muscular dystrophy. Cardiac failure and respiratory insufficiency associated with Duchenne muscular dystrophy usually lead to death by 25 years of age (107). Numerous case reports attest to the anesthetic difficulties in patients with Duchenne dystrophy (66,81,97). Cardiac arrest during anesthesia has been reported frequently, probably as a manifestation of both the cardiac and the respiratory involvement. In addition, intraoperative problems related to hyperkalemia and malignant hyperthermia appear to occur more frequently in patients with Duchenne dystrophy. Myocardial muscle necrosis occurs as the muscular dystrophy progresses and cardiac infiltration with fatty tissue can be detected by electrocardiogram abnormalities. The additive cardiodepressant effects of volatile anesthetics often compound hemodynamic depression in this patient population.

Progressive weakness of respiratory muscles prevents an effective cough, and pulmonary infection in the postoperative period due to retained secretions is a major cause of perioperative morbidity. Aggressive bronchopulmonary toilet decreases the risks for postoperative pneumonic problems. Postoperative ventilation for 24 hours or longer after a major spinal procedure is often the most appropriate management, particularly if bed rest in the supine position is required. A progressive decrease in vital capacity is anticipated with muscular dystrophy. Preoperative pulmonary function testing may help detect patients with a vital capacity of less than 15 mL/kg who will most likely require mechanical ventilation postoperatively.

Increased intraoperative bleeding is a frequent problem in patients with friable osteopenic bone due to neuromuscular disease. Blood requirements are frequently increased in these patients, who may not tolerate a low hematocrit (less than 25%) in the perioperative period.

Diagnostic Radiology

Sophisticated diagnostic procedures, such as computed tomography (CT) and magnetic resonance imaging (MRI), produce high-resolution images of the body that are useful in the evaluation of a variety of orthopaedic conditions. Although not painful, CT scanning and MRI may cause discomfort or distress in children because of the noise generated by the scanning equipment and the claustrophobic sensation that occurs when a patient is placed inside the scanner. In addition, it is difficult for young children to remain motionless for the long periods required to complete a successful study. Consequently, some type of sedation or anesthesia is often required (17).

In an effort to avoid general anesthesia, orthopaedic surgeons and radiologists often use a "lytic cocktail" to sedate children. Although many recipes are available, there is no single drug or combination of drugs that will safely and consistently sedate all children (46). Infants up to about 6 months of age may be adequately immobilized by simply bundling them in a blanket. School-aged children usually do well with reassurance and an oral sedative like chloral hydrate or a benzodiazepine (41,82) given before the procedure, but young children from 1 to 6 years of age often need deep sedation or general anesthesia if an adequate study is to be obtained.

If adequate sedation is not achieved with oral, rectal, or intramuscular medications, general anesthesia may be required. Many different anesthetic techniques have been used successfully, including intramuscular ketamine, pure intravenous techniques (e.g., thiopental, midazolam, propofol), or volatile anesthetics with or without nitrous oxide (131). During these types of diagnostic procedures, it is desirable to obtain intravenous access, and the same standard of monitoring is required whether the child receives general anesthesia or sedation (3,4).

MRI introduces a number of unique problems for the anesthesiologist that are related to the imager's powerful magnetic field and the radiofrequency pulses it emits (11). First, any object containing ferromagnetic material, including gas cylinders and anesthesia machines, will be attracted to the magnetic fields and can be violently pulled into the scanner. Second, many electronic monitors do not function properly when brought into the magnetic field produced by the imager. Finally, metallic equipment and electronic monitors near the patient may emit radiofrequency waves that affect the scanning procedure and result in degraded, nondiagnostic images.

In addition to the anesthetic problems that can occur during MRI, there are other hazards that can affect patients or personnel working near the unit. People with implanted metallic devices, such as cerebrovascular clips or pacemakers, are at substantial risk because the magnetic forces exerted on them by the scanner can cause displacement or dislodgment. Demand pacemakers may be converted to the asynchronous mode by the static magnetic field, or radiofrequency waves generated by the imager can suppress pacemaker activity (94). The changing magnetic field can also cause heating of metal objects, such as orthopaedic prostheses or external wire leads, causing severe burns.

After sedation or general anesthesia for a diagnostic procedure, children require the same standard of postanesthesia care that they would have received postoperatively. This can occur in the radiology suite, or the patient may be transferred to the postanesthesia care unit in the main operating room. After recovery, the same discharge criteria used for surgical patients also apply to children who receive sedation or anesthesia for diagnostic procedures (3,4).

Malignant Hyperthermia

Malignant hyperthermia is a rare genetic syndrome characterized by a fulminant, hypermetabolic response of skeletal muscle to the administration of potent, halogenated anesthetic agents (usually halothane) or the depolarizing muscle relaxant succinylcholine (19). Because most susceptible patients presenting for surgery exhibit no signs or symptoms of the disease, and because no simple diagnostic test is available, it is critical that early manifestations of the disease be recognized quickly so that triggering agents can be stopped and therapy initiated. Although new noninvasive biochemical tests for malignant hyperthermia are being evaluated, a specific diagnosis can be made only by performing a muscle biopsy and caffeine contracture test (73,105).

Clinical Manifestations

Muscle rigidity after the administration of a triggering agent, particularly succinylcholine, is perhaps the most common sign of malignant hyperthermia (Table 4). It is more common in children, and although any muscle group may be affected, the rigidity frequently occurs in the muscles of the jaw. This muscle rigidity persists for several minutes and is quickly followed by other manifestations of the disease if the triggering agents are continued (104).

Other early signs and symptoms of malignant hyperthermia are related to the fulminant hypermetabolic response that occurs

TABLE 4. CLINICAL SIGNS OF MALIGNANT HYPERTHERMIA

Tachycardia
Tachypnea
Respiratory acidosis
Metabolic acidosis
Central venous desaturation
Fever
Muscle rigidity
Cyanosis

in skeletal muscle exposed to a triggering inhalation agent or succinylcholine. A defect in release of calcium from the sarcoplasmic reticulum results in a marked rise in the concentration of calcium within the muscle cell. This increase in intracellular cytoplasmic calcium activates aerobic and anaerobic metabolism, increases oxygen consumption and hydrolysis of adenosine triphosphate, and produces massive quantities of lactic acid, carbon dioxide, and heat. As the disease progresses, oxidative phosphorylation with mitochondria becomes uncoupled, further increasing oxygen consumption, lactic acidosis, and heat production. As the production of adenosine triphosphate falls, membrane integrity begins to be lost. At this point, the malignant hyperthermia rapidly becomes fatal.

Hypercarbia is one of the early signs of malignant hyperthermia and should always be carefully evaluated. Tachycardia, tachypnea, muscle rigidity, fever, hypercarbia, and central venous deoxygenation are other primary signs of a malignant hyperthermia crisis (104). As the disease progresses, the clinical picture may be further complicated by cardiac dysrhythmias, hypertension or hypotension, hyperkalemia, disseminated intravascular coagulation, and left ventricular failure. When first described in 1960, malignant hyperthermia was almost invariably fatal. Now, with prompt diagnosis and treatment, mortality in the most fulminant forms of the disease is less than 15% and continues to decrease (19).

Treatment of the Acute Crisis

When a diagnosis of malignant hyperthermia is made, specific aggressive treatment must be initiated immediately (Table 5).

TABLE 5. TREATMENT OF ACUTE MALIGNANT HYPERTHERMIA CRISIS

1. Stop all triggering agents, and end surgery as quickly as possible.
2. Hyperventilate with 100% oxygen.
3. Administer dantrolene.
4. Cool with ice, cold intravenous fluid, and cold irrigants.
5. Correct metabolic acidosis with bicarbonate.
6. Treat hyperkalemia, if present.
7. Treat arrhythmias with procainamide.
8. Monitor arterial and venous blood gases, arterial pressure, central venous pressure, end-tidal CO_2, urine output, K^+, Ca^+, lactate, creatine phosphokinase, urine myoglobin, prothrombin time, partial thromboplastin time, platelets, and temperature.
9. Maintain urine output with fluid and diuretics.
10. Transfer to intensive care unit for continued monitoring for 24–48h.

The triggering anesthetic agents must be stopped and the surgery concluded as rapidly as possible. The patient should be hyperventilated with 100% oxygen, and any potential source of even trace amounts of a volatile anesthetic agent should be removed. Cooling of the patient should be started with intravenous iced saline, lavage of body cavities, and surface cooling with a blanket or ice. Acidosis and hyperkalemia should be treated with bicarbonate and glucose, and arterial blood gases must be obtained frequently to assess the early response to therapy.

Dantrolene must be administered immediately after a diagnosis of malignant hyperthermia has been made (19). By acting directly on the sarcoplasmic reticulum and inhibiting the release of calcium, dantrolene can quickly abort a malignant hyperthermia crisis. The initial dose is 2.5 mg/kg and additional doses should be given (up to 10 mg/kg) until all signs of the crisis have abated. Because dantrolene can cause significant muscle weakness and prolong the duration of neuromuscular blocking drugs, it is important that ventilation be monitored carefully and supported, if necessary, to prevent respiratory failure.

Cardiac dysrhythmias occur frequently during a malignant hyperthermia crisis and may persist despite aggressive treatment with dantrolene. These dysrhythmias can be treated with 3 to 15 mg/kg of procainamide. While initiating specific treatment, aggressive monitoring should also be established, including an arterial line, central venous or pulmonary artery catheter, and urinary catheter. Arterial and venous blood gases, acid-base balance, serum potassium, calcium lactate, creatinine phosphokinase, and coagulation times should be checked frequently. Urine output should be stimulated with volume expansion, mannitol, and furosemide, if necessary. The patient should be observed in an intensive care setting for 24 to 48 hours to monitor for a relapse of the crisis or other late complications.

Anesthetic Management of Susceptible Patients Having Elective Surgery

Children may present for elective surgery with a anesthetic history or family history that suggests susceptibility to malignant hyperthermia. In most cases, a diagnostic muscle biopsy will not have been done and is usually unnecessary. It is important, however, that this type of patient be treated as being susceptible to malignant hyperthermia and that specific steps be taken to avoid anesthetic triggering agents, to establish appropriate intraoperative monitoring, to ensure the immediate availability of emergency supplies and support personnel, and to arrange for an appropriate period of postanesthetic recovery.

Although no anesthetic technique can be considered absolutely safe, there are a variety of general anesthetic techniques that will minimize the risk of triggering an acute crisis. All triggering agents must be avoided, including succinylcholine and the volatile anesthetics—halothane, enflurane, isoflurane, desflurane, and sevoflurane. Nitrous oxide and all the intravenous anesthetics, including barbiturates, benzodiazepines, ketamine, propofol, and the narcotics, are considered safe in susceptible patients, as are the nondepolarizing muscle relaxants. Local anesthetics are also safe, and regional anesthesia is an acceptable alternative in these patients. The prophylactic use of dantrolene is not recommended in children because of the potentially serious side effects. However, it must be immediately available for use if an acute crisis should occur. If no complications are encountered during surgery or after several hours in the postanesthesia care unit, the patient can be discharged from the hospital.

Diseases Associated with Malignant Hyperthermia

A variety of myopathies have been associated with malignant hyperthermia and, although in most cases the association is weak, the relationship between malignant hyperthermia and central core disease appears to be well established (52). Patients with Duchenne muscular dystrophy (20,21,97) and osteogenesis imperfecta (101) have also been reported to manifest signs and symptoms of malignant hyperthermia during surgery. Various other syndromes, including arthrogryposis, hyperkalemia periodic paralysis, myotonia congenita, and neuroleptic malignant syndrome are also believed to be related to malignant hyperthermia, but these associations are controversial (20).

ANESTHETIC COMPLICATIONS

Morbidity and Mortality in Anesthesia

In 1846, William Morton demonstrated that ether could be safely administered to provide anesthesia during surgery. Within months of this report, inhalation techniques with nitrous oxide, chloroform, or ether were used to provide pain relief for a wide variety of surgical procedures. Less than 2 years after Morton's administration of ether at Massachusetts General Hospital, the first death during anesthesia was reported (117). Hannah Greener, a 15-year-old girl, aspirated and died during removal of an ingrown toenail. Although anesthesia is extremely safe today, outcome studies continue to identify the complications that most commonly contribute to anesthetic morbidity and mortality (68,111). The incidence of cardiac arrest attributed to anesthesia has steadily decreased over the years, but children still experience a three times higher incidence of morbidity and mortality during anesthesia (25,68,111), primarily because of a higher frequency of intraoperative cardiovascular and respiratory complications.

Keenan and Boyan (68) surveyed anesthetic morbidity in one institution and noted an overall incidence of cardiac arrest of 1.7 per 10,000 infants. Tiret and colleagues (125) noted a similar incident of cardiac arrest and confirmed a greater propensity for serious cardiorespiratory events in anesthetized children, particularly infants younger than 1 year of age. Although cardiac arrest and death are the most serious outcome, other significant cardiac and respiratory events also occur more commonly in children and are almost five times as common in infants younger than 12 months of age (40 per 10,000) (Fig. 9) (126).

A variety of factors may be responsible for the increased anesthetic morbidity and mortality in children when compared with that in adults. The anatomy of the infant airway differs from that of the adult and results in a greater likelihood of airway obstruction. In addition, children have a higher oxygen consumption but a diminished respiratory reserve. Therefore, hypoxia develops rapidly when apnea or airway obstruction occurs. Interpreting cardiorespiratory measurements is also more diffi-

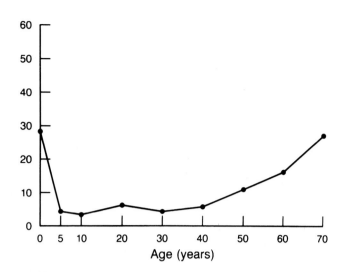

FIGURE 9. Anesthetic morbidity related to age: Major cardiovascular and respiratory anesthetic complications during anesthesia per 10,000 anesthetics. Neonates have the highest incidence of complications in the perioperative period. (From Tiret L, Desmonts JM, Hatton F, et al. [1986]: Complications associated with anesthesia: a prospective survey in France. *Can Anaesth Soc J* 33:336–344, with permission.)

cult because physiologic and pharmacologic data derived from adult studies may not be reliable when applied to children (88), yet comparatively little clinical or basic science anesthetic research has been done in children.

An approach to anesthesia management in this diverse patient population encompassing neonates through adolescents requires an understanding of anatomic, physiologic, pharmacologic, and physiologic differences related to growth and development. Age-related differences, special requirements related to underlying pediatric disease, and the intended operative procedure all need to be considered when developing an anesthetic plan.

Anesthetic complications can occur during the preoperative, intraoperative, and postoperative time periods (Table 6). Case reports from the earliest anesthetic experiences indicate that such complications evolve through stages of recognition, evaluation of frequency and etiology, and finally solution. When all complications and side effects are considered, the frequency of perioperative problems in children approaches 30% (25). Nausea and vomiting account for a relatively high proportion of postoperative side effects (70%).

Many anesthetic complications have had a slow period of recognition and continue to be unresolved. Asphyxic deaths reported throughout the first 100 years of anesthesia included all types of respiratory and cardiovascular complications, including hypoxic gas mixtures due to equipment failure, airway obstruction, unrecognized esophageal intubation, aspiration of gastric contents, pulmonary edema, anesthetic overdose, and gas emboli. Better equipment design with integrated monitoring devices and audible alarms has helped decreased hypoxic insults cause by unrecognized equipment failure, and monitoring standards have been adopted to help prevent hypoxic gas mixtures from being administered to patients. Today, the major causes of hypoxia during anesthesia are respiratory complications, such as aspiration, bronchospasm, or pulmonary embolism.

TABLE 6. COMPLICATIONS OF ANESTHESIA IN CHILDREN

Preinduction
  Hypoglycemia secondary to NPO period
  Preoperative sedative or narcotic overdose leading to respiratory depression
  Idiosyncratic or anaphylactic reaction to premedicant
  Hyperthermia secondary to dehydration or anticholinergic drugs
Anesthesia induction
  Hypoventilation secondary to anesthetic drugs, upper airway obstruction, or laryngeal spasm
  Failure to intubate, or esophageal intubation
  Mechanical failure of anesthetic equipment leading to hypoventilation
  Anaphylaxis with bronchospasm
  Anesthetic overdose leading to circulatory arrest
  Aspiration of gastric contents
  Dental injury
Anesthesia maintenance
  Hypoventilation
    Bronchospasm
    Obstruction of tracheal tube
    Failure to recognize tracheal tube disconnection or extubation
    Pneumothorax
    Air emboli
  Anaphylaxis
  Hypotension secondary to hypovolemia or anesthetic overdose
  Peripheral nerve injuries secondary to positioning
  Inadvertent hypothermia
  Pressure injuries secondary to positioning (skin, cornea, eye)
Postoperative (early and late)
  Hypoventilation
    Airway obstruction
    Laryngeal spasm
    Croup or stridor secondary to subglottic edema or laryngeal injury
  Aspiration
  Vomiting
  Hoarseness or recurrent stridor secondary to laryngeal injury or subglottic stenosis
  Nightmares or changes in behavior
  Subglottic stenosis

Aspiration

In 1946, Mendelson recognized the relationship between aspiration and severe pneumonitis in obstetric patients who required cesarean section (79). Endotracheal intubation as a means of protecting the airway of unconscious patients has helped decrease the incidence of aspiration pneumonitis, but this remains a serious anesthetic complication. Aspiration pneumonitis may occur when gastric contents are present, laryngeal reflexes are depressed by drugs or disease, mechanisms to prevent reflux of gastric contents fail, and aspiration of acid or particulate matter lead to chemical pneumonitis (130).

The preoperative fasting period, particularly for solid foods and dairy products, can decrease the presence of particulate matter in the stomach. Under normal circumstances, gastric emptying occurs in 2 to 3 hours, but stress in the form of anxiety or pain may delay it. One percent of all elective surgery patients who have observed traditional fasting guidelines still have particulate matter in their stomachs at anesthesia induction. Gastric fluid with a low pH is also capable of causing a severe chemical pneumonitis. More than 60% to 70% of children undergoing elective surgery have acidic gastric fluid after fasting. A variety of approaches have been taken to decrease gastric volume (anticholinergics), increase gastric pH (antacids, histamine-2 receptor blockers), and promote gastric emptying (metoclopramide). Under normal circumstances, regurgitation of gastric contents is prevented by esophagogastric sphincter mechanisms, but increased intraabdominal pressure from coughing or increased intragastric pressure from gastric dilation can disrupt sphincter mechanisms and allow gastric contents to reflux into the esophagus. Techniques to achieve tracheal intubation before anesthesia induction or rapid tracheal intubation after anesthesia induction lessen the chance of aspiration in patients at high risk. In neonates, infants, and children who have low oxygen reserves and increased oxygen consumption, hypoxia occurs more rapidly after intravenous anesthesia induction than in adults; hence, rapid induction techniques are more frequently associated with hypoxia in this age group.

Treatment of aspiration pneumonitis is primarily supportive. If particulate matter has been aspirated, rigid bronchoscopy to remove large particles is indicated. If the aspirate is acidic, the acid is neutralized almost immediately upon contact with tracheal mucosa; thus, tracheal lavage has no role in decreasing the extent of chemical pneumonitis and may extend the pulmonary damage. The initial pulmonary aspiration is often associated with bronchospasm; later, over the course of 6 to 12 hours, a severe pneumonitis often develops. Steroid use may contribute to later superinfection and does not modify the course of pneumonitis. Antibiotic use may lead to superinfection by resistant bacteria. Positive-pressure ventilation with oxygen and positive end-expiratory pressure are the mainstays of supportive therapy and should be continued until the pneumonic process resolves.

Bronchospasm

Failure of ventilation during anesthesia can encompass a variety of mechanical and patient factors. One of the most difficult intraoperative problems is bronchospasm. When it is severe, bronchospasm can lead to an inability to ventilate, followed by hypoxia and death. Preoperative evaluation of asthmatic patients to prevent an exacerbation of bronchospasm is a major concern in preoperative preparation. Bronchodilators must be tailored to decrease asthmatic symptoms. Asthmatic patients should not have elective surgery if significant bronchospasm remains uncontrolled before the operation. Bronchospasm may occur in asthmatic patients during tracheal intubation; hence, intubation and extubation under deep anesthesia are advocated by many to lessen the frequency of bronchospasm. Occasionally, healthy patients with no allergic or asthmatic history respond to anesthesia and operative events with severe bronchoconstriction, leading to the inability to ventilate. Other causes of bronchospasm or wheezing include pneumothorax, anaphylaxis, pulmonary edema, congestive heart failure, and endobronchial intubation.

Air or Gas Emboli

Air can enter the venous circulation when veins are open and a pressure gradient favors air entrainment. During major spine surgery, the conditions that can lead to air emboli are frequently present. With better techniques for recognizing air in the venous circulation, such as echocardiography or end-tidal gas monitoring, the frequency of air emboli appears to be much higher than previously recognized. Fortunately, even though air can be visualized entering the venous circulation and right atrium during a variety of operative procedures, it only infrequently leads to clinical symptoms. Posterior spinal stabilization procedures are characterized by the opening of multiple venous channels above the level of the heart, and significant air emboli may occasionally occur.

If air enters the pulmonary artery, ventilation in the absence of pulmonary perfusion leads to dead space ventilation. If pulmonary circulation is impaired by air embolism, hypoxia may occur. When air entrainment is massive, right ventricular pressure markedly increases, and a combination of hypoxia and hypotension is frequently observed. The constellation of hypoxia, hypercarbia, and decreased end-tidal carbon dioxide despite adequate ventilation should suggest the possibility of gas emboli.

POSTOPERATIVE ANALGESIA

The treatment of pain in children has received considerable attention in recent years as it has become increasingly apparent that postoperative pain in children is a common problem that is often inadequately treated. Besides causing discomfort and distress for the patient, it may also have a detrimental effect on morbidity and mortality (8,9,77). There are a variety of reasons that a child's pain may not be adequately treated, including the physician's attitude toward pain in pediatric patients, the reluctance of nursing staff to administer potent analgesics to children, and the inability or reluctance of children to communicate their discomfort if it results in an intramuscular injection to relieve the pain.

Assessment of Pain

Pain is a sensory perception to tissue injury that is modulated by physiologic and psychological factors and by the patient's previous experience with pain (100). To a great extent, pain is a subjective phenomenon, making measurement or quantification of pain difficult. Because there is no physiologic measure of pain intensity, we must rely on more indirect measurement techniques, including cardiorespiratory or endocrine responses to pain, behavior changes, or self-reporting of the intensity of pain.

Marked increases in blood pressure and heart rate occur in infants and children subjected to painful procedures. Although these reactions are a common response to pain, they may also be a reaction to other factors, such as the anxiety the child experiences when placed in a clinical environment. Frequently, these cardiovascular responses can be markedly reduced by providing adequate analgesia before the procedure.

There are also changes in the plasma concentrations of catecholamines, cortisol, aldosterone, growth hormone, and glucagon in children undergoing surgical procedures. This endocrine stress response increases the breakdown of proteins, carbohy-drates, and fats, resulting in increased nitrogen losses, hyperglycemia, and elevated levels of lactate and free fatty acids. The hormonal response to surgery can be reduced or eliminated by providing analgesia or deep anesthesia. In addition, at least in some neonates, the incidence of postoperative morbidity and mortality also appeared to decrease when deeper anesthesia and postoperative analgesia were provided (9).

In children younger than 4 years of age who may be unable to express themselves verbally, pain scales incorporating changes in heart rate, blood pressure, and behavioral responses, such as withdrawal, facial expression, and crying, have been used to assess pain and the child's response to analgesia. Between 4 and 7 years of age, children are often able to understand a visual scale that uses "smiley faces," numbers, or colors to quantify pain. Agreement between this type of self-reporting and behavioral assessments can be significant in this age group. In children older than 6 or 7 years of age, a standard visual analogue scale using a 10-cm line representing "no pain" at one end and "worst possible pain" at the other end can be used to assess pain. It is important to remember, however, that if any type of scale is used to measure pain, the child must be exposed to the scale before surgery and understand how it is to be used.

Choice of Analgesics

The management of postoperative pain can employ nonnarcotic analgesics, narcotics, or local anesthetics.

Nonnarcotics

Acetaminophen and nonsteroidal antiinflammatory drugs given orally or rectally are useful analgesics in children experiencing mild or moderate pain. In the usual recommended doses, adverse affects from acetaminophen are rare. The nonsteroidal antiinflammatory agents, although safe, have been associated with gastritis and hepatic or renal dysfunction when used for prolonged periods.

Unlike the narcotics, these drugs do not produce sedation, tolerance, or dependence; however, the analgesic effect is limited, and it is unlikely that these agents alone will provide adequate analgesia after a major spinal operation.

Narcotics

For many years, narcotics have been the medication of choice in the treatment of postoperative pain, and morphine is the standard by which all other analgesics are judged. When given in adequate doses and in a way that maintains plasma levels at or above analgesic concentrations, morphine provides excellent pain relief (42). Side effects of morphine are common and include itching, nausea and vomiting, urinary retention, and histamine release. Meperidine produces similar side effects and, with prolonged administration, can cause dysphoric reactions as a result of accumulation of active metabolites. Cardiovascular side effects are infrequent.

Respiratory depression is always a concern when narcotics are used for pain relief, and it appears that neonates and young infants are more sensitive to the depressant effects of morphine. In addition, the clearance of morphine is delayed in newborns and the elimination half-life is prolonged (74). Therefore, when morphine is used in infants younger than 1 year old, close cardiovascular monitoring is required for at least 12 hours after the morphine has been discontinued.

Traditionally, narcotics have been administered intramuscularly using a fixed drug dose given at regular intervals. This approach to postoperative analgesia often results in alternating periods of inadequately controlled pain and excessive narcosis. Attempts to improve the reliability of analgesia in the postoperative period have resulted in the use of continuous infusion of morphine. These continuous infusions achieve superior pain relief when compared with intermittent intramuscular injections and are not associated with any significant increase in the incidence of side effects or complications. Another advantage of continuous infusion is that some children deny pain rather than submit to an intramuscular injection.

Patient-controlled analgesia (PCA) can be used by children as young as 6 years of age to provide effective postoperative analgesia (102). PCA allows a patient to administer an intravenous dose of a narcotic by manually activating a small drug pump. The major advantage of PCA is that it allows the patient to determine the optimal time for drug administration. After delivering a dose of narcotic, the pump activates a preset lockout time during which the patient cannot administer another dose. When a patient is placed on PCA, the bolus dose, the lock-out time, and a time-limited maximal dose are selected by the physician. The flexibility of PCA allows the patient to anticipate when more analgesia may be required and prophylactically self-medicate, for example, before chest physiotherapy or ambulation. It also allows the patient to titrate the analgesic requirement against the sedation or side effects that can occur with the use of morphine. Although other potent synthetic narcotics are available, including fentanyl, sufentanil, and alfentanil, their short duration of action makes them useful postoperatively only when administered by infusion (71) with continuous respiratory monitoring.

Narcotics, particularly morphine, have also been administered into the epidural or subarachnoid space to provide postoperative analgesia (129). The advantages of this method of pain control are that very small doses of narcotic can provide up to 24 hours of analgesia. If a catheter is placed into the epidural space, a continuous infusion or intermittent bolus doses can prolong pain control for several days. Pruritus, nausea and vomiting, and urinary retention are the most common side effects, and these can usually be controlled with small doses of naloxone, if necessary, without losing the analgesic effect. A more serious potential problem is respiratory depression, which may occur more frequently in children than in adults. Children receiving epidural or spinal narcotics must be monitored closely for signs of excessive sedation and receive continuous cardiorespiratory monitoring for 12 to 24 hours after the last dose of narcotic.

Local Anesthetics

Long-acting local anesthetics, such as bupivacaine, can also be used to provide effective postoperative analgesia. Local infiltra-

tion of the incision or specific nerve blocks have been shown to provide excellent postoperative pain relief without many of the side effects associated with narcotics (10). In children undergoing thoracotomy for anterior spinal surgery, intercostal nerve block performed under direct vision by the surgeon before wound closure can be a useful technique for providing analgesia.

Local anesthetics can also be administered epidurally through a thoracic, lumbar, or caudal approach for control of postoperative pain (40). If long-term analgesia is required, a continuous infusion of bupivacaine through an epidural catheter can be used. Although effective for pelvic or lower limb surgery, the usefulness of this technique after spinal surgery has not been established.

Effective postoperative analgesia is an integral part of the anesthetic management of children. Although assessing pain and determining the adequacy of analgesia are difficult in young children, it is an aspect of their care that must be neglected. New techniques and new drugs have provided physicians with many effective ways of controlling postoperative pain, and no child should suffer unnecessarily because of inadequate postoperative pain control.

REFERENCES

1. Alanay A, Acaroglu E, Özdemir O, et al. (1999): Effects of deamino-8-D-arginine vasopressin on blood loss and coagulation factors in scoliosis surgery. *Spine* 24:877.
2. Aitken D, West D, Smith F, et al. (1977): Cyanide toxicity following nitroprusside induced hypotension. *Can Anaesth Soc J* 24:651–660.
3. American Academy of Pediatrics (1985): Committee on Drugs, Section on Anesthesiology: Guidelines for the elective use of conscious sedation, deep sedation and general anesthesia in pediatric patients. *Pediatrics* 76:317–321.
4. American Academy of Pediatrics (1992): Committee on Drugs: Guidelines for monitoring and management of pediatric patients during and after sedation for diagnostic and therapeutic procedures. *Pediatrics* 89:1110–1115.
5. American Society of Anesthesiologists (1963): New classification of physical status. *Anesthesiology* 24:111.
6. American Society of Anesthesiologists (1994): *Manual for anesthesia department organization and management.* Park Ridge, IL: pp. 59–62.
7. American Society of Anesthesiologists Task Force on Preoperative Fasting (1999): Practice guidelines for preoperative fasting and the use of pharmacologic agents to reduce the risk of pulmonary aspiration: application to healthy patients undergoing elective procedures. *Anesthesiology* 90:896–905
8. Anand KS, Hickey PR (1987): Pain and its effects in the human neonate and fetus. *N Engl J Med* 317:1322.
9. Anand KJS, Sippele WG, Aynsley-Green A (1987): Randomized trial of fentanyl anaesthesia in preterm babies undergoing surgery. *Lancet* 1:243–247.
10. Arthur DS, McNicol LR (1986): Local anaesthetic techniques in paediatric surgery. *Br J Anaesth* 58:760–778.
11. Bark NS (1989): Anesthesia for magnetic resonance imaging. *Anesthesiol Clin North Am* 7:707–721.
12. Barker S, Tremper K (1987): Pulse oximetry application. *Int Anesthesiol Clin* 25:155–178.
13. Bell GR, Gurd AR, Orlowski JP, et al. (1986): The syndrome of inappropriate ADH secretion following spinal fusion. *J Bone Joint Surg (Am)* 26:720–723.
14. Dabbagh S, Ellis D, Gruskin AB (1996): Regulation of fluids and electrolytes in infants and children. In: Motoyami E, Davis P, eds. *Anesthesia for infants and children.* St. Louis: CV Mosby, pp. 105–113.
15. Borgeat A, Popovic V, Meier D, et al. (1990): Comparison of propofol

and thiopental/halothane for short-duration ENT surgical procedures in children. *Anesth Analg* 71:511–515.

16. Bourke DL, Smith TC (1974): Estimating allowable hemodilution. *Anesthesiology* 41:609–612.

17. Boyer RS (1992): Sedation in pediatric neuroimaging: the science and art. *AJNR* 13:777–783.

18. Boylan JF, Klinck JR, Sandler AN, et al. (1996): Tranexemic acid reduces blood loss, transfusion requirements, and coagulation factor use in orthotopic liver transplantation. *Anesthesiology* 85:1043–1048.

19. Britt BA (1985): Malignant hyperthermia. *Can J Anaesth* 32:666–677.

20. Brownell AKW (1988): Malignant hyperthermia: relationship to other diseases. *Br J Anaesth* 60:303–308.

21. Brownell AKW, Paasuke RT, Elash A, et al. (1983): Malignant hyperthermia in Duchenne's muscular dystrophy. *Anesthesiology* 58:180–182.

22. Cameron CV, Robinson S, Gregory GA (1984): The minimum anesthetic concentration of isoflurane in children. *Anesth Analg* 63:418–420.

23. Chapler CK, Cain SM (1986): The physiologic reserve in oxygen carrying capacity: studies in experimental hemodilution. *Can J Physiol Pharmacol* 64:7–12.

24. Ciavarella D, Reed RL, Counts RB, et al. (1987): Clotting factor levels and the risk or diffuse microvascular bleeding in the massively transfused patient. *Br J Haematol* 67:365–368.

25. Cohen MM, Cameron CB, Duncan PG (1990): Pediatric anesthesia morbidity and mortality in the perioperative period. *Anesth Analg* 70:160–167.

26. Consensus Conference (1985): Fresh-frozen plasma, indications and risks. *JAMA* 253:551–553.

27. Consensus Conference (1988): Perioperative red cell transfusion. *JAMA* 260:2700–2703.

28. Consensus Conference (1987): Platelet transfusion therapy. *JAMA* 257:1777–1780.

29. Cook DR (1981): Muscle relaxants in infants and children. *Anesth Analg* 60:335–343.

30. Copley LAB, Richards BS, Safaui LZ, et al. (1999): Hemodilution as a method to reduce transfusion requirements in adolescent spine fusion surgery. *Spine* 24:219–222.

31. Coté CJ, Goudsouzian NG, Liu LMP, et al. (1981): The dose response of intravenous thiopental for the induction of general anesthesia in unpremedicated children. *Anesthesiology* 55:703–705.

32. Coté CJ, Goudsouzian NG, Liu LMP, et al. (1982): Assessment of risk factors related to the acid aspiration syndrome in pediatric patients: gastric pH and residual volume. *Anesthesiology* 56:70–72.

33. Coté CJ, Liu LMP, Szyfelbein SK, et al. (1985): Changes in serial platelet counts following massive blood transfusion in pediatric patients. *Anesthesiology* 62:197–201.

34. Crawford M, Lerman J, Christensen S, et al. (1990): Effects of duration of fasting on gastric fluid pH and volume in healthy children. *Anesth Analg* 71:400–403.

35. Cullen JJ, Murray DJ, Kealey GP (1989): Changes in coagulation factors in patients with burns during acute blood loss. *J Burn Care Rehabil* 6:517–523.

36. Cushing (1917): *Tumors of the nervus acusticus.* Philadelphia: WB Saunders.

37. Delphin E, Jackson D, Rothstein P (1987): Use of succinylcholine during elective pediatric anesthesia should be reevaluated. *Anesth Analg* 66:1190–1192.

38. des Hollander JM, Hennis PJ, Burm AGL, et al. (1988): Alfentanil in infants and children with congenital heart defects. *J Cardiothorac Anesth* 2:12–17.

39. DeSoto H, Patel RI, Soliman IE, et al. (1988): Changes in oxygen saturation following general anesthesia in children with upper respiratory infection signs and symptoms undergoing otolaryngological procedures. *Anesthesiology* 68:276–279.

40. Desparmet J, Meistelman C, Barre J, et al. (1987): Continuous epidural infusion of bupivacaine for postoperative pain relief in children. *Anesthesiology* 67:108–110.

41. Diament MJ, Stanley P (1988): The use of midazolam for sedation of infants and children. *AJR Am J Roentgenol* 150:377–378.

42. Dilworth NM, MacKellar A (1987): Pain relief for the pediatric surgical patient. *J Pediatr Surg* 22:264–266.

43. Du Toit G, Relton JES, Gillespie R (1978): Acute hemodilutional autotransfusion in the surgical management of scoliosis. *J Bone Joint Surg Br* 60:178–180.

44. Eger EI III, Saidman LJ (1965): Hazards of nitrous oxide anesthesia in bowel obstruction and pneumothorax. *Anesthesiology* 26:61–66.

45. Feld LH, Champeau MW, van Steennis CA, et al. (1989): Preanesthetic medication in children: a comparison of oral transmucosal fentanyl citrate versus placebo. *Anesthesiology* 71:374–377.

46. Fisher DM (1990): Sedation of pediatric patients: an anesthesiologist's perspective. *Radiology* 175:613–615.

47. Fisher DM, Robinson S, Brett CM, et al. (1985): Comparison of enflurane, halothane and isoflurane for diagnostic and therapeutic procedures in children with malignancies. *Anesthesiology* 63:647–650.

48. Forbes RB, Murray DJ (1990): The effect of anesthetic agents on cardiovascular function in infants and children. *Circ Cont* 11:301–309.

49. Forbes RB, Murray DJ, Dillman JB, et al. (1989): Pharmacokinetics of two per cent rectal methohexital in children. *Can J Anaesth* 36:160–164.

50. Forbes RB, Murray DJ, Dull DL, et al. (1989): Haemodynamic effects of rectal methohexitone for induction of anaesthesia in children. *Can J Anaesth* 36:526–529.

51. Forbes RB, Vandewalker GE (1988): Comparison of two and ten per cent rectal methohexitone for induction of anaesthesia in children. *Can J Anaesth* 35:345–349.

52. Frank JP, Harate Y, Butler IJ (1980): Central core disease and malignant hyperthermia syndrome. *Ann Neurol* 7:11–17.

53. Friis-Hansen B (1961): Body water compartments in children: changes during growth and related changes in body composition. *Pediatrics* 28:169–181.

54. Furman EB, Roman DG, Lemmer LAS, et al. (1975): Specific therapy in water, electrolyte and blood-volume replacement during pediatric surgery. *Anesthesiology* 42:187–193.

55. Gauntlett I, Barnes J, Brown TCK, et al. (1985): Temperature maintenance in infants undergoing anaesthesia and surgery. *Anaesth Intens Care* 13:300–304.

56. Goldthorn J, Badgwell JM (1986): Upper airway obstruction in infants and children. *Int Anesthesiol Clin* 24:133–144.

57. Gregory GA, Eger EI, Munson ES (1969): The relationship between age and halothane requirement in man. *Anesthesiology* 30:488–491.

58. Gronert GA, Theye RA (1975): Pathophysiology of hyperkalemia induced by succinylcholine. *Anesthesiology* 43:89–99.

59. Gross JB (1983): Estimating allowable blood loss: correction for dilution. *Anesthesiology* 58:277–280.

60. Grundy BL, Nash CL Jr, Brown RH (1982): Deliberate hypotension for spinal fusion: prospective randomized study with evoked potential monitoring. *Can Anaesth Soc J* 29:452–461.

61. Guay J, Reinberg C, Poitras B, et al. (1992): A trial of desmopressin to reduce blood loss in patients undergoing spine fusion for idiopathic scoliosis. *Anesth Analg* 75:405–410.

62. Hackel A (1986): Preoperative anesthesia. In: Gregory GA, ed. *Pediatric anesthesia.* New York: Churchill Livingstone, pp. 501–521.

63. Hannallah RS, Baker SB, Casey W, et al. (1991): Propofol: effective dose and induction characteristics in unpremediated children. *Anesthesiology* 74:217–219.

64. Hannallah RS, Rosales JK (1983): Experience with parents' presence during anaesthesia induction in children. *Can Anaesth Soc J* 30:286–289.

65. Henderson JM, Brodsky DA, Fisher DM, et al. (1988): Pre-induction of anesthesia in pediatric patients with nasally administered sufentanil. *Anesthesiology* 68:671–675.

66. Henderson WAV (1984): Succinylcholine-induced cardiac arrest in unsuspected Duchenne muscular dystrophy. *Can Anaesth Soc J* 31:444–446.

67. Kafer ER (1980): Respiratory and cardiovascular function in scoliosis and principles of anesthetic management. *Anesthesiology* 52:339–351.

68. Keenan RL, Boyan CP (1985): Cardiac arrest due to anesthesia: a study of incidence and causes. *JAMA* 253:2373–2377.

69. Kingston HG (1986): Halothane and isoflurane anesthesia in pediatric outpatients. *Anesth Analg* 65:181–184.

70. Knill RL (1978): Ventilatory responses to hypoxia and hypercapnia during halothane sedation and anesthesia in man. *Anesthesiology* 49:244–251.

71. Koehntop DE, Rodman JH, Brundage DM, et al. (1986): Pharmacokinetics of fentanyl in neonates. *Anesth Analg* 65:227–232.

72. Krane EJ, Davis PJ, Smith RM (1996): Preoperative preparation. In: Motoyama EK, Davis PJ, eds. *Smith's anesthesia for infants and children,* 6th ed. St. Louis: CV Mosby, pp. 213–226.

73. Levitt RC (1992): Prospects for the diagnosis of malignant hyperthermia susceptibility using molecular genetic approaches. *Anesthesiology* 76:1039–1048.

74. Lynn AM, Slattery JT (1987): Morphine pharmacokinetics in early infancy. *Anesthesiology* 66:136–139.

75. Malhotra N, Roizen MF (1991): Laboratory testing. In: McGough EK, Monroe MC, eds. *Preoperative evaluation. Part I. Problems in anesthesia,* vol 5. New York: Churchill Livingstone, pp. 575–590.

76. Marcel RJ, Stegall WC, Suit CT, et al. (1996): Continuous small-dose aprotinin controls fibrinolysis during orthotopic liver transplantation. *Anesthesiology* 82:1122–1125.

77. Mather L, Mackie J (1983): The incidence of postoperative pain in children. *Pain* 15:271–282.

78. McNeil TW, DeWald RL, Ken NK (1979): Controlled hypotensive anesthesia in scoliosis surgery. *J Bone Joint Surg Am* 56:1167–1172.

79. Mendelson CL (1946): The aspiration of the stomach contents into the lungs during obstetric anesthesia. *Am J Obstet Gynecol* 52:191–205.

80. Messmer K (1975): Hemodilution. *Surg Clin North Am* 55:659–678.

81. Miller ED, Sanders DB, Rowlingson JC, et al. Anesthesia-induced rhabdomyolysis in a patient with Duchenne's muscular dystrophy. *Anesthesiology* 48:146–148.

82. Mitchell AA, Louik C, Lacouture P, et al. (1982): Risks to children from computed tomographic scan premedication. *JAMA* 247:2385–2388.

83. Miyasaka K, Edmonds JF, Conn AW (1976): Complications of radial artery lines in the paediatric patient. *Can Anaesth Soc J* 23:9–14.

84. Moore RA, Yang SS, McNicholas KW, et al. (1985): Hemodynamic and anesthetic effects of sufentanil as the sole anesthetic for pediatric cardiovascular surgery. *Anesthesiology* 62:725–731.

85. Murray DJ, Forbes RB (1989): Neonatal physiology and pharmacology. *Hosp Formul* 24:140–152.

86. Murray DJ, Forbes RB, Dillman JB, et al. (1989): Haemodynamic effects of atropine during halothane or isoflurane anaesthesia in infants and small children. *Can J Anaesth* 36:295–300.

87. Murray DJ, Forbes RB, Dull DL, Mahoney LT (1991): Hemodynamic responses to nitrous oxide during inhalation anesthesia in pediatric patients. *J Clin Anesth* 3:14–19.

88. Murray DJ, Forbes RB, Mahoney LT (1992): Comparative hemodynamic depression in neonates and infants: an echocardiographic study of halothane versus isoflurane. *Anesth Analg* 74:329–337.

89. Murray DJ, Forbes RB, Murphy K, et al. (1988): Nitrous oxide: cardiovascular effects in infants and small children during halothane and isoflurane anesthesia. *Anesth Analg* 67:1059–1064.

90. Murray DJ, Mehta MP, Forbes RB, et al. (1990): Additive contribution of nitrous oxide to halothane MAC in infants and children. *Anesth Analg* 71:120–124.

91. Murray DJ, Olson J, Strauss R, et al. (1988): Coagulation changes during packed red cell replacement of major blood loss. *Anesthesiology* 69:839–845.

92. Murray D, Vandewalker G, Matherne GP, et al. (1987): Pulsed Doppler and two-dimensional echocardiography: comparison of halothane and isoflurane on cardiac function in infants and small children. *Anesthesiology* 67:211–217.

93. Murray D (1999): Hemodilution: reducing transfusion requirements. *Spine* 24:223–224.

94. New PF, Rose BR, Brady TJ, et al. (1983): Potential hazards and artifacts of ferromagnetic surgical and dental materials and devices in nuclear magnetic resonance imaging. *Radiology* 217:139.

95. O'Brien RT, Pearson HA (1971): Physiology anemia of the newborn infant. *J Pediatr* 79:132–138.

96. O'Connor ME, Drasner K (1990): Preoperative laboratory testing of children undergoing elective surgery. *Anesth Analg* 70:176–180.

97. Oka S, Igarashi Y, Takagi A, et al. (1982): Malignant hyperthermia and Duchenne's muscular dystrophy: a case report. *Can Anaesth Soc J* 29:627–629.

98. Owall A, Gordon E, Lagerkranser M, et al. (1987): Clinical experience with adenosine for controlled hypotension during cerebral aneurysm surgery. *Anesth Analg* 66:229–234.

99. Park SC, Mathews RA, Zuberbuhler JR, et al. (1977): Down syndrome with congenital heart malformation. *Am J Dis Child* 131:29–33.

100. Raja SN, Meyer RA, Campbell N (1988): Peripheral mechanisms of somatic pain. *Anesthesiology* 68:571–590.

101. Rampton AJ, Kelly DA, Shanahan EC, et al. (1984): Occurrence of malignant hyperpyrexia in a patient with osteogenesis imperfecta. *Br J Anaesth* 56:1443–1446.

102. Rodgers BM, Webb CJ, Stergios D, et al. (1988): Patient-controlled analgesia in pediatric surgery. *J Pediatr Surg* 23:259–262.

103. Rohrer MJ, Michelotti MC, Nahrwold DL (1988): A prospective evaluation of the efficacy of preoperative coagulation testing. *Ann Surg* 208:554–557.

104. Rosenberg H (1988): Clinical presentation of malignant hyperthermia. *Br J Anaesth* 60:268–273.

105. Rosenberg H, Reed S (1983): In vitro contracture tests for susceptibility to malignant hyperthermia. *Anesth Anal* 62:419–420.

106. Rosenberg H, Gronert G (1992): Intractable cardiac arrest in children given succinylcholine. *Anesthesiology* 77:1054.

107. Rowland LP (1976): Pathogenesis of muscular dystrophies. *Arch Neurol* 33:315–321.

108. Roy WL, McIntyre BG (1991): Is preoperative haemoglobin testing justified in children undergoing minor elective surgery? *Can J Anaesth* 38:700–703.

109. Royston D (1993): Drugs for surgical blood loss. *Lancet* 341:1629.

110. Salanitre E, Rackow H (1969): The pulmonary exchange of nitrous oxide and halothane in infants and children. *Anesthesiology* 30:388–394.

111. Salem MR, Bennett EJ, Schweiss JF, et al. (1975): Cardiac arrest related to anesthesia: contributing factors in infants and children. *JAMA* 233:238–241.

112. Salem MR, Wong, AY, Bennett EJ, et al. (1974): Deliberate hypotension in infants and children. *Anesth Analg* 53:975–981.

113. Schulman JL, Foley MJ, Vernon DTA, et al. (1967): A study of the effect of the mother's presence during anesthesia induction. *Anesth Analg* 39:111–114.

114. Sebel PS, Lowdon JD (1989): Propofol: a new intravenous anesthetic. *Anesthesiology* 71:260–277.

115. Shimosato S (1983): Blood pressure pulse. In: Shimosato S, ed. *Anesthesia and cardiac performance in health and disease.* Springfield, IL: Charles C. Thomas, pp. 80–99.

116. Sieber FE, Smith DS, Traystman RJ, et al. (1987): Glucose: a re-evaluation of its intraoperative use. *Anesthesiology* 67:72–81.

117. Sim JM (1877): Discovery of anesthesia. *Va Med Monthly* 4:81–99.

118. Smith RM (1996): History of pediatric anesthesia. In: Motoyama E, Davis P, eds. *Anesthesia for infants and children,* 6th ed. St. Louis, CV Mosby, pp. 909–921.

119. Soliman IE, Broadman LM, Hannallah RS, et al. (1988): Comparison of the analgesic effects of EMLA to intradermal lidocaine infiltration prior to venous cannulation in unpremedicated children. *Anesthesiology* 68:804–806.

120. Steward DJ (1994): Psychological preparation and premedication. In: Gregory GA, ed. *Pediatric anesthesia,* 3rd ed. New York: Churchill Livingstone, pp. 179–182.

121. Tait AR, Knight PR (1987): Intraoperative respiratory complications in patient with upper respiratory tract infections. *Can J Anaesth* 34:300–303.

122. Tait AR, Knight PR (1987): The effects of general anesthesia on upper respiratory tract infections in children. *Anesthesiology* 67:930–935.

123. Tellez LT, Galvis AG, Storgion SA, et al. (1991): Dexamethasone in the prevention of post extubation stridor in children. *J Pediatr* 18: 289–294.

124. Thompson GE, Miller RD, Stevens WC, et al. (1978): Hypotensive anesthesia for total hip arthroplasty: a study of blood loss and organ function (brain, heart, liver, kidney). *Anesthesiology* 48:91–96.

125. Tiret L, Desmonts JM, Hatton F, et al. (1986): Complications associated with anesthesia: a prospective survey in France. *Can Anaesth Soc J* 33:336–344.

126. Tiret L, Nivoche Y, Hatton F, et al. (1988): Complications related to anaesthesia in infants and children: a prospective survey of 40,240 anesthetics. *Br J Anaesth* 61:263–269.

127. Troll GF, Dohrmann GJ (1975): Anaesthesia of the spinal cord injured patient: cardiovascular problems and their management. *Paraplegia* 13:162–171.

128. Turnbull JM, Buck C (1987): The value of preoperative screening investigations in otherwise healthy individuals. *Arch Intern Med* 147: 1101–1105.

129. Valley RD, Bailey AG (1991): Caudal morphine for postoperative analgesia in infants and children: a report of 138 cases. *Anesth Analg* 72:120–124.

130. Warner MA, Warner MG, Warner DQ, et al. (1999): Perioperative pulmonary aspiration in infants and children. *Anesthesiology* 90: 66–71.

131. Weston G, Strunin L, Amundson GM (1985): Imaging for anaesthetists: a review of methods for anaesthetic implications of diagnostic imaging techniques. *Can Anaesth Soc J* 32:552–561.

132. White PF, Way EL, Trevor AJ (1982): Ketamine: its pharmacology and therapeutic uses. *Anesthesiology* 56:118–136.

133. Williams JO, Somerville GM, Miner ME, et al. (1987): Atlantoaxial subluxation and trisomy-21: another perioperative complication. *Anesthesiology* 67:253–254.

134. Wilton NC, Leigh J, Rosen DR, et al. (1988): Preanesthetic sedation of preschool children using intranasal midazolam. *Anesthesiology* 69: 972–975.

135. Wood RA, Hackelman RA (1991): Value of the chest x-ray as a screening test for elective surgery in children. *Pediatrics* 67:445–452.

136. Wodey E, Pladys P, Copin C, et al. (1997): Comparative hemodynamic depression of sevoflurane versus halothane infants. *Anesthesiology* 87:795–800.

137. Yaster M, Simmon RS, Rolo VT, et al. (1986): A comparison of nitroglycerine and nitroprusside for inducing hypotension in children: a double-blind study. *Anesthesiology* 65:175–179.

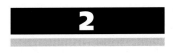

BLOOD SALVAGE

THOMAS E. BAILEY, JR

The idea of salvaging blood, or reclaiming blood before or during surgical procedures, is not new. Even before 1900, surgeons reclaimed blood during surgery (6,18,32). The advent of blood banks and the development of improved preservation techniques have made storage of a patient's own blood a reality (2,27,36,44,45). Newer techniques and advancing technology make possible the preoperative collection of large amounts of blood for future use, as well as the salvage and reclamation of blood lost intraoperatively and postoperatively. The primary concern of patients and surgeons today is the safety of receiving someone else's blood (50). This chapter informs the spinal surgeon of alternative approaches to reduce the need for homologous blood replacement.

TRANSFUSION AND DONATION

The real issue confronting patients and surgeons currently is the potential transmission of blood-borne diseases during transfusion of homologous blood or administration of blood components. Even with today's safeguards in the selection of donors and the processing of blood and blood components, whole blood, packed red blood cells, plasma, platelets, and cryoprecipitates still have the potential for transmitting disease, whereas albumin, gamma globulin, factor VIII, and factor IX are currently handled or manufactured in such a way as to be safe and effective (11). Associated with transfusion of homologous blood are allergic reactions, febrile reactions, hemolytic reactions, isosensitization, and bacteremia. Of even greater threat are the viral diseases, such as cytomegalovirus, human immunodeficiency virus (HIV), and hepatitis C (11). Though the major fear is that of contracting HIV, hepatitis C virus causes much more illness and many more deaths of patients and health care workers (11). Many physicians believe that the use of autologous blood significantly reduces these concerns.

The attitudes of surgeons toward the practicalities of autologous blood transfusion must be addressed specifically as to who can and should donate blood preoperatively. Rules of the Red Cross and the American Association of Blood Banks (AABB) concerning blood donations have been modified for most autologous deposit programs (3,12,37). No longer do patients have to meet strict age and weight requirements (37). Many patients weighing between 25 and 50 kg can give weekly autologous donations of half units (250 cm^3) in many blood banks in anticipation of future surgery (3,45).

When considering spinal reconstructive surgery, as well as some pelvic and femoral osteotomies, the surgeon must be the prime motivator. The surgeon must assess the potential blood requirements of the patient undergoing spinal surgery and use the available methods to store preoperatively, conserve and salvage intraoperatively, and reclaim postoperatively the patient's own blood.

The patient's religious beliefs may be a factor in planning conservation and salvage techniques. Jehovah's Witnesses do not accept predonated blood, either autologous or homologous (11). However, they may accept cell saver blood and blood collected immediately preoperatively through hemodilution methods. These considerations are a necessary part of the evaluation of infants, children, and teenagers when major elective reconstructive surgery is being contemplated.

Preoperative donation of the patient's own blood for future elective surgery has become popular in the past 15 years (3,31,45,47). The advent of new blood banking techniques, particularly storage solutions, allows for storage up to 35 days using citrate phosphate dextrose with adenine (CPDA-1). The use of adenine, dextrose, and mannitol (Adsol, Fenwald Laboratories, Deerfield, IL) can extend the storage time to 42 days, thereby giving patients the opportunity to donate up to six units of autologous blood preoperatively (3,36,37,45).

Finch et al. (21) and Hamstra and Block (35) reported that patients who had adequate stores of iron demonstrated a fourfold to fivefold increase in hematopoiesis when undergoing serial phlebotomies. These studies suggest that obtaining blood on a weekly basis is safe. It has been the author's experience that most young patients undergoing surgery for spinal deformity who are otherwise healthy tolerated weekly or near-weekly preoperative donations quite well (3,45).

PREOPERATIVE PREPARATION AND DONATION

The surgeon prepares the patient for preoperative autologous donations by prescribing iron, usually ferrous sulfate, at the time

T. E. Bailey, Jr: Department of Orthopaedic Surgery, University Hospital, and Medical College of Georgia, Augusta, Georgia 33901-2668.

TABLE 1. ALTERNATIVE IRON PREPERATIONS

Iron Preparation	Elemental Iron (mg)
Ferrous sulfate 325 mg	65
Ferrous gluconate 325 mg	38
Ferrous sulfate drops 75 mg/0.6 cm³	15
Ferrous sulfate syrup 90 mg/5 cm³	18
Ferrous sulfate elixir 220 mg/5 cm³	44

surgery is scheduled. Inasmuch as it takes 6 weeks to obtain the maximum amount of blood and 2 weeks to prepare for the potentially weekly autologous donations, surgery is usually scheduled 2 to 3 months in advance (21,46). In most otherwise normal teenagers, a dosage of 325 mg ferrous sulfate (65 mg of elemental iron) administered orally three times a day is tolerated quite well. In smaller children the optimum dose is 5 mg/kg/day of elemental iron (Table 1).

The patients are then referred to the local blood bank where his or her weight, blood pressure, hemoglobin, and general medical information are recorded and evaluated by blood bank personnel. The patient/donor returns to the blood bank on a weekly basis, starting 6 weeks before the scheduled surgery. If the patient/donor's condition permits, either a half or a whole unit of blood is taken. If the patient/donor's condition does not permit donation because of low hemoglobin or for other medical reasons, the patient returns the following week for reevaluation and possible donation. This procedure is continued until 5 days before the scheduled surgical procedure (1). This method has been well received by patients, their families, and the local blood banks (3) (Fig. 1).

Preoperatively donated autologous blood can be frozen and stored. This method is particularly useful for storing blood of rare type in patients with immunologic problems that make cross-matching difficult. The donated blood must be frozen within 10 days of phlebotomy and stored at −65 to −85°C. It can be stored for 7 to 20 years, depending on technique. Preparing the frozen red cells for use (thaw and deglycerolize) requires 30 to 60 minutes. The blood must be transfused within 24 hours. Whereas geographic considerations may make this method desirable in some areas, the high cost of freezing red cells, the routine preservation of red cells for 42 days using Adsol, the short shelf life (24 hours) of thawed red cells, and increased networking and cooperation among blood banks have made the use of predonated frozen red cells rare (37).

Preparation of predonated autologous blood is usually slightly more expensive than preparation of homologous blood, principally because of increased administrative costs. However, these donation programs have been well accepted in most communities. Bailey and Mahoney (3) reported only one missed appointment in 205 scheduled visits for preoperative autologous donations (Fig. 1).

Acute normovolemic hemodilution is another method of obtaining autologous blood preoperatively. By controlled dilution through phlebotomy and replacement of volume with crystalloid and/or colloid—aiming for a hematocrit of 20% to 25%—the number of red cells lost through surgical bleeding is reduced. The blood that ends up on the sponges and in the suction bottle has a lower hematocrit. The blood obtained by phlebotomy provides a source of fresh autologous blood for replacement later in the procedure (4,65). From 400 to 900 mL of autologous blood may be made available by this technique. Because the

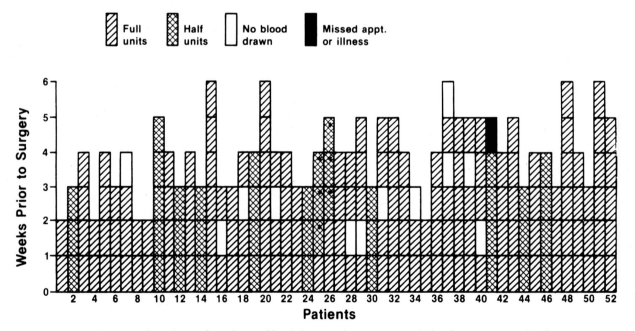

FIGURE 1. The volume of autologous blood that was drawn preoperatively. There was one missed appointment out of 205 scheduled visits. Forty-five of 193 (21%) units drawn were half units. (From Bailey TE Jr, Mahoney OM [1987]: The use of banked autologous blood in patients undergoing surgery for spinal deformity. *J Bone Joint Surg Am* 69:329–332, with permission.)

autologous blood, phlebotomized earlier in the procedure, is kept in continuity with the patient's circulation, this technique is usually acceptable to Jehovah's Witnesses (53).

INTRAOPERATIVE TECHNIQUES

Intraoperatively, hypotensive anesthesia has been available for many years (27), and reclaiming blood loss during surgery via cell saver has been an acceptable practice for over 15 years (23). Several simple techniques that should be part of the regular routine can supplement these specific procedures. First, the patient is positioned appropriately for the procedure. Steps are taken to minimize pressure points on the body and to reduce intraabdominal pressure on the vena cava; this lessens engorgement of the valveless epidural veins of Batson's plexus. This care decreases intraoperative bleeding. Second, the surgeon should have adequate surgical assistance. Decreasing operating times will lessen blood replacement needs. Third, meticulous surgical technique must be used, including intradermal and subcutaneous infiltration of epinephrine solution (1:500,000), judicious packing with sponges, and careful use of electrocautery. These simple techniques may seem excessively time consuming to the inexperienced surgeon; however, with careful attention to these details throughout every surgical procedure, the average operating time and blood loss will decrease.

Hypotensive Anesthesia

Hypotensive anesthesia was suggested by Goldstein (27) in 1966 as a method of reducing blood loss. In 1974, McNeill et al. (48) reported a decreased need for blood replacement and a 40% reduction in total blood loss using hypotensive anesthesia. Hypotension can be induced intraoperatively in many ways. In the past, it was most frequently accomplished pharmacologically using sodium nitroprusside (42,48,49,71). Now that arterial lines, Foley catheters, spinal cord monitors, and pulse oximeters are part of modern anesthesia monitoring routines, no additional monitoring is needed. Birch and Boyce (5) demonstrated the safety of sodium nitroprusside hypotensive anesthesia, especially as related to renal blood flow, as long as adequate hydration exists. Kling et al. (43) used a dog model to evaluate spinal cord blood flow. Using halothane and nitroprusside-induced hypotension, they reduced the mean arterial pressure by half. After an initial significant fall in spinal cord blood flow, mean arterial pressure returned to normal within 30 minutes. Spinal distraction during the induced hypotension did not cause further reduction in spinal cord blood flow. Jacobs et al. (38) confirmed these findings in a similar study. They also established a linear relationship between the partial pressure of carbon dioxide, P_{CO_2}, and spinal cord blood flow; as P_{CO_2} decreased, the spinal cord blood flow decreased. Presently, newer pharmacologic agents are used for inducing and maintaining hypotensive anesthesia.

These investigations demonstrated that with modern anesthesia monitoring techniques, excellent hydration, avoidance of oligemia, hyperventilation, hypocarbia, induced hypotensive anesthesia maintained within established limits (mean arterial pressure no lower than 50 mm Hg) is a safe technique. Hypotensive anesthesia is most appropriate for the healthy adolescent undergoing elective spinal surgery; however, it is contraindicated in the older patient with renal, hepatic, cerebrovascular, or coronary disease and some cardiac diseases (4).

Cell Saving

In selected patients, intraoperative autotransfusion (IAT) is a necessary and complimentary addition to the above mentioned techniques. Intraoperative autotransfusion via cell saving technique is particularly useful when preoperative phlebotomy techniques fall short of expected needs and when there is more than the anticipated blood loss.

Acid citrate dextrose (ACD) solution or a dilute solution of heparin is mixed with the aspirated blood and debris at the tip of a tonsil tip suction catheter (negative pressure less than 100 mm Hg). The aspirate is passed through a 140-μm filter and then roller-pumped into a disposable bowl housed in a portable centrifuge. Centrifugal force separates the healthy red blood cells from the waste products, including plasma, most white cells, platelets, hemolyzed red cell casings, tissue debris and stroma, free hemoglobin, phospholipids, and other potential pulmonary arteriole–irritating substances (22,76,61). This suspension of red blood cells in saline is roller-pumped into a blood bag without anticoagulant. The end product is a unit of washed, packed red blood cells. The red blood cells are then transfused to the patient by gravity through a 20- to 40-μm filter.

Essential to the cell saver-washer is the centrifuge bowl. This bowl usually comes in two sizes; adult 225 mL and pediatric 125 mL. The pediatric bowl is usually preferred in smaller patients because the bowl must be filled before washing.

Approximately 50% of shed red cells entering the wound can be salvaged (23,61). These harvested red cells, when labeled with chromium 51, survive equally with normal red cells—approximately 50% survival at 24 days (61).

Hemoglobinuria as well as pulmonary and coagulopathy complications have been reported with use of a cell saver. Flynn reported no pulmonary complications in 382 cases. Factors causing irritation of pulmonary arterioles, such as free phospholipids from cell lyses and tissue debris, are discarded in the wash (22,23,61). If the saline wash volume is seven times that of the bowl, the free hemoglobin is removed with the saline. If insufficient wash is used, the urine appears disconcertingly red due to the presence of free hemoglobin. This is usually harmless in well-hydrated patients (7,23,60). Coagulopathy complications may occur from loss of fibrinogen and platelets if the volume of blood loss is high. Jacobs et al. (39) showed that blood loss greater than 80 mL/kg during spinal surgery resulted in falling values of coagulation factors, including platelets and fibrinogen, as well as a decrease in the arteriolar/alveolar oxygen tension ratio. Flynn et al. (23) reported only one patient who had a minor coagulopathy that was easily reversed with fresh frozen plasma. Current recommendations require that patients be given one unit of fresh frozen plasma for each 900 mL (4 cycles × 225 mL) of washed red blood cells (55,56). Also, after 10 adult units has been given, the platelet count should be determined and platelets administered according to need as reflected in counts below 85,000 (14,23). The major contraindications to IAT are malignancy, infection, and gross wound contamination.

Jehovah's Witness patients have accepted the use of the cell saver when assured that the circuit of wound suction, centrifuge, and transfusion bag are made complete with an intravenous line returning the washed cells to the patient. Use of cell saver centrifuge units requires the knowledge of a well-trained technician. In most institutions, the cell saver usage charge is approximately two to three times the charge for a unit of either predonated autologous or homologous blood.

POSTOPERATIVE BLOOD SALVAGE

Blood loss and blood replacement during spinal surgery in children have long been major concerns (23,39,73). Segmental instrumentation techniques, accompanying posterior spinal fusion for spinal deformity, add to blood loss because of the need to decorticate before placement of instrumentation. The active bone bleeding continues longer than with Harrington instrumentation, in which the decortication is performed at the end of the procedure. After the wound is closed the bleeding continues. In fact, significant blood loss may occur, as evidenced by the drop in hematocrit on the first and second postoperative days. The drop in the hematocrit is more than can be accounted for by hemodilution. Historically, when a drain was used, the drainage was discarded and the blood it contained was lost.

Because preoperative deposit of autologous blood and intraoperative blood salvage are practiced in many centers (22,23,31,64,75), a logical third step of harvesting shed blood from the drainage of postoperative scoliosis wounds warrants consideration. A recent study showed a saving of one unit postoperatively; this was returned to the patient (24).

A controversy exists as to the salvage of autologous red blood cells from postoperative drainage involving the use of washed versus unwashed cells. Activated complements A3 and A5 are found in the drainage along with injured platelets and other toxic substances. They may precipitate a disseminated intravascular coagulopathy (DIC) or pulmonary distress syndrome. Surgeons favoring the use of unwashed cells have eliminated the anticoagulant. They contend that the drainage blood is defibrinated and does not clot. The collection vesicle is simply turned upside down and the drainage blood administered intravenously to the patient through a 20- to 40-μm filter (20). No untoward results have been reported by surgeons favoring the use of unwashed cells. Reinfusion of unwashed filtered autologous blood has been shown to be cost-effective in decreasing the need for allogeneic blood transfusion (69). Most reports favoring the use of unwashed cells have been from cases of total joint surgery and not primarily spine surgery (14,20,25,34,68,72).

Washing of postoperative drainage blood requires either a portable cell washer, as mentioned earlier, or the collected drainage blood must be transported to the blood bank for processing. Either method of washing postoperative drainage challenges the cost-effectiveness of this technique (25,66).

"Transfusion Trigger"

Until recently, surgeons had arbitrarily defined a hemoglobin level below 10 g/dL, and a hematocrit of less than 30%, as unacceptable. Although there is no physiologic basis for this so-called transfusion trigger (54), concerns for transfusions of allogeneic blood have caused a reconsideration of these historical hemoglobin and hematocrit levels. The rate of drop of the hemoglobin and hematocrit and the overall medical condition of the patient are much better determinants of transfusion needs. Many young, otherwise healthy, patients can tolerate a slow drop (over 3 to 4 days) of the hemoglobin to 6 to 8 g/dL. In cases of acute blood loss, decreased blood pressure, or symptomatic anemia resulting in tachycardia, mental status changes, cardiac ischemia, or dyspnea, no single measure can replace sound clinical judgment as the basis for decisions regarding perioperative transfusions (15,33,57,69).

Recombinant Human Erythropoietin

Erythropoietin is a hematopoietic growth factor produced mostly in the kidney. Through recombinant DNA technology, erythropoietin is now available commercially as epoetin alfa (rhEPO). Prior to 1990, most of the experience in using rhEPO was gained in treating the chronic anemia of renal failure patients. Pediatricians have been using rhEPO in the treatment of neonatal anemia, anemia secondary to leukemia, as well as renal failure patients. Goodnough et al. (28,29) reported the effectiveness of rhEPO to augment a patient's ability to donate blood preoperatively in anticipation of total joint surgery and spinal surgery. The hypothetical risks of rhEPO therapy, such as hypertension, myocardial infarction, and deep venous thrombosis, are, for all practical purposes, not a concern in the usually healthy pediatric orthopaedic surgical patient (63).

Many centers are now using rhEPO therapy routinely in concert with other conservation techniques mentioned earlier. rhEPO can be used in either the preoperative preparation or the perioperative treatment of the patient. Patients are usually given ferrous sulfate 325 mg two or three times per day. Preoperative rhEPO therapy consists of using 300 to 600 IU per kilogram of body weight per week for 3 to 4 weeks before surgery. In the perioperative setting, rhEPO 300 IU per kilogram of body weight is given daily for 15 days, starting 10 days before surgery (40). The physiologic benefits of rhEPO-accelerated erythropoiesis include improved tissue oxygenation and reduced need for allogeneic blood transfusion, secondary to increased hemoglobin concentration (40). Although rhEPO is relatively expensive, its use has become routine in all orthopedic surgery including pediatric spine surgery. The author feels that rhEPO has a definite role in management of certain major pediatric spine cases. As experience with rhEPO increases, particularly in conjunction with other conservation techniques, such as preoperative autologous donation, acute normovolemic hemodilution, hypotensive anesthesia, and cell saving, its cost-effectiveness will be better defined.

Artificial Blood

The high cost of acquisition, screening, storage, transport, and administration of blood plus the forecasted shortage of available red blood cells for transfusion in the coming decades has led to the continued interest in developing artificial red blood cells

(13,16,17,40,74). For the past 35 years, experimental work has proceeded on the development of red blood cell substitutes. Red blood cell substitutes may be divided into fluorocarbons, hemoglobin solutions, and liposome-enveloped hemoglobin (artificial red blood cells).

Fluorocarbons

Fluorocarbons have the capacity to carry oxygen. Experimental work with fluorocarbons first appeared in the 1960s (9), and work reportedly progressed into the late 1970s (10,26,51,67). A commercial preparation called Fulosol, intended for intravenous use in humans, was produced in Japan (52,76); however, there were many difficulties. Emulsions were unstable, and excessive fluorocarbon was stored in organs. Fulosol also had a low oxygen carrying capacity as a result of its low fluorocarbon content. Intravascular time of persistence was short (30), making it of limited value in the treatment of anemia. The U.S. Food and Drug Administration failed to approve it for treatment of anemia (19).

More recently, an improved Fulosol DA 20% underwent clinical trials for treatment of anemia (mainly in Jehovah's Witness patients), but results were disappointing. Though some of those treated survived, most of the severely anemic patients died. The lack of effectiveness continues to be attributable to the short intravascular time of persistence and the rapid elimination (70).

A second-generation fluorocarbon, perflubron emulsion (Oxygent, Alliance Pharmaceutical, San Diego, CA), is currently in Phase II investigation trials. It is reported to be more stable at room temperature, highly concentrated, and well tolerated by humans. In general, the potential wide range of clinical applications as temporary oxygen carriers continues to stimulate the development of fluorocarbons (40,41).

Hemoglobin Solutions

Free hemoglobin protein readily bonds oxygen but to the extent that oxygen is not released to the tissues effectively. A second serious problem that has prevented its use as a blood substitute is that when released from the red cell it breaks from four protein chains into two parts. These are rapidly filtered from the vascular system by the kidney and are nephrotoxic (58). Several new hemoglobin-based oxygen carriers are currently in Phase I and Phase II clinical trials. Early data suggest that many of the adverse effects and limitations of previous hemoglobin-based oxygen carriers have been reduced (40,62). However, the use of hemoglobin-based oxygen carriers has not reached Phase III clinical trials and is still several years away from general clinical use.

Artificial Red Blood Cells

Many years ago, efforts to produce artificial red blood cells in the form of encapsulated hemoglobin met with success (8). The capsule is made from synthetic lecithin-based lipid mixtures. In vivo studies have established that the liposome-encapsulated hemoglobin has a half-life of 16 to 20 hours and can carry oxygen sufficient to sustain life (59). The microencapsulated hemoglobin keeps the hemoglobin in circulation longer and prevents escape of the molecule through the glomeruli. The oxygen affinity of the solution within the capsule is similar to that of whole blood. Oxygen diffuses easily across the membrane, and studies in experimental animals suggest that this substance can keep alive animals that have had more than 90% of their red cells removed. Little is known yet of encapsulated hemoglobin toxicity and, like the other red blood cell substitutes, its use in the clinical setting has not yet begun.

REFERENCES

1. Aach RD, Kahn RA (1980): Post-transfusion hepatitis: current perspectives. *Ann Intern Med* 92:539–546.
2. Bailey DN, Bove JR (1975): Chemical and hematological changes in stored CPD blood. *Transfusion* 15:244–249.
3. Bailey TE Jr, Mahoney OM (1987): The use of banked autologous blood in patients undergoing surgery for spinal deformity. *J Bone Joint Surg Am* 69:329–332.
4. Ben-David B, Haller GS, Taylor PO (1987): Anesthesia for surgery of the spine. In: Bradford DS, Lonstein JE, Moe JH, et al., eds. *Moe's Textbook of scoliosis and other spinal deformities,* 2nd ed. Philadelphia: WB Saunders, pp. 607–628.
5. Birch AA, Boyce WH (1979): Renal blood flow autoregulation during anesthesia (abstract). *Anesthesiology* 51:5123.
6. Blundell J (1818): Experiments on the transfusion of blood by syringe. *Med Clin Trans* 1818:9–56.
7. Brener BJ, Raines JK, Darling RC (1973): Intraoperative autotransfusion in abdominal aortic resections. *Arch Surg* 107:78–84.
8. Chang TM (1998): Pharmaceutical and therapeutic application of artificial cells including microencapsulation. *Eur J Pharm Biopharm* 45(1):3–8.
9. Clark LC, Gollan F (1966): Survival of mammals breathing organic liquids equilibriums with oxygen at atmospheric pressure. *Science* 152:1755–1756.
10. Clark LC (1978): Perfluorodecalin as a red cell substitute. In: Jamieson GA, Greanwalt TE, *Blood substitutes and plasma expanders.* New York: Alan R. Liss, p. 69.
11. Cone J, Day LJ, Johnson GK, Murray DG, Nelson CL (1990): Blood products: optimal use, conservation and safety. *AAOS Instr Course Lect* 39:431–434.
12. Cowell HR, Swichard KW (1974): Autotransfusion in children's orthopaedics. *J Bone Joint Surg Am* 56:908–912.
13. Cumming PD, Wallace EL, Schorr JB, et al. (1989): Exposure of patients to human immunodeficiency virus through the transfusion of blood components that test antibody-negative. *N Engl J Med* 321:941–946.
14. Dainow I (1991): The benefits of using autologous blood with the Solcotrans orthopaedic system. *Orthopaedics* 14:473–476.
15. Dekutoski MD (1999): Blood loss and transfusion management in spinal surgery. *Orthopedics* 22(Suppl): S155–157.
16. Dodd RY (1992): The risk of transfusion-transmitted infection. *N Engl J Med* 327:419–421.
17. Donahue J.G, Munoz A, Ness M, et al. (1992): The declining risk of post-transfusion hepatitis C virus infection. *N Engl J Med* 327:369–373.
18. Duncan J (1886): On re-infusion of blood in primary and other amputations. *Br Med J* 1886:1–192.
19. *FDC Rep* (1983): Oct. 31, p. 12.
20. Faris PM, Ritter MA, Keating EM, et al. (1991): Unwashed filtered shed blood collected after knee and hip arthroplasties. A source of autologous red cells. *J Bone Joint Surg Am* 73:1169–1178.
21. Finch S, Haskins D, Finch CA (1950): Iron metabolism. Hematopoiesis following phlebotomy. Iron as a limiting factor. *J Clin Invest* 29:1078–1086.
22. Flynn JC (1986): Intraoperative transfusion with the cell saver. In: *Proceedings of the 3rd International Congress on Cotrel-Dubousset Instrumentation.* Paris: Sauramps Medical Co., pp. 91–96.
23. Flynn JC, Csencsitz TA, Metzger CR (1982): Intraoperative autotransfusion (IAT) in spine surgery. *Spine* 7:423–435.

24. Flynn JC, Price CT, Zink WP (1991): The third step of total autologous blood transfusion in scoliosis surgery. Harvesting blood from the postoperative wound. *Spine* 16:S328–S329.

25. Gannon DM, Lombardi AV, Mallory TH, et al. (1991): An evaluation of the efficacy of postoperative blood salvage after total joint arthroplasty. A prospective randomized trial. *J Arthroplasty* 1:109–114.

26. Geyer RP (1973): Fluorocarbon polyol artificial blood substitutes. *N Engl J Med* 289:1077–1082.

27. Goldstein LA (1966): Surgical management of scoliosis. *J Bone Joint Surg Am* 48:167–196.

28. Goodnough LT, Rudwick S, Price TH, et al. (1989): Increased preoperative collection of autologous blood with recombinant erythropoietin therapy. *N Engl J Med* 321:1163–1168.

29. Goodnough LT, Rudwick S, Price TH, et al. (1992): Preoperative red cell production in patients undergoing aggressive autologous blood phlebotomy with and without erythropoietin therapy. *Transfusion* 32:441–445.

30. Gould SA, Rosen AL, Sehgal LR, et al. (1986): Fulosol-DA as a red cell substitute in acute anemia. *N Engl J Med* 314:1653–1656.

31. Goulet JA, Bray TJ, Timmerman LA, et al. (1989): Intraoperative autologous autotransfusion in orthopaedic patients. *J Bone Joint Surg Am* 71:3–7.

32. Grant FC (1921): Autotransfusion. *Ann Surg* 74:253–254.

33. Greenburg AG (1995): A Physiologic basis for Red Blood Transfusion decisions. *Am J Surg* 170(Suppl 6A):445–485.

34. Groh GI, Buchert PK, Allen WC (1990): A comparison of transfusion requirements after total knee arthroplasty using the Solcotrans autotransfusion system. *J Arthroplasty* 3:281–285.

35. Hamstra RD, Block MH (1969): Erythropoiesis in response to blood loss in man. *J Appl Physiol* 27:503–507.

36. Heaton A, Miripol J, Aster R, et al. (1984): Use of Adsol Preservation solution for prolonged storage of low viscosity AS-1 red blood cells. *Br J Haematol* 57:467–478.

37. Holland PV, ed. (1989): *Standards for blood banks and transfusion services,* 13th ed. Arlington, VA: American Association of Blood Banks.

38. Jacobs HK, Lieponis JV, Bunch WH, et al. (1982): The influence of halothane and nitroprusside on canine spinal cord hemodynamics. *Spine* 7:35.

39. Jacobs RR, Asher MA, Gilbert JL (1980): Correlation of coagulopathy and pulmonary insufficiency with blood transfusion in spinal fusions. *Spine* 5:1–3.

40. Keating EM (1999): Current options and approaches for blood management in orthopaedic surgery. *AAOS Instr Course Lect* 48:655–665.

41. Keipert E (1978): Use of Oxygent, a perfluoro chemical-based oxygen carrier, as an alternative to intraoperative blood transfusion. *Artif Cells Blood Subst Immobil Biotechnol* 23:381–394.

42. Khambatta HJ, Stone JG, Matteo RS, et al. (1978): Hypotensive anesthesia for spine fusion with sodium nitroprusside. *Spine* 3:171.

43. Kling TF, Fergusson N, Leach AW, et al (1984): The effect of induced hypotension and spine distraction in spinal cord blood flow in dogs. *Orthop Trans* 8:144.

44. Latham JT, Bove JR, Welrich FL (1982): Chemical and hematologic changes in stored CPDA-1 blood. *Transfusion* 22:158–159.

45. MacEwen GD, Bennett E, Girille JT (1990): Autologous blood transfusion in children and young adults with low body weight undergoing spinal surgery. *J Pediatr Orthop* 10:750–753.

46. McCurdy PR (1965): Oral and parenteral iron therapy. *JAMA* 191:859–862.

47. McKittrick JE (1974): Banked autologous blood in elective surgery. *Am J Surg* 128:137–142.

48. McNeill TW, DeWald RL, Kuo KN, et al. (1974): Controlled hypotensive anesthesia in scoliosis surgery. *J Bone Joint Surg Am* 56:1167–1172.

49. Michenfelder JD, Theye RA (1977): Canine systemic and cerebral effects of hypotension induced by hemorrhage, trimethaphan, halothane or nitroprusside. *Anesthesiology* 46:188–195.

50. Myhre BA (1980): Fatalities from blood transfusion. *JAMA* 244:1333–1335.

51. Naito R, Yokoyama K (1975): On the perfluorodecalin/ phospholipid emulsion as the red cell substitute. *Proceedings of the 10th International Congress Nutr Symp PCF Artif Blood,* pp. 55–72.

52. Naito R, Yokoyama K (1978, 1981): *Perfluorochemical blood substitutes. FC-43 emulsion Fulosol-DA. 20% and 35%.* Technical Information Series No.5. Osaka: Green Cross Corp., p. 7.

53. Nelson CL, Bowen WS (1986): Total hip arthroplasty in Jehovah's Witness without blood transfusion. *J Bone Joint Surg Am* 68:350–353.

54. Nelson CL, Nelson RL, Cone J (1990): Blood conservation techniques in orthopaedic surgery. *AAOS Instr Course Lect* 39:425–429.

55. Orr M (1991): University of Texas Health Science Center, San Antonio, Texas, personal communication.

56. Orr MD, Blenko JW (1978): Autotransfusion of concentrated washed red cells from the surgical field. A biomechanical and physiological comparison with hemologous cell transfusion. In: *Proceedings of Blood Conservation Institute.*

57. Perioperative red blood cell transfusion. NIH Consensus Development Conference Consensus statement. *JAMA* 260:2700–2703.

58. Pool R (1990): Slow going for blood substitutes. *J Sci* 250:1655–1656.

59. Rabinovici R, Rudolph AS, Ligler FS, et al. (1990): Liposome-encapsulated hemoglobin: an oxygen-carrying fluid. *J Circ Shock* 32:1–17.

60. Rains J, Bluth J, Brewster JC, et al. (1976): Intraoperative autotransfusion equipment, protocol and guidelines. *J Trauma* 16:616–623.

61. Ray JM, Flynn JC, Bierman AH (1986): Erythrocyte survival following intraoperative autotransfusion in spinal surgery: an in vivo comparative study and 5-year update. *Spine* 11:879–882.

62. Roberge JQ (1996): Search narrows for blood substitutes. *Biotech Lab Inst* 6.

63. Roye DP (1999): Recombinant human erythropoietin and blood management in pediatric spine surgery. *Orthopedics* 22: S 158–S160.

64. Semkiw LB, Schurman DJ, Goodman SB, et al. (1989): Post-operative blood salvage using the cellsaver after total joint arthroplasty. *J Bone Joint Surg Am* 71:823–827.

65. Singler RC (1983): Special techniques: deliberate hypotension, hypothermia, and acute normovolemic hemodilution. In: Gregory GA, ed. *Pediatric anesthesia.* New York: Churchill Livingstone, pp. 553–577.

66. Slagis SV, Benjamin JB, Volz RG, et al. (1991): Postoperative blood salvage in total hip and knee arthroplasty: a randomized controlled trial. *J Bone Joint Surg Br* 73B:591–594.

67. Slovieter HA, Kamimoto T (1976): Erythrocyte substitute for perfusion of brain. *Nature* 216:458–460.

68. Spence, R.K. (1995): Surgical Red blood cell transfusion practice policies. *Am J Surg* 170(Suppl 6A):3S–15S.

69. Spence RK, Carson JA, Poses R, et al. (1990): Elective surgery without transfusion: influence of preoperative hemoglobin level and blood loss on maturity. *Am J Surg* 159:320–324.

70. Spence RK, McCoy S, Costabile J, et al. (1990): Fulosol DA 20 in the treatment of severe anemia: randomized, controlled study of 46 patients. *J Crit Care Med* 18:1227–1230.

71. Thompson GE, Miller RO, Stevens WC, et al. (1978): Hypo-tensive anesthesia for total hip arthroplasty. *Anesthesiology* 48:91.

72. Trammell TR, Fisher D, Brueckmann FR, et al. (1991): Closed-wound drainage systems. The Solcotrans Plus versus the Stryker-CBC Consta-Vac. *Orthop Rev* 20:536–542.

73. Tredwell SJ, Sawatsky B (1989): The use of fibrin sealant to reduce blood loss during Cotrel-Dubousset instrumentation for idiopathic scoliosis. Presented at the annual meeting of the Scoliosis Research Society, Amsterdam, Sept 1989.

74. Vamvakas EC, Taswell HF (1994): Epidermiology of blood transfusion. *Transfusion* 34:464–470.

75. Wilson WJ (1989): Intraoperative autologous transfusion in revision total hip arthroplasty. *J Bone Joint Surg Am* 71:8–14.

76. Yokoyama K, Yamanouchi K, Suyama T (1983): Recent advances in a perfluoro-chemical blood substitute and its biomedical application. *Life Chem Rep* 2:35–93.

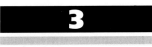

NERVE CONDUCTION STUDIES AND ELECTROMYOGRAPHY

MARK A. ROSS

Disorders of the peripheral nervous system are frequently evaluated with nerve conduction studies and needle electromyography (EMG). The information obtained with these electrophysiologic studies helps to confirm suspected clinical diagnoses and allows more precise localization of clinical abnormalities. Such studies facilitate diagnosis of most disorders of the peripheral nervous system and can localize focal peripheral nerve abnormalities to specific nerve segments. In many cases, these tests can help determine if the pathophysiologic process affecting nerve is due to axonal injury or demyelination.

ANATOMY

The cell bodies of motor and sensory nerves are within the anterior horn of the spinal cord and the dorsal root ganglion, respectively. After leaving the spinal cord, the motor and sensory rootlets join to form spinal nerves. The 31 pairs of spinal nerves include 8 cervical, 12 thoracic, 5 lumbar, 5 sacral, and 1 coccygeal. After exiting the intervertebral foramen, the spinal nerve divides into anterior and posterior primary rami. The posterior rami innervate the skin of the back and the paraspinal muscles. The anterior rami of the cervical spinal nerves enter the brachial plexus, and those of the lumbosacral spinal nerves enter the lumbosacral plexus. Within each plexus, the spinal nerves reorganize into individual nerves that provide sensory and motor function to the limbs. The anterior rami of the thoracic spinal nerves form intercostal nerves, which innervate the abdominal and intercostal muscles and skin of the thoracic and abdominal areas. Table 1 lists the major muscles and their peripheral nerve and segmental innervation.

The peripheral nerve consists of thousands of individual axons arranged in multiple fascicles supported by connective tissue. Schwann cells, arranged linearly along the axon, are connected by a continuous basal lamina to form a conduit for the axon, called the Schwann cell tube. Myelin, the Schwann cell membrane, wraps around the axon in spiral fashion, forming multiple layers called myelin lamellae. Myelin completely covers the axon except at the junctions between Schwann cells—called

nodes of Ranvier—which are free of myelin. Unmyelinated axons are not spirally wrapped by myelin but are individually encased, with other unmyelinated axons, within a small portion of a Schwann cell membrane. Myelinated fibers comprise the somatic motor and large-diameter sensory fibers, collectively known as type A fibers, and the preganglionic autonomic fibers, known as type B fibers (26). Unmyelinated fibers include small-diameter sensory fibers and postganglionic autonomic fibers, which are known collectively as type C fibers (26). Most nerve conduction studies performed in the EMG lab assess the function of the large myelinated fibers.

PHYSIOLOGY

Membrane Potential

Nerve and muscle tissues are unique in their capability of transmitting electrical signals for substantial distances along their cell membranes. The inherent excitability of these tissues depends on a transmembrane potential, which is maintained by separation of different charged ions across a semipermeable membrane. Measured with an intracellular recording electrode, the resting membrane potential for nerve and skeletal muscle is approximately -70 to -90 mV (48). In the resting state, the membrane is permeable to potassium. A high intracellular potassium concentration is maintained by negatively charged anions that prevent potassium from diffusing from the cell. In addition, the sodium-potassium pump actively pumps potassium into the cell in exchange for sodium.

Action Potential

If the nerve or muscle cell membrane is depolarized by 15 to 25 mV, the membrane becomes permeable to sodium ions (23). This change, called *threshold potential,* results in an action potential. For skeletal muscle, the process of depolarization begins at the neuromuscular junction, where the motor nerve fibers synapse with the skeletal muscle. When a nerve action potential reaches the presynaptic part of this synapse, a synchronized release of acetylcholine occurs. Acetylcholine diffuses across the synapse and activates receptors on the postsynaptic muscle membrane. As a result, sodium ions enter the muscle cell, causing

M. A. Ross: Department of Neurology, University of Kentucky, Lexington, Kentucky 40536-0284.

TABLE 1. MAJOR MUSCLES

Upper Extremity Muscles			Lower Extremity Muscles		
Muscle	**Nerve**	**Segments**	**Muscle**	**Nerve**	**Segments**
Sternocleidomastoid	Spinal accessory	C2, C3	Extensor digitorum minimi	Radial	C7, C8
Upper, midtrapezius	Spinal accessory	C3, C4	Abductor pollicis longus	Radial	C7, C8
Lower trapezius	Cervical plexus	C3, C4	Extensor pollicis longus	Radial	C7, C8
Diaphragm	Phrenic	C3, C4	Extensor pollicis brevis	Radial	C7, C8
Levator scapulae	Dorsal scapular	C4, C5	Extensor indicia proprius	Radial	C7, C8
Rhomboid major	Dorsal scapular	C4, C5	Iliopsoas	Femoral	L2, L3, L4
Rhomboid minor	Dorsal scapular	C4, C5	Sartorius	Femoral	L2, L3, L4
Subclavius	N to subclavius	C4, C5, C6	Quadriceps	Femoral	L2, L3, L4
Supraspinatus	Suprascapular	C5, C6	Gracitis	Obturator	L2, L3, L4
Infraspinatus	Suprascapular	C5, C6	Adductor longus	Obturator	L2, L3, L4
Subscapularis	Upper subscapular	C5, C6	Adductor brevis	Obturator	L2, L3, L4
Subscapularis	Lower subscapular	C5, C6	Adductor magnus	Obturator, tibial	L3, L4, L5
Teres major	Lower subscapular	C5, C6	Obturator externus	Obturator	L3, L4
Teres minor	Axillary	C5, C6	Obturator internus	Obturator internus	L5, S1, S2
Deltoid	Axillary	C5, C6	Inferior gemellus	Quadratus femoris	L4, L5, S1
Biceps brachii	Musculocutaneous	C5, C6	Superior gemellus	Obturator internus	L5, S1, S2
Coracobrachialis	Musculocutaneous	C5, C7	Piriformis	N to piriformis	S1, S2
Serratus anterior	Long thoracic	C5, C6, C7	Gluteus medius	Superior gluteal	L4, L5, S1
Pectoralis major, clavicular	L Ant thoracic	C5, C6	Gluteus minimus	Superior gluteal	L4, L5, S1
Pectoralis major, sternocostal	M Ant thoracic	C7, C8, T1	Tensor fasciae latae	Superior gluteal	L4, L5, S1
Pectoralis minor	M, L Ant thoracic	C6, C7, C8	Gluteus maximus	Inferior gluteal	L5, S1, S2
Latissimus dorsi	Thoracodorsal	C6, C7, C8	Quadratus femoris	N to quad femoris	L4, L5, S1
Pronator teres	Median	C6, C7	Semitendinosus	Sciatic (tibial)	L5, S1, S2
Flexor carpi radialis	Median	C6, C7, C8	Semimembranosus	Sciatic (tibial)	L5, S1, S2
Palmaris longus	Median	C7, C8, T1	Biceps femoris long head	Sciatic (tibial)	L5, S1, S2
Flexor digitorum superficialis	Median	C7, C8, T1	Biceps femoris short head	Sciatic (peroneal)	L5, S1, S2
Flexor digitorum profundus 1, 2	Median	C7, C8	Tibialis anterior	Deep peroneal	L4, L5
Flexor policis longus	Median	C7, C8, T1	Extensor digitorum longus	Deep peroneal	L5, S1
Pronator quadratus	Median	C7, C8, T1	Extensor digitorum brevis	Deep peroneal	L5, S1
Abductor pollicis brevis	Median	C8, T1	Peroneus tertius	Deep peroneal	L5, S1
Flexor pollicis brevis, short head	Median	C8, T1	Extensor hallucis longus	Deep peroneal	L5, S1
Opponens pollicis	Median	C8, T1	Extensor hallucis brevis	Deep peroneal	L5, S1
Lumbricals 1, 2	Median	C8, T1	Peroneus longus	Sup peroneal	L5, S1
Flexor carpi ulnaris	Ulnar	C7, C8, T1	Peroneus brevis	Sup peroneal	L5, S1
Flexor digitorum profundus 3, 4	Ulnar	C7, C8	Tibialis posterior	Tibial	L5, S1
Flexor digiti minimi	Ulnar	C8, T1	Popliteus	Tibial	L5, S1
Abductor digiti minimi	Ulnar	C8, T1	Flexor digitorum longus	Tibial	L5, S1, S2
Opponens digiti minimi	Ulnar	C8, T1	Flexor hallucis longus	Tibial	L5, S1, S2
Adductor pollicis	Ulnar	C8, T1	Gastrocnemius medial head	Tibial	S1, S2
Flexor pollicis brevis, deep head	Ulnar	C8, T1	Gastrocnemius lateral head	Tibial	S1, S2
Palmar interossei	Ulnar	C8, T1	Soleus	Tibial	L5, S1, S2
Dorsal interossei	Ulnar	C8, T1	Flexor digitorum brevis	Medial plantar	S1, S2
Lumbricals 3, 4	Ulnar	C8, T1	Flexor hallucis brevis	Medial plantar	S1, S2
Triceps	Radial	C7, C8, T1	Abductor hallucis	Medial plantar	S1, S2
Brachioradialis	Radial	C5, C8	Abductor digiti minimi	Lateral plantar	S1, S2
Extensor carpi radialis	Radial	C6, C7	Abductor hallucis	Lateral plantar	S1, S2
Anconaus	Radial	C7, C8	Flexor digiti minimi	Lateral plantar	S1, S2
Supinator	Radial	C5, C6	Interossei	Lateral plantar	S1, S2
Extensor carpi ulnaris	Radial	C6, C7, C8	Quadratus plantae	Lateral plantar	S1, S2
Extensor digitorum communis	Radial	C7, C8			

Ant, anterior; L, lateral; M, medial; N, nerve; Sup, superior.

further membrane depolarization and a brief reversal of the membrane potential from negative to positive, known as the action potential. The intracellular current flow associated with the action potential depolarizes adjacent membrane segments and causes bidirectional propagation of the action potential along the membrane. The action potential of a single muscle fiber is called muscle fiber action potential (MFAP). This depolarization spreads along the muscle fiber membrane and deep within the muscle fiber into structures called transverse tubules. Depolarization of the transverse tubules leads to release of calcium from the sarcoplasmic reticulum, which triggers muscle contraction. The process of an electrical signal (MFAP) leading to physical contraction of muscles is known as *excitation-contraction coupling.*

The resting membrane potential physiology for peripheral nerve is similar to that described for skeletal muscle. The nerve action potential (NAP) differs from the MFAP primarily in the mechanism and speed with which it propagates along the cell membrane. In myelinated peripheral nerves, virtually all of the sodium channels of the axon membrane are located at the nodes of Ranvier (35). Because current traverses the membrane via sodium channels in the nodal regions and myelin prevents passage of current through the internodal nerve segments, action potentials travel along myelinated nerves by jumping from node to node. This process, known as saltatory conduction (18,39), results in much faster conduction of action potentials along myelinated peripheral nerves than unmyelinated nerves or skeletal muscle. The speed of conduction for myelinated fibers is 40 to 60 m/s, whereas that for unmyelinated fibers is about 1 to 2 m/s (22).

NERVE CONDUCTION STUDIES

Nerve Stimulation

Application of an electrical stimulus of sufficient intensity and duration near a peripheral nerve depolarizes the nerve and generates a NAP. This is accomplished with two surface electrodes placed on the skin directly over the nerve. With a surface stimulus of 0.1 millisecond duration, a healthy nerve can usually be fully activated with 5 to 40 mA or 100 to 300 V (26). Activation of a diseased or inordinately deep nerve may require 60 to 75 mA or 400 to 500 V (26). When a nerve is directly stimulated (e.g., during intraoperative monitoring or when a stimulating needle electrode is placed close to a nerve), considerably less current is needed to fully activate the nerve. In these situations, the stimulus duration is decreased to 0.05 millisecond and the current or voltage is limited to 5 to 8 mA or 25 to 30 V, respectively (9).

Recording Nerve Responses

In clinical practice, two electrodes are used to record nerve responses. One electrode is called active (G1) and the other is called *reference* (G2). Each electrode is connected to a separate input of a differential amplifier, which amplifies only the difference in electrical potential between the two electrodes. Potentials common to each electrode are eliminated. The amplifier output is displayed on an oscilloscope screen, with voltage plotted vertically and time horizontally. By convention, if the electrical potential at the G1 electrode is positive relative to G2, the vertical deflection on the oscilloscope is downward. If G1 is negative relative to G2, the deflection is upward. A downward waveform deflection is referred to as *positive* and an upward deflection as *negative.*

Once initiated by electrical stimulation, the NAP travels along a nerve and can be recorded at a distant site. For sensory fibers, the NAP is recorded with electrodes placed directly over a sensory nerve branch and is called the sensory nerve action potential (SNAP). Normal amplitude values of SNAPs are in the range of 10 to 100 μV. In the case of motor nerve fibers, the NAP recording is made indirectly, with muscle acting as intermediary. The summated potential of all the depolarized muscle fibers is called the compound muscle action potential (CMAP). The amplitude of the CMAP is normally in the range of 3 to 20 mV.

Nerve conduction velocity is calculated by dividing the distance the NAP travels from the stimulus to the recording electrode by the response latency. Nerve conduction velocities vary with age, reaching adult values of approximately 50 to 70 m/s by age 3 to 5 years (11,21,41). Normal values for infants and young children (11,32) are listed in Table 2.

Routine nerve conduction studies assess the distal and midportions of the peripheral nerve. Special studies that include conduction through the proximal or central nerve segments may reveal abnormalities not evident on routine studies. These tests are often classified as "late responses" because the response latencies are generally much longer than those obtained with conventional studies. Common late-response studies are F wave and H reflex investigations.

The F wave is a late-occurring muscle potential resulting from "backfiring" of antidromically activated anterior horn cells. When a motor nerve is stimulated, orthodromic impulses descend, producing a CMAP, and antidromic impulses ascend proximally toward the spinal cord. In some anterior horn cells, the antidromic impulses depolarize the cell body, creating a new orthodromic impulse that descends and produces the F wave. The F wave is recorded from the same electrodes used to measure the CMAP. Compared with the CMAP, the F wave has smaller and more variable amplitude, more variable waveform morphology, and a longer and more variable latency. Because the F wave latency varies from trial to trial, multiple trials are performed and the shortest latency is reported. Values for infants and young children differ considerably from those for older children and adults (32).

The H reflex is a monosynaptic spinal reflex elicited by electrical stimulation of 1A afferent fibers. In the first year of life, the H reflex can be elicited in most nerves (32). In older children and adults, the H reflex can be routinely elicited only in the soleus and flexor carpi radialis muscle (19,24). In clinical practice, the H reflex is determined only in the calf muscle, providing information regarding the S1 reflex arc. To elicit the H reflex, a submaximal, long-duration (1 millisecond) stimulus is given to the tibial nerve in the popliteal fossa. As the stimulus intensity is increased gradually, the H reflex amplitude increases, and a CMAP is also recorded. The H reflex is recorded bilaterally, and

TABLE 2. RANGE OF NORMAL VALUES FOR NERVE CONDUCTION STUDIES IN CHILDREN

	No. Subjects	Amplitude (mV/μV)	Conduction Velocity (m/s)	Distal Latency (ms)	Distance (cm)
Neonate					
Motor					
Ulnar	56	1.6–7.0	20.0–36.1	1.3–2.9	1.0–3.4
Median	4	2.6–5.9	22.4–27.1	2.0–2.9	1.9–3.0
Peroneal	4	1.8–4.0	21.0–26.7	2.1–3.1	1.9–3.8
Sensory					
Median	10	7–15 (A)	25.1–31.9	2.1–3.0	3.8–5.4
	1	8–17 (O)			
Sural	8		—	3.3	5.5
MedPlantar	3	10–40	—	2.1–3.3	4.4–5.8
1–6 months					
Motor					
Ulnar	22	2.5–7.4	33.3–50.0	1.1–3.2	1.7–4.4
Median	6	3.5–6.9	37.0–47.7	1.6–2.2	2.1–4.1
Peroneal	10	1.6–8.0	32.4–47.7	1.7–2.4	2.5–4.1
Sensory					
Median	11	13–52 (A)	36.3–41.9	1.5–2.3	4.3–6.3
		9–26 (O)			
Sural	2	9–10	—	1.7–2.3	5.8
MedPlantar	2	17–26	35.4–35.7	1.5–1.9	4.5–5.5
7–12 months					
Motor					
Ulnar	28	3.2–10.0	35.0–58.2	0.8–2.2	1.9–4.6
Median	13	2.3–8.6	33.3–46.3	1.5–2.8	1.9–4.3
Peroneal	19	2.3–6.0	38.8–56.0	1.4–3.2	2.2–5.5
Sensory					
Median	15	14–64 (A)	39.1–60.0	1.6–2.4	5.5–6.8
		11–36 (O)			
Sural	5	10–28	40.6	1.7–2.5	5.8–7.6
MedPlantar	6	15–38	39.4–40.3	1.9–2.7	6.5–7.9
13–24 months					
Motor					
Ulnar	53	2.6–9.7	41.3–63.5	1.1–2.2	2.4–4.8
Median	16	3.7–11.6	39.2–50.5	1.8–2.8	2.2–4.3
Peroneal	36	1.7–6.5	39.2–54.3	1.6–3.5	2.2–5.8
Sensory					
Median	29	14–82 (A)	46.5–57.9	1.7–3.0	5.7–9.1
		7–36 (O)			
Sural	9	8–30	—	1.4–2.8	4.5–8.6
MedPlantar	12	15–60	42.6–57.3	1.8–2.5	6.1–9.3

A, antidromic sensory potential; O, orthodromic sensory potential; MedPlantar, medial plantar nerve.
(From Miller RG, Kuntz NL [1986]: Nerve conduction studies in infants and children. *J Child Neural* 1:19–26, with permission.)

the results of the two sides are compared. Unilateral absence, or prolongation of H reflex latency by 1.5 millisecond compared with the normal side, suggests an abnormality in the S1 reflex pathway.

PITFALLS OF NERVE CONDUCTION STUDIES: PHYSIOLOGIC FACTORS

Physiologic factors affecting the interpretation of nerve conduction studies include patient age, limb temperature, and nerve anomalies (21). Although age does not affect results in young and middle-aged adults, it may have a major effect on tests involving the very young and the elderly. For premature infants, nerve conduction velocities can be as slow as 15 to 25 m/s. Full-term infants have nerve conduction velocity values of 21 to 39

m/s for the ulnar nerve (41). Adult values (approximately 50 to 70 m/s) are reached by age 3 to 5 years (11,21,41). By the sixth to eighth decades of life, nerve conduction velocities decrease by less than 10 m/s compared with young-adult values (33). Individuals over the age of 60 frequently lose lower-extremity SNAPs and H-reflex responses.

Temperature may profoundly affect nerve conduction study results because cool temperatures prolong latencies and slow nerve conduction velocities. The nerve conduction velocity of the median and ulnar nerves has been shown to change linearly by 2.4 m/s per degree C over the temperature range of 29 to 38°C (17). Median and ulnar nerve wrist latencies increase by 0.3 m/s per degree when the hand is cooled (21). To avoid interpretative error, skin temperature should be measured before the study is begun; if it is less than 34°C, the patient should be warmed. An alternative approach is to attempt to adjust the nerve conduction velocity values for temperature by adding 5% of the calculated velocity for each degree below 34°C (21).

ELECTROMYOGRAPHY

The EMG Examination

The EMG examination involves recording electrical signals from muscle with an intramuscular needle-recording electrode. Four assessments are made during the examination: insertional activity, spontaneous activity, motor unit potential (MUP) characteristics, and MUP recruitment. The first two assessments are made simultaneously with the muscle relaxed. The needle is advanced into the muscle in increments of 1 to 2 mm, held still for several seconds between each advancement. Multiple advancements are made in each of four directions. Insertional activity is assessed as the needle moves, and spontaneous activity is monitored while the needle is stationary. MUP assessment involves measuring individual MUPs generated during minimal voluntary muscle contraction. The recruitment pattern refers to the pattern of activation of additional MUPs as the patient contracts the muscle with gradually increased effort.

Insertional Activity

When an EMG needle is placed in normal muscle, a discharge of electrical activity, called insertional activity, results from mechanical stimulation of muscle fibers. This is normally several hundred microvolts in amplitude and lasts several hundred microseconds. Normal insertional activity lasts only slightly longer than the needle movement. Increased insertional activity may occur as a prolonged train of positive sharp waves or negative spikes or as a mixture of positive sharp waves and negative spikes. Increased insertional activity may be the only electrophysiologic abnormality in the early stages of either a neuropathic or a myopathic disorder. Increased insertional activity may also occur in some normal individuals (44,45). Decreased insertional activity is usually seen in a severely diseased muscle that has undergone replacement by fibrous or fatty tissue.

Spontaneous Activity

When the EMG needle electrode is held stationary in a normal muscle, no spontaneously occurring electrical discharges occur. Exceptions to this rule include end plate potentials (potentials recorded only in the end plate region) and fasciculation potentials. Fasciculation potentials are discussed below. Fibrillation potentials are the most common form of abnormal spontaneous activity.

A fibrillation potential is an abnormal, spontaneous depolarization of an individual muscle fiber that occurs when a muscle fiber is dissociated from its nerve supply. This may be a physical dissociation, from disease affecting either the axon or the muscle fiber. Fibrillation potentials may also develop secondary to botulinum toxin, severe myasthenia gravis, or prolonged neuromuscular pharmacologic blockade. Fibrillation potentials do not appear immediately after a muscle fiber has been isolated from

its nerve supply; they develop several days to weeks later (3). Fibrillation potentials generally signify disease within the motor unit (the lower motor neuron, its axon, or muscle fibers). Fibrillation potentials occur in two forms: negative spikes and positive sharp waves, which have the same clinical significance. Fibrillation potentials are graded on a scale of 0 to 4, where 0 indicates none and 4 indicates abundant fibrillation potentials at all sites.

A fasciculation potential represents a spontaneous discharge of a group of muscle fibers belonging to either a motor unit or a subset of it. Fasciculation potentials occur irregularly. They may originate in the motor neuron or anywhere along its axon (43). Fasciculation potentials occur in normal individuals (benign fasciculation potentials) as well as in a variety of neurogenic or metabolic disease states. The complexity of the waveform and any other evidence of abnormality, such as fibrillation potentials, distinguish those associated with neurogenic disease from the benign type. Neurogenic conditions causing fasciculation potentials include disorders of anterior horn cells, nerve roots, plexuses, and peripheral nerves. Metabolic conditions causing fasciculation potentials include thyrotoxicosis, tetany, and anticholinesterase toxicity (10).

Complex Repetitive Discharges

Complex repetitive discharges represent groups of MFAPs activated ephaptically that fire sequentially in a monotonously repetitive pattern. These discharges have been described in neurogenic conditions such as motor neuron disorders, radiculopathies, and chronic neuropathies and in muscle disorders such as inflammatory myopathies, muscular dystrophies, myxedema, and the Schwartz-Jampel syndrome (10).

Myokymic Discharges

Myokymic discharges are bursts of repetitively firing MUPs arising from single or multiple motor units. Myokymic discharges may be associated with clinical myokymia, an involuntary, continuous, undulating movement of the skin surface attributable to nonuniform muscle contractions. Myokymia occurs in generalized and focal forms (37). Generalized myokymic discharges have been observed in Guillain-Barré syndrome, uremia, and thyrotoxicosis, and may be hereditary or idiopathic. Focal myokymia can involve the limbs or the face. Facial myokymia suggests multiple sclerosis or brain stem glioma, but it may also occur with other pontine mass lesions, facial nerve palsy, vertebrobasilar insufficiency, and a variety of other neurologic disorders (34,37). Limb myokymia occurs infrequently with compressive nerve lesions but commonly with radiation plexopathy (13).

Motor Unit Potential Assessment

When a muscle is minimally contracted voluntarily, MFAPs belonging to a single motor unit can be recorded with a needle electrode. Their summated electrical activity is a MUP. The MUP is typically a triphasic wave with initial positivity, a negative spike, and subsequent positivity. MUPs may also be monophasic, biphasic, or have three or more phases. The MUP is derived from only those fibers that are discharging within the recording radius of the needle electrode; therefore, it does not reflect all of the muscle fibers of the motor unit. The presence of fewer than 20 muscle fibers within a 1-mm radius of the needle tip contributes to the negative spike (40). Presence of fibers of the motor unit at greater distances from the needle tip contributes to the initial and subsequent positive components of the MUP. MUPs may have numerous profiles, depending on the relationship of the needle to different fibers of the motor unit. A slight movement of the needle while recording changes the appearance of the MUP, even though the individual fibers of the motor unit have not changed their firing. MUPs are described by several parameters, including rise time, amplitude, duration, number of phases, stability, and firing pattern. Multiple factors influence MUP characteristics, including distance of the recording needle from the fibers, size of individual muscle fibers, synchrony of firing of fibers of the motor unit, patient age, the muscle being studied, temperature, the degree of effort of muscle contraction, and the type of needle used (10,27).

Motor Unit Potentials in Disease States

Neuromuscular disease processes may alter the motor unit structure and, hence, produce changes in normal MUP characteristics. To determine if a MUP is abnormal, one must know normal MUP values, which vary with the specific muscle and the age of the patient (2,4–6,36). Both neurogenic and myopathic disorders produce changes in the motor unit structure. Neurogenic disorders often cause loss of whole motor units, whereas myopathies cause random loss of fibers from the motor unit. These different pathologic processes may produce distinct MUP changes, allowing EMG to help differentiate a muscle disease from a neurogenic disorder (1,14,15). However, some overlap of MUP abnormalities may occur (8,28).

Lower Motor Neuron Disorders

In neurogenic disorders—disorders of the lower motor neuron or its axon—the usual pathologic event is loss of entire motor units. As a consequence, surviving axons may develop sprouts that reinnervate the denervated fibers; thus, the surviving axon acquires an expanded motor unit in terms of total number of muscle fibers and the distribution of fibers within the muscle. The EMG correlate of this process is an increase in amplitude and duration of the MUP. The amplitude increases because fiber density increases. The duration may increase because of an increased number of fibers or a loss of synchrony of discharging fibers in the motor unit. An increased percentage of polyphasic MUPs may occur because of decreased synchrony of firing of individual muscle fibers within the motor unit. This may be a result of varied lengths of axon terminals in the restructured motor unit or impaired neuromuscular transmission in newly formed synapses. MUPs in neurogenic disorders may show some (but not necessarily all) of the above abnormalities.

Myopathic Disorders

In myopathic disorders, MUPs are typically of short duration and low amplitude (8,28,46). The random loss of muscle fibers

from the motor unit that occurs in myopathy decreases motor unit territory. Because some muscle fibers distant from the needle no longer contribute to the initial and terminal MUP components, the MUP duration is decreased. Loss of muscle fibers from the motor unit also reduces fiber density; thus, fewer fibers near the recording electrode contribute to the MUP amplitude. Despite the fact that the total MUP duration is decreased in myopathies, MUPs often show increased polyphasia. In general, polyphasia is attributed to desynchronized firing of muscle fibers of the unit (27). This may be caused by increased variation in the conduction time of action potentials along intramuscular terminal nerve branches or diseased muscle fiber membranes. In addition, reinnervated split fibers and regenerating fibers may contribute to desynchronized muscle fiber firing because of differential slowing of conduction in their terminal nerve branches. This may be due either to variable lengths of new axon terminals or to impaired transmission in immature neuromuscular junctions.

Recruitment Pattern Assessment

Normal Recruitment

Motor units are activated according to the Henneman size principle, which indicates that motor neurons recruit in an orderly manner, beginning with small motor neurons (16). With a minimal voluntary contraction, small type 1 fibers belonging to type 1 motor neurons are activated first. One or several motor units discharge, producing MUPs that fire at a frequency of 5 to 7 Hz. The pattern of voluntary MUP firing is distinctive and has been referred to as semirhythmic because of its gradually speeding, then gradually slowing, pattern (10). With increasing effort, the initially firing MUP fires faster and additional MUPs begin firing. The frequency of firing of the initial MUP when an additional MUP begins firing is called the *recruitment frequency*. The normal recruitment frequency is generally 5 to 15 Hz (10). With increasing levels of contraction, many MUPs begin to fire, and it becomes impossible to identify individual MUPs. This is called the *interference pattern*.

Abnormal Recruitment Patterns

When disease results in loss of motor units, the firing frequency of the remaining motor units is increased relative to the number of motor units firing. This abnormal pattern of recruitment is called *reduced recruitment* (10). A single MUP firing at greater than 35 Hz is always considered abnormal and is definite evidence of reduced recruitment. The pattern of reduced recruitment is usually seen in neurogenic disorders that result in loss from the muscle of whole motor units. An incomplete interference pattern without rapidly firing MUPs may be seen in upper motor neuron disorders or when the patient's effort is reduced.

The recruitment pattern in myopathies is characterized by activation of more motor units than expected for the degree of force exerted. This pattern has been referred to as either *early recruitment* (28) or *rapid recruitment* (10). The basis for this pattern is that the random loss of fibers within motor units prevents individual motor units from generating the normal degree of tension associated with their activation. To compensate, additional motor units are recruited, producing an interference pattern of many MUPs firing. Despite this rally, the force generated remains low. The recruitment frequency in this pattern is normal. Only the examiner, who can feel the degree of force the patient is exerting, appreciates the pattern of early recruitment.

SINGLE-FIBER ELECTROMYOGRAPHY

Single-fiber EMG is a selective EMG recording technique performed with a special needle that allows measurement of action potentials from individual muscle fibers. Two major categories of information are obtained with single-fiber EMG studies: *fiber density* and *jitter*. Fiber density refers to the number of muscle fibers belonging to one motor unit within the 300-μm recording radius of the needle. The fiber density is determined by counting the number of muscle fiber potentials at 20 different sites, using several skin insertions. The fiber density is measured as the mean value of the number of MFAPs at these 20 sites. Normal fiber density values are roughly between 1 and 2, but they vary for different muscles and increase with age. Fiber density is increased when muscle reinnervation occurs.

Jitter, measured in microseconds, is the variation in the interpotential interval between pairs of action potentials from two or more muscle fibers activated by a single motor unit (38). Jitter is a normal phenomenon occurring secondary to variation in the rise time of the muscle end plate potentials. Normal jitter values are defined based on patient age and specific muscles. Jitter increases beyond the normal range when impaired neuromuscular transmission produces reduced-amplitude end plate potentials, which have a slower rise time to reach threshold. To analyze jitter, the recording electrode must be positioned such that action potentials are recorded from two or more muscle fibers belonging to the same motor unit.

INTERPRETATION

Electrophysiologic Classification of Nerve Injury

Abnormal nerve conduction studies results must be correlated with the patient's clinical condition. This usually reveals if the patient has peripheral nerve disease and if it is focal (mononeuropathy) or diffuse (polyneuropathy). Next, the type of nerve injury is classified as demyelinating or axonal, based on the electrophysiologic findings.

Demyelinating Injury

Manifestations of a demyelinating nerve injury include conduction block, temporal dispersion, prolonged latencies, and slow nerve conduction velocities. Loss of myelin from peripheral nerve interferes with saltatory conduction of impulses through the region of demyelination. The depolarizing current dissipates in the demyelinated region and either becomes insufficient to depolarize subsequent nerve segments or does so in a much de-

layed fashion (29). The electrophysiologic manifestation of failure of the impulse to conduct due to loss of myelin is conduction block. Conduction block is recognized when the amplitude of the CMAP is significantly reduced compared with that with distal stimulation. Conduction block suggests that a demyelinating nerve injury is acquired because it is usually not seen in the hereditary demyelinating polyneuropathies (29,31). The exception is hereditary liability to pressure palsies, which may have conduction block.

When the impulse is delayed in the demyelinated region but is still conducted, the electrophysiologic findings include temporal dispersion, prolonged latencies, and slow nerve conduction velocities. Temporal dispersion indicates that the CMAP is abnormally long duration, and often the waveform becomes irregularly contoured.

Slow nerve conduction velocities and prolonged latencies occur as a consequence of slow conduction through demyelinated regions. The functional and electrophysiologic outcomes of demyelination are determined by how severely individual axons are demyelinated, the number of axons affected at a given site of demyelination, and the number of sites along the course of the nerve that are demyelinated.

Axonal Injury

The SNAP and CMAP amplitudes are proportional to the number of conducting axons. Axonal injury and subsequent degeneration reduce the number of conducting axons, causing the SNAP and CMAP amplitudes to decline. Depending on the nature and severity of the disorder causing nerve injury, there may be selective involvement of sensory or motor fibers. As a general rule, slowing of nerve conduction velocity with axonal nerve injury is mild in comparison with that seen with demyelinating nerve injury. Loss of large numbers of fast-conducting fibers may reduce the velocity to 70% to 80% of the lower normal limit (30). If roughly 50% or more of the fast-conducting fibers remain, slowing of nerve conduction velocity due to axonal injury is estimated to result in a velocity that is 80% to 90% of the lower normal limit (30).

The other major finding with axonal injury of motor fibers is evidence of muscle fiber denervation on the needle examination (EMG). Fibrillation potentials develop in muscles about 7 to 10 days after axonal injury (3). Fibrillation potentials do not occur in purely demyelinating nerve lesions, but they may be seen when a primarily demyelinating nerve lesion has associated axonal degeneration.

The electrophysiologic changes of axonal injury are seen with either axonotmesis or neurotmesis. If CMAPs and SNAPs are completely lost immediately following axonal nerve injury, it cannot be determined whether this represents severe axonotmesis or neurotmesis. If reduced-amplitude CMAPs and/or SNAPs continue to be obtained many weeks after the onset of nerve injury, neurotmesis can be excluded, as this would be expected to produce complete loss of responses. An exception occurs in nerve root avulsion, in which the SNAPs remain normal despite neurotmesis (42). This occurs because the injury involves the preganglionic dorsal root ganglion fibers. The postganglionic dorsal root ganglion fibers, which are assessed with sensory nerve conduction studies, remain in continuity with the dorsal root ganglion and function normally.

Other Causes of Abnormal Nerve Conduction Studies

In addition to primary peripheral nerve disease, other neuromuscular disorders may produce abnormal results. Reduced-amplitude CMAPs may be seen with anterior horn cell disorders (6), radiculopathies (47), plexopathies, certain neuromuscular transmission disorders (20), and some myopathies (25). With anterior horn cell disorders, radiculopathies, plexopathies, and neuropathies, reduced-amplitude CMAPs are caused by axonal degeneration of motor nerve fibers. With neuromuscular transmission disorders and myopathies, motor nerve axons are generally normal, and the reduced-amplitude CMAPs result from disease involving the neuromuscular junction and the muscle fiber, respectively.

As a general rule, SNAPs remain normal in anterior horn cell diseases, radiculopathies, neuromuscular transmission disorders, and myopathies. With anterior horn cell disorders, neuromuscular transmission disorders, and myopathies, the underlying disease process largely spares the peripheral sensory system. Plexopathies and neuropathies are the only categories of neuromuscular diseases that typically show reduced amplitude of both CMAPs and SNAPs.

CLINICAL DISORDERS

Anterior Horn Cell Disorders

The anterior horn cell disorders are a diverse group of conditions (12). Because these disorders cause degeneration of the anterior horn cell and its axon, the EMG findings of the various entities are similar. Nerve conduction studies in anterior horn cell disorders typically show reduced amplitude CMAPs but preserved SNAPs (7). Nerve conduction velocities are usually normal in anterior horn cell disorders, although slowing of motor conduction velocities may occur when CMAP amplitudes are significantly reduced. The EMG exam shows either ongoing muscle fiber denervation or previous muscle fiber denervation and subsequent reinnervation. Evidence of denervation consists of fibrillation potentials and positive sharp waves. Fasciculation potentials are commonly seen. Evidence of reinnervation consists of MUPs that are large amplitude, excessively polyphasic, long duration, or some combination of these abnormal features. Recruitment of MUPs in anterior horn cell disorders is reduced.

Radiculopathy

Nerve conduction studies are generally normal in radiculopathy. If a root lesion results in significant motor fiber axonal injury, there may be a reduction in the amplitude of the CMAP of nerves receiving fibers from the affected root. In contrast, the SNAP amplitude is maintained. This occurs because the dorsal root ganglion is a bipolar cell and the site of the nerve injury in radiculopathy is typically the preganglionic fibers (sensory fibers that travel proximally from the dorsal root ganglion) (47). The distal fibers of the dorsal root ganglion are tested with sensory nerve conduction studies, and these remain intact. The H reflex may be lost or delayed on the affected side with S1 radiculopathy.

The EMG examination is the most important electrophysiologic test for diagnosing radiculopathy. A diagnosis of radiculopathy is established by demonstrating fibrillation potentials restricted to the distribution of a single myotome. In practice, this means involvement of two or more limb muscles of the same myotome and the corresponding paraspinal muscles.

Plexopathy

Electrodiagnostic studies play a critical role in the evaluation of plexopathy because they can confirm and localize plexus involvement and estimate the severity and type of plexus injury. To evaluate suspected plexus lesions, extensive nerve conduction studies and EMG must be performed. Plexus lesions that produce axonal injury show reduced-amplitude CMAPs and SNAPs when compared with the homologous nerve on the unaffected side. Reduction or loss of SNAPs is an important electrodiagnostic feature of plexopathy and helps distinguish plexopathy from radiculopathy. If the EMG exam reveals fibrillation potentials in limb muscles but not paraspinal muscles, a diagnosis of plexopathy is favored. An extensive EMG exam must be performed to evaluate a suspected plexopathy. This includes paraspinal muscles innervated by the spinal segments contributing to the plexus and multiple muscles of the affected limb. Fibrillation potentials in paraspinal muscles exclude the diagnosis of plexopathy because the posterior primary ramus supplying the paraspinal muscles departs from the spinal nerve proximal to the formation of the plexus. The pattern of muscle involvement is analyzed to determine the site(s) of abnormality within the plexus.

Neuropathy

Disease of the peripheral nerve may occur diffusely (polyneuropathy), focally (mononeuropathy), or in an intermediate pattern in which several noncontiguous peripheral nerves are affected either simultaneously or in sequence (mononeuritis multiplex). Nerve conduction and EMG studies help to confirm the presence of polyneuropathy and to distinguish if the pathophysiologic process is due to demyelination or axonal loss, as discussed above.

Neuromuscular Transmission Defects

Neuromuscular transmission defects are usually assessed by repetitive nerve stimulation or, less often, with single-fiber EMG. However, conventional nerve conduction studies may provide clues to a neuromuscular transmission disorder. For example, in the appropriate clinical setting, low-amplitude CMAPs should raise the possibility of botulism or Lambert-Eaton myasthenic syndrome. Fibrillation potentials occur commonly in botulism, beginning during or after the second week of illness. Fibrillation potentials are not a feature of Lambert-Eaton syndrome or myasthenia gravis. MUPs may show variation in amplitude in neuromuscular transmission disorders.

In neuromuscular transmission disorders, single-fiber EMG shows increased jitter or blocking. If the end plate potential of one of the muscle fibers being studied does not reach threshold, the single-fiber action potential will not appear. This is called *blocking*. Blocking represents a more severe defect in neuromuscular transmission than abnormal jitter and tends to occur when jitter values reach the range of 80 to 100 μs (38). If blocking is excessive, jitter cannot be calculated. Blocking is expressed as the percentage of potential pairs in which it occurs. Blocking in more than one of 20 pairs of MFAPs is considered abnormal.

Myopathy

Conventional nerve conduction studies are usually normal in myopathies. The CMAP amplitude may be reduced when recorded from proximal muscles, such as the deltoid or quadriceps. The amplitude of CMAPs from distal hand and foot muscles is usually normal. However, in some myopathies (hereditary and sporadic forms of distal myopathy, inclusion body myositis, and myotonic dystrophy), CMAPs from distal muscles may be reduced. This may also occur with other myopathies in advanced stages. Sensory nerve conduction studies remain normal in myopathy.

Depending on the type, severity, and stage of the pathologic process, the EMG exam may show different results. Insertional activity is increased in many myopathies, but when myopathy is advanced, muscle fibrosis and fatty replacement create decreased insertional activity (10,28). Myotonic discharges or complex repetitive discharges occur in several myopathic disorders (8,10,28,46). Fibrillation potentials are also seen in many myopathies. In general, fibrillation potentials provide an indicator of the degree of activity of the myopathic process, profuse fibrillation potentials are suggestive of an active or ongoing myopathic process, and infrequent fibrillation potentials are suggestive of relatively inactive disease (46). MUPs in myopathy are typically of low amplitude and short duration. Mild metabolic and endocrine myopathies often show little change in MUPs (28).

LIMITATIONS OF ELECTROMYOGRAPHY

The clinician should remember that negative EMG studies do not exclude pathology of the peripheral nervous system. Failure to study the appropriate nerves and muscles for a given clinical problem may result in a false-negative EMG study. Even when appropriate muscles are selected for study, false-negative EMG studies may occur if the disease process is so focal that abnormalities escape detection. Timing of the study too early in the evolution of the disorder may also give a false-negative result. EMG performed in the first few days after an incomplete axonal injury may be deceptively normal, as it takes 7 to 10 days for fibrillation potentials to develop. Negative EMG studies may also occur because certain neuromuscular disorders simply do not manifest abnormalities on conventional EMG studies. Examples include a radiculopathy involving predominantly sensory fibers, exclusively small-fiber neuropathies, and some myopathies.

REFERENCES

1. Black JT, Bhatt GP, DeJesus PV, et al. (1974): Diagnostic accuracy of clinical data, quantitative electromyography and histochemistry in neuromuscular disease: a study of 105 cases. *J Neurol Sci* 21:59–70.
2. Buchthal F (1957): *An introduction to electromyography.* Copenhagen: Scandinavian University Books.
3. Buchthal F (1982): Fibrillations: clinical electrophysiology. In: Culp WJ, Ochoa J, eds. *Abnormal nerves and muscles as impulse generators.* New York: Oxford University Press, pp. 632–662.
4. Buchthal F, Guld C, Rosenfalck P (1954): Action potential parameters in normal human muscle and their dependence on physical variables. *Acta Physiol Scand* 32:200.
5. Buchthal F, Pinelli P, Rosenfalck P (1954): Action potential parameters in normal human muscle and their physiological determinants. *Acta Physiol Scand* 32:219–229.
6. Buchthal F, Rosenfalck P (1955): Action potential parameters in different human muscles. *Acta Psychiatr Neurol Scand* 30:125–140.
7. Daube JR (1982): *EMG in motor neuron disease* (Minimonograph 18). Rochester, MN: American Association of Electromyography and Electrodiagnosis, p. 6.
8. Daube JR (1986): Electrodiagnosis of muscle disorders. In: Engel AG, Banker BQ, eds. *Myology.* New York: McGraw-Hill, pp. 1081–1122.
9. Daube JR (1989): *Intraoperative monitoring of cranial nerves* (Course B). Rochester, MN: American Association of Electromyography and Electrodiagnosis, p. 10.
10. Daube JR (1991): Needle examination in clinical electromyography. *Muscle Nerve* 14:685–700.
11. Gamstorp I (1963): Normal conduction velocity of ulnar, median and peroneal nerves in infancy, childhood and adolescence. *Acta Paediatr* 146(Suppl):68–76.
12. Gomez MR (1986): Motor neuron diseases in children. In: Engel AG, Banker BQ, eds. *Myology.* New York: McGraw-Hill, pp. 1993–2012.
13. Gutmann L (1991): Facial and limb myokymia. *Muscle Nerve* 14:1043–1049.
14. Hausmanowa-Petrusewicz I, Jedrzejowska H (1971): Correlation between electromyographic findings and muscle biopsy in cases of neuromuscular disease. *J Neurol Sci* 13:85–106.
15. Hausmanowa-Petrusewicz I, Wasowicz B, Kopec A (1967): Electromyography in neuromuscular diagnostics. *Electromyography* 7:203–225.
16. Henneman E (1957): Relations between size of neurons and their susceptibility to discharge. *Science* 126:1345–1347.
17. Henrikson JD (1956): Conduction velocity of motor nerves in normal subjects and patients with neuromuscular disorders. PhD thesis, University of Minnesota.
18. Huxley AF, Stampfli R (1949): Saltatory transmission of the nervous impulse. *Arch Sci Physiol* 3:435–448.
19. Jabre JF (1981): Surface recording of the H-reflex of the flexor carpi radialis. *Muscle Nerve* 4:435–438.
20. Keesey JC (1989): Electrodiagnostic approach to defects of neuromuscular transmission. *Muscle Nerve* 12:613–626.
21. Kimura J (1984): Principles and pitfalls of nerve conduction studies. *Ann Neurol* 16:415–429.
22. Kimura J (1989): Anatomy and physiology of the peripheral nerve. In: Kimura J, ed. *Electrodiagnosis in diseases of nerve and muscle: principles and practice,* 2nd ed. Philadelphia: FA Davis Co.,, pp. 55–77.
23. Kimura J (1989): Electrical properties of nerve and muscle. In: Kimura J, ed. *Electrodiagnosis in diseases of nerve and muscle: principles and practice,* 2nd ed. Philadelphia: FA Davis Co., pp. 25–36.
24. Kimura J (1989): H, T, masseter, and other reflexes. In: Kimura J, ed. *Electrodiagnosis in diseases of nerve and muscle: principles and practice,* 2nd ed. Philadelphia: FA Davis Co., pp. 356–374.
25. Kimura J (1989): Myopathies. In: Kimura J, ed. *Electrodiagnosis in diseases of nerve and muscle: principles and practice,* 2nd ed. Philadelphia: FA Davis Co., pp. 535–557.
26. Kimura J (1989): Principles of nerve conduction studies. In: Kimura J, ed. *Electrodiagnosis in diseases of nerve and muscle: principles and practice,* 2nd ed. Philadelphia: FA Davis Co., pp. 78–102.
27. Kimura J (1989): Techniques and normal findings. In: Kimura J, ed.

Electrodiagnosis in diseases of nerve and muscle: principles and practice, 2nd ed. Philadelphia: FA Davis Co., pp. 227–248.

28. Kimura J (1989): Types of abnormality. In: Kimura J, ed. *Electrodiagnosis in diseases of nerve and muscle: principles and practice,* 2nd ed. Philadelphia: FA Davis Co., pp. 249–274.

29. Kimura J (1991): *Pathophysiology in demyelinating neuropathy* (Course B). Rochester, MN: American Association of Electrodiagnostic Medicine, pp. 7–11.

30. Kimura J (1993): Nerve conduction studies and electromyography. In: Dyck PJ, Thomas PK, eds. *Peripheral neuropathy,* 3rd ed. Philadelphia: WB Saunders, pp. 598–644.

31. Lewis RA, Sumner AJ (1982): The electrodiagnostic distinctions between chronic familial and acquired demyelinative neuropathies. *Neurology* 32:592–596.

32. Miller RG, Kuntz NL (1986): Nerve conduction studies in infants and children. *J Child Neurol* 1:19–26.

33. Norris AH, Shock NW, Wagman IH (1953): Age changes in the maximum conduction velocity of motor fibers of human ulnar nerves. *J Appl Physiol* 5:589–593.

34. Radu EW, Skorpil V, Kaeser HE (1975): Facial myokymia. *Eur Neurol* 13:499–512.

35. Ritchie JM, Rogart RB (1977): The density of sodium channels in mammalian myelinated nerve fibers and the nature of the axonal membrane under the myelin sheath. *Proc Natl Acad Sci USA* 74:211–215.

36. Sacco G, Buchthal F, Rosenfalck P (1962): Motor unit potentials at different ages. *Arch Neurol* 6:366.

37. Sivak M, Ochoa J (1987): Positive manifestations of nerve fiber dysfunction: Clinical, electrophysiologic, and pathologic correlates. In:

Brown WF, Bolton CF, eds. *Clinical electromyography.* Boston: Butterworth, pp. 1–30.

38. Stalberg E, Trontelj J (1979): *Single fibre electromyography.* Old Woking, Surrey, UK: Mirvalle Press Limited, p. 75.

39. Stampfli R (1981): Overview of studies on the physiology of conduction in myelinated nerve fibers. In: Waxman SG, Ritchie JM, eds. *Demyelinating disease: basic and clinical electrophysiology.* New York: Raven Press, pp. 11–23.

40. Thiele B, Bohl A (1978): Number of spike-components contributing to the motor unit potential. *Z EEG-EMG* 9:125–130.

41. Thomas JE, Lambert EH (1960): Ulnar nerve conduction velocity and H-reflex in infants and children. *J Appl Physiol* 15:1–9.

42. Warren J, Gutmann L, Figueroa AF, et al. (1969): Electromyographic changes of brachial plexus root avulsion. *J Neurosurg* 31:137–140.

43. Wettstein A (1979): The origin of fasciculations in motor neuron disease. *Ann Neurol* 5:295–300.

44. Wiechers DO (1977): Mechanically provoked insertional activity before and after nerve section in rats. *Arch Phys Med Rehabil* 58:402–495.

45. Wilbourn AJ (1982): An unreported, distinctive type of increased insertional activity. *Muscle Nerve* 5:S101–S105.

46. Wilbourn AJ (1987): *The EMG examination in myopathies* (Course A). Rochester, MN: American Association of Electromyography and Electrodiagnosis, pp. 7–20.

47. Wilbourn AJ, Aminoff MJ (1988): The electrophysiologic examination in patients with radiculopathies. *Muscle Nerve* 11:1099–1114.

48. Woodbury JW (1965): Action potential: properties of excitable membranes. In: Ruch TC, Patton HD, Woodbury JW, et al., eds. *Neurophysiology,* 2nd ed. Philadelphia: WB Saunders, pp. 26–57.

Pediatric Spine Surgery, 2nd ed., edited by Stuart L. Weinstein. Lippincott Williams & Wilkins, Philadelphia © 2001.

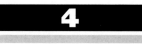

SPINAL CORD MONITORING

MASAFUMI MACHIDA
THORU YAMADA

Electrophysiologic monitoring techniques have come to play an increasingly important role in the identification of potentially reversible damage and the prevention of neurologic complications during spinal or spinal cord surgery. The efficacy of any monitoring technique is based on a number of factors. First, it is presumed that neural injury occurs in a measurable fashion that can be detected by particular monitoring techniques being used. Second, for a monitoring technique to be beneficial, it must be capable of detecting changes at a point at which they are potentially reversible. It follows that reversal of the alterations detected during monitoring is predictive of a good neurologic outcome. Finally, the monitoring technique must be capable of detecting injury to the pathways that are at risk during a given procedure.

Neurologic impairment can be caused by factors such as circulatory disturbance or excess compression by retraction, bone structures, hematoma, or mechanical stretching. Monitoring provides assurance to the surgeon that no identifiable complication has occurred up to that point, allowing the surgeon to proceed and provide a more through surgical intervention than could not have been carried out in the absence of monitoring. Some high-risk patients, including those with onset of scoliosis before age 10 years, rapid progression of the curve, clinical symptoms such as back pain or headache, neurologic symptoms or signs, or an atypical curve pattern, may be candidates for surgical procedures only if monitoring is available.

Intraoperative neurophysiologic monitoring has increased in popularity during the past several decades. Spinal cord monitoring and scoliosis surgery leads in these applications. The techniques of somatosensory monitoring for scoliosis were developed initially more than two decades ago and have become standard during the past 15 years (13,18,19,22,38,58–60,69,77,81,89, 96). New inroads are being made into motor pathway monitoring (8–10,20,31,43,50,61,80,97,99). This new technique involves stimulation of the spinal cord or motor cortex, with monitoring of the pyramidal pathways. This may replace somatosensory monitoring in the future. A substantial number of animal and human studies demonstrated that these techniques, when used in expert hands, have a high degree of sensitivity.

Several methods have been employed for intraoperative monitoring of descending motor pathways (Table 1). The wake-up test has been considered to be the gold standard technique (1,30,37,89,101–108). Other methods of monitoring motor pathways include either direct or transcranial electrical stimulation of the cortex (8,55,56,70,76, 86,104). More recently, the activation has focused on transcranial magnetic stimulation (20,31,43,50,76,104). Recordings can be made from lower-limb muscles or from spinal cord below the operation site. It is also possible to stimulate the spinal cord electrically by epidural electrodes and record the response from the pyramidal tract (53,54) or the compound muscle action potential (CMAP) from the muscles (61–66,72,75). Recently, reports have described the use of motor evoked potentials (MEPs) as an electrophysiologic technique to monitor spinal cord motor pathways; they were found to be extremely sensitive to mild cord injury. In humans, it is possible to record MEPs intraoperatively under anesthesia for early detection of any changes in conduction of the motor pathway. There is no doubt that further advances in magnetic stimulation techniques or other technical improvements in monitoring motor systems will aid in ensuring safe spinal or spinal cord surgery.

CLINICAL EVALUATION OF SPINAL CORD FUNCTION DURING SURGERY

Wake-Up Test

The wake-up test was originally described in 1973 by Vauzelle et al. (101,107) and later by Hall et al. (30) and others (1,37,92). It measures gross motor function of the upper and lower extremities. The test consists of decreasing the anesthetic state so that the patient can respond to verbal commands. The patient is asked to squeeze the hand, thereby demonstrating that he or she is responding, and then to move feet and toes. If the patient is unable to move the feet after achieving a sufficient level of wakefulness, the distraction is reduced and the test repeated until a safe level of distraction can be demonstrated (89).

Inhalation anesthetics make timing of a wake-up test difficult. An opioid with nitrous oxide or ketamine anesthesia is widely used to allow reliable testing (6,79). Substitution of nitrous oxide with oxygen usually results in awakening within 5 minutes.

The advantages of the wake-up test are that it is simple to perform and requires no additional equipment or personnel,

M. Machida: Department of Orthopaedic Surgery, Nihon University School of Medicine, Tokyo, Japan.

T. Yamada: Department of Neurology, University of Iowa College of Medicine, Iowa City, Iowa 52242.

TABLE 1. TECHNIQUES FOR MONITORING CORTICAL–SPINAL FUNCTION

Clinical technique
  Wake-up test
  Ankle clonus test
Neurophysiologic technique
  Stimulation (electrical or magnetic)
    Motor cortex
    Spinal cord
    Spinal root
  Recording
    Spinal cord
    Peripheral nerve
    Muscle

making it inexpensive. Removal or modification of the spinal instrumentation within 3 hours of onset of a neurologic deficit decreases the risk of permanent neurologic sequelae (52,108).

Risks associated with the wake-up test include accidental extubation, dislodgement of instrumentation, self-injury, bronchospasm, recall of intraoperative events, psychological trauma, air embolism, and cardiac ischemia. An intraoperative death following the wake-up test has been reported (6). The cause of death was thought to be cardiac ischemia precipitated by the wake-up test. Another drawback of the wake-up test is that the test can be performed only once and does not function as an ongoing monitoring tool during surgery. The wake-up test is also not likely to detect isolated nerve root injury or sensory changes. False-negative findings are possible because a motor deficit may be delayed in onset rather than an immediate sequela of overdistraction (5,92). The test cannot be used with patients who are mentally retarded, deaf, or very young, and it may be contraindicated in patients with coronary artery disease. Despite these shortcomings, the benefits of the wake-up test far outweigh its disadvantages.

Ankle Clonus Test

Hoppenfeld et al. reported using the ankle clonus test as an alternative form of intraoperative spinal cord monitoring (33). The ankle clonus reflex is normally absent in the awake state, but it appears when the level of anesthesia is light. The test is based on the assumption that with cord injury there should be flaccidity; the absence of ankle clonus suggests loss of the central inhibitory mechanism secondary to the cord damage. The test is ambiguous, and its validity has not been confirmed.

SPINAL CORD MONITORING WITH SOMATOSENSORY EVOKED POTENTIALS

Scalp-Recorded SEPs

Nash et al. pioneered the early development of scalp-recorded cortical somatosensory evoked potentials (SEPs) for spinal cord monitoring (78), and their measurement now constitutes the most widely used spinal cord monitoring technique. The recording of cortical SEPs during surgery correctly predicts major

postoperative neurologic deficits (7,14,18,19,22,26,40,49,73, 81,96).

The signal introduced by electrical stimulation travels by means of the peripheral nerve through the plexus to the nerve root and the ipsilateral dorsal column. The signal crosses over at the level of the brain stem and progresses rostrally to the thalamus and on to the primary sensory cortex via thalamocortical projections.

From the scalp, with the ear as reference, an early positive potential after stimulation of the tibial nerve at the ankle is recorded at about 31 milliseconds, followed by a small negative (N35) and subsequent sizable positive potential at about 40 milliseconds (P40) (Fig. 1). P31 arises from the brain stem, and P40 is of cortical origin. For the peroneal nerve stimulation at the knee, latencies are usually about 6 milliseconds shorter. The scalp peaks of P31 and P40 are markers for intraoperative monitoring. We recommend measuring P31 because this peak is much more consistent and resistant to anesthetic agents than the P40 (Fig. 2). To record P31, the scalp electrode (Cz) must be referenced to the ear or cervical spine (C5S). Commonly used scalp reference recording cancels P31 and does not register P31. If the instrument has two available channels, we recommend recording C′z-Fz (Fpz) derivations simultaneously. For cervical cord surgery, SEPs of median or ulnar nerve stimulation are commonly used. Technically, upper-extremity SEPs are much easier to record and give better defined responses than lower-extremity SEPs. The SEPs are recorded from the scalp electrode (C′3 or C′4) contralateral to the side of stimulation, with the reference electrode at the ear or forehead (Fz or Fpz). With ear reference recording, the subcortical brain stem potential of P14

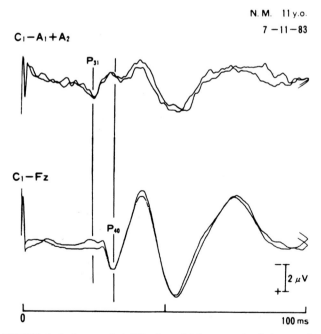

FIGURE 1. Scalp-recorded SEP after tibial nerve stimulation at the ankle. When the ear served as a reference, P31 was recorded. With Fz or Fpz reference recording, P31 was absent, but P40 was generally better defined than with the ear reference recording.

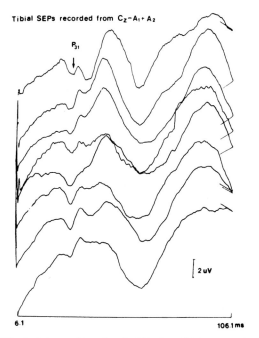

Tibial SEPs recorded from C_z–A_1 + A_2

P_31

2 uV

6.1   106.1 ms

FIGURE 2. Serial recording of scalp SEP after tibial nerve stimulation during scoliosis surgery. Well-defined and stable P31 was recorded; subsequent peaks, including P40, varied in latency and amplitude.

and the cortical potential of N20 are measured; only N20 is registered with the Fpz reference. We recommend the ear reference recording because P14, similar to P31 of the tibial nerve SEP, is a subcortical potential and the most consistent component, and is resistant to various anesthetic agents.

A series of later peaks can be seen, depending on the recording conditions. However, these peaks are less useful for intraoperative purposes. Their latencies and amplitude vary considerably, depending on temperature change, level of anesthesia, electolytes, blood pressure, and other ill-defined factors.

Nerves to Be Stimulated

The tibial nerve at the ankle is usually chosen as the site for stimulation (13). Alternately, stimulation of peroneal nerve at the knee produces comparable scalp SEPs. Although the peroneal nerve can be easily stimulated by surface electrodes, a slight change of leg positioning may adversely affect the consistency of stimulus delivery. Other cutaneous nerves, such as the sural nerve at the ankle or various dermatomal areas, are available as sites of stimulation, but the appropriate delivery of stimulus and stimulus sites are difficult to verify under anesthetic state and are generally not suitable for intraoperative stimulation sites except in special cases.

SEP amplitude of lower-limb stimulation is doubled when both limbs are stimulated simultaneously, as compared with unilateral stimulation; therefore, bilateral stimulation can be used when the response to independent unilateral stimulation is of low amplitude and poorly defined. However, Molaie reported that simultaneous bilateral stimulation may fail to detect a significant change from baseline if half the cord is impaired and the

other half is still functioning well (74). Therefore, unilateral stimulation is usually used, with stimuli alternated between legs. Alternating left and right unilateral stimulation and recording of the separate responses would be ideal to evaluate the sensory pathways from both extremities within the same time frame. In contrast, bilateral stimulation in the upper extremities may reveal asymmetry between the C'3 and C'4 responses if sensory input from one side is impaired (108,109).

Stimulus Intensity and Rate

Up to a certain point, the amplitude of the SEPs increases as the stimulus intensity increases. Beyond that point, there is little or no gain in SEP amplitude with further increases in the stimulus intensity (supramaximal stimulus intensity). In theory, it would be appropriate to define for each patient the stimulus intensity that is just barely sufficient to reach maximum SEP amplitude. The supramaximal intensity differs among patients and among various nerves within the same patient. In an awake patient, supramaximal intensity is generally reached at about two to three times the motor threshold (58). This corresponds to a stimulation intensity of roughly 15 to 30 mA by consistent current or 80 to 150 V by consistent-voltage stimulator. The amount of current varies, depending on the impedance of stimulus electrodes if a constant-voltage stimulator is used; the constant-current stimulator delivers a predetermined fixed-current stimulator. Therefore, it is preferable to use the constant-current stimulator. The motor threshold should be defined before neuromuscular junction blockade is initiated. In the absence of noticeable motor movement, a proper stimulus intensity can still be found by increasing the intensity gradually until the SEP amplitude no longer increases with further increase of stimulus intensity.

There is an inherent trade-off in trying to determine the optimum stimulus rate. Because one of the purposes of spinal cord monitoring during surgery is to identify and report neurologic complications as soon as possible, a faster stimulus rate is preferable. However, the SEP amplitude tends to decrease with a faster stimulus rate. Therefore, the appropriate stimulus rate must be a compromise between the two competing trends. The trade-off point for stimulus rate is often at about five per second or less for scalp-recorded SEPs (81). The stimulus rate can be varied, so that if a patient has a particularly low-amplitude response, a lower rate of stimulation may be tried. Conversely, if a patient has a very large and well-defined evoked potential, faster rates of stimulation can be employed. Generally, averaging of more than 500 responses is required to yield a measurable and reliable response, especially for lower-extremity SEPs.

Filters

Appropriate use of a band pass filter is essential to remove unwanted artifacts while keeping most of the desired signal. The artifacts include muscle, movement, electrocardiogram, and various electrical interferences that are inherent in the operating room. If wide-open filters with an autorejection or editing mode are used, it may take too much time to accumulate acceptable responses. Filter setting differs, depending on the response of interest, and finding the appropriate filter setting is important.

Generally, low filter settings of 15 to 30 Hz and high filter settings of 1 to 3 kHz are used. One should be aware that changing filters alters the latency and amplitude of the response.

Recording Electrodes

The cortical representation of leg and foot regions is located in the interhemispheric fissure. As a result, the generators of the cortical evoked potentials from those regions are not as accessible to recording electrodes as are those of the hand region, which lies over the lateral convexity of the hemisphere. Cortical SEPs of the leg stimulation have the maximum amplitude at the vertex or hemisphere ipsilateral to the side of stimulation. This phenomenon has been described as "paradoxical localization" (16). This has been explained by cortical representation of distal leg recording on the mesial surface of the hemisphere; P40 field is directed radially and obliquely toward the ipsilateral hemisphere, thus being registered better at midline or ipsilateral electrode (93). N20 of a median SEP is "properly" registered at contralateral hemisphere because the cortical representation of the hand is located on the lateral convexity of the hemisphere.

With the 10–20 system for electrode placement, the location of the foot region of the central fissure is situated roughly halfway between electrodes Cz and Pz. Reference electrodes may be forehead (Cz, Fpz), ear, neck, or shoulder. Using a noncephalic reference, such as neck or shoulder, has some advantage in that it registers subcortical far-field potentials generated at the spinal cord and brain stem. However, these noncephalic reference recordings are often prone to technical difficulties and are practically impossible to use, especially in the electrically "noisy" environment of the operating room. Scalp-to-scalp bipolar recording (C'3- or C'4-Fpz for median SEPs and C'z-Fpz for tibial SEPs) makes it easier to achieve satisfactory recordings, especially in the operating room, but it records only N20 of median or P40 of tibial SEPs and does not register subcortical potentials. Monitoring of subcortical potentials is advantageous because they are stable and consistent even in anesthetized patients. Cortical potentials (N20 of median SEPs, P40 of tibial SEPs) are greatly affected by anesthetic agents. We recommend ear reference recording, which registers the subcortical potential of P14 for median and P31 for tibial SEPs. These subcortical potentials serve as useful markers for intraoperative monitoring (Fig. 3).

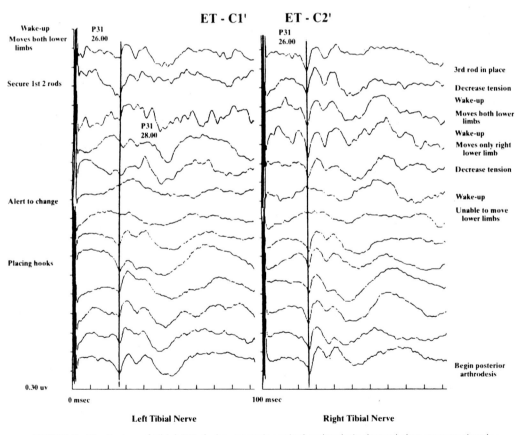

FIGURE 3. Monitoring of tibial SEP during posterior spinal arthrodesis showed that sensory signals could no longer be obtained after placement of the long rod on the left side of the curve. After the distraction on the short and long rods on the left side had been decreased slightly, monitoring showed sensory signals on the right side but prolonged latency on the left side. After all distraction forces had been released, monitoring revealed a return of all signals and normal latency on the both sides. (From Potenza V, Weinstein SL, Neyt J [1998]: Dysfunction of the spinal cord during spinal arthrodesis for scoliosis: recommendations for early detection and treatment: a case report. *J Bone Joint Surg Am* 80: 1679–1683, with permission.)

Effect of Anesthesia

Pharmacologic intervention and cardiovascular changes introduce variability in the SEPs that may not be distinguished from the changes indicating spinal cord compromise. The significant increase in latency and decrease in amplitude seen at reportedly acceptable concentrations of inhalation agents make waveform recognition difficult, decreasing the specificity and sensitivity of the monitoring. The effect of anesthetics appears to be dose-related, with increasing doses of anesthetic agents producing greater alteration of the evoked response, until no response is recorded. The volatile anesthetics are notorious in their effect on SEP amplitude. However, a study conducted to determine the effect of volatile anesthetics on SEPs showed that with 0.5 minimum alveolar concentration (MAC) of halothane or up to 1.0 MAC of isoflurane or enflurane (each with 50% nitrous oxide), scalp-recorded SEPs can be generated that are adequate for spinal cord monitoring during scoliosis surgery (84). One study concluded that enflurane or isoflurane offers better conditions for monitoring than 50% nitrous oxide (79).

Another key to successful monitoring of SEPs is maintenance of a physiologically stable condition, which involves maintaining the patient's temperature, oxygenation, hematocrit, glucose, circulating blood volume, and blood pressure.

SEPs by Dermatomal Stimulation

SEPs elicited by stimulation of dermatomal or segmental fields have been examined in an effort to improve the ability to determine single nerve root involvement. This method assists in the evaluation of lumbar radiculopathy and is used to monitor nerve root function during reduction of spondylolisthesis or decompression of spinal stenosis. Dermatomal or segmental stimulation theoretically provides a more selective study for single root involvement as compared with multisegmental activation, such as with tibial nerve stimulation (67). Nevertheless, the study by Aminoff et al. found that dermatomal SEPs are disappointing for the diagnosis of radiculopathy (2). One must also be aware that scalp SEPs are not always specific for the diagnosis of radiculopathy because any dysfunction of the brain, spinal cords, spinal root, or plexus may result in a prolonged latency.

SEPs by Pudendal Nerve Stimulation

Haldeman et al. recorded evoked potentials over spine and scalp after stimulation of the pudendal nerve in humans (28,29). The response was elicited by stimulating the pudendal nerve with ring electrodes at the base of the penis in men or with surface electrodes straddled over the clitoris in women. If a spinal potential is recorded at the lumbar spine, it allows the examiner to determine the time required by the nerve impulse to travel from the lumbar spine to the cortex. This measure, known as the central conduction time, provides information about the integrity of the peripheral and central segments of this neural pathway. Unfortunately, the recording of spinal potentials from surface electrodes after stimulation of the pudendal nerve is often unsuccessful.

Neuwirth et al. used scalp SEPs from stimulation of the pu-

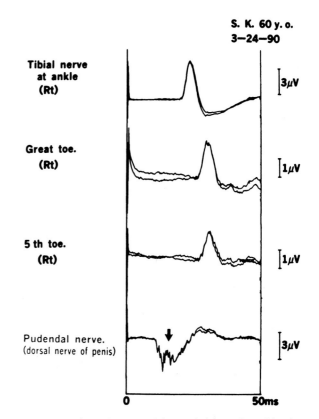

FIGURE 4. Cauda equina potential recorded from the epidural space at the L1–2 spinal level in response to stimulation of tibial nerve, great toe, or fifth toe and pudendal nerve. This method allows detailed evaluation of a cauda equina lesion affecting limited nerve roots.

dendal nerve to monitor the integrity of S2 to S4 segments during surgery in 16 patients (78). We recorded cauda equina potential directly from the epidural space in response to pudendal nerve stimulation and found that the method is useful for diagnosis of the level of a cauda equina lesion (67) (Fig. 4).

Spinal Evoked Potentials after Peripheral Nerve Stimulation

Several investigators have described the techniques for recording the response from the spinal cord with electrodes placed in the subarachnoid space, epidural space, interspinous ligament, or spinous processes of the vertebrae. These methods measure spinal cord function more directly than scalp-recorded SEPs and generally yield stable responses that are resistant to anesthetic agents.

Epidural Recording

Using stainless steel wire electrodes inserted into the epidural space, Shimoji et al. pioneered spinal evoked potential (SpEP) recording after stimulation of peripheral nerves in humans (45,94). Jones et al. reported their success with this technique in monitoring 115 operations for scoliosis (38).

There are two types of SpEPs: segmental and conductive

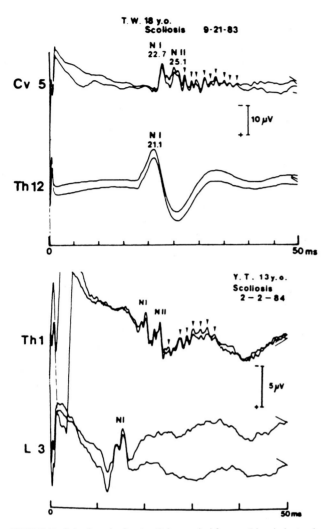

FIGURE 5. Spinal evoked potential recorded from epidural electrodes in response to tibial nerve stimulation in two patients during scoliosis surgery. At the conus medullaris (T12) to cauda equina (L3), a biphasic (segmental) potential was recorded. At the high thoracic to cervical cord, polyphasic (conductive) waves followed major negative peaks NI and NII. (From Machida M, Weinstein SL, Yameda T, et al. (1985): Spinal cord monitoring: electrophysiological measure of sensory and motor function during spinal surgery. *Spine* 10:407–413.

evoked potentials. In segmental evoked potentials, SpEPs consist of bi- or triphasic waves (Fig. 5). Conductive evoked potentials are polyphasic and generally consist of two major negative peaks (N1 and N2) and subsequent multiple rippling. The evoked potential becomes progressively smaller in amplitude and more polyphasic at the higher spine levels. Jones et al. (38) and Macon and Poletti (69) found that SpEPs consist of at least three components with different activation thresholds and conduction velocities; the fastest activity was 65 to 68 m/s, and the slowest was 30 to 50 m/s.

SpEPs recorded from the epidural space are considered more useful than scalp-recorded SEPs because of their greater consistency and less susceptibility to anesthetic agents and fluctuation of blood pressure. SpEPs can be recorded at much faster stimulation rates than scalp-recorded cortical responses, thus yielding

a result more quickly. SpEPs may be potentially more sensitive and specific in evaluating spinal cord function than scalp-recorded SEPs, especially if neural pathways from different components of the SpEP are elucidated in more detail. One technical difficulty is securing electrode position in the epidural space. Epidural electrodes may carry potential risk, such as infection or cord trauma associated with placement. However, no case of such damage has been reported in the literature.

Recently, the use of the pedicle screw has been associated with risk of injury of spinal nerve roots. Specifically, postoperative monoradiculopathies resulting from malpositioned pedicle screws can occur. Several studies have reported the use of dermatome somatosensory evoked potential (DSEP) for monitoring individual nerve root function during surgeries that use transpedicular instrumentation (68,83). Unlike scalp-recorded DSEPs, DSEPs recorded from spinal cord were found to be sensitive to mechanical irritation or displacement of nerve roots. Severe mechanical irritation or displacement of a nerve root can easily result in the total disappearance of a response.

Interspinous Ligament Recording

Lueders et al. developed a technique for recording from the interspinous ligaments (58). The needle electrodes are placed both rostral and caudal to the surgical maneuver site. In contrast to epidurally recorded SpEPs, which generally require averaging of fewer than 50 responses, interspinous ligament recording requires an average of 400 to 1,000 trials to yield a measurable response. The amplitude of the potentials depends on how close the recording electrode is to the spinal cord.

Spinous Process Recording

Maccabee et al. described a technique for recording from electrodes implanted in the spinous processes of vertebrae (60). Electrodes were inserted and secured in bone by using a threaded Steinmann pin or Kirschner wire. They suggested placing the reference electrode rostrad to the vertebra and 6 to 8 cm lateral, usually on the right to the minimize electrocardiogram artifacts. The recording electrodes were placed at several vertebral levels.

Effect of Anesthesia

SpEPs can be affected by anesthetic agents, although they are less vulnerable than cortical SEPs. Intravenous administration of thiamylal sodium (5 mg/kg) increased the amplitude of the major negative peak by 35%, with a slight latency increase during the first several minutes after an intravenous bolus (95). Diazepam (0.2 mg/kg) reduced early P1 amplitude by 20% but increased N1 amplitude by 10%.

SpEPs after Spinal Cord Stimulation

A group of investigators in Japan pioneered techniques for recording SpEPs over the spinal cord after direct stimulation of the spinal cord through epidural electrodes (42,46,100). As a result of direct stimulation of the spinal cord rostral to the surgi-

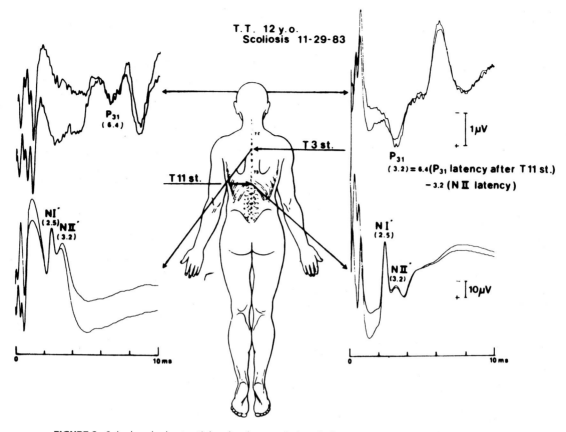

FIGURE 6. Spinal evoked potential and scalp-recorded cortical potentials after stimulation of the spinal cord. *Bottom* tracings are spinal potentials; *left* is the potential recorded at T3 after stimulation of the spinal cord at T11 (ascending conduction), and *right* is the potential at T11 after T3 stimulation (descending conduction). Both potentials were similar, consisting of NI and NII, which had the same latencies in ascending and descending conduction. (From Machida M, Weinstein SL, Yameda T, et al. (1985): Spinal cord monitoring: electrophysiological measure of sensory and motor function during spinal surgery. *Spine* 10:407–413.

cal site, an evoked signal is conducted downward through both ascending (antidromic conduction) and descending (orthodromic conduction) tracts, and the response is recorded from the caudal spinal cord. Conversely, the stimulus can be delivered via the caudal electrodes by reversing stimulus and recording electrodes (Fig. 6). The waveforms and latencies of the different peaks do not differ by either method, but the amplitude is greater with rostral stimulation. A possible explanation for this is the activation of larger tracts in rostral stimulation than in caudal stimulation.

This recording method has the advantage that SpEP amplitude is much greater than that produced by peripheral nerve stimulation. Thus, it is possible to record the response without averaging (i.e., with a single stimulation). This is a great advantage in the electrically noisy environment of the operating room. If averaging is necessary, the stimulus rate can be increased up to 30 to 50 pulses per second without attenuation of SpEPs, resulting in a new averaged wave every few seconds. Such high rates of stimulation are possible because the pathways used in this technique do not involve synaptic transmission. The signal is also very stable and resistant to anesthetic agents.

In animals, SpEPs were found to consist of two negative peaks following direct cord stimulation (34,47,105). The typical SpEP signal is likely transmitted solely by the posterior and lateral cord, with no contribution from the anterior cord. The first negative peak was markedly attenuated by lateral column transection; transection of the posterior column resulted in attenuation of the second negative peak. These studies suggested that N1 may arise from the spinocerebellar tract and N2 from the dorsal column. In humans, SpEPs after stimulation of the spinal cord also consisted of two negative peaks, N1 and N2, but whether they represent the same pathways as those found in animals has not been proved. Unlike SpEPs of peripheral nerve stimulation, no polyphasic wave following N1 and N2 was recorded by antidromic or orthodromic recording. The waveform may be different from case to case, possibility being influenced by the location of stimulating and recording electrodes.

SpEPs may be recorded at several levels to localize a lesion in the spinal cord. Loss of negative peak with a remaining positive potential (killed-end effect) rostral to the level of injury and abrupt degradation of the peak amplitude are common findings

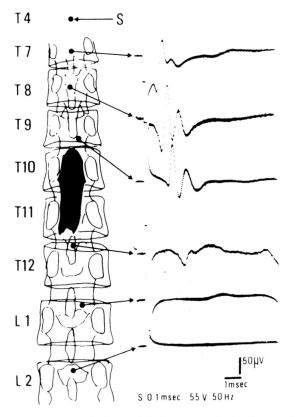

FIGURE 7. Spinal evoked potential (SpEP) in a patient with metastatic tumor at the T10–11 level. Well-defined SpEPs were recorded rostral to the lesion, from T7 to T9, after stimulation at the T4 level. The only positive potential due to killed-end effect was recorded at T12. (From Tsuyama N, Tsuzuki N, Kurokawa T, et al. [1978]: Clinical application of spinal cord action potential measurement. *Int Orthop* 2:39–46, with permission.)

that indicate the location of impaired neural transmission (105) (Fig. 7). Compressive and destructive insults to the spinal cord and anoxic injury tend to affect both amplitude and latency. Increased latency without noticeable change in amplitude can be observed as an effect of cooling of the spinal cord or the whole body. In general, amplitude attenuation implies potential neurologic complication (102,110). False-negative cases involving postoperative motor deficit following unchanged SpEPs have been reported (34,45). This could occur because the SpEPs are primarily mediated through the posterior or lateral column pathways rather than reflecting anterior cord function.

In summary, SpEP monitoring is an effective but incomplete means of monitoring spinal cord function, as is scalp-recorded SEP monitoring. The relative advantages and disadvantages will be weighted differently in each institution's decision about whether to use SpEP and/or SEP monitoring. Neither method is sensitive for detection of motor dysfunction.

SPINAL CORD MONITORING WITH MOTOR EVOKED POTENTIALS

There have been case reports of postoperative deficits despite unchanged intraoperative SEP (4,12,26,34,51), although in

some of these cases the deficits may have occurred after monitoring was terminated. For most patients, paralysis would be a more devastating postoperative sequel than loss of sensation, and this has provided much of the motivation to develop techniques that can detect dysfunction in motor pathways. In animal experiments, motor pathways have been reported to be more susceptible than sensory pathways to spinal cord traction and ischemia; therefore, identifiable motor dysfunction commonly might be expected to precede sensory dysfunction.

Intraoperative monitoring of corticospinal function is no longer an experimental technique and is a routine procedure in a number of centers. The corticospinal system can be activated by transcranial stimulation of the motor cortex (8–10,20,31,43,48,55–57,70,76,80,86,97,98,103,104,111) or by direct stimulation of the spinal cord (53,54,61–63,75) with electrical or magnetic stimuli delivered singly or as double or multiple pulse. The evoked activity may be recorded directly from the spinal cord using epidural electrode, or from the motor axons as a postsynaptic volley ("neurogenic motor evoked potentials"), or from innervated muscles as a compound muscle action potential (CMAP).

Monitoring Motor Function in Response to Brain Stimulation

A method of stimulating the motor cortex through the skull (transcranial stimulation) using electrical current was described by Merton and Morton (71). They used a brief high-voltage electric shock to activate the motor cortex, which gives rise to a brief muscle response in the extremities. This has been designated a motor evoked potential (MEP). Rossini et al. (90) and Levy et al. (55) modified the technique and successfully recorded MEPs in experimental animal studies and in clinical applications in humans. Undoubtedly, its painful nature and patients' fear of brain stimulation by high-voltage electricity are negative aspects of this technique.

More recently, magnetic stimulation was introduced by Barker et al. (3), and such a stimulator is now available commercially. A magnetic pulse is generated by the passing of a brief high-current pulse through the magnetic coil. Unlike electrical stimulation, magnetic stimulation is painless. It promises to provide a substantial impetus to the clinical assessment of conduction in central motor pathways. It can also be used to stimulate peripheral nerves, including those at deep sites that are inaccessible to conventional surface electrical stimulation.

For monitoring purposes, examination of the D wave elicited by electrical stimulation appears to be the most practical method and has several advantages over magnetic stimulation. Magnetic stimuli can activate corticospinal axons both directly and indirectly (producing "D" and "I" waves, respectively), although this depends on coil orientation (39,76). In addition, the I-wave activity appears to be more prominent than in electrically evoked volleys (10). The D wave results from direct stimulation of corticospinal axons, whereas I waves are generated by transsynaptic activation of corticospinal neurons. D waves, particularly when evoked by stimuli two to three times threshold, are resistant to volatile anesthetics, but I waves are extremity sensitive.

The MEP elicited by magnetic stimulation varies considerably, depending on the position of the coil; a slight change in coil position alters the response altogether. Magnetic stimulation requires that a large coil with a thick heavy cable be held over precisely the same scalp region throughout the operation to prevent inadvertent coil movements that might lead to less effective motor cortex stimulation. Also, the neurophysiologic equipment could interfere with the workspace for anesthesiologists' territory. With electrical stimulation, the stimulating electrodes are fixed in place preoperatively and effective stimulus delivery is more consistent, so that the responses are more stable than those generated by magnetic stimulation. Furthermore, focal activation of a particular region of the motor cortex is much easier with electrical stimulation.

In awake subjects, magnetic stimulation has an advantage over electrical stimulation because it produces minimal discomfort, but pain is no longer problematic in anesthetized patients. We therefore prefer electrical stimulation for intraoperative monitoring; in particular, multipulse stimulation is effective in eliciting MEPs under anesthetic conditions.

Electrical Stimulation

Two types of electrical stimulation have been proposed (91). One is bifocal or bipolar montage, which utilizes two stimulating electrodes placed on the scalp region overlying the motor cortex. With this bifocal technique, a special stimulator capable of discharging high current intensity is required (70). The other type is unifocal or unipolar montage, which gives essentially the same results as bifocal but requires a consistently lower current intensity to deliver the effective stimulation (90). For this purpose, a pericranial cathode using a belt or consisting of several (usually six to eight) interconnected electrodes is located on the scalp overlying the motor cortex. In either method, the anodal impulse is superior to the cathodal impulse in eliciting MEPs. The variation proposed by Levy et al. (55), with an anode on the scalp and a cathode on the soft plate, supposedly creates a larger electrical field through the brain. These anodal stimulation methods are effective in exciting the deep gray matter of superficial levels of the subcortical white matter.

Recently, most investigators have preferred electrical stimulation for intraoperative monitoring (41,70,76,85,99,104). Electrical stimulation of motor cortex is easy to carry out in the operating room. It requires that surface electrodes be glued to the scalp with collodion or that needle electrodes be inserted in the scalp. Dislodgement of stimulating electrodes is rare, and the leads do not interfere with the anesthetist's access to the head. The motor response obtained after each cortical stimulation yields an unaveraged signal that can be easily and rapidly reproduced.

Limitations of this technique are essentially related to the type of anesthesia. Anesthesia modifies the conditions of stimulation and recording. Some authors reported that only electrical stimulation is possible during anesthesia (21), whereas others claim that with appropriate anesthesia magnetic stimulation of the cortex is feasible as well (20,25). We believe that magnetic stimulation has no advantages over electrical stimulation.

Magnetic Stimulation

The magnetic stimulator uses a magnetic field created by a high-intensity pulse current by discharging capacitors through a magnetic coil. Transcranial depolarization of corticospinal neurons is possible because of Faraday's law, which states that a time-varying or changing magnetic field induces an electrical field, which in turn impedes the original magnetic field. The core of this concept is the term *changing* because a stationary magnetic field does not induce an electrical field. If the induced electrical field is produced within a conductive medium, such as the brain, electrical current will flow. If the induced current is of sufficient duration and/or amplitude, neuronal activation occurs. The flow of electrical current through the electromagnetic coil generates the magnetic field, which is represented by invisible lines of magnetic flux. The magnitude of the induced electrical field and ultimately the induced current is proportional to the total magnetic flux. The total magnetic flux is represented by the integral of the flux density (in tesla) over the area containing the flux. The total flux generated by the stimulating coil is dependent on the area of and number of turns in the coil as well as the current flowing in each turn of coil. It was found that circular coils induced an electrical field of maximal intensity directly beneath the border of the coil and of minimal intensity in the center. Indeed, for a perfectly round coil, the induced electrical field is exactly zero at the geometrical center of the coil. Tightly wound coils generate a more localized field with a more acute declination of the field adjacent to the border of the coil than do spiral coils. The peak field at the scalp is generally about 1.6 T, and the peak field at the cortex is approximately 1.4 T, assuming that the brain surface is more than 10 mm below the plane of the coil.

The coil is placed flat on the top of the head, with its center close to the vertex; the edges overlie the regions of the C3 or C4 electrode (in proximity to the hand motor area). For leg stimulation, the coil is placed more posteriorly than for upper extremity stimulation. Greater intensity is required to stimulate the leg motor area, probably because cortical somatotopic organization lies deep in the interhemispheric fissure.

When magnetic stimulation is performed, the muscle to be activated can be at rest or voluntarily contracted. The muscle response—the compound muscle action potential (CMAP)—is recorded from the muscle belly referenced to the nearby tendon. The CMAP amplitude increases with a higher intensity of stimulation and often does not reach a plateau within the range of stimulator intensity clinically used. When the amplitude reaches a plateau or is near the maximal output of the stimulator, the amplitude of the CMAP or MEP is typically about half the value obtained with direct nerve stimulation. Contraction of the muscle not only facilitates the amplitude of the response but also shortens the latency of the MEP by about 2.5 milliseconds.

The results of magnetic stimulation of the brain are similar to those of electrical stimulation. One difference is that the latency of the response, either at rest or with voluntary muscle contraction, is shorter with electrical stimulation. The explanation for this difference appears to be related to the nature of the descending volley in the corticospinal tract produced by stimulation. With electrical stimulation, but typically not with magnetic stimulation, there is an early D wave that reflects direct activation of the descending axons. With both electrical and magnetic stimulation, there is a series of later I waves that apparently reflect transsynaptic activation of the corticospinal pathways.

Within the range of clinical application, no adverse effects of magnetic stimulation have been reported. The physical properties of the magnetic stimulus do not damage tissue. It seems that stimulation does cause transient brain dysfunction, at least focally, for a period of milliseconds. This has been demonstrated by brief visual impairment after stimulation of the occipital cortex, but the impairment may be too brief to be noticed by the subject (15). No long-term psychological or intellectual deficits have been observed. A theoretical concern might be whether the stimulation causes kindling—the development of an epileptogenic focus at the site of stimulation. There are many reasons to believe that this does not occur.

Magnetic stimulation is contraindicated, or should at least be performed with caution, in patients with implanted metal or electronic devices in the brain or the body and in patients having cardiac procedures. The magnetic stimulation may precipitate seizures in the epileptic patients (32). In the United States, the Food and Drug Administration has not approved magnetic stimulation in humans. The use of magnetic stimulation, especially to the brain, must be approved by each institution's research review committee.

Epidural Recording after Brain Stimulation

Several investigators described corticospinal potentials (CSPs) of the spinal cord evoked by direct or transcutaneous motor cortex stimulation (8,41,86). Transcranial stimulation results in depolarization of cortical cells or axons, which produce descending volleys consisting of an initial D (direct) wave and the later I (indirect) waves (88). Because of the unidirectional nature of synaptic transmission, no signal is propagated via sensory axons to the spinal cord. Transmitted impulses pass down the corticospinal tract, cross at the pyramid, and proceed on to the lateral corticospinal tract. A small portion may enter uncrossed fibers of the ventral corticospinal tract. Lesioning studies confirmed the corticospinal tract as the major pathway for transcranial MEPs. The D wave can be excited at low stimulus intensity and is often preceded by a small positive wave, which probably reflects the approaching volley of corticospinal tract. At high stimulus intensity, several I waves follow a D wave.

Direct or transcranial stimulation of the cerebellum yields a nonpyramidal motor signal probably conducted via vestibulospinal, rubrospinal, fastigospinal, and reticulospinal pathways (56,57). These cerebellar evoked potentials (CeEPs) are not diminished by pyramidectomy (56). Because these pathways probably reflect cerebellar function, CeEP monitoring may complement MEP or CSP monitoring.

Effect of Anesthesia

There have been a number of studies of the motor tract potentials recorded from the thoracic and low cervical spinal cord after electrical or magnetic stimulation. However, Thompson et al. experienced difficulty recording descending spinal potentials resulting from magnetic brain stimulation and the later waves resulting from electrical brain stimulation in anesthetized subjects (104). Recording from the cervicomedullary junction during deep anesthesia without a muscle paralysis agent revealed an initial negative potential (D wave) with electrical stimulation (Fig. 8). This was followed by a muscle potential that obscured any later waveforms. The early waves from magnetic stimulation during deep anesthesia had a latency that was 1 to 2 milliseconds longer than the earliest potential from electrical stimulation. After the anesthetic was lightened and the muscle relaxant decreased, a series of later negative potentials (I waves) was more clearly seen from both electrical and magnetic stimulation. The

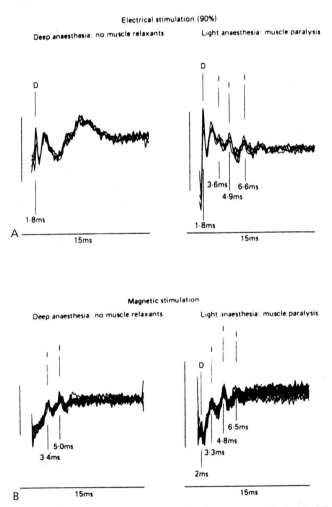

FIGURE 8. Cervicomedullary potentials after transcranial electric **(A)** and magnetic **(B)** stimulations to the brain. With electrical stimulation, a prominent D wave was recorded, but I waves were more clearly evident when a muscle relaxant was used. Without muscle paralysis, I waves were obscured by the muscle artifacts. The magnetic stimulation elicited I waves without the use of a muscle relaxant. A small D wave could be elicited with the use of a stronger intensity magnetic stimulation and muscle relaxant. (From Thompson PD, Day BL, Crockard HA, et al. (1991): Intra-operative recording of motor tract potentials at the cervico-medullary junction following scalp electrical and magnetic stimulation of the motor cortex. *J Neurol Neurosurg Psychiatry* 54:618–623.

the eddy current field, enabling the delivery of sufficient current to the spinal cord (68).

It has been demonstrated that magnetic stimulation over the vertebral column leads to activation of the ventral motor roots 2 to 4 cm distal to the cell body of the alpha motor neuron (72). This roughly corresponds to the region where the ventral root enters the neural foramen. Magnetic stimulation preferentially stimulates the root, which is generally not an easily accessible site for electrical stimulation by surface or needle electrodes, and this characteristic can be used to evaluate conduction of proximal nerve segments. For example, a circular coil centered at the posterior temporal region on the scalp stimulates the proximal portion of the facial nerve where the nerve is still in the facial canal. This makes it possible to examine the proximal portion of facial nerve conduction.

Monitoring Nerve Root Function to Nerve Root Stimulation

The use of transpedicular screw fixation for achieving rigid immobilization of the lumbosacral spine has increased in recent years. Unfortunately, there have been reports of relatively high complication rates associated with this procedure because of incorrect screw placement (23,24). Failure of pedicle screw placement was defined as any cortical perforation on any side of the pedicle, inside or outside the spinal canal. Roentgenography resulted in unacceptably high rates of false-positive and false-negative findings regarding accuracy of pedicle screw placement.

Surgical maneuvers, such as creating the pedicle hole, probing the pedicle with a pedicle finder, or placing the pedicle screw, can put a nerve root at risk. They can result in nerve root irritation or varying degrees of damage to the nerve root.

To avoid these complications, neurophysiologic procedures that monitor the functional status of nerve roots are administered. To be effective, the neurophysiologic response must demonstrate adequate nerve root specificity as well as sensitivity to any instantaneous changes in nerve root function. There are three electrophysiologic procedures that could be used during surgery: (a) DSEP recorded from epidural space (Fig. 4); (b) mechanically elicited electromyogram (EMG); (c) electrically elicited compound muscle action potential (CMAP) (Fig. 11).

A mechanically elicited EMG can only be elicited by nerve root irritation (83). EMGs were recorded from muscles innervated by nerve roots at risk; quadriceps femoris for L4 root, tibialis anterior for L5 root, medial gastrocnemius for S1 root. To record the EMGs from the legs bilaterally, pairs of subdermal needle electrodes were placed in the muscle. Reference electrode was placed subdermally, and active electrode was placed approximately 1 in. away in belly of muscle. The acquisition parameters used to record the spontaneous EMGs are used filter for 5 to 5,000 Hz, sensitivity for 50 to 100 μV, and time base for 50 milliseconds. If the pedicle wall is intact, no EMG activity will be elicited at a searching intensity level. However, if the pedicle wall has been fractured or pedicle has been contacted to the nerve root, an EMG response will be elicited. Owen et al. reported that there was no false-positive and false-negative rate when this method was used (83).

For electrically elicited CMAP, a gas-sterilized cable with an

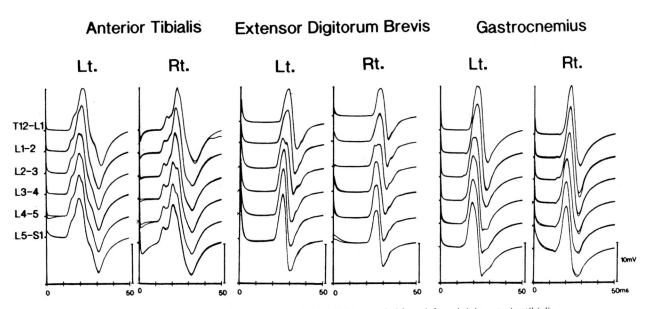

FIGURE 11. Compound muscle action potentials (CMAPs) recorded from left and right anterior tibialis, extensor digitorum brevis, and gastrocnemius muscles after electrical stimulation was given percutaneously from L5–S1 to T12–L1 levels. Each potential from caudal to rostral stimulation was recorded as a traveling wave.

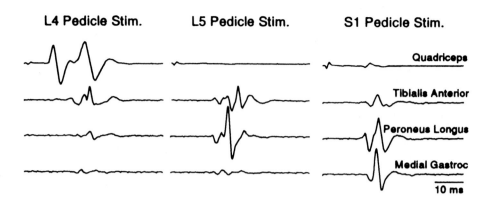

FIGURE 12. Compound muscle action potentials (CMAPs) to stimulation through screws placed in the L4, L5, and S1 pedicles in the same patient. These responses were in each case to stimulus intensities 1 to 2 mA above the threshold (minimum) intensity for evoking responses, which were 18, 22, and 23 mA for the L4, L5, and S1 screws, respectively. (From Calancie B, Madsen P, Lebwohl N [1994]: Stimulus evoked EMG monitoring during transpedicular lumbosacral spine instrumentation. *Spine* 19:2780–2786, with permission.)

alligator clip on one end formed the cathode lead, the other end of which was passed off the field and connected to the stimulator cable. The anode lead was a self-adhesive bovie pad placed on the skin between the scapulas. Calancie et al. stimulated through each of the devices used to make the hole and through the screw during placement (11). Monophasic square-wave stimuli of 200 microseconds duration were delivered at 3 Hz. The range of stimulus intensities used for direct nerve root stimulation was up to 6 mA. The range of stimulus intensities used for the screw once implanted was up to 40 mA (Fig. 12). Calancie reported that the false-negative rate with this procedure was 0% but that the false-positive rate was 13%.

SUMMARY

There are two clinical reasons for monitoring neurologic function during surgical operations: to detect inadvertent damage early when the resulting dysfunction might still be reversible, and to guide the surgeon with regard to the extent of safe operative maneuvers as effective and successful treatment. For these roles, the ideal neurophysiologic techniques should have high sensitivity and specificity, should provide real-time feedback, should not intrude physically into the operative field, should not hinder access for the anesthetist, should not prolong the operation unduly, should not be subject to artifactual changes that could be misinterpreted as incipient or actual neural dysfunction, and should be equally useful in patients with and without preexisting neurologic deficits.

Several monitoring methods have been introduced to evaluate spinal cord function during surgery under anesthesia. The most commonly used method is the scalp-recorded SEP following stimulation of the peripheral nerve. The scalp SEP can also be recorded by stimulation of the distal spinal cord via epidural electrodes. SpEPs are recorded from epidural electrodes placed at the rostral spinal cord following stimulation of the peripheral

nerves. All of these methods require averaging techniques and thus take several minutes to obtain measurable responses. The recording of the SpEP following stimulation of the spinal cord has an advantage because no averaging (or at least fewer averaged responses) is required, yielding a quick response. The response can be recorded from the rostral spinal cord after stimulation of the distal spinal cord or vice versa.

The aforementioned methods primarily reflect the function of the sensory system. To evaluate motor function during surgery, electrically or magnetically elicited transcranial stimulation to the brain has been used. Transcranial stimulation elicits motor responses (compound muscle action potentials) from the limb muscles, thus reflecting descending motor pathways. With transcranial stimulation, however, it is generally difficult to elicit a measurable response during anesthesia. The motor response or compound muscle action potential from the lower limb can also be recorded after stimulation of the rostral spinal cord. The same stimulation also elicits the potential over the peripheral nerve. These responses are less sensitive to anesthesia than those elicited by transcranial stimulation and are fairly consistently recordable during surgery. Recording of the muscle response clearly reflects the motor pathway, but the peripheral nerve response may include the antidromic sensory pathway. One should also be aware of the significant effect of anesthesia on the responses. The medication, level of anesthesia, anesthetic technique, body temperature, blood pressure, and technical problem can all affect the response.

Each of these methods has advantages and disadvantages. The selection of the method depends on the institution's choice or the individual case-by-case conditions. The monitoring procedure should be set up so that both somatosensory and motor evoked potential can be recorded, ideally at the same time and preferably from more than one level (Fig. 13). This should increase the sensitivity of the monitoring procedure and provide accurate assessment of motor and sensory functions during surgery.

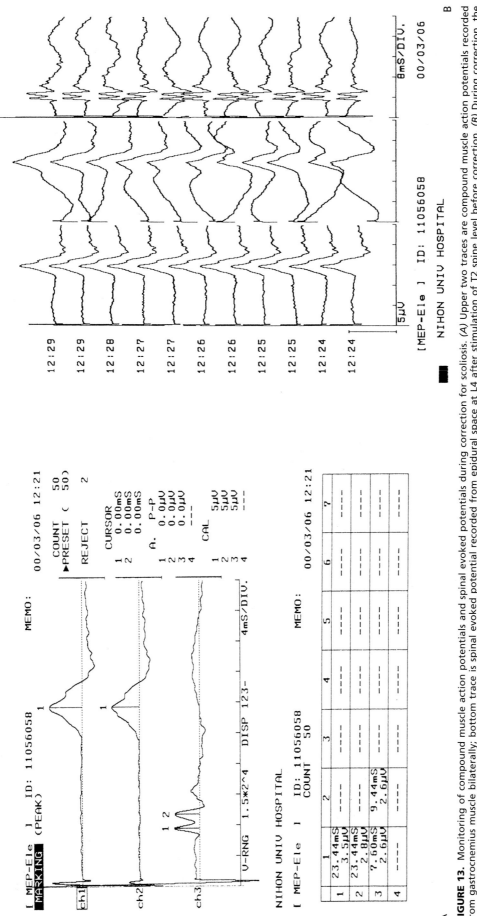

FIGURE 13. Monitoring of compound muscle action potentials and spinal evoked potentials during correction for scoliosis. (*A*) Upper two traces are compound muscle action potentials recorded from gastrocnemius muscle bilaterally; bottom trace is spinal evoked potential recorded from epidural space at L4 after stimulation of T2 spine level before correction. (*B*) During correction, the compound muscle action potentials of bilateral gastrocnemius muscles (left & middle columns) and spinal evoked potentials (right column) were recorded simultaneously. The amplitude of the compound muscle action potential from the right side (middle column) decreased transiently, but subsequently recovered to the baseline.

REFERENCES

1. Abott ET, Bently CO (1980): Intraoperative awakening during scoliosis surgery. *Anaesthesia* 35:298–302.
2. Aminoff MJ, Goodin DS, Barbaco NM, Weinstein PR, Rosenblum HL (1985): Dermatomal somatosensory evoked potentials in unilateral lumbosacral radiculopathy. *Ann Neurol* 17:171–176.
3. Barker AT, Freeston IL, Jalinous R, jarrat JA (1986): Clinical evaluation of conduction measurements in central motor pathways using magnetic stimulation of the human brain. *Lancet* 1:1325–1326.
4. Ben-David B, Haller GS, Taylor PD (1987): Anterior spinal fusion complicated by paraplegia: a case report of false negative somatosensory evoked potential. *Spine* 12:536–539.
5. Ben-David B, Taylor PD, Haller GS (1987): Posterior spinal fusion complicated by posterior column injury: a case report of false negative wake-up test. *Spine* 12:540–543.
6. Ben-David B (1988): Spinal cord monitoring. *Orthop Clin N Am* 19:427–448.
7. Berenstein A, Young W, Ransohoff J, et al. (1984): Somatosensory evoked potentials during spinal angiography and therapeutic transvascular embolization. *J Neurosurg* 60:777–785.
8. Boyd SG, Rothwell JC, Cowan JMA, et al. (1986): A method of monitoring function in corticospinal pathways during scoliosis surgery with a note on motor conduction velocities. *J Neurol Neurosurg Psychiatry* 49:251–257.
9. Burke D, Hicks RG, Stephen JPH, et al. (1992): Assessment of corticospinal and somatosensory conduction simultaneously during scoliosis surgery. *Electroencephalogr Clin Neurophysiol* 85:388–396.
10. Burke D, Hicks RG (1998): Surgical monitoring of motor pathways. *J Clin Neurophysiol* 15:194–205.
11. Calancie B, Madsen P, Lebwohl N (1994): Stimulus evoked EMG monitoring during transpedicular lumbosacral spine instrumentation. *Spine* 19:2780–2786.
12. Chatrian GE, Berger MS, Wirch AS (1988): Discrepancy between intraoperative SSEP's and postoperative function. *J Neurosurg* 69:450–454.
13. Chiappa KH (1980): *Evoked potentials in clincal medicine.* New York: Raven Press, 1–340.
14. Coles JG, Wilson GJ, Sima AF, Klement P, Tait GA (1982): Intraoperative detection of spinal cord ischemia using somatosensory evoked potentials during thoracic occlusion. *Ann Thorac Surg* 34:299–306.
15. Cracco R RQ (1987): Evaluation of conduction in central motor pathways: techniques, pathophysiology, and clinical interpretation. *Neurosurgery* 20:199–203.
16. Cruse R, Klem G, Lesser RP, Lueders H (1982): Paradoxical lateralization of cortical potentials evoked by stimulation of posterior tibial nerve nerve. *Arch Neurol* 36:402–406.
17. Djindjian R (1970): Arterial supply of the spinal cord. In: Djindjian R, ed. *Angiography of the spinal cord.* Paris: Masson, pp. 3–26.
18. Dinner DS, Lueders H, Lesser RP, et al. (1986): Intraoperative spinal somatosensory evoked potential monitoring. *J Neurosurg* 65:807–814.
19. Dorfman LJ, Perkash I, Bosely TM, et al. (1980): Use of cerebral evoked potentials to evaluate spinal somatosensory function in patients with traumatic and surgical myelopathies. *J Neurosurg* 196:285–296.
20. Edmonds HL, Paloheimo MPJ, Backmann MH, et al. (1989): Transcranial magnetic motor evoked potentials (tc MMEP) for functional monitoring of motor pathways during scoliosis surgery. *Spine* 14:683–686.
21. Eisen A (1988): Clinical experiences with cortical magnetic stimulation. In: *Proceedings of the American Electroencephalographic Society Symposium on Magnetic Coil of the Human Nervous System,* San Diego, October 5, 1988. Atlanta: American EEG Society, pp. AEE 1–3.
22. Engler GL, Spielholz NI, Bernhard WN, et al. (1978): Somatosensory evoked potentials during Harrington instrumentation for scoliosis. *J Bone Joint Surg Am* 60:528–532.
23. Esses SI, Sacks BL (1992): Complications of pedicle screw fixations. *Orthop Trans* 16:160.
24. Gertzbein SD, Robbins SE (1990): Accuracy of pedicular screw placement in vivo. *Spine* 15:11–14.
25. Ghaly RF, Stone JL, Levy WJ, et al. (1980): The effect of etomidate on motor evoked potentials induced by transcranial magnetic stimulation in the monkey. *Neurosurgery* 9:962–965.
26. Ginsberg HH, Shetter AG, Raudzens PA (1985): Postoperative paraplegia with preserved intraoperative somatosensory evoked potentials. *J Neurosurg* 13:296–300.
27. Haghighi SS, York DH, Gaines RW, et al. (1994): Monitoring of motor tracts with spinal cord stimulation. *Spine* 19:1518–1524.
28. Haldeman S, Bradley WE, Bhatia NN, et al. (1982): Pudendal evoked responses. *Arch Neurol* 39:280–283.
29. Haldeman S, Bradley WE, Bhatia NN, et al. (1982): Cortical evoked potentials on stimulation of pudendal nerve in women. *Urology* 21:590–593.
30. Hall JE, Levine CR, Sudhir KG (1978): Intraoperative awakening to monitor spinal cord function during Harrington instrumentation and spinal function. *J Bone Joint Surg Am* 60:533–536.
31. Herdmann J, Lumenta CB, Huse KO (1993): Magnetic stimulation for monitoring of motor pathways in spinal procedures. *Spine* 18:551–559.
32. Homberg V, Netz J. (1989): General seizures induced by transcranial magnetic stimulation of motor cortex. *Lancet* 18:1223.
33. Hoppenfeld S, Cross A, Andrews C (1984): The ankle clonus test: an alternative to the Stagnara wake-up test and somatosensory evoked potentials in the assessment of spinal cord damage in the treatment of scoliosis with Harrington rod damage in the treatment of scoliosis with Harrington rod instrumentation. Presented at the Scoliosis Research Society Meeting, Orlando, FL, September.
34. Ihaya A, Morioka K, Noguchi H, et al. (1990): A case report of descending thoracic aortic aneurysm associated with anterior spinal artery syndrome despite no marked ESP change. *Thorac Surg* 43:843–846.
35. Imai T (1976): Human electrospinogram evoked by direct stimulation on the spinal cord through epidural space. *J Jpn Orthop Assoc* 50:1037–1056.
36. Jellinek D, Platt M, Jewkers D, et al. (1991): Effects of nitrous oxide on motor evoked potentials recorded from skeletal muscle in patients under total anesthesia with intravenously administered propofol. *Neurosurgry* 29:558–567.
37. Jones ET, Matthews LS, Hensinger RN (1982): The wake up technoque as a dual protector of spinal cord function during spinal fusion. *Clin Orthop* 168:113–118.
38. Jones SJ, Edgar MA, Ransford AO (1982): Sensory nerve conduction in the human spinal cord: epidural recording made during scoliosis surgery. *J Neurol Neurosurg Psychiatry* 45:446–451.
39. Kaneko K, Kawai S, Fuchigami Y, et al. (1996): The effect of current direction induced by transcranial magnetic stimulation on the corticospinal excitability in human brain. *Electroencephalogr Clin Neurophysiol* 101:478–482.
40. Kaplan BJ, Friedman WA, Alexander JA, et al. (1986): Somatosensory evoked potential monitoring of spinal cord ischemia during aortic operations. *Neurosurgery* 19:82–89.
41. Katayama Y, Tsubokawa T, Maejima S, et al. (1988): Corticospinal direct response in humans: identification of the motor cortex during intracranial surgery under the general anesthesia. *J Neurol Neurosurg Psychiatry* 51:50–59.
42. Kimura J, ed. (1989): *Electrodiagnosis in diseases of nerve and muscle: principles and practice.* Philadelphia: FA Davis Co, pp 408–409.
43. Kitagawa H, Nakamura H, Kawaguchi Y, et al. (1995): Magnetic-evoked compound muscle action potential neuromonitoring in spine surgery. *Spine* 20:2233–2239.
44. Kobayashi M (1985): On the origin of spinal cord potentials evoked by peripheral nerve stimulation and its clinical meaning. Part 1: clinical study. *J Jpn Orthop Assoc* 59:27–38.
45. Komatu S, Kikuchi S, Sasaki T, et al. (1985): Detection of spinal cord ischemia in surgery of the thoracoabdominal aorta using spinal cord potentials. *Surg Treat* 53:214–215.
46. Kurokawa T (1972): Spinal conduction potentials evoked by epidural

stimulation of cord: a report of human and animal record. *Jpn J Electorencephalogr Electromyogr* 1:64–66.

47. Kurokawa T (1979): Clinical application of the evoked electrospinogram. *Adv Neurol Sci* 23:409–420.

48. Kurokawa T (1979): Measurement of spinal evoked potentials for spinal cord monitoring. *Clin Electroencephalogr* 22:464–470.

49. Laschinger JC, Cunningham JN, Cadnella FP, et al. (1982): Detection and prevention of intraoperative spinal cord ischemia after cross-clamping of the thoracic aorta: Use of somatosensory evoked potentials. *Surgery* 92:1109–1117.

50. Lee WY, Hou WY, Yang LH, et al. (1995): Intraoperative monitoring of motor function by magnetic motor evoked potentials. *Neurosurgery* 36:493–500.

51. Lesser RP, Raudzens P, Lueders H, et al. (1986): Postoperative neurological deficits may occur despite unchanged intraoperative somatosensory evoked potentials. *Ann Neurol* 19:22–25.

52. Letts RM, Hollenberg C (1977): Delayed paresis following spinal fusion with harrington instrumentation. *Clin Orthop* 125:45–48.

53. Levy WJ (1983): Spinal evoked potentials from the motor tracts. *J Neurosurg* 58:38–44.

54. Levy WJ, York DL (1983): Evoked potentials from the motor tracts in humans. *Neurosurgery* 12:422–429.

55. Levy WJ, McCafrey M, York DL (1984): Motor evoked potentials from transcranial stimulation of the motor cortex in humans. *Neurosurgery* 15:287–302.

56. Levy WJ, McCaffrey M, Goldman D, et al. (1986): Nonpyramidal motor activation produced by stimulation of the cerebellum, direct or transcranial: a cerebellar evoked potential. *Neurosurgery* 19:163–176.

57. Levy WJ (1987): Clinical experience with motor and cerebellar evoked potentials monitoring. *Neurosurgery* 20:169–182.

58. Lueders H, Gurd A, Hahn J, et al. (1982): A new technique for intraoperative monitoring of spinal cord function: multichannel recording of spinal cord and subcortical evoked potentials. *Spine* 7: 110–115.

59. Lueders H, Lesser RP, Dinner DS, et al. (1985): Optimizing stimulating and recording parameters in somatosensory evoked potential studies. *J Clin Neurophysiol* 2:383–396.

60. Maccabee PJ, Levine DB, Pinkasov EI (1983): Evoked potentials recorded from scalp and spinous process during spinal column surgery. *Electroencephal Clin Neurophysiol* 55:569–582.

61. Machida M, Weinstein SL, Yamada T, et al. (1985): Spinal cord monitoring: electrophysiological measure of sensory and motor function during spinal surgery. *Spine* 10:407–413.

62. Machida M, Weinstein SL, Yamada T, et al. (1986): Motor potentials after stimulation of the spinal cord in human and cat. *J Pediatr Orthop* 6:375.

63. Machida M, Weinstein SL, Yamada T, et al. (1988): Monitoring of muscle action potentials after stimulation of spinal cord. *J Bone Joint Surg Am* 70:911–918.

64. Machida M, Weinstein SL, Yamada T, et al. (1988): Dissociation of muscle action potentials and spinal somatosensory evoked potentials after ishemic damage of spinal cord. *Spine* 13:1119–1124.

65. Machida M, Weinstein SL, Imamura Y, et al. (1989): Compound muscle action potentials and spinal evoked potentials in experimental spine maneuver. *Spine* 14:687–691.

66. Machida M, Yamada T, Ross M, et al. (1990): Effect of spinal cord ischemia on compound muscle action potentials and spinal evoked potentials following spinal cord stimulation in the dog. *J Spinal Disord* 3:345–352.

67. Machida M, Hasue M, Toriyama T, et al. (1991): Level diagnosis with cauda equina action potentials in herniated lumbosacral disc and lumbar spinal stenosis. Presented at the International Society for the Study of the Lumbar Spine, Heidelberg, Germany, May.

68. Machida M, Kimura J, Yamada T, et al. (1992): Magnetic coil stimulation of the spinal cord in the dog: effect of removal of the bony strucure on eddy current. *Spine* 17:1405–1408.

69. Macon JB, Poletti CE (1982): Conducted somatosensory evoked potentials during spinal surgery. Part 1. Control conduction velocity measurements. *J Neurosurg* 57:349–353.

70. Matsuda H, Kondo M, Hashimoto T, et al. (1984): The prediction of the surgical prognosis of the compression myelopathy. *Osaka City Med J* 30:91–112.

71. Merton PA, Morton HB (1980): Stimulation of the cerebral cortex in the intact human subject. *Nature* 285:227.

72. Mills KR, Murray NMF (1986): Electrical over human vertebral column: which neural elements are excited? *Electroencephalogr Clin Neurophysiol* 62:582–589.

73. Mizrahi EM, Cawford ES (1984): Somatosensory evoked potentials during reversible spinal cord ischemia in man. *Electrophysiol Clin Neurophysiol* 58:120–126.

74. Molaie M (1986): False negative intraoperative somatosensory evoked potentials with stimutaneous bilateral stimulation. *Clin Electrocephalogr* 17:6–9.

75. Nagle KJ, Emerson RG, Adams DC, et al. (1996): Intraoperative monitoring of motor evoked potentials: a review of 116 cases. *Neurology* 47:999–1004.

76. Nakamura H, Kitagawa H, Kawaguchi T, et al. (1996): Direct and indirect activation of human corticospinal neurons by transcranial magnetic and electrical stimulation. *Neurosci Lett* 210:45–48.

77. Nash CL Jr, Loring RA, Shatzinger LA, et al. (1977): Spinal cord monitoring during operative treatment of the spine. *Clin Orthop* 126: 100–105.

78. Neuwirth MG, Nainzadeth NK, Bernstein RL (1989): The use of pudendal nerve in monitoring lower sacral roots (S2-S4) during anterior and/or posterior spinal stabilization. *Orthop Trans* 13:89.

79. Nielson CH (1991): Anesthesia for spinal surgery. In: Bridwell KH, Dewald RL, eds. *The textbook of spinal surgery*. Philadelphia: JB Lippincott, pp. 19–29.

80. Noel P, Deltenre P, Lamoureux J, et al. (1994): Neurophysiologic detection of a unilateral motor deficit occurring during the noncritical phase of scoliosis surgery. *Spine* 19:2399–2402.

81. Nuwer MR, Dawson E (1984): Intraoperative evoked potential monitoring of the spinal cord: enhanced stability of cortical recordings. *Electroencephalogr Clin Neurophysiol* 59:318–327.

82. Owen JH, Lashinger J, Bridwell KH, et al. (1988): Sensitivity and specificity of somatosensory and neurogenic-motor evoked potentials in animals and humans. *Spine* 12:1111–1118.

83. Owen J, Kostuik JP, Gornet M, et al. (1994): The use of mechanically elicited electromyograms to protect nerve roots during surgery for spinal degeneration. *Spine* 19:1704–1710.

84. Pathak KS, Annadio BS, Kalamchi MD, et al. (1987): Effect of halathane, enflurane and isoflurane on somatosensory evoked potentials during nitous oxide anesthesia. *Anesthesiolgy* 66:753–754.

85. Pechstein U, Cedzich C, Nadstawek J, et al. (1996): Transcranial high-frequency repetitive electrical stimulation for recording myogenic motor evoked potentials with the patient under general anesthesia. *Neurosurgery* 39:335–344.

86. Pelosi L, Caruso G, Balbi P (1988): Characteristics of spinal potentials to transcranial motor cortex stimulation: intraoperatve recording. In: Rossini P, Marsden CD, eds. *Non-invasive stimulation of brain and spinal cord*. New York: Alan R. Liss, pp. 297–304.

87. Pereon Y, Bernard JM, Delecrin J, et al. (1995): Could neurogenic motor evoked potentials be used to monitor motor and somatosensory pathways during scoliosis surgery? (letter) *Muscle Nerve* 18: 1214–1215.

88. Phillips CG, Porter R (1977): Corticospinal neurons. Their role in movement. London: Academic Press, pp. 65–77.

89. Potenza V, Weinstein SL, Neyt J (1998): Dysfunction of the spinal cord during spinal arthrodesis for scoliosis: recommendations for early detection and treatment: a case report. *J Bone Joint Surg Am* 80: 1679–1683.

90. Rossini PM, DiStefano E, Stanzione P (1985): Nerve impulse propagation along central and peripheral fast conduction motor and sensory pathways in man. *Electroencephal Clin Neurophysiol* 60:320–334.

91. Rossini PM, Caramia MD (1988): Methodological and physiological consideration on the electrical or magnetic transcranial stimulation. In: Rossini P, Marsden CD, eds. *Non-invasive stimulation of brain and spinal cord: fundamentals and clinical applications*. New York: Alan R. Liss, pp. 37–65.

92. Schmitt EW (1978): Post-instrumentation paraplegia and a negative

Stagnara test—a case report. Presented at the Annual Meeting of the Scoliosis Research Society, Boston, September.

93. Seyal M, Emerson RG, Pedley TA (1983): Spinal early scalp-recorded components of the somatosensory evoked potential following stimulation of the posterior tibial nerve. *Electroencephalogr Clin Neurophysiol* 55:320–330.

94. Shimoji K, Higashi H, Kano T (1971): Epidural recording of spinal electrogram. *Electroencephalgr Clin Neurophysiol* 30:236–239.

95. Shimoji K, Kano T (1975): Evoked electrospinogram: Interpretation of origin and effects of anesthetics. *Int Anesthesiol Clin* 13:171–189.

96. Spielholz NI, Benjamin MV, Engler GL, et al. (1979): Somatosensory evoked potentials during decompression and stabilization of the spine: methods and findings. *Spine* 4:500–505.

97. Stephen JP, Sullivan MR, Hicks RG, et al. (1996): Cotrel-Dubousset instrumentation in children using simultaneous motor and somatosensory evoked potential monitoring. *Spine* 21:2450–2457.

98. Su CF, Haghighi SS, Oro JJ, et al. (1992): "Backfiring" in spinal cord monitoring: high thoracic spinal cord stimulation evokes sciatic response by antidromic sensory pathway conduction, not motor tract conduction. *Spine* 17:504–508.

99. Tabaraud F, Boulesteix JM, Moulies D, et al. (1993): Monitoring of the motor pathway during spinal surgery. *Spine* 18:546–550.

100. Tamaki T, Yamashita T, Kobayashi H (1972): Spinal cord monitoring. *J Electroencephalogr Electromyogr* 1:196.

101. Tamaki T, Tsuji H, Inoue S, et al. (1981): The prevatention of iatrogenic spinal cord injury utilizing the evoked spinal potential. *Int Orthop* 4:313–317.

102. Tamaki T, Takano H, Nakagawa T (1986): Evoked spinal cord potential elicited by spinal cord stimulation and its use in spinal cord monitoring. In: Cracco RQ, Bodies-Wollner I, eds. *Evoked potentials.* New York: Alan R. Liss, pp. 428–436.

103. Thompson PD, Dick JPR, Asselman P (1987): Examination of motor function in lesions of the spinal cord by stimulation of the motor cortex. *Am Neurol* 21:389–396.

104. Thompson PD, Day BL, Crockard HA, et al. (1991): Intra-operative recording of motor tract potentials at the cervico-medullary junction following scalp electrical and magnetic stimulation of the motor cortex. *J Neurol Neurosurg Psychiatry* 54:618–623.

105. Tsuyama N, Tsuzuki N, Kurokawa T, et al. (1978): Clinical application of spinal cord action potential measurement. *Int Orthop* 2:39–46.

106. Vauzelle C, Stagnara P, Jouvinroux P (1973): Functional monitoring of spinal cord activity during spinal surgery. *Clin Orthop* 93:173–178.

107. Vauzelle C, Stagnara P, Jourinroux P (1973): Functional monitoring of spinal cord activity during spinal surgery. *J Bone Joint Surg Am* 55:441.

108. Waldman J, Kaufer H, Hensinger RN, et al. (1977): Wake-up technique to avoid neurologic sequela during Harrington rod procedure: a case report. *Anesth Analg* 56:733–735.

109. Yamada T, Dickins S, Machida M, et al. (1986): Somatosensory evoked potentials to simultaneous bilateral median nerve stimulation in man: Method clinical application. In: Cracco RQ, Bodis-Wollner I, eds. *Evoked potentials: frontiers of clinical neurosciences*, Vol. 3. New York: Alan R. Liss, pp. 45–57.

110. York DH (1987): Review of descending motor pathways involved with transcrinical stimulation. *Neurosurgery* 20:70–73.

111. Zentner J (1989): Noninvasive motor evoked potential monitoring during neurosurgical operations on the spinal cord. *Neurosurgery* 24: 709–712.

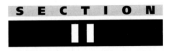

TRACTION AND CASTING

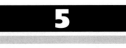

TRACTION

HAEMISH CRAWFORD

Traction is one of the oldest methods used for the correction of spinal deformity. Traction was initially thought to stretch out the shortened tissue on the concave side of the deformity; however, when the deformity recurred after cessation of traction, other methods of correction came into use.

Casting once the curve had been corrected by traction was devised by Sayre in the late nineteenth century (Fig. 1). He used gravity-assisted traction before the application of the plaster of Paris cast. A number of modifications of casting techniques evolved, including the turnbuckle cast by Hibbs, later modified by Risser in 1927. These early casting and traction techniques coincided with the advent of surgical treatment of spinal deformity by Hibbs in 1911. Surgeons then had to decide on the best combination of casting, traction, or surgery to correct the deformity and prevent it from recurring. "Internal traction" was provided with the use of the Harrington distraction rod in the 1950s. Newer generation internal fixation devices have led to a decrease in the use of traction in spinal deformity.

Traction has remained a mainstay of treatment for cervical spine trauma. With the evolution of the skull tong initially described by Crutchfield in 1933 and later developed by Vinke in 1948 and Gardner in 1973, skeletal traction has been used to reduce cervical spine fractures and dislocations. The halo device was devised by Nickel and Perry in 1959; it controls the head more effectively than tongs, thereby providing increased stability to the cervical spine by having more fixation points to the child's skull. The halo can also be more easily converted into a vest or plaster jacket once reduction and stability have been achieved.

The belief of some surgeons that preoperative traction permits more correction and possibly decreases neurologic complications in operative cases had been disproved (13,14,20,46, 68,79). Despite the fact that traction is rarely used today, it does remain an important option for the treatment of children with spinal disorders.

BIOMECHANICS

There are six degrees of freedom at each motion segment in the spine, and forces can be applied to correct each one of these

components (77a). Distraction by traction or instrumentation alone corrects the deformity only in the coronal plane and does not correct the sagittal plane or correct rotation. This has been one of the complications of the use of Harrington rod distraction with the development of the "flatback" (1,58). Distraction is a force-limited correction that is useful in decreasing the magnitude of a large curve. However, huge distractive forces are required to correct a curve more than 55 degrees in magnitude due to the change in force vectors (89). The correction moment equals the distraction force $\times$ the distance of the apical vertebra from the midline, so the correction moment decreases as the curve gets smaller (Figure 11 in 77a). Transverse forces have been shown to be more efficient than distraction alone at correcting these curves of smaller magnitude. White et al. showed that when the curve was less than 53 degrees the transverse forces were most efficient (89). These distractive forces described above have been largely investigated using the Harrington distraction apparatus. If halo-pelvic or halo-femoral traction is used to achieve this degree of distraction, greater forces must be applied to overcome the viscoelastic forces from the "normal tissue" cephalad and caudad to the area of the curve to be straightened. This can lead to excessive hip joint distraction or cervical spine injury. Also, the surface on which the patient lies offers frictional resistance to the distraction, which must also be overcome.

The ligaments, vertebrae, and discs of the spinal column behave as a viscoelastic material that can be qualitatively analyzed on stress/strain and load/deformation graphs. Curve correction by traction results in the gradual increase in deformation, the tissues then undergo creep with sustained correction, and unless some other intervention is initiated (e.g., casting, orthosis, or surgery), unloading will result in the gradual return to the pre-correction deformity (Figures 3 and 4 in 77a). Traction alone will not correct the deformity, as our pioneers found out. The maximum correction obtainable usually occurs within the first week of its application, and prolonged traction only results in an increase in complications without any marked improvement in correction.

TRACTION METHODS
Halter

Traction is applied with one limb of the halter around the mandible and the other around the occiput, with weights exerting

H. Crawford: Department of Orthopaedic Surgery, Starship Children's Hospital, Auckland, New Zealand.

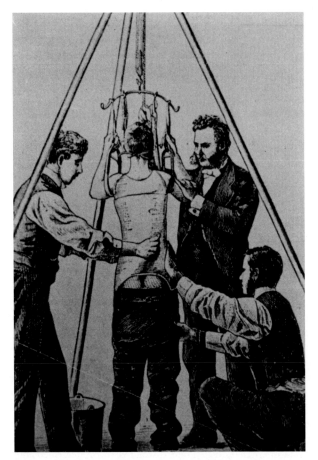

FIGURE 1. Sayre's traction and cast application in the treatment of scoliosis (From Sayer LA (1876): *Orthopaedic surgery and disease of the joints.* New York: Appleton and Colleguos).

a direct pull over the edge of the bed. This relatively simple device is used mainly in reducing the rotatory deformity of C1 on C2 in atlantoaxial subluxation when more conservative measures have been unsuccessful (9,24,66). Halter traction can uncomfortable for children due to the irritating action of the straps on the facial skin. If prolonged traction is required, the halter may have to be replaced by halo traction.

Depending on the size and age of the child in halter traction, 5 to 8 lb of weight is the most that can be tolerated for any length of time.

Halter traction should never be used for cervical spine instability because rigid immobilization is not attained and subsequent neurologic compromise could occur.

Simple halter traction was modified by Cotrel in the 1960s to include a pelvic strap with trochanteric pads so that countertraction could be applied over the edge of the bed (Fig. 2). This was advocated for preoperative correction in adolescent scoliosis. Weights can be added daily, up to a maximum of 16 lb divided evenly between the halter and pelvic traction devices.

Tongs and Halo

In considering the use of skeletal traction for immobilization of the cervical spine or for applying longitudinal traction to the spine, one must first consider the unique anatomy of the child's skull.

In the child younger than 2 years, cranial interdigitations may not be complete and the fontanels may still be open. The anterior fontanel closes at around 18 months of age, the posterior at around 6 months of age. A Minerva cast may be more appropriate in this age group.

Skull thickness varies considerably between the ages of 2 and

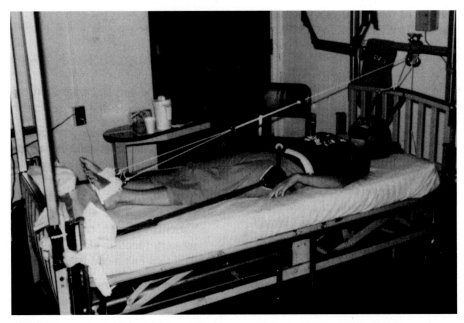

FIGURE 2. Cotrel dynamic traction using head halter and pelvic sling. (Photo courtesy of Stuart L. Weinstein, M.D.)

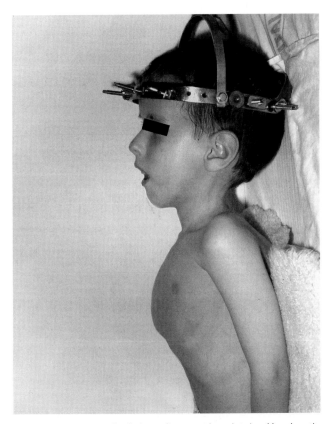

FIGURE 3. Correct sagittal plane alignment is maintained by elevating the shoulders with folded towels. This keeps the external auditory meatus aligned with the shoulder.

6 and becomes increasingly thick between ages 10 and 16 (28,45). Wong has shown that children up to the age of 10 can have a skull thickness of only 2 mm in some areas of pin placement (92). The average antero-lateral thickness is 3.7 mm at 1 to 2 years and 6.1 mm at 5 to 12 years. The average posterolateral thickness is 3.9 mm between 1 and 2 years and 5.9 mm at 5 to 12 years (28). Letts found that a 2-mm-thick skull could be penetrated by a halo pin if a 160-lb force is applied to it (less than the torque pressure recommended for adult skulls) (45). This has led to use of multiple pins and less torque pressure in the application of halo devices in the child.

The child's head is also disproportionately larger than the torso when compared with adult anatomy. Despite the fact that the head reaches 50% of its final size by the age of 18 months, the trunk is not half its size until the age of 8 years. To maintain correct sagittal alignment and prevent flexion of the cervical spine, the external auditory meatus should be aligned with the shoulder when traction is applied. This can usually be achieved by elevating the shoulders with folded towels (Fig. 3).

Crutchfield first described the use of tongs for the treatment of fracture-dislocations of the cervical spine in 1933. However, the Gardner-Wells tongs have now taken over as the most commonly used device (Fig. 4). Their use is restricted to the adolescent and adult patient rather than the child. Although the tongs allow more weight to be applied to the traction than when the halter is used, they do not confer as much stability as the halo device and cannot be readily incorporated into a vest or plaster jacket.

Gardner-Wells tongs can be applied under general or local anesthesia. The pins should be placed inferior to the equator of the skull, in line or 1 cm posterior to the external auditory canal just above the pinna. If the pins are placed anterior to the auditory canal the head will extend with traction, and if they are placed posteriorly the head will flex. The pins are tightened by hand until the indicator on the pin protrudes 1 cm. The pins should be retightened 24 hours later so that the indicator is flush with the spring-loaded pins (Fig. 4).

The halo is an excellent device for applying axial skeletal traction and stabilization of the cervical spine in children. However, traction through the halo can be dangerous as overdistraction of the elastic cervical spine tissue in children can lead to neurologic complications. The halo can be better used as a reduction and holding device that can be incorporated into a cast or vest to maintain the head position relative to the trunk. Garfin et al. found that the complication rate associated with use of the halo in children was 39%, compared with 8% in adults, and that most of the complications were related to the pins (29). In a child, consideration must be given to the underlying cause of the condition being treated. For example, in Down syndrome, the skull is often very thin. In hydrocephalus or skeletal dyspla-

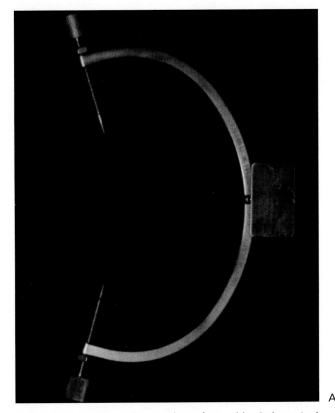

A

FIGURE 4. A: Gardner-Wells tongs (manufactured by Codman, Inc.). *(Figure continues.)*

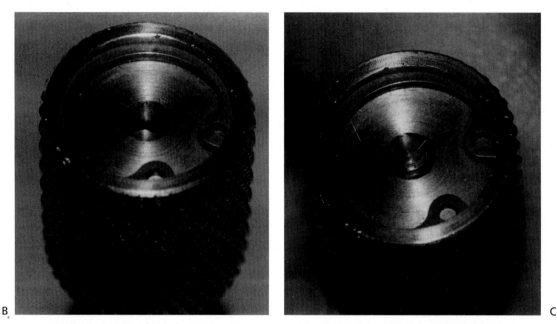

B   C

FIGURE 4. *Continued.* **B:** Spring indicator unloaded. **C:** Spring indicator protruding, indicating adequate tension of the tongs.

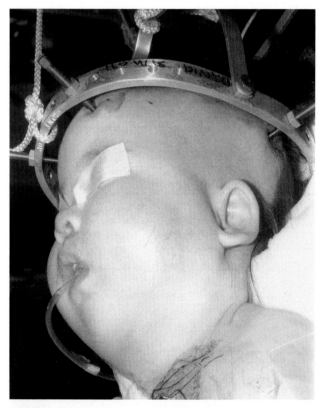

FIGURE 5. This patient required a custom-made halo because of abnormal skull morphology. Only four pins could be used due to the thin skull.

sias, the head may be asymmetrical, making ring size and pin placement difficult (Fig. 5).

HALO APPLICATION

The halo can be applied under general anesthesia in younger children but preferably under local anesthesia in older patients so that they can "splint" their neck with voluntary muscle control and can warn the physician of any change in neurologic status. The halo ring is selected to facilitate 1 to 2 cm of clearance from the skull to allow for edema and enhance pin site care. If magnetic resonance imaging (MRI) is required after its application, the rings should be manufactured from compatible material. The ring is positioned 1 to 2 cm above the eyebrows and helix of the ear, just below the maximum diameter of the skull, so that any pressure or traction on the ring after its application will not cause it to slip off (Fig. 6). The ring can be temporarily held using the manufacturer's base plates and positioning screws. The rings should be horizontal in the anterior and lateral planes, so that a flexion or extension moment is not applied to the neck.

It is paramount that an assistant hold the head on a cupped-metal extension board while the surgeon applies the halo. Because of the disproportionately large size of the head relative to the trunk, the assistant must hold the head to prevent its going into flexion.

Pin placement is carried out under sterile conditions. Antiseptic lotion is applied to the skin, which need not be shaved. Three to four milliliters of local anesthetic without adrenaline is infiltrated down to the periosteum (Fig. 7). The anterior screws are inserted perpendicular to the skin in the hairline,

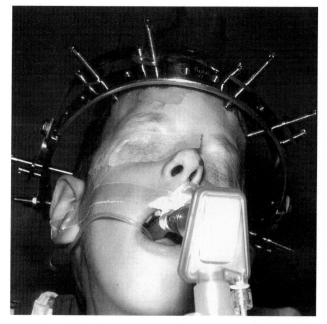

FIGURE 6. The halo position. One to two centimeters above the eyebrows and helix of the ear. Note that the ring is placed below the maximum diameter of the skull to prevent its migrating cephalad with traction.

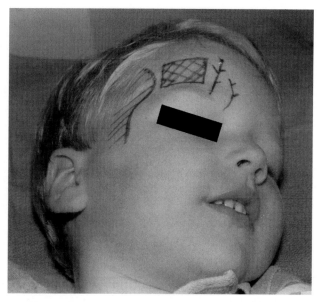

FIGURE 8. Anterior pins should be placed in the crossed area to avoid the supraorbital and supratrochlear nerves. Pins placed in the temporalis muscle (*diagonal lines*) should also be avoided.

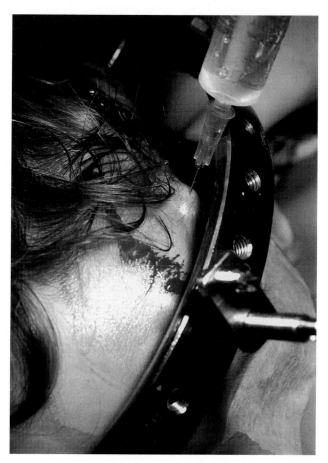

FIGURE 7. Local anesthetic infiltration.

above the lateral two thirds of the orbit and just below the greatest circumference of the skull. A pin inserted too posteriorly will interfere with temporalis muscle function, and the bone in the temporal region is very thin. A pin placed too anteriorly runs the risk of entering the frontal sinus or damaging the supraorbital or supratrochlear nerves (Fig. 8). Garfin et al. found the anterolateral and posterolateral skull to have the thickest bone (28). The posterior screws should be inserted in the hairline as close as possible to 180 degrees from the anterior screws. To prevent skin necrosis, no adrenaline is used with the local anesthetic and the screws should be backed off a quarter turn when fully tightened (7). How many screws to insert has been a matter of debate, but in a child more is better than fewer. Catler suggests using a Minerva cast or brace attached to a helmet in children younger than 2 years, 6 to 8 screws in children between 2 and 6, and 4 pins (as in an adult) in children older than 8 years (51). Mubarak recommends using 10 to 12 screws in children between 2 and 6 years of age (57). The screws should be finger-tightened or no more than 2 in.-lb in infants and young children. A child 8 years or older can be treated as an adult; however, if there is altered skull morphology, a preapplication computed tomography (CT) scan is useful in showing the thickness of the skull bones (7,45,51,57). Two diagonally opposite screws should be tightened simultaneously to maintain the desired ring position, and once tightened the screws should be secured with the appropriate lock nuts or set screws (Fig. 9). The traction can then be applied or a vest attached according to the clinical scenario. The screws should be retightened in the first 48 hours but not weekly as in the adult because in the child this can lead to screw penetration. Loose screws promote infection and also lead to ring displacement. Retighten the screws by hand. A torque screw driver should not be used as this can lead to screw penetration. Screw care consists of the daily use of hydrogen

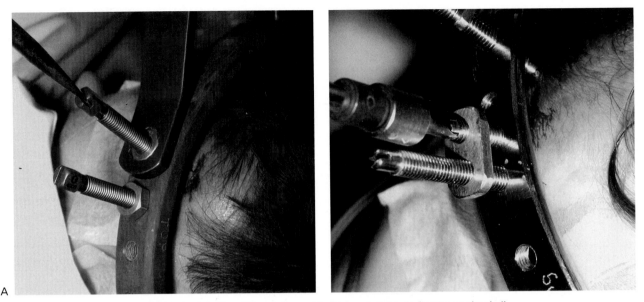

A

B

FIGURE 9. A,B: Two different types of locking nuts for halo fixation to the skull.

peroxide or povidone-iodine to remove the crusts around the screws. The hair and scalp should be washed at least once a week. In the event of infection or if there is concern about screw penetration, the screw can be removed and a new one inserted close by, with awareness of the anatomy of the child's skull. Oral antibiotics usually suffice for early skin infections. Osteomyelitis and intracranial abscesses have been reported with use of the halo (57).

Halo-Pelvic Traction

Halo-pelvic traction was first described by DeWald and Ray in 1970 for the treatment of severe scoliosis in four patients (16). The halo part of the device is applied as in the previous section. Threaded external fixator pins are inserted into the pelvis through stab wounds just lateral and inferior to the anterior superior iliac spine and are directed to the posterior iliac spine (Fig. 10). They are inserted so that the pelvis and the rods are parallel to the floor after the entire device has been constructed (16). To avoid possible laceration of the perineum or bowel perforation, some surgeons have recommended placing the patient in the lateral decubitus position and performing subperiosteal dissection so that the pin path can be visualized (40,42). Distraction forces up to 40 N could be generated by the device (15).

Advantages of using halo-pelvic traction over previous forms of treatment for scoliosis were thought to be as follows:

1. Patients could remain ambulatory before and after surgery, especially those with poor pulmonary function.
2. Pelvic obliquity could be corrected.
3. Deformity could be corrected gradually.
4. Halo-pelvic traction could provide stability when the spine is collapsing, such as in poliomyelitis, spinal muscular atro-

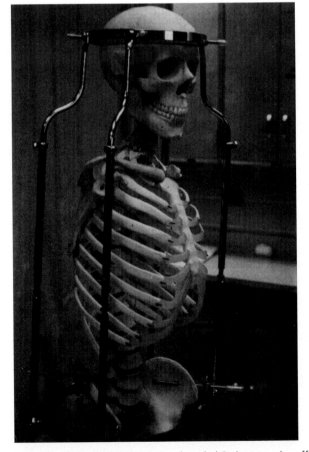

FIGURE 10. Halo-pelvic device. Large threaded Steinmann pins affix the ring to the iliac crest. (Photo courtesy of Daniel Benson, M.D.)

phy, or severe tuberculosis where there is a collapsing kyphosis.

5. Anterior and posterior access for surgery would be easy.

The main reason for finding alternatives to the halo-pelvic distraction apparatus was its high complication rate. Dove et al. found that 53% of the patients they reviewed had significant cervical complications after a minimum 5-year follow-up. These complications included radiologic degenerative changes with and without pain, avascular necrosis of the dens, loss of movement, and spontaneous fusion (18,82,83). In their analysis of 150 consecutive patients treated by this method, Kalamchi et al. concluded that "the apparatus should be reserved for severe deformities when other means of traction or stabilization are inadequate" (38). Complications are more likely to occur if the halo-pelvic apparatus is applied for more than 6 months, if the patient is 15 years of age or older, the curve is stiff, or the curve is a tuberculous kyphosis (18). When used for 2 to 8 weeks postoperatively, and with traction forces less than 50% of body weight, some of these complications have been avoided (25,36,70,71). Halo-pelvic traction is rarely used today as orthotics and surgical techniques have evolved.

Halo-Femoral Traction

Halo-femoral traction was first reported by Kane et al. in 1967 for the preoperative correction of severe scoliotic curves (39) (Fig. 11). The distal femoral pins are inserted with fluoroscopic guidance under sterile conditions. Small stab incisions are made

in the skin followed by blunt dissection with a hemostat down to the periosteum. A large-diameter threaded Steinmann pin is then inserted at least 1 cm proximal to the distal femoral physis. No more than half of the patient's body weight should be applied to the halo and femoral pins. One half of the traction weight is applied to the halo, and a quarter of the weight is applied to each femur. Pelvic obliquity can be corrected by applying asymmetrical weights to each femur. The traction must overcome the static friction between the patient and the bed to be effective, and this can be aided by the use of a split mattress or a skid applied to the halo.

Halo-Gravity Traction

Stagnara is credited with the development of halo-gravity traction in scoliosis. It has been used both in the preoperative assessment of patients potentially having surgery and in the perioperative treatment of persons with spinal deformity. The halo device is applied by the technique already described and the appropriate weight suspended from it. The patient's own weight is used as a counterbalance. This is achieved by the patient using modified walkers or wheelchairs (Fig. 12). When a wheelchair is used a counterbalance often must be fixed to the footrest to prevent the chair from tipping backward. When the patient is lying down, countertraction can be applied with a pelvic sling, or femoral pins can be inserted and cervical traction applied. Depending on the patient's size, an initial traction weight of 10 to 15 lb is applied, with daily additions of 2 lb up to a maximum of 30% to 50% of body weight.

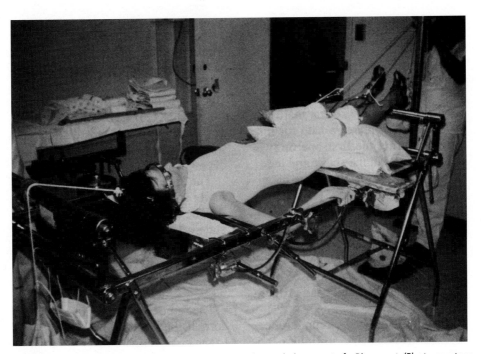

FIGURE 11. Halo-femoral traction. Preoperative traction and placement of a Risser cast. (Photo courtesy of Daniel Benson, M.D.)

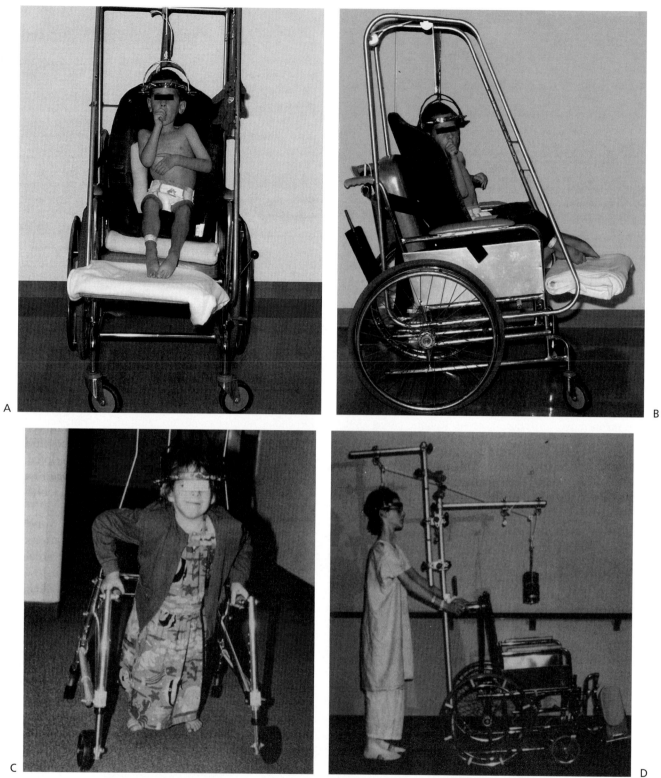

FIGURE 12.   Halo-gravity traction. **A, B:** This modified wheelchair with a car-seat inserted allows the patient to be upright during the day. The traction was used preoperatively for pulmonary assessment and for 2 weeks between staged anteroposterior surgery. **C:** Halo-walker traction allows patients to be ambulatory during the daytime. (Photo courtesy of Richard Haynes, M.D.) **D:** Halo-wheelchair traction in a patient after anterior release for severe kyphosis. (Photo courtesy of Stuart L. Weinstein, M.D.)

CLINICAL INDICATIONS FOR TRACTION

The indications for traction in spinal deformity and trauma have decreased with time as success with newer surgical techniques has evolved. Following is a summary of areas where traction is still useful in clinical practice. More detailed descriptions of the treatment alternatives for each condition can be found in the appropriate chapter.

Cervical Spine

Cervical spine trauma is the most common clinical indication for traction. Children younger than 10 years most commonly have cervical spine trauma above C3 and children older than 10 more typically have cervical spine injuries below this level. The most important complication to avoid in treating these patients is overdistraction and hence they must be monitored very closely radiographically and neurologically while being treated (37). No more than 2- to 3-lb increments should be used. Ten minutes after the application of each increment a lateral radiograph should be taken; if there is any overdistraction at the fracture or dislocation site, weight should be removed and a repeat radiograph taken.

For fractures from the occiput to C2, only 2 to 5 lb of weight is required to obtain a safe reduction. Often this is the weight of the tongs (or halo) and the weight holder. For fractures below C2, 5 lb of weight usually needs to be added for each level. Five pounds of weight is applied at 10-minute intervals, after which a lateral radiograph should be taken and a neurologic examination performed. If there is any change in neurologic function or if there is more than 7 to 10 mm of distraction at the injury site, the weight should be decreased and the examinations repeated.

Occipitoatlantal Dislocation

Traction can be applied using Gardner-Wells tongs or a halo. Only 2 to 5 lb of weight should be applied due to the extensive ligament disruption that has occurred in this injury. A halo vest, Minerva jacket, or surgical stabilization procedure should be performed as soon as the child is medically stable due to the high risk of overdistraction. If surgery is performed, the halo vest can be kept on postoperatively to aid stability (56,61,64,88).

Odontoid Fracture

Halo traction aids in the reduction of an odontoid fracture in a child. Extension and posterior translation helps to reduce the fracture; then the halo can be incorporated into a jacket or vest as surgical intervention is usually not required (22,31,75,76).

C2 Fracture

The traumatic spondylolisthesis of C2 or "hangman's fracture" can be reduced with extension of the cervical spine with gentle traction. This is followed by immobilization in a Minerva jacket or halo vest for 8 to 10 weeks (47,67).

C3–7 Fracture

The main use of skeletal traction in injuries from C3–7 is when there is a fracture subluxation or dislocation of one vertebra on another. This is the most common injury to the cervical spine in children older than 10 years (26,53). The traction can be applied with Gardner-Wells tongs or halo, as described above. The patient has to be monitored carefully both radiographically and neurologically (10,78). For reductions performed under a general anesthetic, spinal cord monitoring has been recommended by some (53). If there is any change in neurologic status, the traction should be reduced and MRI performed to evaluate the spinal canal and look for any herniated disc contents or bony fragments (21).

Cervical Spine Deformity

The major cause of cervical spine deformity requiring traction is atlantoaxial rotatory subluxation or fixation. Fielding and Hawkins reported on the use of preoperative skeletal traction in 17 patients with atlantoaxial rotatory fixation. They recommended the use of skeletal traction for 2 to 3 weeks to achieve as much correction of the deformity as possible before C1–2 arthrodesis (24). In young children, 7 to 8 lb of weight was recommended, and if necessary traction can be increased by 1 to 2 lb every 3 or 4 days, up to a maximum of 15 lb. Adolescents and adults were treated with an initial weight of 15 lb, and a 20-lb maximum was recommended.

Atlantoaxial subluxation is a less severe form of rotatory displacement. Phillips and Hensinger proposed a treatment algorithm in 1987 based on the duration of the deformity. Patients with less than 1 week of symptoms were treated with bed rest and a soft collar. Patients failing this treatment regimen or having symptoms for longer than a week and less than a month were admitted to the hospital and treated with chin-halter traction. Patients with symptoms greater lasting longer than a month were treated in a manner similar to that of Fielding and Hawkins group. Three to five pounds of weight was applied to the halter traction depending on the patient's size. Oral analgesics and muscle relaxants were administered as needed. Skeletal traction with a halo was utilized if the halter was not tolerated by the patient. All patients had postreduction immobilization in a cervical collar (66).

Thoracic Spine

Scoliosis

Historically, skeletal traction has been used in the management of scoliosis for the following reasons:

1. Preoperative
   a. Assessment of pulmonary function
   b. Assessment of spine flexibility
   c. Improve curve correction and decrease the intraoperative complications
2. Perioperative
   a. Between first- and second-stage surgery to maintain or increase correction

b. Control the position of an unstable spine between first- and second-stage surgeries
3. Postoperative
   a. To maintain the correction if internal fixation has been unable to stabilize the correction

Swank et al. have shown that the use of preoperative halo-gravity wheelchair traction was an important predictor of the success of spinal surgery in paralyzed patients. They found that if the patient's vital capacity, partial pressure of oxygen in the alveoli (P_{AO_2}), and partial pressure of carbon dioxide (P_{ACO_2}) improved with traction, then surgical stabilization can often be successfully accomplished. In addition, they warned that if these parameters did not improve then surgery should not be contemplated (79).

In the preoperative assessment of flexibility of spinal curves greater than 70 degrees, radiographs obtained with the patient in Cotrel traction has been a useful predictor of curve correction (19,55,59) (Fig. 2). The most accurate and standardizable technique for evaluating curve flexibility is described by Winter (90), who recommends using longitudinal traction of approximately 50% body weight on a Risser or Cotrel table with a laterally directed force as well.

A number of authors have reported on preoperative halo-femoral or Cotrel traction to improve curve correctability prior to Harrington instrumentation (3,12,39,41,55,77). Nachemson and Nordwell reviewed 206 patients undergoing Harrington distraction and fusion for curves less than 90 degrees and found no significant difference in immediate surgical correction obtained between the patients having Cotrel traction and those who did not. Edgar et al. found similar results in patients with curves up to 100 degrees (20). Preoperative halo-femoral traction does not increase the surgical correction achieved when Harrington rods are used (13,14,46,68,79).

With these results in mind, along with the improvement in operative techniques and implants in scoliosis surgery, the need for preoperative traction has been questioned. The "power" of correction and stability of second- and third-generation fixation devices has increased, and surgeons are increasingly performing anterior releases in addition to posterior spinal fusions for severe curves. This has allowed greater correction at the time of surgery than has historically been achieved.

When staged surgery is planned, traction between the procedures will be beneficial for patient comfort, especially if spinal stability is a concern. Traction can also maintain or even improve the correction from the first-stage release. Nachemson and Nordwell recommended halo-pelvic or halo-femoral traction between stages in patients 20 years or older with curves greater than 90 degrees (59). Cummine et al. used halo-femoral traction in 43 patients undergoing two-stage surgery for failed scoliosis fusion and found an improvement in both thoracic and lumbar curves (13). Toledo et al. have used halo traction and a Circolectric bed between stages without instrumentation and reported good correction (80). Halo-femoral traction is also useful in the management of neuromuscular patients, especially those with athetoid cerebral palsy requiring staged procedures (43,48, 52,63). Asymmetrical weights can be used during this period if pelvic obliquity needs correction as well. The use of halo-gravity traction between stages has the added advantage of keeping the patient mobile and upright, improving respiratory function and decreasing the risks of urinary tract infections (9). The use of traction between surgeries has decreased recently as two-stage procedures are usually performed in one sitting; however, it remains an important treatment option when the second stage cannot be carried out on the same day due to unforeseen surgical or anesthesia-related complications.

Traction has been effective postoperatively if instrumentation has not been used (80). Halo-femoral traction can also be used to control the patient to prevent hook dislodgement as an alternative to immediate postoperative casting under anesthesia (87).

Kyphosis

Traction for sagittal plane deformity is complicated by potential neurologic risks to the patients if the spinal cord is "stretched" across a rigid kyphotic segment (50,52,91). Therefore, traction is only indicated in flexible deformities or when the spine has been made flexible by an anterior release of the kyphosis. The most common indication is between staged procedures for Scheuermann kyphosis when anterior and posterior surgery is not carried out in the same setting (6). Halo-femoral traction can be used, with a sling or bolster supporting the apex of the kyphotic region, or, more commonly, halo-gravity traction can be used, allowing the child to ambulate between procedures.

Halo traction has been used preoperatively in patients with neurofibromatosis and cervical kyphosis that measures greater than 45 degrees (7). The halo can then be attached to a vest for postoperative immobilization. Halo-gravity traction has also been used preoperatively in progressive cervical thoracic kyphosis post laminectomy, with complete resolution of the neurologic symptoms (87).

Lumbar Spine

Spondylolisthesis

Halo-pelvic and halo-femoral traction have been used in the past for the reduction of high-grade (III–V) spondylolisthesis but is now rarely indicated due to the high complication rate associated with this method of treatment (4,5,32,33,34,60,65). The current recommendation for the treatment of high-grade slips in children and adolescents is to perform an in situ posterolateral lumbar sacral fusion followed by a reduction maneuver 5 to 10 days later with the patient awake, as described by Scaglietti (72a).

COMPLICATIONS

Complications as a result of traction are not uncommon. Attention to detail in the application of the traction apparatus and close clinical observation of the patient in traction will eliminate the more serious ones.

Neurologic Complications

Spinal traction can result in injury to the spinal cord, cranial nerves, brachial plexus, or peripheral nerves. The injury can result in partial or complete paraplegia and quadriplegia.

The spinal cord is most likely to be injured in patients with cervical spine injuries (due to overdistraction) and in patients with a rigid thoracic kyphosis between T4 and T9. It is important to recognize these two high-risk groups and treat them appropriately. In cervical spine injuries, the skull must not be hyperflexed, and traction weight must be applied every 10 minutes followed by close clinical and radiologic monitoring. Consideration should be given to early conversion to a halo vest or Minerva jacket.

Dommisse showed the spinal cord is at greatest risk of vascular compromise between T4 and T9 (17). In this area the spinal cord not only has the least number of perforating blood vessels but also the least excursion (8). In a kyphotic deformity, the spinal cord tries to occupy the shortest distance across the deformity, which results in its being pressed against the posterior bodies of the vertebrae involved in the deformity. When traction is applied distraction occurs proximal and distal to the rigid deformity and the cord is further compressed against the vertebral bodies, resulting in circulatory changes and edema.

The first clinical symptoms of impending paraplegia are urinary retention, a heavy feeling in the legs, dysesthesias, and ankle clonus. MacEwen et al. reported a 32% neurologic complication rate in patients with congenital scoliosis and kyphosis treated by traction (49).

Intracranial injuries can occur as a complication of pin placement in the halo fixation. Infected pin sites can be cleaned or pin placement changed. However, if pin penetration has occurred, intracranial abscess can result (57,85). This complication should be suspected in a patient with a halo who has onset of headache, fever, focal neurologic signs, or change in mental status. If the dura has been perforated, cerebrospinal fluid may be visible around the offending pins.

Cranial nerve palsies can also occur secondary to traction to correct spinal deformities. The abducens (VI) is commonly affected due to its long intracranial course over the petrous temporal bone. Stretching of this nerve leads to loss of lateral gaze and is usually unilateral (62). The lower cranial nerves can also be stretched where they exit the skull bone. Paralysis of the ninth to twelfth nerves can lead to alterations in speech, swallowing, even respiratory arrest (62,81).

Brachial plexus palsies can occur by excessive traction. The most common roots involved are C6, C7, and T1 because of their course. C6 and C7 have a near-vertical direction, which makes them more susceptible to traction neuropraxias. T1 is injured due to its course over the first rib. Motor function is affected first, followed by sensory changes in the arms.

These neurologic changes can be very subtle clinically; hence, there is no substitute for thorough examination of patients in traction paying attention to both the central and peripheral nervous systems. Any detection of neurologic change should alert the physician to decrease traction weight until the symptoms or signs resolve.

Dermatologic Complications

Pressure sores, especially over bony prominences, can become a major problem in a patient who has to be recumbent in traction for a long time. It is therefore vital to prevent pressure sores from occurring. This is often made more difficult by the fact that some patients have insensate skin and others are unable to communicate if they have pain. The bed should have foam on top of the mattress. Bony prominences should have extra padding or a "donut" cushion for support, and the patient should be rolled every 2 to 4 hours. In the event of skin breakdown, additional pressure-relieving measures should be carried out; conversion to halo-wheelchair traction or even cessation of this method of treatment may be considered. The patient's back should be inspected with each rolling to look for any red areas that may forewarn the staff that pressure is occurring.

Gastrointestinal Complications

The third part of the duodenum can be compressed by the superior mesenteric artery (SMA) when spinal curvature is corrected by traction (2,23,30,69,74). This occurs most commonly in thin, undernourished patients and can occur after correction in a cast, brace, surgery, or traction. It has been termed SMA or "cast" syndrome, and it leads to distention of the stomach and subsequent nausea, vomiting, and epigastric fullness. The abdomen is usually soft to palpation, with normal bowel sounds. Prolonged obstruction leads to dehydration and hypokalemic alkalosis, which can result in death. The diagnosis can be made clinically if the above signs or symptoms are recognized. This can be confirmed with upper gastrointestinal radiographs with or without contrast. The obstruction can usually be treated nonoperatively by releasing the traction, positioning the patient in the left decubitus position, giving intravenous fluids, administering nasogastric suction, and closely monitoring the electrolytes. General surgical consultation should be considered early.

Vascular Complications

Deep Veinous Thrombosis

Deep veinous thrombosis is an uncommon complication in children that may be underdiagnosed because it is overlooked. There have been reports of associated fatal pulmonary emboli (13,54,84). Leslie et al. performed bilateral venography on 54 children treated with halo-femoral traction for an average of 28 days and found the incidence of thrombosis to be 3.7% (44). There were no clinically silent cases. When halo-femoral traction is used for prolonged periods, prophylactic measures, including antiembolic stockings, foot pumps, and pharmaceutical agents (e.g., aspirin or low molecular weight heparin) should be considered to avoid this uncommon but potentially life-threatening complication.

SUMMARY

Although traction is rarely used today, it remains an important option in the treatment of children with spinal deformities. The most common indications for traction are as follows:

1. For preoperative assessment of respiratory function
2. To confer perioperative stability when two-stage procedures cannot be carried out on the same day

3. Postoperatively, to maintain the correction if internal fixation cannot stabilize the correction
4. For treatment of occipioatlantial dislocation
5. For treatment of cervical spine trauma.

In all forms of traction, there must be attention to detail in terms of application of the devices and close monitoring to minimize potential complications that can arise from its use.

REFERENCES

1. Aaro S, Ohlen C (1983): The effect of Harrington instrumentation on the sagittal configuration and mobility of the spine in scoliosis. *Spine* 8:570–574.
2. Bisla RS, Louis HJ (1975): Acute vascular compression of the duodenum following cast application. *Surg Gynecol Obstet* 140:563–566.
3. Bonnett C, Perry J, Brown JC, et al. (1992): Halofemoral distraction and posterior spine fusion for paralytic scoliosis. *J Bone Joint Surg Am* 54:202.
4. Boxali D, Bradford DS, Winter RB, Moe JH (1969): Management of severe spondylolisthesis in children and adolescents. *J Bone Joint Surg Am* 61:479–485.
5. Bradford DS (1979): Treatment of severe spondylolisthesis: a combined approach for reduction and stabilization. *Spine* 4:423–429.
6. Bradford DS, Ahmed KB, Moe JH, et al. (1980): The surgical management of patient with Scheuermann's disease: a review of 24 cases. Managed by combined anterior and posterior spine fusion. *J Bone Joint Surg Am* 62:705–712.
7. Bradford DS, Lonstein JA, Moe JH, et al., eds (1994): *Moe's Textbook of scoliosis and other spinal deformities.* Philadelphia: WB Saunders.
8. Breig A (1966): *Biomechanics of the central nervous system.* Stockholm: Almquest and Wiksell.
9. Burkus JK, DePonte RJ L(1986): Chronic atlantoaxial rotatory fixation correction by cervical traction, manipulation, and bracing. *J Paediatr Orthop* 6:631–635.
10. Cotler M, Herbison AJ, Nasuti JF, et al. (1993): Closed reduction of traumatic cervical spine dislocation using traction weight up to 140 pounds. *Spine* 18:386–390.
11. Cotrel Y, D'Amore M (1968): Spinal traction in scoliosis. In: Zosab P, ed. *Proceedings of the Second Symposium on Scoliosis.* London: Churchill Livingstone, pp. 37–43.
12. Cotrel Y, Seringe, Plais PY, et al. (1980): Spinal traction in scoliosis. In: Zorab PA, Siegler D, eds. *Scoliosis 1979.* New York: Academic Press.
13. Cummine JL, Lonstein JE, Moe JH, et al. (1979): Reconstructive surgery in the adult for failed scoliosis fusion. *J Bone Joint Surg Am* 61:1151–1161.
14. Curtis RL, Dickson JH, Harrington PR, et al. (1979): Results of Harrington instrumentation in the treatment of severe scoliosis. *Clin Orthop* 144:128–134.
15. DeWald RL, Mulcahy TM, Schultz AB (1973): Force measurement studies with the halo-hoop application in scoliosis. *Orthop Rev* 2:17.
16. DeWald RL, Roy RD (1970): Skeletal traction for the treatment of severe scoliosis. *J Bone Joint Surg Am* 52:233–238.
17. Dommisse GF (1974): The blood supply of the spinal cord. *J Bone Joint Surg Br* 56:225–235.
18. Dove J, Hsu Lc, Vau AC (1980): The cervical spine following halo-pelvic traction. *J Bone Joint Surg Br* 62:158–161.
19. Edgar MA, Chapman RA, Glasglow MM (1982): Preoperative correction in adolescent idiopathic scoliosis. *J Bone Joint Surg Br* 64:531.
20. Edgar MA, Chapman RA, Glasglow MM (1982): Preoperative correction in adolescent idiopathic scoliosis. *J Bone Joint Surg Br* 64:530–535.
21. Eismont FJ, Arena MJ, Green BA (1991): Extrusion of an intervertebral disk associated with trauma subluxation or dislocation of cervical facets. *J Bone Joint Surg* 73:1555–1560.
22. Ewald FC (1971): Fracture of the odontoid process in a seventeen month old infant treated with a halo. *J Bone Joint Surg Am* 53:1636–1640.
23. Ewarts CM, Winter RB, Hall JE (1971): Vascular compression of the duodenum associated with the treatment of scoliosis. *J Bone Joint Surg Am* 53:431–444.
24. Fielding JW, Hawkins RJ (1977): Atlantoaxial rotatory fixation. *J Bone Joint Surg Am* 59:37–44.
25. Fielding JW, Waugh TL (1962): Postoperataive correction of scoliosis. *JAMA* 182:541–544.
26. Finch GD, Barnes MJ (1998): Major cervical spine injuuries in children and adolescents. *J Pediatr Orthop* 18(6):811–814.
27. Gardner WJ (1973): The principal of spring-loaded points for cervical traction. *J Neurosurg* 39:543–544.
28. Garfin Sr, Botte MJ, Centeno RS, et al. (1985): Osteology of the skull as it affects halo pin placement. *Spine* 10:696–698.
29. Garfin SR, Botte MJ, Waters RL, et al. (1986): Complications in the use of the halo fixation device. *J Bone Joint Surg Am* 68:320–325.
30. Gray SW, Akin JT, Milsap JH, et al. (1976): Vascular compression of the duodenum. *Contemp Surg* 9:37–39.
31. Griffiths SC 1972): Fracture of the odontoid process in children. *J Pediatr Surg* 7:680–683.
32. Harrington PR, Tullos HS (1971): Spondylolisthesis in children: observations and surgical treatment. *Clin Orthop* 79:75–84.
33. Harris RI (1951): Spondylolisthesis. *Ann R Coll Surg Engl* 8:259–297.
34. Hensinger RN, Lang JR, MacEwen GD (1976): Surgical management of spondylolisthesis in children and adolescents. *Spine* 1:207.
35. Herzenberg JE, Hensinger RN, Dedrick DK, et al. (1989): Emergency transport and positioning of young children who have an injury of the cervical spine. The standard backboard may be hazardous. *J Bone Joint Surg Am* 71:15–22.
36. Hume M, Nachemson A, Tornvall A, et al. (1981): Halo pelvic traction: a long term clinical and radiographic evaluation with emphasis on the cervical spine. Presented at the Annual Meeting of the Scoliosis Research Society of Minneapolis.
37. Jeanneret B, Mager IF, Ward JC (1991): Over distraction: a hazard of traction in the management of acute injuries of the cervical spine. *Arch Orthop Trauma Surg* 110:242–245.
38. Kalamchi A, Vau AC, O'Brien JP, et al. (1976): Halo pelvic distraction apparatus. *J Bone Joint Surg Am* 58:1119–1125.
39. Kane WJ, Moe JH, Lai CC (1967): Halo-femoral pin distraction in the treatment of scoliosis. *J Bone Joint Surg Am* 49:1018–1019.
40. Kostuik J (1973): Halo-pelvic traction in the medical management of adult scoliosis. *J Bone Joint Surg Br* 55:232.
41. Kostuik JP, Isreal J, Hall JE (1973): Scoliosis surgery in adults. *Clin Orthop* 93:225–234.
42. Kostuik J, Tooke M (1983): The application of pelvic pins in the halo-pelvic distraction. An anatomic study. *Spine* 8:35–38.
43. Leong JC, Wilding K, Mock MA, et al. (1981): Surgical treatment of scoliosis following poliomyelitis. A review of 110 cases. *J Bone Joint Surg Am* 63:726–740.
44. Leslie EJ, Dorgan JC, Bentley G, et al. (1981): A prospective study of deep vein thrombosis of the leg in children on halofemoral traction. *J Bone Joint Surg Br* 63:168–170.
45. Letts M, Kaylos D, Couw A (1988): A biomechanical analysis of halo fixation in children. *J Bone Joint Surg Br* 70:277–279.
46. Letts RM, Palakar B, Bobecko WP (1975). Preoperative skeletal traction in scoliosis. *J Bone Joint Surg Am* 57:616–619.
47. Levine AM, Edwards CC L (1985): The management of traumatic spondylolisthesis of the axis. *J Bone Joint Surg Am* 67:217–226.
48. Lonstein JE, Akbarnia BA (1983): Operative treatment of spinal deformities in patients with cerebral palsy or mental retardation. *J Bone Joint Surg Am* 65:43–55.
49. MacEwan GD, Bunnel WP, Sriram K (1975): Acute neurological complications in the treatment of scoliosis. A report of the Scoliosis Research Society. *J Bone Joint Surg Am* 57:404–408
50. Malcolm BW, Bradford DS, Winter RS, et al. (1981): Post traumatic kyphosis. Review of 48 surgically treated patients. *J Bone Joint Surg Am* 63:891–899.
51. Marks RM, Cotler JM (1996): Early closed reduction for pediatric fracture-dislocations. In: Betz RR, Mulcahel MJ, eds. *The child with a spinal cord injury.* Park Ridge, IL: AAOS.
52. Mayer PJ, Dove J, Ditmonson M, et al. (1981): Post poliomyelitis

paralytic scoliosis. A review of curve patterns and results on surgical treatment in 118 consecutive patients. *Spine* 6:573–582.

53. McGrory BJ, Klassen RA, Chao EY. et al. (1993): Acute fractures and dislocations of the cervical spine in children and adolescents. *J Bone Joint Surg Am* 75:988–995.

54. Moe JN (1967): Complications of scoliosis treatment. *Clin Orthop* 53: 21–30.

55. Moe JN (1972): Methods of correction and surgical technique in scoliosis. *Orthop Clin N Am* 2:17–48.

56. Montane I, Eismont FJ, Green BA (1991): Traumatic occipitoatlantal dislocation. *Spine* 16:112–116.

57. Mubarak SJ, Camp JF, Vuletich W, et al. (1989): Technique: halo application in the infant. *J Bone Joint Surg Am* 73:1547–1554.

58. Nachemson A, Elfstrom C (1976): Intravital wireless telemetry of axial forces in Harrington distraction rods in patients with ideopathic scoliosis. *J Bone Joint Surg Am* 53:445.

59. Nachemson A, Nordwell A (1977): Effectiveness of preoperative Cotrel traction for correction of ideopathic scoliosis. *J Bone Joint Surg Am* 59: 504.

60. Newman PH (1965): A clinical syndrome associated with severe lumbrosacral subluxation. *J Bone Joint Surg Br* 47:472–481.

61. Newman P, Sweetman R (1969): Occipito-cervical fusion: an operative technique and its indications. *J Bone Joint Surg Br* 51:423–431.

62. O'Brien JP (1975): The halo-pelvic apparatus. *Acta Orthop Scand* 163(Suppl):79.

63. O'Brien JP, Yau ACMCD, Gertzbein S, et al. (1975): Combined staged anterior and posterior correction and fusion of the spine in scoliosis following poliomyelitis. *Clin Orthop* 110:81–89.

64. Page CP, Story JL, Wissinger JP, et al. (1973): Traumatic atlantoccipital dislocatoin: case report. *J Neurosurg* 39:384–397.

65. Phalen GS, Dickson JA (1961): Spondylolisthesis and tight hamstrings. *J Bone Joint Surg Am* 43:505–512.

66. Phillips WA, Hensinger RN (1989): The management of rotatory atlanto-axial subluxation in children. *J Bone Joint Surg Am* 71:664.

67. Pizzutillo PD, Rocha EF, D'Astous J, et al. (1986): Bilateral fracture of the pedicle of the second vertebra in the young child. *J Bone Joint Surg Am* 68:892–896.

68. Ponder RC, Dickson JH, Harrington PR, et al. (1975): Results of Harrington instrumentation and fusion in the adult idiopathic scoliosis patient. *J Bone Joint Surg Am* 57:797–801.

69. Puronik SR, Keiser RP, Gilbert MG (1972): Anteriomesentoic duoderal compression in children. *Am J Surg* 124:334–339.

70. Ronford AAO, Manning CW (1975): Complications of halo-pelvic distraction. *J Bone Joint Surg Br* 57:131–137.

71. Rozario RA, Stein BM (1986): Complications of halo-pelvic traction. *J Neurosurg* 45:716–718.

72. Sayre LA (1876): *Orthopaedic surgery and disease of the joints.* New York: Appleton and Colleagues.

72a. Scaglietti O (2001): In: Weinstein SL, ed. *The pediatric spine: principles and practice,* 2nd ed. Philadelphia: Lippincott Williams & Wilkins, pp. xx–xx.

73. Scaglietti O, Frontino A, Bastolozzi P (1976): Technique of anatomical reduction of lumbar spondylolisthesis and its surgical stabilization. *Clin Orthop* 117:164.

74. Shadling B (1976): The so-called superior mesenteric artery syndrome. *Am J Dis Child* 130:1371–1373.

75. Sherk HH, Schut C, Lane JM (1976): Fractures and dislocations of the cervical spine in children. *Orthop Clin N Am* 7:593–604.

76. Sherk HH, Nicholson JT, Chung SM (1978): Fractures of the odontoid process in young children. *J Bone Joint Surg Am* 60:921–924.

77. Stagnavap, Jouvinroux P, Peloux J, et al. (1969): Cypho- Scolioses Essentielles de l'Adult. Foimes Severes de Plus de 100 degrees. In: *Redressement Partial et Arthrodese X1 SICOT Congress,* Mexico City, pp. 206–233.

77a. Stokes IAF (2001): Spinal biomechanics. In: Weinstein SL, ed. *The pediatric spine: principles and practice,* 2nd ed. Philadelphia: Lippincott Williams & Wilkins, pp. xx–xx.

78. Stor AM, Jones AA, Cotler JM, et al. (1990): Immediate closed reduction of cervical spine dislocations using traction. *Spine* 15:1068–1072.

79. Swank SM, Winter RB, Moe JH (1982): Scoliosis and cor pulmonale. *Spine* 7:343–354.

80. Toledo LC, Toledo CH, MacEwen AD (1982): Halo traction with the circolectric bed in the treatment of severe spinal deformitie: a preliminary report. *J Paediatr Orthop* 2(5):554–559.

81. Transfeldt EE (1994): In: Lonstein JE, Bradford DS, Winter RB, et al., eds. *Textbook of scoliosis and other spinal deformities.* Philadelphia: WB Saunders.

82. Tredwell SJ, O'Brien JP (1975): Avascular necrosis of the proximal end of the dens. A complication of halo-pelvic distraction. *J Bone Joint Surg Am* 57:332–336.

83. Tredwell SJ, O'Brien JP (1980): Apophyseal joint degeneration in the cervical spine following halo pelvic distraction. *Spine* 5:497–501.

84. Uden A. (1979): Thromboembolic complications following scoliosis surgery in Scandinavia. *Acta Orthop Scand* 50:175–178.

85. Victor DI, Bresnan MJ, Keller RB (1973): Brain abscess complicating the use of halo traction. *J Bone Joint Surg Am* 55:635–639.

86. Ward TW, Doyle S (1996): Management of the upper cervical spine injuries: occiput to C3. In: Betz RR, Mulcahej MJ, eds. *The child with a spinal cord injury.* Park Ridge, IL: AAOS.

87. Weinstein SL (1985): Role of traction in the management of spinal deformities. In: Hensinger RM, Bradford DS, eds. *The pediatric spine.* New York: Thieme-Stratton.

88. Wertheim SB, Bohlman HH (1987): Occipitocervical fusion: indications, technique and long-term results in thirteen patients. *J Bone Joint Surg Am* 69:833–836.

89. White AA, Panjali MM (1978): *Clinical biomechanics of the spine.* Phaveadelphia: JB Lippincott, p. 105.

90. Winter RB (1983): *Congenital deformities of the spine.* New York: Thieme-Stratton.

91. Winter RB, Moe JH, Lonstein JE (1985): The surgical treatment of congenital kyphosis: a review of 94 patients age 5 years or older with 2 years or more follow-up in 77 patients. *Spine* 10:224–231.

92. Wong WB, Haynes RJ (1994): Osteology of the paediatric skull: considerations of halo pin placement. *Spine* 19:1451–1454.

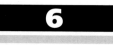

6

CASTING

VITTORIO SALSANO *(Deceased)*
ANTONELLO MONTANARO
FRANCESCO TURTURRO

The idea of using bandages impregnated with plaster of Paris to immobilize limbs first occurred in 1852 and is generally attributed to Antonius Mathijsen. It marked a milestone in the history of orthopaedics. At the same time, the use of plaster of Paris as a body cast was introduced.

The history of plaster jackets is intimately linked with the history of the treatment of spinal deformities. In 1877, Lewis A. Sayre (23) described a method of treating scoliosis by means of plaster jackets prepared with the patient standing and in cervical traction.

Around the turn of the century, the foundations for all of the contemporary techniques of body casting were laid. These resulted from a mixture of attempts—some imaginative but useless, others scientifically based and clinically valid.

In 1902, Wullstein and Schulthess (32) reported the results of a technique for preparing the cast in which the patient was held in the correct position by axial traction and lateral thrusts. Abbott (1), in 1911, described correction obtained on a frame that is still widely used today (after Cotrel's modifications). Risser perfected the turnbuckle in 1927.

But it was only in the 1950s, with the popularity of the localizer cast (developed by Risser) and the elongation derotation flexion (EDF) cast (developed by Cotrel), that treatment with body casts achieved success (22). This was due in part to improved methods of application but mostly to modifications in indications for treatment that developed from a better understanding of the natural history of spinal deformities.

MATERIALS

Plaster

The plaster used in medical practice is purified calcium sulfate hemihydrate, obtained by heating the dihydrate to 120°C. Addition of water to the dehydrated plaster allows the plaster to return to the crystalline state. The crystals are formed rapidly and are tightly interlocked. This interlocking gives plaster its mechanical resistance to loads and traction.

Movement disturbs or interrupts the formation of the interlock and decreases the strength of the plaster. Therefore, it is important in clinical practice to avoid any further molding or movement of the plaster once bonds start to form between the crystals.

Excess water is eliminated by evaporation, and in its final condition the plaster has a water content of 21%. Most of the water is lost in a few hours, but the plaster attains its final state over the course of a few days—rarely less than 24 hours (11,30).

Plaster Substitutes

Of the many replacements for plaster suggested in recent years, the latest generation of synthetic bandages is the most valid alternative. These bandages consist of fiberglass or other synthetic materials, such as polypropylene, impregnated with polyurethane resin. Preparation is not complicated as it was for the first synthetic materials (water at high temperatures, fixing liquids, etc.) and is no different from traditional plaster preparation.

Synthetic substitutes are light, radiotransparent, porous, and wettable, and their mechanical and preparation characteristics are similar to those of plaster. However, they have one major disadvantage: they are not as moldable as plaster. Plaster is safe (fire-proof), nonallergenic, and cheap, but it is heavy and partially radiopaque and loses its strength if it gets wet. Nevertheless, plaster is still preferred to its substitutes for the preparation of jackets, chiefly because of its unsurpassed moldability.

BIOMECHANICAL PRINCIPLES OF BODY CASTING

The long bones of the lower and upper limbs can easily be surrounded over their whole circumference by casts. Because only skin and muscles interpose themselves between the plaster and the bone, forces can easily be applied by such casts. However, the spine can be reached for part of its circumference with only paravertebral muscles interposed. The rest is hidden, as in a cage, by the ribs, abdominal viscera, and muscles. This prevents application of forces or pressures directly on the spine. Correction or immobilization of the spine therefore depends on the

V. Salsano, A. Montanaro, and F. Turturro: Second Division of Orthopedic Surgery, Children's Hospital (Ospedale Bambino Gesu), Rome, Italy.

possibility of transmitting forces through the structures that surround it. This possibility is a function of the rigidity of the structures concerned. A visceral structure, for example, is not rigid; any force applied deforms it, and little or nothing is transmitted. It is therefore easier to apply a force at the level of the thoracic rather than the lumbar spine because the ribs are more rigid than the abdominal muscles and viscera (31).

The forces applied may be classified according to their direction: horizontal (bending) and longitudinal (distraction). One must also consider the force of abdominal compression, even though its resultant can always be reduced to a longitudinal vector. Compression applied to the system formed by the abdominal wall, the pelvic floor, and the diaphragm creates a hydraulic effect of abdominal pressurization (as two equal and opposite horizontal forces applied to a football cause its deformation), which appears as increased axial compression strength of the spine.

The form of the jacket and its holds and pressures therefore results not only from the need to fit the anatomical conformation of the spine like a glove but chiefly from the need to apply these forces. Thus, some jackets leave the spine completely free, not surrounding any part of it (e.g., the elongation plaster or halo-pelvic cast), but nonetheless effectively immobilizing and correcting it.

The spine affords two different holds: the pelvic girdle and the occipitomandibular ring. The lower and more important is the pelvic hold, which exploits the powerful sacroiliac articulation to immobilize the sacrolumbar spine. In addition, pelvic anti- and retroversion movements can modify the sagittal aspect of the spine. The upper occipitomandibular hold is less efficient mechanically. It exploits the occipitoatlantoid articulation to block the cervical spine.

The pelvic girdle and occipitomandibular ring are the two points of application of traction to the spine; they can also be the upper and lower points of a three-point system for the application of horizontal forces.

Horizontal forces are transmitted to the spine through the ribs at the thoracic level and through the erector spinae muscle at the lumbar level. The thoracic thrust must be applied not at the level of the chosen vertebra but along the rib that joins it. It must be applied posterolaterally rather than laterally so as not to increase rib deformation. Anterolateral counterthrusts are always necessary in the thrust areas. Other pressure areas can be created at the pubic level to exploit the hydraulic effects of abdominal pressurization.

BASIC CASTING TECHNIQUE

Plaster application requires good practical skill and a full set of tools and materials.

The tubular stockinette is applied without folds and serves to protect the skin from contact with the plaster. Water-repellent cotton is then applied on the stockinette in a single layer with the same type of turn that will be used later for the plaster bandages (Fig. 1). The protection of the zones most at risk for pressure sores—the bony prominences, especially in thin patients—is completed by a layer of cotton or felt with a hole cut in the center so that it surrounds the base of the protrusion.

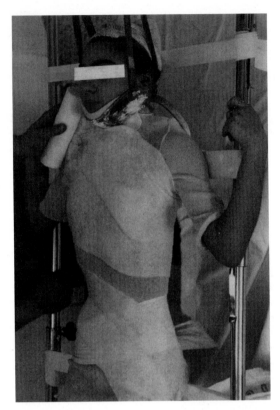

FIGURE 1. Application of cotton with the same oblique turn as used for the plaster bandage.

This serves to level the protrusion and ensures that the plaster bandages can cover it without irritating or compressing it (Fig. 2).

After the cotton and the felts have been applied, the plaster bandages are wound. The plaster bandages should be wound in the caudad-craniad direction with the ball of the hand, not with the thumb. In this way, the force will be distributed uniformly over the whole width of the bandage, avoiding asymmetrical tension that could provoke wrinkling or tightness.

The first plaster bandage must be wound from the pelvis anteriorly, hooking an iliac crest from the front to the rear and returning anteriorly to complete the first turn on the abdomen. From here one proceeds obliquely toward the armpit on the same side as was first hooked, circling it posteriorly and then returning anteriorly, passing over the opposite shoulder. The subsequent plaster bandages are wound in alternating directions to produce a uniform layer of plaster.

Finally, the plain bandage is applied to dry the cast more quickly. At this point, molding of the holds and maneuvers to correct the components of the deformity are performed, as will be described in detail below. Molding, thrusts, and counterthrusts must be performed as soon as the plaster has started to set but before it has dried completely.

Molding of the important zones (e.g., waist, subclavicular fossa, subaxillary zones) should be performed with the ulnar side of the forearm and edge of the hand until the cast is completely set (Fig. 3). Thrusts and counterthrusts are aimed at correcting the deformity and, according to the type of cast, can be effected

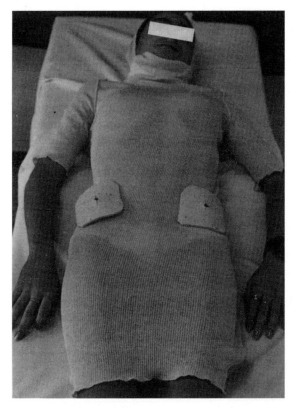

FIGURE 2. Felts protect bony prominences.

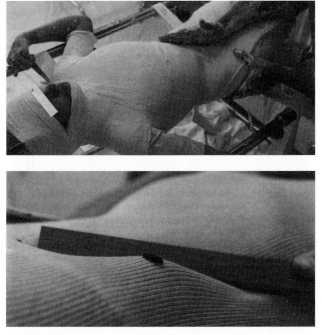

FIGURE 3. A: Molding of the pelvic area is performed with the ulnar edge of the hand and forearm. **B:** This is done medial to the anterior superior iliac spine *(black dot)*, thus avoiding direct compression.

manually, with devices (e.g., straps, pressers), or both. They must therefore be applied at the most favorable mechanical points for correction of the individual deformities.

After the cast has been completed it is trimmed. Windows can be opened in the front or back to permit chest expansion or application of felt padding.

GENERAL INDICATIONS FOR THE USE OF CASTS

Spinal Injuries

Vertebral fractures and dislocation are rare in adolescents and exceptional in infants on account of the great flexibility of the spine. The cervical level is affected most often; the thoracic and lumbar levels more rarely.

Fractures occur only as a result of major trauma. Cervical fractures in particular are often associated with medullary lesions (2). In children, the skeletal lesion most commonly affects the upper cervical segment: occiput dislocation, atlantoaxial lesions (traumatic ligament disruption, odontoid epiphyseal separation), and subluxation of C2 on C3. At the thoracic and lumbar levels, compression fractures are more common (7).

If the lesion is stable, conservative treatment (reduction and immobilization) is sufficient. In cases of instability, spinal fusion must be performed. However, surgical treatment is rarely required because such lesions are uncommon, and most are stable.

The type of cast needed varies according to the level of the fracture. In lumbar fractures, an underarm cast is applied; in thoracic fractures from T4 to T12, a cast with shoulder straps is preferred. Immobilization of the high thoracic segment requires an occipitomandibular extension. For cervical fractures, a Minerva jacket or halo cast is required.

Spinal Deformities

Scoliosis

Conservative treatment of idiopathic scoliosis is indicated in persons with curves between 30 and 45 degrees (Cobb angle) who have not achieved bone maturity; in persons with curves of 20 to 30 degrees before the onset of puberty, who demonstrate progression (at least 5 degrees in 6 months); and in persons with curves of 40 degrees who have infantile or juvenile scoliosis in order to postpone surgery.

The rationale for the use of casts is that because they apply greater force, they provide a better correcting and molding effect and permit more effective countering of progression of the scoliosis as well as better stabilization.

For curves between 30 and 50 degrees, Stagnara (26) used the Milwaukee brace up to the growth spurt and then applied a plaster jacket with successive reapplication every 2 months. After casting, a brace was employed. We still prefer to start treatment with casts and move on to a brace after 3 months in the case of curves with indications for conservative treatment. Such curves have the following characteristics: high clinical and radiologic structuralization, marked rigidity in bending films, and a very pronounced hump. Casts are also used when bracing has failed to halt curve progression or to provide satisfactory correction.

Kyphosis

As in the case of idiopathic scoliosis, use of plaster jackets in the treatment of idiopathic kyphosis and Scheuermann kyphosis should be restricted to curves with indications for conservative treatment that display marked rigidity on radiographic examination in hyperextension. We use a plaster jacket when the angle in hyperextension exceeds 40 degrees and the correction does not exceed 20% of the initial angle. The casts are reapplied every 45 days for a total of 3 months and are followed by a brace, which is used until bone maturity is achieved.

Inflammatory Diseases

Nonspecific infections of the intervertebral disc may occur in infants but are less common in children older than 5 to 7 years. Antibiotic therapy associated with immobilization in a plaster jacket for about 3 months, depending on clinical conditions, is indicated. The type of plaster jacket (underarm, with shoulder straps, or Minerva) depends on the site of the problem.

COMPLICATIONS

Pressure Sores

There can be various complications of casts, but the only ones of significance in terms of frequency are pressure sores (14). The sores generally form at bony protuberances (e.g., the anterior superior iliac spine, sacrum, ribs at the level of the hump, spinous process at the level of the apex of the kyphosis, mandible, occiput) where zones of point contact are created during preparation of the cast. Reduction of the surface in contact inevitably produces an increase in cutaneous pressure if the force applied remains the same.

In normal subjects, the mean tolerable skin pressure is about 1.5 lb/in.^{2} (25). When this is exceeded, an erythema appears in the zones affected. If the pressure persists, a localized ischemia is produced in the affected skin. The initial pain decreases gradually as ischemic damage to the sensory nerve progresses. A necrosis of the skin then occurs and, depending on the amount and duration of the pressure, may extend from the surface layer of the derma to the lower layers and, in the most serious cases, to the muscle layer. Prevention is largely a matter of careful preparation of the casts and only secondarily of monitoring the skin under the plaster.

As has already been emphasized in the section on technique, good molding of the holds when the cast is being prepared is essential, and the contact area should be as large as possible.

In the initial phase of monitoring in the days following application of the cast, much attention is paid to pain or reddening reported by the patient. The areas affected are explored, and windows may be cut in the plaster to facilitate examination and care.

Cast Syndrome

A gastric dilatation secondary to vascular compression of the duodenum may occur following application of plaster jackets in traction; it is much rarer in the absence of traction. Correction of the curve may cause a trapping of the third part of the duodenum between the aorta posteriorly and the emergence of the superior mesenteric artery anteriorly, where it is drawn by the ligament of Treitz (6,10,13,14,15). The symptoms are nausea, persistent vomiting, gastric distention, and reduction—but not cessation—of peristalsis. Direct radiography of the abdomen reveals gastric and duodenal dilatation with liquid and gas. Contrast radiography shows occlusion of the third part of the duodenum. The vomiting produces dehydration, hypovolemia, and loss of electrolytes and, if not treated, may lead to irreversible shock.

Treatment should be prompt. The sooner it begins the greater the probability of eliminating the occlusion without recourse to surgery. A nasogastric probe is inserted, and electrolyte and acid-base equilibrium and water balance are evaluated. Water and electrolyte losses are restored by endovenous perfusion. The patient is placed in the left lateral decubitus position with a slight Trendelenburg positioning. If the symptoms do not disappear, the plaster is removed rather than windowed because the cause of the compression on the duodenum is the correction, not abdominal compression. If the above measures are taken promptly, the occlusion is generally resolved in 2 to 3 days.

If conservative treatment is ineffective, the patient must undergo surgery to release the ligament of Treitz or must have a duodenojejunostomy.

In our experience, it has never been necessary to resort to surgery for an occlusion secondary to a cast, though it may be required for vascular compressions of the duodenum secondary to surgical distraction instrumentation or other surgical procedures.

An additional gastrointestinal complication is peptic esophagitis. This is due to an increased intraabdominal pressure caused by the cast, which can promote gastroesophageal reflux (9).

Neurologic Complications

A minor neurologic complication is compression of the femoral cutaneous nerve. The femoral cutaneous nerve reaches the thigh by passing over (or, less frequently, under) the sartorius muscle, about 2.5 cm distal to the anterior superior iliac spine. If the nerve is very near the surface and the anterior superior iliac spine is protuberant, the cast may compress the nerve and provoke paresthesia or anesthesia of the anterior thigh. To prevent this problem, molding of the cast over the iliac crests must be continued forward to the pubis and maintained medially to the anterior superior iliac spine, thus avoiding direct compression. When this problem does occur, a window should be opened over the anterior superior iliac spine to eliminate the pressure.

It is unusual for major neurologic complications to result from casts used for conservative treatment of deformities. In the presence of previously unnoticed neurologic abnormalities (e.g., diastematomyelia, tethered cord, syringomyelia), neurologic complications can occur when traction is applied (3).

Thrombophlebitis

Thrombophlebitis occurs rarely in adolescents, usually in patients who require prolonged immobilization in bed (e.g., those in elongation casts, halo-pelvic casts, and particularly leg extension casts). The thrombophlebitis is caused by the complete immobilization of the limb, associated with a possible stretching of the vessels. Preventive measures include exercise and minimizing the period of immobilization. When possible, the limb to be immobilized can be alternated (14,21).

Psychological Problems

Problems of two different types may result from use of a cast: those associated with application of the cast, and those linked directly to the characteristics (e.g., dimensions, bulk) of the jacket. The latter are felt to be obstacles to human relationships, especially in adolescent patients. The cast makes them "different," which might lead to their exclusion from group activities (8,26).

Fear associated with the cast application may precipitate a dramatic reaction, particularly in young patients. They should be given a full explanation that includes the use of illustrative material, such as videotapes.

TREATMENT OF SCOLIOSIS

Risser's localizer cast and Cotrel's EDF cast are the most widely used plaster jackets and have been the basis of nonsurgical treatment for scoliosis for 40 years (4,19,22,26). The so-called Risser-Cotrel cast is a combination of the two techniques (14). We use Cotrel's method for the correction of curves with an apical vertebra higher than T8. For reduction of scoliosis with an apical vertebra at T8 or below, we use an original correction technique, developed by Salsano, based on a cast without longitudinal traction. This type of plaster jacket is well tolerated by the patient, and the incidence of complications is low (24,28).

The various casting techniques described below give similar angular correction. One cannot be said to be clearly better than another. Rather, each individual operator must find the technique that best suits him or her. Experience gained with a method invariably leads to personal modifications of the basic technique.

EDF Cast

On the basis of the principles for reduction of scoliosis described by Abbot, Cotrel perfected his frame and developed the EDF plaster jacket (4). The jacket was adopted by Stagnara in 1954 (26).

The patient is placed supine on a Cotrel frame (Fig. 4A). The pelvis is positioned on the special metal support, and the trunk lies on a longitudinal canvas strap 20 cm wide, which is removed when the patient has been placed in traction. A sling for occipitomandibular traction is applied and connected to a windlass at the head of the bed; the straps for pelvic traction are applied, and the legs are placed in the special support. The straps are connected to the windlasses at the foot of the frame, thus permitting traction to be applied to the pelvis. The patient is then gradually put in traction (Fig. 4B).

Some equipment is fitted with a dynamometer, but generally the appropriate traction force (which must never exceed the body weight) can be determined with a minimum of clinical experi-

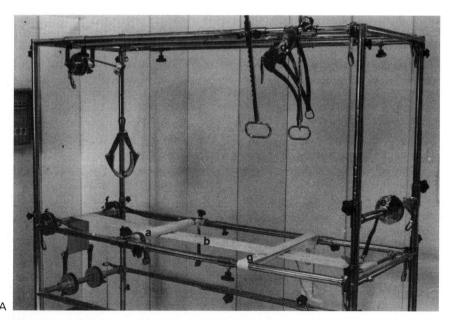

FIGURE 4. A: A Cotrel frame consisting of *(a)* sacral bar, *(b)* longitudinal strap, *(c)* foot board, *(d)* occipitomandibular sling, *(e)* windlass for cervical traction, *(f)* windlasses for pelvic traction, and *(g)* shoulder bar. *(Figure continues.)*

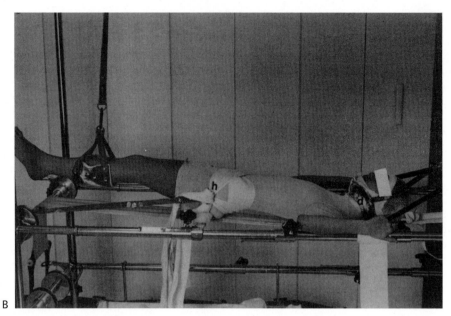

FIGURE 4. *Continued.* **B:** After application of pelvic straps *(h)* and of the occipitomandibular sling *(d),* traction is commenced before the longitudinal strap is removed.

ence. The longitudinal strap that supported the patient before traction was applied is removed. The correction maneuvers are then performed, applying the appropriate straps. Then the plaster bandages are applied, as described in the section on general technique, incorporating the straps. Many people, ourselves included, prefer to apply the correction straps after the plaster bandages have been applied. This procedure allows more mold-

ing of the jacket and reduces the possibility of wrinkles, but it requires very fast work.

Corrective Maneuvers

When the plaster bandages have been wound, the first derotating strap is applied. If there is only one curve, the strap is applied

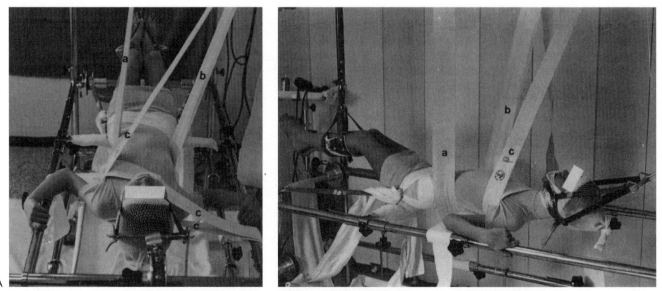

FIGURE 5. Correction with an EDF (elongation derotation flexion) cast, consisting of *(a)* lumbar derotation strap, *(b)* thoracic derotation strap, and *(c)* Y-shaped strap. **A:** Frontal view. **B:** Lateral view. A three-point system is formed by *(b)* on the convex side and *(a)* and *(c)* on the concave side.

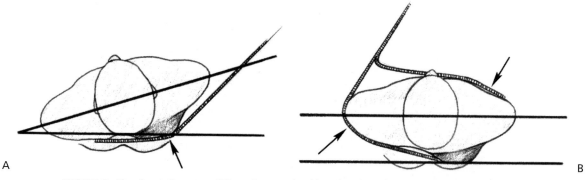

FIGURE 6. The derotation strap **(A)** produces a shoulder elevation; the Y-shaped strap **(B)** corrects shoulder imbalance.

on the convexity in such a way as to include the apical vertebra (Fig. 5). The strap is fixed with one end at the horizontal tube of the frame, on the side opposite the convexity. The strap passes around the rib hump from behind, comes forward, and is fixed to the tube on the other side of the superstructure so as to exit very laterally, pressing on the posterolateral part of the convexity and leaving the lateral part free.

The Y-shaped strap is then applied under the armpit on the concavity side. The two short arms of the Y encompass the armpit, passing under and over the trunk, respectively, and are fixed to the bed on the side opposite the armpit. The long arm is fixed to the superstructure, again on the side opposite the armpit (Fig. 5).

When the straps have been positioned, the windlasses are used to rotate the tubes of the Cotrel frame. As they rotate, they wind the straps around them and put the straps in tension.

Correction Mechanism

The reduction is obtained from the three forces that give their name to the cast: elongation, derotation, and flexion. Elongation is obtained by occipitopelvic traction. Derotation is obtained by the tension applied to the derotation strap fixed to the higher upright, using the Y-shaped strap as counterthrust. The pressure exerted on the ribs in a posteroanterior direction provokes rotation of the trunk in a direction opposite to that of the deformity; by acting with the Y-shaped strap, the rotation induced on the scapular band is balanced (Fig. 6). It is advisable to avoid applying the strap in such a way that the pressure is exerted on the lateral part of the ribs; this could lead to aggravation of rib deformity (Fig. 7).

Flexion is obtained by putting the thoracic strap in horizontal tension, thus producing translation of the trunk that is opposed by the Y-shaped strap and the pelvic traction or, in the case of a double curve, the lumbar strap. A three-point system is thus created (Fig. 5).

When the cast has been completed, it is trimmed with an anterior expansion window, with care taken to ensure that the anterior counterthrust on the chondrocostal zone of the side opposite the convexity is maintained; this makes the derotation

more effective. Posteriorly, windows are opened in the side opposite the convexity to permit felt application and provide further additional expansion zones. The window should be oblique, following the direction of the ribs (Fig. 8).

Localizer Cast

In the localizer cast, devised by Risser in 1946, correction is obtained by combining longitudinal traction and flexion, with the addition of localized pressure on the convexity. The patient, wearing a stockinette tube, is put on a Risser frame lying on the longitudinal canvas strap, with the pelvis on the sacral seat and the lower limbs on the footboard. The bony protrusions are protected by shaped felts. The pelvic part of the cast is applied with careful molding on the iliac crests. The patient is then placed in longitudinal traction. The lower traction is applied by straps that hold the pelvic cast. The upper traction is applied with the occipitomandibular sling. Initially traction is weak because it

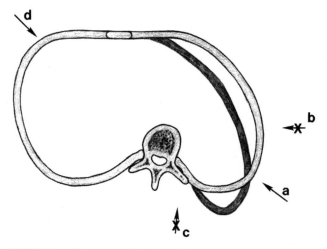

FIGURE 7. *a,* The correct direction of thrust is posterolateral. *b,* An excessively lateral thrust increases the rib hump. *c,* An excessively posterior thrust causes or increases lordosis. *d,* An anterolateral counterthrust facilitates correction of vertebral rotation.

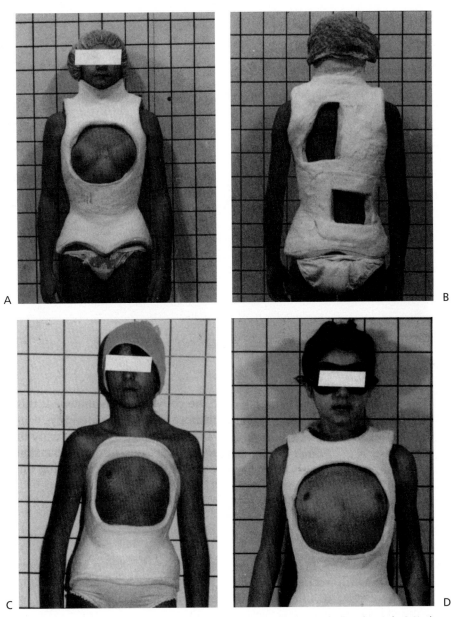

FIGURE 8. **A–D:** EDF (elongation derotation flexion) cast. **A** and **B:** Cast including the neck. **C:** Underarm cast. **D:** Cast with shoulder straps.

serves only to immobilize the patient. A cervical cast is made with molding on the mandible and occiput. After withdrawal of the occipitomandibular sling, cervical traction is applied by means of straps that hook the cervical cast. A localized pressure-application device is then applied, corresponding to the apex of the convexity. The presser is mounted on a threaded rod connected to a metal arc on which it can slide, altering its angle. Pressure is applied by advancing this rod.

Special attention is required in positioning the presser, which must act in a lateroposterior direction to be effective in vertebral derotation. In thoracic curves, the presser must be at right angles to the line tangential to the apex of the rib hump. If excessively lateral, it deforms the ribs and accentuates the hump. If exces-

sively posterior, it provokes thoracic lordosis (Fig. 7). In lumbar curves, the presser must be positioned on the paravertebral muscle masses. If it is excessively lateral, the force is exhausted on the abdominal wall. If excessively posterior, it accentuates lumbar lordosis.

Correction is obtained by combining pressure and traction. When the best correction possible has been obtained, the body cast is completed. Trunk alignment must be checked. The cast is then trimmed.

Body Cast without Traction

This is the type of cast we currently use for conservative treatment of scoliosis (24,28). Its principal characteristic is elimina-

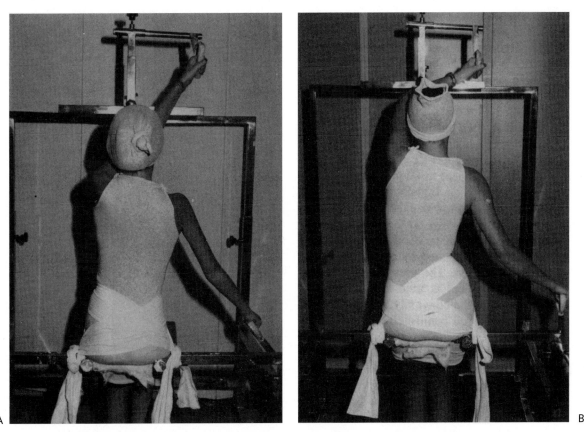

FIGURE 9. A: Thoracic scoliosis. The patient is placed in the bending position; the pelvic straps are fixed symmetrically to the bar. **B:** Lumbar scoliosis. The pelvic straps are fixed asymmetrically.

tion of any form of longitudinal traction; correction of the curve is obtained by a bending maneuver associated with a localized pressure.

We use a specially constructed metal frame, but any device that allows the patient to be appropriately positioned can be used. The patient, wearing a stockinette tube, sits on the cross-bar, which is adjustable in height, with 80 degrees of hip flexion to reduce lumbar lordosis. The pelvis is fixed to the bar with two textile straps passed over the iliac crests and crossed (Fig. 9). The patient is placed in the bending position. The operator sits behind the patient, with an assistant seated in front. After a layer of water-repellent cotton has been applied, the cast is executed. During hardening of the plaster, a strong force is applied to the convexity directly with the hand.

Thoracic Scoliosis

The straps that fix the pelvis are applied symmetrically (Fig. 9A). Manual pressure on the convexity, applied during hardening, should not go past the rib corresponding to the apical vertebra. With the other hand, the operator applies a counterpressure under the armpit, thus creating a three-point system (pelvis and armpit on the side of the concavity, and pressure on the ribs on the convex side) (Fig. 10). The assistant applies a thoracic force anteriorly to complete the derotation action and rebalance the

rotation of the shoulders provoked by the posterior thrust (Fig. 11A).

Lumbar and Thoracolumbar Scoliosis

The straps on the pelvis are applied asymmetrically (Fig. 9B). On the concave side, the strap is placed slightly lower, so as not to oppose the thrust on the convexity. The waist needs molding only on the convex side. The thrust must act on the paravertebral muscles and not go beyond the apex of the curve. The assistant executes an anterior abdominal-pelvic counterthrust.

Double Major Scoliosis

The cast can be applied in two stages, correcting first the lumbar and then the thoracic curve. When the lumbar curve is very flexible, the cast can be applied in one operation. In this case, the pelvic straps are applied asymmetrically, and correction of the lumbar curve is obtained by molding of the flank and by hand pressure. The thoracic curve is corrected with bending and hand pressure.

Trimming

Trimming is done as for an underarm cast. A window is opened anteriorly on the thorax and posteriorly on the concave side of

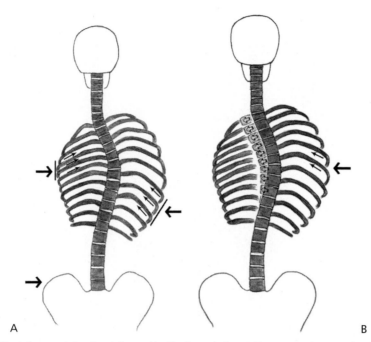

A   B

FIGURE 10.   A three-point system is formed by the thoracic thrust, the counterthrust under the armpits, and the pelvic hold. **A:** The thoracic thrust must be applied not to the apex vertebra but along the rib that joins it. **B:** If the thoracic thrust is too high, it causes an increase of the curve.

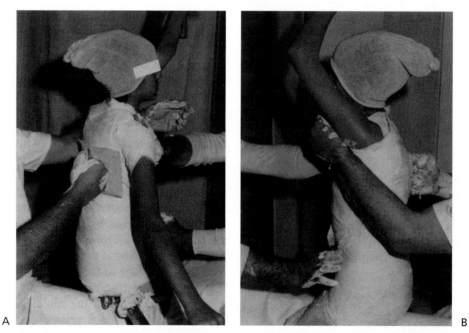

A   B

FIGURE 11. A: Pressure on the rib hump is applied. A counterthrust is applied below the armpits. Anterior counterthrusts and shoulder balance are provided by the assistant. **B:** Felt padding.

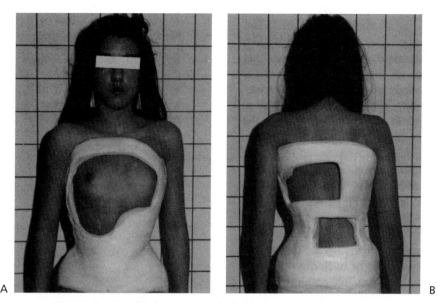

FIGURE 12. **A** and **B:** Body cast applied without traction after trimming.

each curve. Posterior windows are opened so that felt padding can be inserted that corresponds with the apex of the convexity (Fig. 11B). This is an important step: the felt must be thick enough to exert a molding action on the convexity but not so thick as to cause pressure problems for the patient (Fig. 12). At the thoracic level, the felt must be positioned to cover a long part of the ribs; the felt must never go beyond the rib that joins the apical vertebra.

Preoperative and Postoperative Casts

Until the late 1970s the rationale for using postoperative casts (e.g., Risser, Risser-Cotrel, EDF) was to achieve and maintain the correction after a vertebral arthrodesis without instrumentation. When a spinal instrumentation was applied, such as a Harrington rod, postoperative casts were used to protect and support stability.

Preoperative casts (e.g., Stagnara's elongation cast, halo-pelvic) were used to correct high-angle rigid spinal deformities.

The great advantage of preoperative casts was that they permitted adaptation of the vascular and nervous structures of the spinal cord with slow, gradual correction of the curves, thereby considerably reducing the risks associated with intraoperative correction and improving the final result.

In the 1980s, the advent of new spine instrumentation (e.g., Luque, Cotrel-Dubousset, Texas Scottish Rite Hospital) considerably improved the operative outcome of correction and stability of scoliosis. As a result, the use of preoperative and postoperative casts became obsolete.

Elongation Cast

Devised by Stagnara (26), the elongation cast is based on the cast of Donaldson and Engh (5), but it differs in the absence of armpit thrusts and the presence of an occipitomandibular

support. It has upper and lower parts connected by Donaldson screws, which have metal fins at the ends for fixing to the cast (Fig. 13A).

Symmetrically elongation is commenced when the plaster is completely dry (after 24 to 48 hours), first rapidly (two to three turns a day), then more slowly (one turn per day).

The cast does not prevent walking, which is easy in the first few days but becomes increasingly difficult as distraction develops.

This type of cast is well tolerated initially, but tolerance decreases as distention develops.

The most common neurologic disturbances are those affecting the lower limbs. Arm disturbances are rare and are caused by compression of the armpit by the subaxillary rings rather than by distraction of the brachial plexus. Daily checking of the deep-tendon reflexes and muscular strength and sensation is required. If disturbances appear, elongation should be stopped or reduced.

Halo Cast

The halo cast is a device that can be used both to immobilize the spine and to distract the spine. It is applied to immobilize the spine after fractures have occurred, especially in the cervical and upper thoracic spine, or after spinal fusion, cervical or cervicothoracic arthrodesis, or spinal instrumentation believed to be unstable (12,16). A body cast with shoulder straps is generally applied, and the halo is connected to it. A pelvic cast can be applied when it is advisable to keep the thorax completely free (Fig. 13B).

As a distraction system the halo cast was applied in major, rigid scoliosis, when a gradual preoperative correction was desired. In such cases, a pelvic cast was always applied.

When the halo cast is used as a distraction system, typical halo traction–related complications occur, such as infected pins

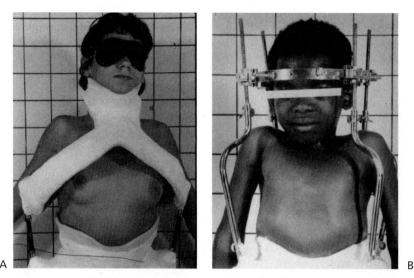

FIGURE 13. **A:** Elongation cast. **B:** Halo-pelvic cast.

or neurologic problems (e.g., paraplegia, cranial nerve lesions, lesions of the brachial plexus, halo slippage, necrosis of the dens epistrophei, diastasis of the atlantoaxial joint, and degeneration of the posterior joints) (13,14,17,18,20,27,29).

TREATMENT OF KYPHOSIS

Correction of a kyphotic curve is possible using two different types of force: traction and bending. There are two types of casts most commonly used in the treatment of kyphosis: the hyperextension cast, which uses both forces; and the two-stage cast, which uses only bending.

In regular kyphoses with the apex up to T8, both jackets give similar angular corrections. In high kyphoses with the apex above T7 and in posttraumatic angular kyphoses, the hyperextension cast is more effective. The hyperextension cast can be used for all types of kyphosis regardless of the height of the apex, but there are some disadvantages: The traction is poorly tolerated by patients, the cast cannot be applied on an outpatient basis, and complex equipment (a Cotrel or Risser-Cotrel frame) is required to apply it.

The two-stage cast can be used only for kyphoses with the apex up to T8. It is well tolerated by patients, can be applied on an outpatient basis, and does not require complex equipment for its application. In reality, because most kyphoses have their apex around T8, either type could be used. We generally prefer the two-stage cast because it is well tolerated, inexpensive, and simple to apply.

Hyperextension Jacket

After being enveloped in a stockinette tube that covers the neck and the trunk, the patient is placed supine on a Cotrel frame and put gradually in traction. The cast is prepared, as described in "EDF Cast," with occipitomandibular support or with only sternal support.

The correction is made through both traction and bending. Traction is provided by the windlasses connected to the occipito-mandibular sling and pelvic straps; bending is obtained from a U-shaped strap passing over the apex of the kyphosis and fixed to the superstructure of the frame (Fig. 14). The strap is put under tension by two windlasses until the patient—held on the frame by pelvic and cranial traction—is lifted slightly. This results in a three-point system with a fulcrum on the apex of the kyphosis, which provokes hyperextension of the thoracic spine. It is essential to remember that the hyperextension provided in this phase by the U-shaped strap produces an alteration in the traction; the extent of the traction must be constantly checked and appropriate corrections made.

The jacket is trimmed craniad with a sternal hold; if the apex is high or there is significant forward projection of the head, the neck is included. The thorax should be extensively windowed.

Two-Stage Jacket

The patient is placed in a half-sitting position. With hip flexion to 80 degrees and forward bending of the trunk, a reduction in the lumbar lordosis is obtained. The patient is asked to keep arms abducted to 90 degrees with the hands on the specific supports. It may be useful, though not essential, to fix the pelvis to the bar with straps. The cotton is applied first, followed by the plaster bandages. It is advisable to adequately pad not only the crests but also the apex of the kyphosis (Fig. 15A). The jacket must include the trunk up to the apex of the kyphosis posteriorly and up to the lower margin of the thoracic cage anteriorly. Molding must be performed while the plaster is set-

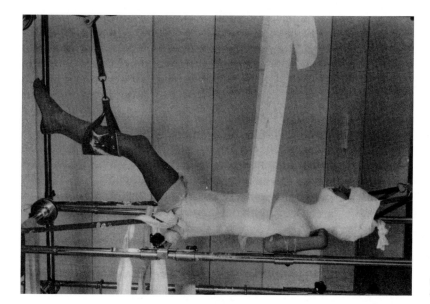

FIGURE 14. Kyphosis correction with U-shaped strap on a Cotrel frame.

ting. The waist must be molded and a pubic thrust executed to reduce the lordosis.

When the cast has set, it is trimmed posteriorly to the level of the apex. The patient is then placed supine on a frame in such a way that the trunk protrudes (Fig. 15B). A correction in hyperextension is thus obtained by gravity, using the apex of the kyphosis as a fulcrum without using traction (Fig. 16). The second stage of the jacket is executed in this position and consists of completion of the anterior part. The pectoral region is left free, and the cast is molded carefully at the level of the sternoclavicular

joints and the sternum, where the thrust is created (Fig. 15B). The patient is put upright and the effectiveness of the thrust is checked. If it is insufficient, felt padding is added as necessary.

Complications secondary to plaster casts have already been discussed extensively. At this point, we mention only some specific problems. In thin patients with very little vertebral muscle mass, the apex of the spinous process may be particularly protuberant. In such cases, the thrust applied to the apex may be poorly tolerated or cause a pressure sore. This problem can be solved by means of two felt pads, one on either side of the spine,

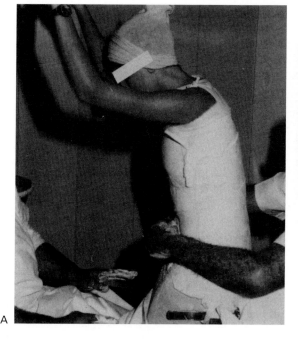

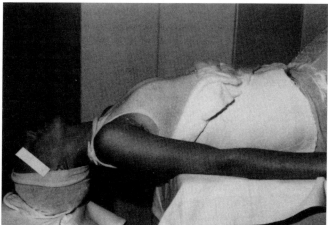

FIGURE 15. Two-stage cast. **A:** First stage. **B:** Second stage—correction of kyphosis by gravity; a sternal thrust fixes the correction.

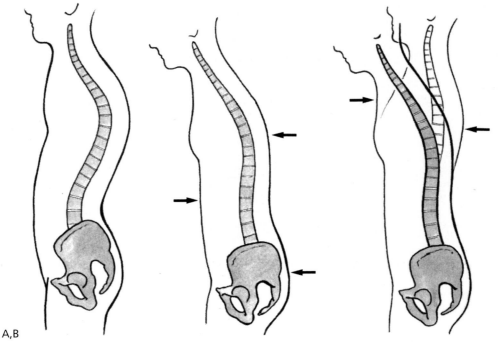

FIGURE 16. Two-stage cast. **A:** Hyperkyphosis. **B:** First stage—forward bending of the trunk and hip flexion produce a reduction in the lordosis. A further reduction is obtained with a three-point system formed by abdominal pressure and by two posterior thrusts on the sacrum and at the kyphosis apex. **C:** Second stage—the correction in hyperextension, obtained by gravity, is fixed by the sternal thrust.

to redistribute the force over a larger area, leaving the spinous process free.

SUMMARY

To achieve successful outcomes using the casts described in this chapter, a great deal of attention to detail is required. Application techniques are demanding. Potential complications must be detected and treated promptly.

ACKNOWLEDGMENT

Dr. Vittorio Salsano died in November 1998. We will miss him.

REFERENCES

1. Abbott EG (1911): Simple rapid and complete reduction of deformity in fixed lateral curvature of the spine. *N Y Med* 63(25):1208–1219.
2. Birney TJ, Hanley EN Jr (1989): Traumatic cervical spine injuries in childhood and adolescence. *Spine* 14(12):1277–1282.
3. Bradford DS, Moe JH, Winter RB (1975): Scoliosis. In: Rothman RH, Simeone FA, eds. *The spine*. Philadelphia: WB Saunders, pp. 271–386.
4. Cotrel Y, Morel G (1964): Le technique de l'E.D.F. dans la correction des scolioses. *Rev Chir Orthop* 50:59–75.
5. Donaldson J, Engh OA (1938): Correction of scoliosis by distraction apparatus. *J Bone Joint Surg* 20:405–410.
6. Evarts CM, Winter RB, Hall JE (1971): Vascular compression of the duodenum associated with the treatment of scoliosis. *J Bone Joint Surg Am* 53:431.
7. Fielding WJ, Hensinger RM (1984): Fractures of the spine. In: Rockwood et al., eds. *Fractures in children*. Philadelphia: JB Lippincott.
8. Henry J, Rodot JC (1979): L'avenir socio-professional du scoliotique. In: Adler, ed. *Journees de la scoliose*. Lyon: Association Lyonnaise pour le Développement des Etudes du Rachis.
9. Hoeffel JC, Lascombes P, Schmitt M, et al. (1992): Peptic esophagitis and scoliosis in children. Ann Pediatr Paris 39(9):561–565.
10. Kennedy RH, Cooper MJ (1983): An unusually severe case of the cast syndrome. *Postgrad Med* J 59:539.
11. Luck JV (1944): Plaster of paris cast: an experimental and clinical analysis. *JAMA* 124:23–29.
12. Marks DS, Roberts P, Wilton PJ, et al. (1993): A halo jacket for stabilisation of the paediatric cervical spine. *Arch Orthop Trauma Surg* 112(3): 134
13. Moe JH (1967): Complications of scoliosis treatment. *Clin Orthop* 53: 21.
14. Moe DH, Winter RB, Bradford DS, et al. (1988): *Scoliosis and other spinal deformities*. Philadelphia: WB Saunders, 393–427, 467–484.
15. Munns SW, Morrissy RT, Golladay ES, et al. (1984): Hyperalimentation for superior mesenteric artery (cast) syndrome following correction of spinal deformity. *J Bone Joint Surg Am* 66:1175.
16. Nickel VL, Perry J, Garret A, et al. (1968): The halo. *J Bone Joint Surg Am* 50:1400.
17. O'Brien JP (1975): The halo pelvic apparatus. *Acta Orthop Scand* 163 (Suppl):79.
18. O'Brien JP, Yau AC, Smith TK, et al. (1971): Halo pelvic traction. *J Bone Joint Surg Br* 53:217.
19. Ollier M (1971): *Techniques des platres et corsets des scolioses*. Paris: Masson, pp. 45–74.
20. Perry J (1972): The halo in spinal abnormalities. Practical factors and avoidance of complications. *Orthop Clin N Am* 3:69.
21. Reilmann H, Bosch U, Barthels M (1988): Thromboembolieprophylaxe in der chirurgie. *Orthopade* 17:110.

22. Risser JC (1966): Treatment of scoliosis during the past 50 years. *Clin Orthop* 44:109.
23. Sayre LA (1878): *Spinal disease and spinal curvature.* London: Smith-Elder.
24. Salsano V, Turturro F, Montanaro A (1988): Trattamento della scoliosi con apparecchi gessati senza trazione. *Progressi Patologia Vertebrale* 10:271–277.
25. Scales JT, Lunn HF, Jeneid PA, et al. (1974): The prevention and treatment of pressure sores using air-support systems. *Paraplegia* 12:118–131.
26. Stagnara P (1985): *Les déformations du rachis.* Paris: Masson, 199–239, 240–316, 395–401.
27. Tredwell SJ, O'Brien JP (1975): Avascular necrosis of the proximal end of the dens. *J Bone Joint Surg Am* 57:332.
28. Turturro F, Costici PF, Montanaro A, et al. (1996): Risultati a distanza del trattamento della scoliosi con apparecchi gessati senza trazione. Follow up 2 anni. *Progressi Patologia Vertebrale* 19(Suppl):65–70.
29. Victor DI, Bresnan MJ, Keller RB (1973): Brain abscess complicating the use of halo traction. *J Bone Joint Surg Am* 55:635.
30. Volker ES, James HS (1973): Mechanical properties of orthopedic plaster bandages. *J Biomech* 6:173–185.
31. White AA, Panjabi MM (1977): *Clinical biomechanics of the spine.* Philadelphia: JB Lippincott, 345–373.
32. Wullstein L, Schulthess W (1902): Die Skoliose in inrer Behandlung und Entschung nach klinischen und experimentellen Studien. *Z Orthop Clin* 10:178.

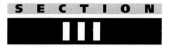

SECTION III

BONE BANKING, GRAFTING, AND SUBSTITUTES

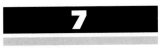

BIOLOGY OF BONE GRAFTING: AUTOGRAFTS, ALLOGRAFTS, SUBSTITUTES

ANDREI A. CZITROM

The use of bone as tissue graft was one of the first surgical transplantation approaches. Throughout the twentieth century, it has been the most commonly performed surgical tissue transfer other than that of skin and blood (19). Bone grafting has a major role in most orthopaedic subspecialties, but its importance and frequency of use are greatest in spinal surgery.

The aim of this chapter is to discuss the basic biology of bone grafting, with special emphasis on how autogenous bone grafts differ from allografts or bone substitutes in terms of healing, incorporation, and remodeling. This comparison is prompted by the increased use of bone allografts and bone substitutes in pediatric and adult spinal surgery. These developments coincide with an unprecedented availability of allografts and substitute materials to the pediatric spine surgeon. The understanding of the basic biology should guide the surgeon when choosing the method of grafting. A critical analysis of current literature on the use of allografts and substitutes is presented to further guide the pediatric spine surgeon in clinical applications.

BONE AUTOGRAFTS

Concept of Clinical Success

From a biologic point of view, the process of "healing" of a bone graft implies the complete union of the graft to the host bed; "incorporation" refers to the complete remodeling of the graft and its integration with host bone. Clinically, these two processes cannot always be well defined or separated. Consequently, the clinical success of a bone graft is often defined as "an ability to withstand physiological load" (51). Clearly, this clinical end result has an underlying biologic explanation in terms of healing and incorporation, but it is important to understand that this end result does not always require a complete remodeling of the graft. On the one hand, a cancellous graft used to fill a bone defect in the metaphysis of a long bone has to heal (unite) and incorporate (remodel) completely before the

construct can withstand load and thus be defined as a clinical success. On the other hand, a cortical intercalary graft used to reconstruct a segmental defect in the diaphysis of a long bone can unite solidly with host bone and represent clinical success despite the fact that it has not incorporated to any significant extent. This distinction brings out the complexity of the biology of bone graft repair and demonstrates that ultimately the clinical success of grafts has to be judged according to the functions they were designed to fulfill. In pediatric spinal surgery, the principal function of bone grafts is to achieve arthrodesis of vertebral segments. This goal requires complete healing (union) and incorporation (remodeling) of the grafts. A clinical success in this situation is a solid fusion of vertebral segments, which would allow the corrected spine to withstand physiological load, in theory without the support of the instrumentation system used initially to achieve the surgical correction. Having an understanding of the healing and incorporation process of bone grafts is a prerequisite for the rational choice of an appropriate graft material to fulfill the goal of clinical success in pediatric spinal fusions.

Unique Biologic Functions

The healing and incorporation of cancellous and cortical bone autografts follow biologic events centered around bone formation and resorption. These events differ importantly for the two types of grafts because of the difference in structure between cancellous and cortical bone. Before discussing these differences, it is appropriate to define and explain those important biologic functions (unique to bone tissue) that allow the successful healing and incorporation of bone grafts: osteogenesis, osteoclastic resorption, osteoconduction, and osteoinduction.

Osteogenesis

Osteogenesis represents the ability of bone to regenerate as a result of the production of new bone by osteoblasts. The process of bone formation after bone grafting may originate from either the host bed or the graft. A significant number of graft osteoblasts survive after transplantation. These osteoblasts are able to

A. A. Czitrom: Clinical Associate Professor of Orthopaedic Surgery, University of Texas Southwestern Medical Center, Medical City Dallas, Dallas, Texas 75230.

produce new bone and contribute to the healing and incorporation of both cancellous and cortical autologous bone grafts (15,16,54).

Osteoclastic Resorption

Osteoclastic resorption is the ability of bone to remove mineral by the activity of osteoclasts. This process is of paramount importance for healing and remodeling after bone grafting because it allows the removal of dead bone and its replacement with live bone (by osteogenesis from osteoblasts). The process of replacement of dead bone with live bone by the combination of osteoclastic resorption and osteogenesis is referred to as *creeping substitution* (91).

Osteoconduction

Osteoconduction is a special property of bone tissue that allows the spatial ingrowth of capillaries, perivascular tissue, and osteoprogenitor cells from the host bed and thus permits the gradual replacement of the graft by new host bone (by the process of creeping substitution). Osteoconduction does not require live cells and works as a scaffold of collagen, noncollagenous proteins, and hydroxyapatite that have the right spatial arrangement for new bone ingrowth. This natural property of bone tissue allows its regeneration after replacement by processed allografts or bone substitutes (56,88,119).

Osteoinduction

Osteoinduction is the unique property of bone tissue to stimulate new bone formation by the differentiation of mesenchymal pluripotential progenitor cells. This property of bone is mediated by bone matrix-derived soluble proteins that are part of the transforming growth factor beta (TGF-β) superfamily, including several bone morphogenic proteins (BMP-2, BMP-4, BMP-5, BMP-6), osteogenin (BMP-3), osteogenic protein (BMP-7), TGF-$\beta_{(1-5)}$, and other TGF-β-like proteins (24,64,78,97). Osteoinduction does not require live cells and is activated when bone is demineralized (49,50,53,103). The process of bone formation by osteoinduction is an orderly process of recruitment of mesenchymal cells that differentiate into cartilage cells, with subsequent bone formation by endochondral ossification (50,96). Given the amplitude of the experimental data available, it is likely that osteoinduction is important in both the healing and incorporation of bone grafts.

Cancellous Bone Autografts

The process of healing and incorporation of cancellous bone autografts follows an orderly sequence of histologically recognizable physiologic events that are similar to those seen in fracture healing (51). In the early phase, which lasts for approximately 3 weeks, inflammation and organization of the hematoma in the area of bone grafting predominate the biologic events. Osteocytes and osteoblasts of the graft that survive the transplantation process are nourished by diffusion from surrounding tissues and

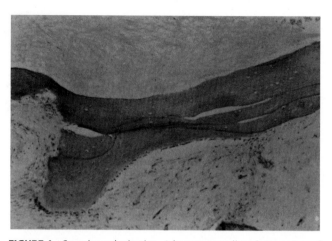

FIGURE 1. Creeping substitution. A human cancellous bone autograft retrieved during the late phase of healing shows the typical histologic features of creeping substitution at the junction of host and graft tissue. The trabecula of the graft is dead, with no surviving cells in the lacunae. Similarly, the marrow spaces of the graft *(top)* are completely necrotic. Host cells have invaded the graft *(bottom)*; osteoblasts are lining the surface of the dead trabecula, producing new bone; and osteoclasts are actively resorbing the necrotic bone *(left)* (hematoxylineosin, ×40). (Courtesy of Rita Kandel M.D., Department of Pathology, Mount Sinai Hospital, University of Toronto, Toronto, Canada.)

are capable of producing new bone (15). Vascular invasion from the host bed occurs quickly and is accompanied by migration of primitive mesenchymal cells into the graft, which differentiate into osteoblasts. Osteoblasts begin to line the edges of the bone trabeculae and produce seams of osteoid that are deposited around central cores of necrotic bone. After a new viable trabecula of bone has formed, osteoclasts resorb the necrotic trabecula. This is the beginning of the process of creeping substitution (51,91,94), which starts during the early phase and continues until the graft is remodeled (Fig. 1). The hallmark of this process is the *simultaneous formation and resorption of bone*, which occurs during the healing and incorporation of cancellous autografts and is not seen with cortical autografts.

The late phase is characterized by ongoing active bone resorption and formation by host cells, and by continuous remodeling and replacement of the graft. This phase relies on the osteoconductive property of the bone graft, which acts as a scaffold for its own replacement with viable host bone. The duration of this phase depends on the depth and surface area of the defect to be remodeled and can last anywhere from 3 months to a year. Eventually, the graft is totally resorbed and replaced by host bone and bone marrow, which remodels according to Wolff's law (66).

Cortical Bone Autografts

The process of healing and incorporation of cortical autografts is different from that of cancellous grafts. The sequence of events during creeping substitution is slower and the replacement process is very limited and prolonged because of the structure of cortical bone. The lamellar nature of cortical bone organized around Volkmann's and haversian canals precludes early vascular invasion and migration of mesenchymal cells into the graft as it occurs in cancellous bone. In cortical bone, the early phase of inflammation and hematoma formation is followed by very slow revascularization. Only at the junction sites with host bone can bone formation occur early by the contribution of surviving graft endosteal cells. At the junction sites, vascular invasion follows, and host osteoclasts and osteoblasts remodel the junction site, leading to union usually within 3 to 6 months. However, within the main substance of the graft, the nutrient canals have to be penetrated by vascular channels before remodeling can begin. This is a slow process that allows osteoclasts to begin resorbing Volkmann's and haversian systems (38,51). Lamellar bone is resorbed very slowly, and only after its resorption can replacement begin. Thus, although the junction sites of cortical grafts unite, their body remains avascular for prolonged periods. The hallmark of this healing and incorporation process is *the obligatory slow resorption of lamellar bone and the lack of simultaneous bone formation* in cortical autografts, unlike the simultaneous formation and resorption seen in cancellous autografts.

The late phase of healing and incorporation of cortical autografts can last indefinitely and represents the ongoing biologic process by which the host attempts to incorporate the graft. During this time, resorption supersedes formation, and cortical autografts become significantly osteoporotic secondary to vascular invasion from the surrounding host bed. Thus, these grafts are weaker than normal bone; the duration of this weakness depends on the size of the graft and persists for years (38,51). In most cases, cortical autografts remain an admixture of dead and live bone indefinitely and continue remodeling over years while protected by internal fixation devices.

The main difference in the healing and incorporation pattern of cancellous and cortical bone grafts is the early formation of new bone on top of necrotic trabeculae before resorption in the former, as opposed to the obligatory resorption of haversian systems followed by formation in the latter. Thus, cancellous grafts do not lose strength during the healing process as cortical grafts do. The healing of cancellous grafts is significantly faster than that of cortical grafts (108). It is for this reason that cancellous and corticocancellous iliac crest autograft is the traditional grafting material used in spinal fusions. It is important to know that vascularized cortical and corticocancellous autografts follow a different and much more rapid course of incorporation than their conventional nonvascularized counterparts because of their ability to remodel independently of the host bed (51,108). Because of this advantage, vascularized bone grafts have special applications in the pediatric spine, as discussed in Chapter 17.

BONE ALLOGRAFTS AND SUBSTITUTES

Fresh Bone Allografts in Heterotopic Transplantation

The differences in the biologic behavior of transplanted autologous (or syngeneic) and allogeneic bone can best be demonstrated in heterotopic models because the contribution of the host bed to the bone formation process can be eliminated. One such model is to transplant finely crushed fragments of syngeneic or allogeneic diaphyseal femoral bone under the kidney capsule in inbred mice. The advantages of this system are the known genetic differences of the inbred mouse strains, the excellent vascularity of the recipient site, and its facilitation of study of the transplanted tissue next to the kidney parenchymal tissue without interference from other mesenchymal tissues. The outcome of such an experiment at 4 weeks after transplantation is shown in Figure 2. The syngeneic bone transplant survives and forms a live ossicle with marrow spaces right next to the kidney

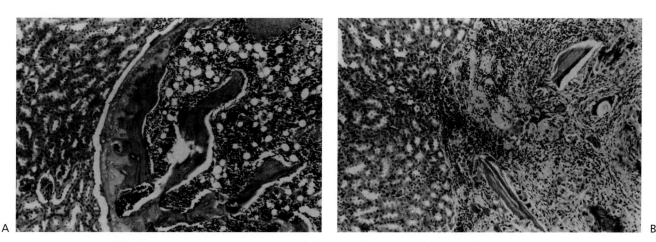

A   B

FIGURE 2. Heterotopic transplantation. Equal amounts of finely crushed diaphyseal femoral bone fragments from DBA (H-2^d) mice were transplanted under the kidney capsule of syngeneic DBA (H-2^d) and allogeneic CBA (H-2^k) recipients. **A:** At 4 weeks after transplantation, the syngeneic graft is alive and has formed an ossicle with marrow spaces adjacent to the normal kidney parenchyma; there is no inflammatory response. **B:** The allogeneic transplant is almost completely resorbed; a violent immune cellular infiltrate is seen, with only a few fragments of necrotic graft remaining (hematoxylin-eosin, ×325). (From Czitrom AA [1989]: Bone transplantation, passenger cells and the major histocompatibility complex. In: Aebi M, Regazzoni P, eds. *Bone transplantation.* Berlin: Springer-Verlag, pp. 103–110, with permission.)

capsule, without any untoward cellular response from the host (Fig. 2A). The allogeneic transplant is violently rejected by a strong lymphocytic infiltrate, there is no bone formation, and the remaining necrotic fragments of bone are almost completely resorbed (Fig. 2B). This result demonstrates the immunogenicity of fresh bone allografts and the profound difference between the biologic behavior of syngeneic bone grafts (equivalent to autologous grafts) and that of allografts. The classic experiments of Chalmers (15,16) analyzed the time sequence of these biologic events, demonstrating that bone formation by autografts starts at 4 days after transplantation, peaks at 16 days, and continues for 6 months; allografts form bone for only 14 days before they are rejected by the immune system. Such experimental data establish that fresh bone allografts are immunogenic in a true sense, as are skin grafts, and that they undergo a true rejection process when transplanted to heterotopic sites. However, bone transplantation is different from the transplantation of other nonvascular tissues because of the unique property of bone tissue that allows regeneration of host bone on the osteoconductive scaffold of its matrix (hydroxyapatite, collagen, and noncollagenous proteins).

Fresh Bone Allografts in Orthotopic Transplantation

When bone allografts are transplanted orthotopically, the rejection process is more subtle and can be detected and quantitated only as a delay in the remodeling process of allografts compared with that of equivalent autografts. This type of observation is illustrated in Figure 3, which shows the remodeling of orthotopic cortical bone grafts in dogs at 20 weeks after transplantation. The remodeling, as measured by serial fluorochrome labeling on both longitudinal (Fig. 3A, C) and transverse (Fig. 3B, D) sections, is significantly more advanced in autografts than allografts. This is an indicator of immunologic recognition of orthotopic fresh bone transplants but does not preclude their use for the purpose of osteoconductive grafts. Indeed, the clinical use of fresh osteochondral allografts has been documented as a means of resurfacing joint defects (73). In this circumstance, fresh grafts are used for the purpose of preserving chondrocyte viability within the articular component (34). The bone components of these grafts are small and, although their live marrow component is rejected, they still function as osteoconductors, with ultimate union and incorporation by the host (87). This illustrates the point made previously that bone is unique among transplanted tissues because of its osteoconductive property, which, at orthotopic sites, allows successful transplantation despite immunologic rejection of the live cellular component.

The Immune Response to Fresh Bone Allografts

Allogeneic organs or tissues that are transplanted without immunosuppression provoke a rejection response by the host immune system. This transplantation response has an afferent arm consisting of the events that trigger and stimulate the immune system (30) and an efferent arm that includes the effector mechanisms that ultimately lead to graft rejection (26). The immune response to bone allografts can be assessed by a variety of methods, including histology (15,16,19,61); in vivo assays of cellular immunity, such as measuring the reaction of regional lymph nodes or skin grafting (9,12,13,15); measurements of humoral immunity (37,46,55,68); and in vitro assays of cell-mediated immunity (44,59,68,83,114). All of these methods indicate that bone allografts, when transplanted fresh, are rejected by the immune system and sensitize the host to alloantigens of the donor. The major immunogenic elements of allograft organs or tissues are marrow-derived cells, commonly referred to as antigen-presenting cells (APCs). These cells express class II major histocompatibility complex (MHC) molecules and are capable of delivering a second signal required to activate the T-lymphocyte system (30,67,107,117). In bone allografts, the majority of immunogenic cells reside in the bone marrow component, as shown conclusively by bone marrow depletion experiments (12,14,83) and radiation chimera repopulation studies (39,70). The APCs in bone marrow are myeloid cells of the granulocyte lineage, which share many properties with dendritic cells in lymphoid organs (25,31,32). Bone cells (osteocytes and osteoblasts) and osteoclasts express class I and class II MHC antigens and have immunogenic properties in vitro (44,59,85,104,105). Knowing that allograft reactivity is triggered by specialized cells and is directed at cell surface alloantigens, it is evident that immune responses generated to matrix components, such as proteoglycans and collagen, are not relevant to immunity in bone transplantation but may be important in autoimmunity (17,113). The living cells expressing cell surface alloantigens in bone allografts are killed or removed by processing of bone tissue, thus decreasing or eliminating its immunogenicity.

Processed Bone Allografts

The principal methods of processing bone allografts are deep-freezing, freeze-drying, and demineralization. Processing of bone allografts allows their preservation and storage for clinical use. The processing of bone allografts is done at regional tissue banks that are accredited by the American Association of Tissue Banks and meet well-documented standards (1,2,81). Donors are screened for acute or chronic infection, malignancy or irradiation, systemic disease of any kind, venereal disease, hepatitis, slow-virus disease, AIDS, drug abuse or toxic substances in tissues, steroid treatment or osteoporosis, immune complex disease, any disease of unknown cause, and unexplained death. This is done by obtaining a detailed medical and social history from the donor or from the next of kin or friends of the deceased. Serologic screening includes testing for syphilis (Venereal Disease Research Laboratory or rapid plasmin reagin test), hepatitis B (antigen and antibody), AIDS (anti-HIV-1 and anti-HIV-2 antibody), and hepatitis C (anti-HCV antibody). The seronegativity for HIV can last for up to 3 years (60,62), but modern tests allow the early pickup and exclusion of positive donors (29,60,81). Sterilization of processed musculoskeletal allograft tissues is an additional safety measure against infection. The most common methods are gas sterilization with ethylene oxide (450 to 1,500 mg/L at 30% to 60% humidity and 21°C) and gamma irradiation (1.5 to 2.5 Mrad from a cobalt-60 source), which has been shown to inactivate HIV (29,65,81,106). Sterili-

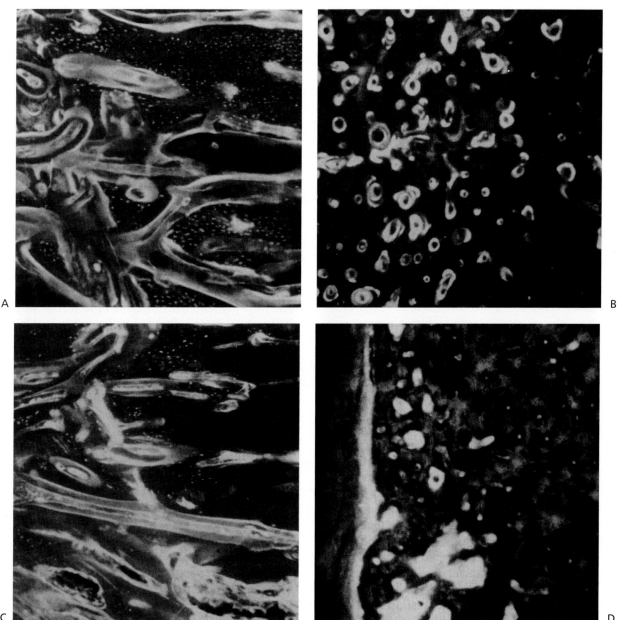

FIGURE 3. Orthotopic transplantation. Diaphyseal autograft and allograft bone segments were transplanted in dogs and assessed at 20 weeks after serial fluorochrome labeling. **A:** Longitudinal section of autologous transplant at the host-graft junction (graft on the *right*) showing both early and extensive remodeling, indicated by the brightly stained areas with an abundance of fluorochromes administered during the first 2 to 4 weeks after transplantation. **B:** Transverse section through the midportion of the autograft showing advanced remodeling (brightly stained osteons) extending from the surface *(left)* toward the medullary canal and spanning two thirds of the cortical diameter. **C:** Longitudinal section of the allograft at the host-graft junction (graft on the *right*) showing late and limited remodeling, indicated by a paucity of early fluorochrome labeling. **D:** Transverse section through the middle of the allograft showing limited remodeling, with brightly stained osteons confined to the outer periphery of the cortex. (Courtesy of Dr. O. Schwarzenbach and Dr. M. Aebi, Inselspital, University of Bern, Bern, Switzerland. From Czitrom AA [1992]: Immunology of bone and cartilage allografts. In: Czitrom AA, Gross AE, eds. *Allografts in orthopaedic practice.* Baltimore: Williams & Wilkins, pp. 15–25, with permission.)

zation is generally used for tissues that are procured in clean but nonsterile operating room type of environments and subsequently processed by freeze-drying or demineralization.

Deep-freezing at −70°C or in liquid nitrogen at −196°C is the simplest method of preserving bone allografts and other connective tissue transplants. The cells in deep-frozen grafts are killed by the freezing process but not removed; therefore, they still contain membrane fragments of cell surface alloantigens. The shelf life of frozen bone stored at −70°C is 5 years; at −20°C it is only 6 months. The method of deep-freezing is employed for the preservation of large-fragment structural grafts used for limb salvage after tumor surgery or in prosthetic hip revision surgery. *Freeze-drying* requires special equipment to remove water in a vacuum and allows the storage of bones and other connective tissues at room temperature. Freeze-drying removes all cells and all water from bone allografts, leaving a composite of collagen, noncollagenous proteins, and hydroxyapatite. This method is particularly useful and is widely employed for preservation of bone that is to be used for morselized grafts, cortical segments, and strut grafts. *Demineralization* is a treatment process that uses hydrochloric acid to remove varying amounts of mineral (hydroxyapatite) for the purpose of preparing bone grafts with osteoinductive properties (49).

Processed bone allografts have limited or no immunogenicity, as demonstrated by several studies (9,13,15,37,45,55,68). However, deep-frozen bone allografts that still contain membrane fragments of MHC alloantigens can stimulate antibody- and cell-mediated immune responses in recipients, resulting in sensitization to donor antigens (35,82,84,110,112). The significance of this immunity to clinical outcome has not been established. Freeze-drying and demineralization removes all living cells; therefore, there is no immunogenic signal to stimulate the host transplantation response. Consequently, these banked allografts heal and incorporate better than fresh allograft bone but are inferior to autografts, the gold standard by which bone grafts are judged in clinical practice. The major disadvantage of processed allografts is the loss of graft osteogenic cells, which in fresh autografts contribute to the early phases of the healing process (15,16,51,54,107). This lack of graft-derived osteogenic potential in deep-frozen and freeze-dried bone allografts is responsible for their slower healing and decreased mechanical strength in comparison with fresh autologous grafts (51,90,94). Under ideal circumstances, allografts would be devoid of immunogenic cells but still contain live osteogenic cells that would be active during the early phases of healing. Examples of experimental approaches that may accomplish this goal include treatment of grafts with specific antibodies or culturing of grafts in vitro before transplantation (101). Although such methods are of great theoretical and possibly clinical interest, they do not address the need for long-term preservation of tissue. Therefore, deep-frozen and freeze-dried bone allografts are, and will remain, the most commonly used transplants in orthopaedic reconstruction.

The healing and incorporation of processed allografts follow the biologic events described in the preceding section for autografts, with the exception that graft-derived osteogenic cells are absent and therefore osteogenesis can only result from the activity of host cells. The biologic differences in the behavior of cancellous versus cortical allografts is the same as described for

autografts. Cancellous allografts placed into host cancellous bone will heal and remodel by concomitant, simultaneous bone formation and resorption following the pattern of creeping substitution (Fig. 1). Complete healing and remodeling of such grafts is somewhat slower than that of autografts, but this difference is not significant in clinical practice. In most cases, cancellous autografts in cancellous beds heal and remodel within 3 to 12 months, depending on the size of the reconstructed defect. Cortical allografts transplanted to cortical bone will heal (unite) by ingrowth from host cells but will not incorporate (remodel) because of the limited ability of the host to resorb the cortical bone organized in a lamellar pattern in haversian systems. The healing of cortical allografts is slower than that of equivalent autografts (38,102). Because in cortical allografts bone formation can only occur after resorption of the lamellar bone, these cortical allografts remain nonviable biologic implants over many years when supported by fixation devices or prosthetic components. In clinical practice, it is desirable to not have vascular invasion and resorption of these grafts because such events would greatly decrease their mechanical strength. It is for this reason that structural cortical allografts are often augmented by methyl methacrylate cement placed in conjunction with prosthetic components. Union at the junction sites of these cortical allografts with host bone occurs in general within 6 months. It is always indicated to graft these junctions with cancellous autograft to avoid nonunions. The biologic principle explaining the limited ability of host bone resorption mechanisms to remove cortical bone is the basis of the clinical practice of reconstructing areas of fibrous dysplasia with cortical rather than cancellous grafts to avoid the reoccurrence of this condition.

Demineralization of bone allografts is a processing step designed to add to the graft the property of osteoinduction. Demineralized bone matrix is available from tissue banks in various forms ranging from granules to cortical cylinders. A commonly used form of demineralized bone matrix product available as gel (in the carrier glycerol), putty, or flex variations is known as Grafton (Osteotech, Inc., Shrewsbury, NJ; Muskuloskeletal Transplant Foundation, Holmdel, NJ) (41,80,99). Although removing the mineral component makes these grafts osteoinductive, it also reduces their structural integrity and mechanical strength. Thus, their principal use is to augment cancellous or cortical autografts or allografts when stimulation of osteoinduction is desirable for union or arthrodesis.

Bone Substitutes

Materials used as a substitute for bone can be classified in the general categories of synthetic or natural matrices, also known as ceramics. The most common *synthetic* bone substitutes are hydroxyapatite, tricalcium phosphate, or a combination of the two. These biomaterials are produced by sintering and high-pressure compaction techniques and are available in porous, nonporous, or granular form. The pore structure of these ceramics is random, and for osteoconduction purposes a pore size of 150 to 500 μm is optimal. Both tricalcium phosphate and hydroxyapatite are resorbed, but parts of these materials remain in the body for a long time (63). A new synthetic bone substitute with interesting prospects is Norian-SRS, a specific mixture of inorganic calcium and phosphate sources that are combined to form a paste. Upon implantation, the mixture solidifies and hardens, forming dahlite (similar to hydroxyapatite of bone) (22). The *natural* matrix that is most available is coralline hydroxyapatite, a repleniform ceramic derived from marine coral. This biomaterial is produced by using a hydrothermal exchange method that replaces the calcium carbonate of the skeleton of sea coral with phosphate replicas and concomitantly removes all organic material (71,118). The pore structure of coralline ceramics is highly organized and resembles that of human bone. There are two pore sizes, depending on the genus of coral used. The smaller pore size material (pores with diameter of 200 μm) comes from organisms of the genus *Porites* and resembles the structure of cortical bone. The larger pore size material (pores with a diameter of 500 μm) comes from organisms of the genus *Goniopora* and resembles the structure of cancellous bone. These two different coralline hydroxyapatites are known as Pro Osteon 200 and Pro Osteon 500 and are available as granules or blocks (Interpore Cross International, Irvine, CA).

The ceramic biomaterials are used for their osteoconduction properties exclusively. These bone substitutes are neither osteogenic nor osteoinductive. Moreover, they are brittle and have very little tensile strength. Their osteoconductive property mimics that of allograft bone as shown in both experimental and clinical studies (7,11,48,58,77). They are not used alone for applications requiring structural support or induction of union or arthrodesis. The desire to add osteogenic and osteoinductive properties to bone substitutes has led to the emergence of *composite grafts*, such as mixtures of tricalcium phosphate or hydroxyapatite with BMP or demineralized bone matrix. Another approach for composites is to use autologous bone marrow cells as a source of osteogenic and osteoinductive properties added to an osteoconductive matrix. The best known composite of this type is Collagraft (Zimmer Corp., Warsaw, IN; Collagen Corp., Palo Alto, CA). Collagraft is a composite of highly purified bovine dermal collagen (a mixture of 95% type I and 5% type III collagen) and a biphasic mixture of 65% hydroxyapatite and 35% β-tricalcium phosphate. The material is available as a sterile kit containing a vial of ceramic granules (with a pore volume of 70% and a size of 0.5 to 1.0 mm) and a syringe of fibrillar collagen that are mixed together and with autologous bone marrow into a paste. The material is also available as soft strips. The advocated use has been for acute, comminuted fractures as a filler of bone defects and substitute for autograft (18,23). Although this composite substitute can and does act as an osteo-conductive filler, its efficacy for osteoinduction or osteogenesis, which would be attributable to the added bone marrow component only, is unknown.

CLINICAL APPLICATIONS IN THE PEDIATRIC SPINE

Properties and Functions of Bone Grafts and Substitutes

The decision whether to use autograft, processed allograft, bone substitute, or a composite in surgical procedures has to start with an understanding of how the *properties* of these bone grafts and alternatives differ in a biologic sense (Table 1). This knowledge will clarify the advantages and disadvantages of the types of grafts to be used in the clinical setting. *Immunogenicity* is not a clinically relevant issue for the grafts and substitutes considered here, which are devoid of cells and therefore are equivalent to fresh autografts in terms of lacking immunogenicity. It is obvious that the *donor site morbidity* associated with the harvesting of autograft bone would be eliminated if one used processed allograft or bone substitute. The *mechanical strength* of fresh autograft is better than that of freeze-dried allograft, whereas demineralized matrix has no structural strength whatsoever. Ceramic substitutes are similar in structural properties and strength to freeze-dried bone. The mechanical properties of composites vary considerably. The *speed of healing* of any allograft or substitute will be slower than that of autograft because of the fundamental differences in the unique biologic functions delivered by the processed materials. *Osteogenesis* can only come from live osteoblasts or their progenitors contained in fresh autograft and, to a lesser extent, in the bone marrow (which is part of composite substitutes such as Collagraft). None of the processed grafts or substitutes are osteogenic on their own, which is by itself a major biologic disadvantage when grafts are used for the induction of union, such as for fusion procedures in pediatric spinal surgery. Processed bone and substitutes used in cancellous applications are *osteoconductive* and therefore allow the ingrowth of host vascular channels and replacement by creeping substitution. As bone formation under these circumstances occurs exclusively from the host side, it is only the osteoconductive property of these materials that allows for healing to proceed, albeit at a slower rate than that of fresh autografts where osteogenesis occurs from both the host and the graft. *Osteoinduction* is a property of noncollagenous proteins contained in the bone matrix.

TABLE 1. PROPERTIES OF VARIOUS BONE GRAFTS AND BONE SUBSTITUTES

	Fresh Autograft	Freeze-dried Allograft	Demin. Allo. Matrix	Ceramic Substitute	Composite Substitute
Immunogenicity	No	No	No	No	No
Donor site morbidity	Yes	No	No	No	No
Mechanical strength	Good	Fair	Poor	Fair	Poor-fair
Healing speed	Fast	Slower	Slower	Slower	Slower
Osteogenesis	Yes	No	No	No	Maybe
Osteoconduction	Yes	Yes	Yes	Yes	Yes
Osteoinduction	Yes	No	Yes	No	Maybe

In the case of fresh autografts or bone marrow (as in composite grafts), live cells are transferred that can provide the appropriate osteoinductive factors. Processed allograft is not osteoinductive unless the mineral is removed and the bone is processed to a small particle size (demineralized bone matrix) for maximal effect (41,50,96). Partially demineralized bone grafts with multiple perforations have also been shown to be active (49,103).

The *function* of a bone graft is the single most important factor determining the choice of autograft, processed allograft, or bone substitute in a particular surgical procedure. An understanding of the intended function in conjunction with knowledge of the biologic properties of the grafts will guide the surgeon toward successful application of autograft and/or alternatives. The knowledge of graft functions in the pediatric spine has to be discussed within the context of general orthopaedic reconstruction (33). The main functions of bone grafts in orthopaedic reconstruction are to replace bone defects, to fill a cavity, to act as a buttress, and to induce or enhance union or arthrodesis. In pediatric spinal surgery, the last function—induction of fusion—is by far the most important and common. Less commonly, there can be a need to replace or buttress a defect in the anterior column after vertebral corpectomy or to fill a cavity after curettage of benign bone lesions.

Replacing Bone Defects

Massive allografts are required to replace bone defects in the long bones and, on rare occasions, in the pediatric spine. The need for such massive replacements usually occurs after the excision of bone tumors (4,28,76). The choice of allografts in this situation is dictated by the massive amount of bone needed. The use of autografts would cause significant morbidity, as these reconstructions usually require large diaphyseal cortical struts. In the pediatric spine, a smart application of massive allograft replacement is the use of fresh-frozen humerus segments after anterior decompression for tuberculosis as described recently by Govender and Parbhoo (52). It is clear that under these circumstances the massive allografts have not only a replacement but also a buttressing function (as described below). An alternative approach for grafting anterior spine defects in children is the use of vascularized autografts, as discussed in Chapter 17.

Filling a Cavity

Morselized allograft bone or ceramic substitute is the ideal choice when the function of the graft is to fill a cavity. The reason for this is the rich vascular supply of a cavity in metaphyseal or trabecular bone, which requires simple filling with osteoconductive material to allow healing by creeping substitution from the host. Morselized allograft bone is frequently used in surgery on long bones after the excision of cysts or benign tumors (27). Because many of these cavities are large and occur in children, it is almost uniformly true that the use of autograft in these situations is associated with too much morbidity and is unnecessary. In pediatric spinal surgery, this function alone is rarely called for (e.g., after curettage of benign tumors in the vertebral body). In almost all cases of vertebral body reconstruction, the need to fill a void is combined with the need to buttress the construct.

Acting as a Buttress

Another function of a bone graft is to prevent collapse of a reconstructed area of the skeleton. In general orthopaedics, an example of such a use is bone grafting procedures following elevation of depressed tibial plateau or calcaneus fractures (27). In spinal surgery, the need to buttress occurs every time the stability of the anterior column is compromised. Therefore, this function is of primary importance in anterior bone grafting procedures. In anterior cervical fusions, anterior lumbar interbody fusions, and anterior thoracic fusions, the role of the bone graft is primarily a buttressing one. In most of these cases, however, an additional aim is to obtain an arthrodesis of the segments involved. This is where the choice between allograft/substitute and autograft gets complicated. Although allografts lack the ability to induce union, they are excellent osteoconductors and can fulfill the role of buttressing the unstable segments. In the anterior spine, the bone grafts are inserted into highly vascular beds in the vertebral bodies. Therefore, cortico-cancellous buttressing allografts with good osteoconductive properties are rapidly replaced by creeping substitution, and arthrodesis occurs without osteogenesis or osteoinduction from the graft. This explains the reported high clinical success rates of anterior cervical and lumbar fusions employing allografts in the adult patient population (10,20,47,72,75,92,98). The major role of the grafts as buttresses and osteoconductors in anterior spinal surgery also explains the clinical success reported in adults with heterografts, such as Kiel bone (42,116). A way to add osteogenesis and osteoinduction to anterior buttressing allografts is the use of composites, such as allograft femoral cortical rings with autograft cancellous dowels in the lumbar spine (100).

Inducing Arthrodesis

Enhancing union, or inducing arthrodesis, requires osteogenesis and osteoinduction provided by the graft. The biology of bone grafting clearly tells us that autografts can fulfill this function best. Thus, in general orthopaedics, allogeneic bone grafts are not indicated for the treatment of nonunion of long bones or in other situations that require the stimulation of osteogenesis, such as enhancing primary union or arthrodesis. The same is true in posterior spinal surgery, where allogeneic morselized bone graft is not a good choice as a primary grafting material for fusions. The most important function of a bone graft in posterior spinal fusions is to induce arthrodesis by osteogenesis and osteoinduction, and this function can best be fulfilled by autograft bone. Another function of posterior spine bone grafts is to act as osteoconductors, and this function can be fulfilled by processed allografts or bone substitutes. Consequently, under circumstances where there is insufficient autograft bone, such as in long spinal fusions for scoliosis or kyphosis, morselized allograft bone can fulfill the special function of *augmenting* the quantity of autograft bone. In these situations, processed allografts or substitutes serve as vehicles to spread limited amounts of autograft bone over large areas, providing osteoconductive material for osteogenesis and osteoinduction derived from the autograft and the host bed. An understanding of these biologic principles explains the contradictory clinical results obtained in various adult clinical studies using allograft bone for posterior spinal fusions (3,21,57,74,86,92,115). The success or failure of such procedures depends on many factors, of which the most important is the vascularity of the host bed. Sufficient vascularity makes it possible for host-derived cells to replace large areas of allograft bone, which has no osteogenic or osteoinductive capability of its own, whereas the vertebral segments are immobilized by instrumentation.

Critical Analysis of Pediatric Clinical Data

The pediatric spinal surgery literature reporting on the use of bone allografts or substitutes for spinal fusions has grown significantly in recent years. The abundance of papers on this subject has helped clarify and lay to rest myths, fears, and misbeliefs related to themes such as immune rejection, introduction of infection, and transmission of viral disease, to name a few. The uniform absence of such complications in all clinical reports confirms what we already know from understanding the biology of processed allografts and substitutes, namely, that they are not immunogenic and not infectious. The studies did not resolve the fundamental biologic question related to the efficacy of allograft or substitute alone acting simply as osteoconductor grafts to achieve spinal fusion in children. The general theme, with some exceptions, is that allograft bone or substitute works in pediatric fusions but the studies are generally not appropriately randomized and are complicated by many variables. While these conclusions are apparent from review of the clinical data, extracting more useful information is difficult. In the following I will critically evaluate the current data with the hope of stimulating readers to take a careful look at the clinical indications for processed grafts and substitutes in their own practice.

Most studies that have been done to date can be organized in the following two broad categories: (a) Fusions using fresh-frozen or freeze-dried allografts (3,5,6,8,40,43,79,95,109,111,120) and (b) fusions utilizing bone substitutes (69,89,93). One study of posterior cervical fusions with freeze-dried cortical bone allografts in seven children showed a 100% nonunion rate, and the authors reasonably argue that this was the result of an incorrect application of these grafts in tension rather than compression (109). All other studies deal with idiopathic or paralytic scoliosis treated with spinal instrumentation. The reasoning of most authors for employing allografts or substitutes is the elimination of donor site morbidity (121), the avoidance of major blood loss (6,43), and the need for ample bone grafts in patients whose pelvis is small and osteoporotic (120). Although all of the fusion procedures are combined with instrumentation, the type of instrumentation varies between studies and even within some studies. In general, the instrumentation employs rigid systems with or without segmental fixation. In some allograft fusion studies, freeze-dried allograft is used alone (111,120); in others, allograft bone is used for augmentation of autograft (5,8,43); and a few studies compare autograft with allograft (3,36,40,79,95). In the category of fusions with bone

substitutes, ceramics are used to either augment autograft bone (69,89) or alone, in direct comparison with autograft (93).

The general results from all these studies indicate at first glance that allografts or substitutes in an augmenting mode or alone may be used with success in pediatric instrumented fusions. However, further analysis shows that the criteria used to measure results in these clinical series are uniformly those related to the pseudarthrosis rate, which is determined by inexact clinical and radiographic evaluations. Based on such methodology, two clinical series comparing allograft with autograft posterior fusion instrumentations found similar pseudarthrosis rates (3,36). A more complex method to evaluate results of spinal fusions in scoliosis is to look for radiographic loss of correction. A nonrandomized study by Montgomery et al. looking at posterior fusions for scoliosis in cerebral palsy patients reported a 46% loss of correction at 3.2 years for the autograft group versus a 38% loss of correction for the freeze-dried allograft group. The authors suggest equal effectiveness of the two graft materials (79). In a recent prospective randomized study by Ransford et al. examining results of fusions for idiopathic scoliosis, the 8% loss of correction at 18 months in the autograft group versus a 3% loss of correction in a matched group of patients receiving a synthetic porous ceramic (Triosite, Zimmer Ltd, Swindon, UK) prompted the authors to suggest equal effectiveness for the two graft types (93). The problem with these evaluation methodologies is the lack of understanding as to when maximal stability of the spine is reached after instrumented fusions to allow assessment of a meaningful end result. Pain, tenderness, and radiographs are unreliable indicators of pseudarthrosis in instrumented spines. Some loss of correction occurs in most cases of instrumented fusions, and though this may be caused by pseudarthrosis, it is by no means a reliable indicator of it or of incomplete fusion. Variables in the instrumentation techniques used in these studies further confound the final evaluation because fixation methods vary widely: Harrington or Luque rods (79), Harrington rods with sublaminar wires, or Cotrel-Dubousset system or Modulok Mark 1 implants with or without additional anterior Zielke or Webb-Morley corrective instrumentation (93). It is apparent that a multitude of surgical techniques compound the variables contributing to the outcome of pseudarthrosis or loss of correction. Modern, rigid instrumentation protects the spine for a prolonged time before pseudarthrosis or incomplete fusion can become apparent. Theoretically, stability is reached when fusion is complete, but it is this very fact that is difficult to demonstrate in the instrumented spine. Even failure of the instrumentation does not necessarily indicate failure of fusion. Surgical exploration has been used for documenting spinal pseudarthrosis but is not practical as an evaluation method.

It is obvious that some uncertainty may arise in the reader's mind at this point as to the validity of studies reporting equally effective fusion rates with processed allograft or bone substitute and autograft when the end result of such studies is difficult to measure with precision. Furthermore, we know from the understanding of the biology of grafting that the best graft for induction of union or fusion is a graft that is osteogenic, osteoinductive, and osteoconductive (autograft). Therefore, it is difficult to accept that processed allograft or bone substitute that is merely osteoconductive would be as effective in this application. A close examination of the methods of surgery in these studies with their multiple variables provides a plausible explanation for the observations. The surgical methods include decortication of the posterior elements and facetectomies of the spine to create a raw, bleeding surgical bed. The bone fragments from these maneuvers and from excised spinal processes are employed locally in addition to exogenous grafts such as allograft or ceramic in both studies referenced under 79 and 93. Consequently, the added exogenous grafts may be simply augmenters of local autograft bone in highly vascular beds of the pediatric spine. This would explain the apparent similar effectiveness of allograft/substitute and autograft in these studies even if one excluded the variables related to evaluation methods or to surgical technique.

It is fair to conclude that despite the fact that safety and decreased morbidity of processed allografts and bone substitutes (79,93) are documented in pediatric spinal fusions by current literature, the efficacy of these osteoconductive grafts alone for instrumented fusions has not been demonstrated. Ideal randomization in a prospective double-blinded fashion using uniform patient populations and uniform surgical technique would be the best way to examine the grafting materials that are becoming available in increasing numbers and in increasingly complex forms. To find the ideal graft for the induction of fusion in the pediatric spine, one must use the knowledge of bone graft biology and of the unique properties of bone tissue. One would predict that future technology will provide the ultimate effective substitute with all of the properties of autologous bone tissue, including osteogenesis, osteoclastic resorption, osteoconduction, and osteoinduction.

REFERENCES

1. American Association of Tissue Banks (1991): *Technical manual for tissue banking musculoskeletal tissues.* McLean, VA: American Association of Tissue Banks.
2. American Association of Tissue Banks (1991): *Standards for tissue banking.* McLean, VA: American Association of Tissue Banks.
3. Aurori BF, Weirman RJ, Lowell HA, et al. (1985): Pseudarthrosis after spinal fusion for scoliosis: a comparison of autogenic and allogeneic bone grafts. *Clin Orthop* 199:153–158.
4. Bell RS, Guest CB (1992): Allografts in pelvic oncologic surgery. In: Czitrom AA, Gross AE, eds. *Allografts in orthopaedic practice.* Baltimore: Williams & Wilkins, pp. 121–146.
5. Blanco JS, Seara CJ (1997): Allograft bone use during instrumentation and fusion in the treatment of adolescent idiopathic scoliosis. *Spine* 22:1338–1342.
6. Bobechko WP (1991): Blood loss in scoliosis surgery. In: Johnson RG, ed. *Spine: state of the art reviews,* vol. 5. Philadelphia: Hanley & Belfus, pp. 75–82.
7. Bucholz RW, Carlton A, Holmes R (1987): Hydroxyapatite and tricalcium phosphate bone graft substitutes. *Orthop Clin N Am* 18: 323–334.
8. Bridwell KH, O'Brien MF, Lenke LG, et al. (1994): Posterior spinal fusion supplemented with only allograft bone in paralytic scoliosis. Does it work? *Spine* 23:2658–2666.
9. Brooks DB, Heiple KG, Herndon AH, et al. (1963): Immunological factors in homogeneous bone transplantation. IV. The effect of various methods of preparation and irradiation on antigenicity. *J Bone Joint Surg Am* 45:1617–1626.
10. Brown MD, Malinin TI, Davis PB (1976): A roentgenographic evaluation of frozen allografts versus autografts in anterior cervical spine fusions. *Clin Orthop* 119:231–236.
11. Buchholz RW, Carlton A, Holmes R (1989): Interporous hydroxyapatite as a bone graft substitute in tibial plateau fractures. *Clin Orthop* 240:53–62.
12. Burwell RG, Gowland G (1961): Studies in the transplantation of bone. II. The changes occurring in the lymphoid tissue after homografts and autografts of fresh cancellous bone. *J Bone Joint Surg Br* 43:820–843.
13. Burwell RG, Gowland G (1962): Studies in the transplantation of bone. III. The immune responses of lymph nodes draining components of fresh homologous cancellous bone and homologous bone treated by different methods. *J Bone Joint Surg Br* 44:131–148.
14. Burwell RG, Gowland G, Dexter F (1963): Studies in transplantation of bone. VI. Further observations concerning the antigenicity of homologous cortical and cancellous bone. *J Bone Joint Surg Br* 45: 597–608.
15. Chalmers J (1959): Transplantation immunity in bone homografting. *J Bone Joint Surg Br* 41:160–178.
16. Chalmers J (1967): Bone transplantation. *Symp Tissue Org Transplant Suppl J Clin Pathol* 20:540–550.
17. Champion BR, Sell S, Poole AR (1983): Immunity to homologous collagen and cartilage proteoglycans in rabbits. *Immunology* 48: 605–616.
18. Chapman MW, Bucholz R, Cornell C (1997): Treatment of acute fractures with a collagen-calcium phosphate graft material. *J Bone Joint Surg Am* 79:495–502.
19. Chase SW, Herndon CH (1955): The fate of autogenous and homogeneous bone grafts. A historical review. *J Bone Joint Surg Am* 37: 801–841.
20. Cloward RB (1980): Gas sterilized cadaver bone grafts for spinal fusion operations. *Spine* 5:4–10.
21. Cloward RB (1985): Posterior lumbar fusion updated. *Clin Orthop* 193:16–19.
22. Constantz BR, Ison IC, Fulmer MT, et al. (1995): Skeletal repair by in situ formation of the mineral phase of bone. *Science* 267:1796–1799.
23. Cornell CN (1992): Initial clinical experience with use of collagraft as a bone graft substitute. *Techniques Orthop* 7:55–63.
24. Cunningham N, Reddi AH (1992): Biologic principles of bone induction: application to bone grafts. In: Habal MB, Reddi AH, eds. *Bone grafts and bone substitutes.* Philadelphia: WB Saunders, pp. 93–98.
25. Czitrom AA (1989): Bone transplantation, passenger cells and the major histocompatibility complex. In: Aebi M, Regazzoni P, eds. *Bone transplantation.* Berlin: Springer-Verlag, pp. 103–110.
26. Czitrom AA (1992): Immunology of bone and cartilage allografts. In: Czitrom AA, Gross AE, eds. *Allografts in orthopaedic practice.* Baltimore: Williams & Wilkins, pp. 15–25.
27. Czitrom AA (1992): Indications and uses of morsellized and small segment allograft bone in general orthopaedics. In: Czitrom AA, Gross AE, eds. *Allografts in orthopaedic practice.* Baltimore: Williams & Wilkins, pp. 47–65.
28. Czitrom AA (1992): Allograft reconstruction after tumor surgery in the appendicular skeleton. In: Czitrom AA, Gross AE, eds. *Allografts in orthopaedic practice.* Baltimore: Williams & Wilkins, pp. 83–119.
29. Czitrom AA (1993): Principles and techniques of tissue banking. In: Heckman JD, ed. *Instructional course lectures.* Park Ridge, IL: American Academy of Orthopaedic Surgeons, pp. 359–362.
30. Czitrom AA (1996): The immune response: the afferent arm. *Clin Orthop* 326:11–24.
31. Czitrom AA, Axelrod T, Fernandes B (1985): Antigen presenting cells and bone allotransplantation. *Clin Orthop* 197:27–31.
32. Czitrom AA, Axelrod TS, Fernandes B (1988): Granulocyte precursors are the principal cells in bone marrow that stimulate allospecific cytolytic T-lymphocyte responses. *Immunology* 64:655–660.
33. Czitrom AA, Gross AE, eds. (1992): *Allografts in orthopaedic practice.* Baltimore: Williams & Wilkins, pp. 1–222.
34. Czitrom AA, Keating S, Gross AE (1990): The viability of articular cartilage in fresh osteochondral allografts after clinical transplantation. *J Bone Joint Surg Am* 72:574–581.
35. Deijkers RLM, Bouma GJ, van der Meer-Prins EMW, et al. (1999): Human bone allografts can induce T cells with high affinity for donor antigens. *J Bone Joint Surg Br* 81:538–544.

36. Dodd CA, Ferguson CM, Freedman L, et al. (1988): Allograft versus autograft bone in scoliosis surgery. *J Bone Joint Surg Br* 78:431–434.

37. Elves MW (1974): Humoral immune response to allografts of bone. *Int Arch Allergy* 47:708–715.

38. Enneking WF, Burchard H, Puhl JJ, et al. (1975): Physiological and biological aspects of repair in dog cortical bone transplants. *J Bone Joint Surg Am* 57:237–252.

39. Esses SI, Halloran PF (1983): Donor marrow-derived cells as immunogens and targets for the immune response to bone and skin allografts. *Transplantation* 35:169–174.

40. Fabri G (1991): Allograft versus autograft bone in idiopathic scoliosis surgery: a multivariate statistical analysis. *J Pediatr Orthop* 4:465–467.

41. Feighan JE, Davy D, Prewett AB, et al. (1995): Induction of bone by demineralized bone matrix gel: a study in a rat femoral defect model. *J Orthop Res* 13:881–891.

42. Fortuna A, Palatinsky E, Di Lorenzo N (1988): Anterior cervical arthrodesis with heterologous bone graft and human fibrin glue in the surgical treatment of myelopathy due to spondylosis. *Clin Neurol Neurosurg* 90:125–129.

43. Fox HJ, Thomas CH, Thompson AG (1997): Spina instrumentation for Duchenne's muscular dystrophy: experience of hypotensive anesthesia to minimize blood loss. *J Pediatr Orthop* 17:750–753.

44. Friedlaender GE, Horowitz MC (1992): Immune responses to osteochondral allografts: nature and significance. *Orthopedics* 15:1171–1175.

45. Friedlaender GE, Strong DM, Sell KW (1975): Studies on the antigenicity of bone. I. Freeze-dried and deep-frozen bone allografts in rabbits. *J Bone Joint Surg Am* 58:854–858.

46. Friedlaender GE (1983): Immune responses to ostechondral allografts: current knowledge and future directions. *Clin Orthop* 174:58–68.

47. Frothingham RE, Solomon A (1988): The use of allografts in anterior cervical interbody fusion. *J Miss Med Assoc* 29:71–74.

48. Gazdag AR, Lane JM, Glaser D, et al. (1995): Alternatives to autogenous bone grafts: efficacy and indications. *J Am Acad Orthop Surg* 3:1–8.

49. Gendler E (1986): Perforated demineralized bone matrix: a new form of osteoinductive biomaterial. *J Biomed Mater Res* 20:687–697.

50. Glowacki J (1992): Tissue response to bone-derived implants. In: Habal MB, Reddi AH, eds. *Bone grafts and bone substitutes.* Philadelphia: WB Saunders, pp. 84–92.

51. Goldberg VM, Stevenson S (1992): Biology of bone and cartilage allografts. In: Czitrom AA, Gross AE, eds. *Allografts in orthopaedic practice.* Baltimore: Williams & Wilkins, pp. 1–13.

52. Govender S, Parbhoo AH (1999): Support of the anterior column with allograft in tuberculosis of the spine. *J Bone Joint Surg Br* 81:106–109.

53. Gupta D, Tuli SM (1982): Osteoinductivity of partially decalcified alloimplants in healing of large osteoperiosteal defects. *Acta Orthop Scand* 53:857–865.

54. Gray JC, Elves MW (1979): Early osteogenesis in compact bone isografts: a comparative study of the contributions of the different graft cells. *Calcif Tissue Int* 29:225–237.

55. Halloran PF, Lee HE, Ziv I, et al. (1979): Orthotopic bone transplantation in mice. II. Studies of the alloantibody response. *Transplantation* 27:420–426.

56. Hench LL (1992): Bioactive bone substitutes. In: Habal MB, Reddi AH, eds. *Bone grafts and bone substitutes.* Philadelphia: WB Saunders, pp. 263–275.

57. Herron LD, Newman MH (1989): The failure of ethylene oxide gas–sterilized freeze-dried bone grafts for thoracic and lumbar spinal fusion. *Spine* 14:496–500.

58. Holmes RE, Bucholz RW, Mooney V (1986): Porous hydroxyapatite as a bone graft substitute in metaphyseal defects. *J Bone Joint Surg Am* 68:904–911.

59. Horowitz MC, Friedlaender GE (1991): Induction of specific T-cell responsiveness to allogeneic bone. *J Bone Joint Surg Am* 73:1157–1168.

60. Horsburgh CR Jr, Ou CY, Jason J, et al. (1989): Duration of human immunodeficiency virus infection before detection by antibody. *Lancet* 2:637–640.

61. Hutchinson J (1952): The fate of experimental bone autografts and homografts. *Br J Surg* 39:552–561.

62. Imagawa DT, Lee MH, Wolinsky SM, et al. (1989): Human immunodeficiency virus type 1 infection in homosexual men who remain seronegative for prolonged periods. *N Engl J Med* 320:1458–1462.

63. Jarcho M (1981): Calcium phosphate ceramics as hard tissue prosthetics. *Clin Orthop* 157:259–278.

64. Joyce ME, Bolander ME (1992): Role of transforming growth factor-beta. In: Habal MB, Reddi AH, eds. *Bone grafts and bone substitutes.* Philadelphia: WB Saunders, pp. 99–111.

65. Kitchen AD, Mann GF, Harrison JF, et al. (1989): Effect of gamma irradiation on the human immunodeficiency virus and human coagulation proteins. *Vox Sang* 56:223–229.

66. Kushner A (1940): Evaluation of Wolff's law of bone formation. *J Bone Joint Surg Am* 22:589–596.

67. Lafferty KJ, Andrus L, Prowse SJ (1980): Role of lymphokine and antigen in the control of specific T cell responses. *Immunol Rev* 51:279–314.

68. Langer F, Czitrom A, Pritzker KP, et al. (1975): The immunogenicity of fresh and frozen allogeneic bone. *J Bone Joint Surg Am* 57:216–220.

69. Le Huec JC, Lesprit A, Delavigne C, et al. (1997): Tri-calcium phosphate ceramicsand allografts as bone substitutes for spinal fusion in idiopathic scoliosis: comparative clinical results at four years. *Acta Orthopaedica Belgica* 63:202–211.

70. Lee WPA, Yaremchuk M, Manfrini M, et al. (1989): Prolonged survival of vascularized limb allografts from chimera donors. *Trans Orthop Res Soc* 14:468.

71. Light M, Kanat IO (1991): The possible use of coralline hydroxyapatite as a bone implant. *J Foot Surg* 30:472–476.

72. Loguidice VA, Johnson RG, Guyer ED, et al. Anterior lumbar interbody fusion. *Spine* 13:366–369.

73. Mahomed MN, Beaver RJ, Gross AE (1992): The long-term success of fresh, small fragment osteochondral allografts used for intraarticular posttraumatic defects in the knee joint. *Orthopaedics* 15:1191–1199.

74. Malinin TI, Brown MD (1981): Bone allografts in spinal surgery. *Clin Orthop* 154:68–73.

75. Malinin TI, Rosomoff HL, Sutton CH (1977): Human cadaver femoral head homografts for anterior cervical spine fusion. *Surg Neurol* 7:249–251.

76. Mankin HJ, Springfield DS, Gebhardt MC, et al. (1992): Current status of allografting for bone tumors. *Orthopedics* 15:1147–1154.

77. Martin RB, Chapman MW, Sharkey NA, et al. (1993): Bone ingrowth and mechanical properties of coralline hydroxyapatite 1 year after implantation. *Biomaterials* 14:341–348.

78. Mizutani H, Urist MR (1982): The nature of bone morphogenetic protein (BMP) fractions derived from bovine bone matrix gelatin. *Clin Orthop* 171:213–223.

79. Montgomery DM, Aronson DD, Lee CL, et al. (1990): Posterior spinal fusion: allograft versus autograft bone. *J Spinal Disord* 3:370–375.

80. Morone MA, Boden SD (1998): Experimental posterolateral lumbar spine fusion with demineralized bone matrix gel. *Spine* 23:159–167.

81. Musclow CE (1992): Bone and tissue banking. In: Czitrom AA, Gross AE, eds. *Allografts in orthopaedic practice.* Baltimore: Williams & Wilkins, pp. 27–45.

82. Muscolo DL, Caletti E, Schajowicz F, et al. (1987): Tissue-typing in human massive allografts of frozen bone. *J Bone Joint Surg Am* 69:583–595.

83. Muscolo DL, Kawai S, Ray RD (1976): Cellular and humoral immune response analysis of bone-allografted rats. *J Bone Joint Surg Am* 58:826–832.

84. Muscolo DL, Ayerza MA, Calabrese ME, et al. (1996): Human leukocyte antigen matching, radiographic score and histologic findings in massive frozen bone allografts. *Clin Orthop* 326:115–126.

85. Muscolo DL, Kawai S, Ray RD (1977): In vitro studies of transplantation antigens present on bone cells in the rat. *J Bone Joint Surg Br* 59:342–348.

86. Nasca RJ, Whelchel JD (1987): Use of cryopreserved bone in spinal surgery. *Spine* 12:222–227.

87. Oakeshott RD, Farine I, Pritzker KPH, et al. (1988): A clinical and histologic analysis of failed fresh osteochondral allografts. *Clin Orthop* 233:283–294.

88. Ono K, Yamamuro Y, Nakamura T, et al. (1988): Apatite-wollastonite containing glass ceramic-fibrin mixture as a bone defect filler. *J Biomed Mater Res* 22:869–885.

89. Passuti N, Daculsi G, Rogez JM, et al. (1989): Macroporous calcium phosphate ceramic performance in human spine fusion. *Clin Orthop* 248:169–176.

90. Pelker RR, McKay J, Troiano N, et al. (1989): Allograft incorporation: a biomechanical evaluation in a rat model. *J Orthop Res* 7: 585–589.

91. Phemister DB (1914): The fate of transplanted bone and regenerative power of its various constituents. *Surg Gynecol Obstet* 19:303–333.

92. Prolo DJ, Pedrotti PW, White DH (1980): Ethylene oxide sterilization of bone, dura mater, and fascia lata for human transplantation. *Neurosurgery* 6:529–539.

93. Ransford AO, Morley T, Edgar MA, et al. (1998): Synthetic porous ceramic compared with autograft in scoliosis surgery. *J Bone Joint Surg Br* 80:13–18.

94. Ray RD (1972): Vascularization of bone grafts and implants. *Clin Orthop* 87:43–48.

95. Recht J, Bayard F, Delloye C, et al. (1993): Freeze-dried bone allograft versus autograft bone in scoliosis surgery. A retrospective comparative study. *Eur Spine J* 2:235–238.

96. Reddi AH, Anderson WA (1976): Collagenous bone matrix-induced endochondral ossification and hemopoiesis. *J Cell Biol* 69:557–572.

97. Reddi AH, Cunningham NS (1990): Bone induction by osteogenin and bone morphogenetic proteins. *Biomaterials* 11:33–34.

98. Rish BL, McFadden JT, Penix JO (1976): Anterior cervical fusion using homologous bone grafts: a comparative study. *Surg Neurol* 5: 119–121.

99. Russell JL, Block JE (1999): Clinical utility of demineralized bone matrix for osseous defects, arthrodesis, and reconstruction: impact of processing techniques and study methodology. *Orthopaedics* 22: 524–531.

100. Salib RM, Graber J (1991): Femoral cortical ring plus cancellous dowel: an alternative in anterior lumbar interbody fusion. In: *Composite grafts in anterior lumbar interbody fusion*. Shrewsbury, NJ: Osteotech, pp. 1–4.

101. Schwarzenbach O, Czitrom AA, Aebi M, et al. (1989): In vitro culture to enhance allogeneic bone grafts. A rat model. *Orthop Trans* 13:340.

102. Schwarzenbach O, Regazzoni P, Aebi M (1989): Segmental vascularized and nonvascularized bone allografts. In: Aebi M, Regazzoni P, eds. *Bone transplantation*. Berlin: Springer-Verlag, pp. 78–81.

103. Sigholm G, Gendler E, McKellop H, et al. (1992): Graft perforations favor osteoinduction. Studies of rabbit cortical grafts sterilized with ethylene oxide. *Acta Orthop Scand* 63:177–182.

104. Skjodt H, Hughes DE, Dobson PRM, et al. (1990): Constitutive and inducible expression of HLA class II determinants by human osteoblast-like cells in vitro. *J Clin Invest* 85:1421–1426.

105. Skjodt H, Moller T, Freiesleben SF (1989): Human osteoblast-like cells expressing MHC class II determinants stimulate allogeneic and autologous peripheral blood mononuclear cells and function as antigen-presenting cells. *Immunology* 68:416–420.

106. Spire B, Dormont D, Barre-Sinoussi F, et al. (1985): Inactivation of lymphadenopathy-associated virus by heat, gamma rays, and ultraviolet light. *Lancet* 1:188–189.

107. Sprent J, Schaefer M (1989): Antigen presenting cells for unprimed T cells. *Immunol Today* 10:17–23.

108. Springfield DS (1992): Autogenous bone grafts: Nonvascular and vascular. *Orthopedics* 15:1237–1241.

109. Stabler CL, Eismont FJ, Brown MD, et al. (1985): Failure of posterior cervical fusions using cadaveric bone graft in children. *J Bone Joint Surg* 67A:370–375.

110. Stevenson S (1987): The immune response to osteochondral allografts in dogs. *J Bone Joint Surg Am* 69:573–582.

111. Stricker SJ, Sher JS (1997): Freeze-dried cortical allograft in posterior spinal arthrodesis: use with segmental instrumentation for idiopathic adolescent scoliosis. *Orthopedics* 20:1039–1043.

112. Strong DM, Friedlander GE, Tomford WW, et al. (1996): Immunologic responses in human recipients of osseous and osteochondral allografts. *Clin Orthop* 326:107–114.

113. Terato K, Hasty KA, Cremer MA, et al. (1985): Collagen induced arthritis in mice. Localization of arthritogenic determinant to a fragment of type II collagen molecule. *J Exp Med* 162:637–646.

114. Tilney NL, Kupiec-Weglinski JW (1989): Advances in the understanding of rejection mechanisms. *Transplant Proc* 21:10–13.

115. Urist MR, Dawson E (1981): Intertransverse fusion with the aid of chemosterilized autolyzed antigen-extracted allogeneic (AAA) bone. *Clin Orthop* 154:97–113.

116. Vich JMO (1985): Anterior cervical interbody fusion with threaded cylindrical bone. *J Neurosurg* 63:750–753.

117. Weaver CT, Unanue ER (1990): The costimulatory function of antigen presenting cells. *Immunol Today* 11:49–55.

118. White E, Shors EC (1986): Biomaterial aspects of interpore-200 porous hydroxyapatite. *Dent Clin N Am* 30:49–67.

119. Yamamuro T, Wilson J, Hench LL, eds. (1990): *CRC handbook bioactive ceramics*. Boca Raton: CRC Press.

120. Yazici M, Asher MA (1997): Freeze-dried allograft for posterior spinal fusion in patients with neuromuscular spinal deformities. *Spine* 13: 1467–1471.

121. Younger EM, Chapman MW (1989): Morbidity at bone graft donor sites. *J Orthop Trauma* 3:192–195.

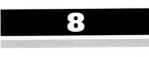

BONE GRAFTING

J. ANDREW SULLIVAN

SOURCES AND METHODS

The goal of spinal arthrodesis is to achieve union of the operated segments by means of formation of a solid mass of bone that obliterates the existing joints. This is achieved by a variety of means, but central to all methods are the following:

1. Meticulous technique with cleaning of all soft tissues from the spine
2. Obliteration of the joints through removal or destruction of the facet joints or discs
3. Spinal immobilization accomplished in most instances through internal fixation or external means
4. Bone grafting to enhance or induce fusion

Albee (2) was a pioneer in the field of bone grafting. In the first decade of this century, he achieved arthrodesis in the spines of dogs by using free grafts from bones of the lower extremities. Albee believed that the same principles involved in the grafting of plants had to be followed, because there is a decrease in adaptability as tissue specificity increases. Although some of Albee's beliefs have been disproved, the following general principles stated in 1944 still apply:

1. The tissue must be applied like to like.
2. The contact must be intimate.
3. The bones must be immobilized in that position.

Autogenous, homogenous, and heterogenous bone grafts all have been used in spinal arthrodesis (16). This chapter deals with the sources of autogenous bone graft, the method for harvesting it, and the complications related to the procedure.

Iliac Crest Autogenous Bone Graft

Although other sites can be used to obtain small grafts, the iliac crest is the most commonly used site for obtaining bone graft. Abbott et al. (1) and Dick (11) have pointed out that the anatomy of the ilium is such that the best place to obtain cancellous bone is in the thickened posterior crest (Fig. 1). Fortunately for surgeons, this is the most accessible area when the patient is prone, and it is the most frequently used. The anterior iliac crest

can be used if the patient has already had posterior harvest of bone, for bicortical grafts, or in situations in which the patient is supine, such as anterior cervical spinal surgery.

Anterior Iliac Crest Technique

An incision is made 1 cm inferior to the crest of the ilium beginning just posterior to the anterior superior iliac spine. By starting at this point, one avoids the possibility of damage to the inguinal ligament, the attachment of the sartorius muscle, or the lateral femoral cutaneous nerve (Fig. 2). One should be aware of anomalous courses of the lateral femoral cutaneous nerve (see later). The incision is carried down through the subcutaneous tissues to the outer table of the ilium. Bone graft can be obtained from the outer table, the inner table, or between the tables. Inner-table grafts are somewhat easier to obtain because of the contour of the ilium. Obtaining tissue from this location may cause less pain immediately after the operation.

For an inner-table graft in a patient with a mature skeleton, the periosteum is incised over the crest of the ilium. For a patient with an immature skeleton, an incision is made just inferior to the iliac apophysis, which is then carefully lifted off the ilium and displaced medially along with the abdominal wall muscles. For outer-table grafts, the periosteum is incised along the crest of the ilium in a patient with a mature skeleton or just inferior to the ilium for patients with an open apophysis. For a patient with an immature skeleton, the apophysis may be left intact during harvest of an outer-table graft. The periosteum is elevated and the muscles reflected either medially or laterally, depending on the table chosen. On the inner crest, when the iliac muscle is being elevated, care must be taken not to penetrate the muscle. Penetration can damage adjacent structures, such as the femoral, ilioinguinal, and femoral cutaneous nerves. A narrow, sharp osteotome is used to outline the incision that will be made in the appropriate table (Fig. 3). A curved osteotome is used to gently elevate the outlined piece of iliac table along with attached cancellous bone. Care should be taken to avoid penetrating the opposite table and thereby producing a full-thickness defect. The remaining cancellous bone can be removed with gouges or curettes.

Several other techniques have been described to remove bone from the anterior crest of the ilium. Wolfe and Kawamoto (32) described a means of obliquely sectioning the crest of the ilium to allow both inner and outer tables to be peeled away from the cancellous bone between them (Fig. 4). The underlying graft of

J. A. Sullivan: Department of Orthopaedic Surgery, University of Oklahoma College of Medicine, Oklahoma City, Oklahoma 73104.

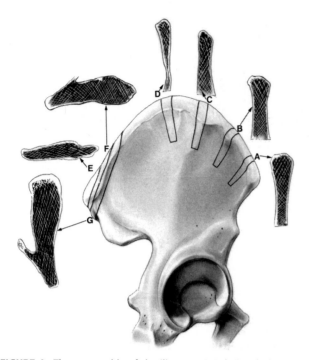

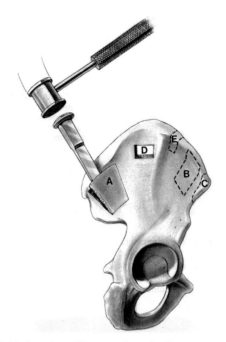

FIGURE 1. The outer table of the ilium. *A–G,* Relative thickness and amounts of cancellous bone available. Most grafts are obtained from *G,* either from the inner or outer table, and give abundant cortico-cancellous graft. Unicortical grafts often are harvested from the area between *A* and *B* from either the inner or outer table. Bicortical graft may be obtained from *A, B, C, D,* or *F.*

FIGURE 3. Various sites of harvest along the iliac crest. *A,* Unicortical graft from the posterior crest. *B,* Unicortical inner-table graft that saves the crest. *C,* Inner-table unicortical graft or bicortical graft. *D* Site for obtaining either a unicortical inner- or outer-table graft. *E* Good source for obtaining a unicortical, bicortical, or tricortical graft while preserving the crest of the ilium.

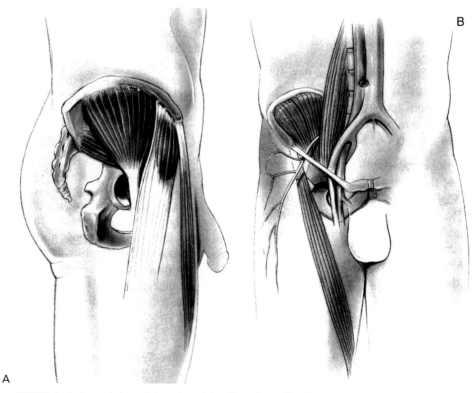

FIGURE 2. **A:** Lateral view of the wing of the ilium shows the gluteus muscle, the tensor fascia lata, and the sartorius muscle. **B:** Anterior view shows the sartorius, the posterior and anterior branches of the lateral femoral cutaneous nerve, and the inguinal ligament.

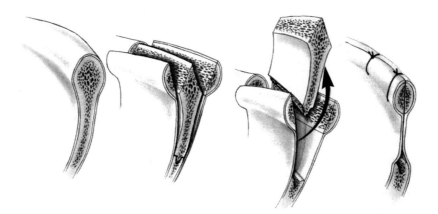

FIGURE 4. Wolfe-Kawamoto technique of harvesting cancellous bone while preserving the entire iliac crest, which is repaired with wire sutures.

cancellous bone can be removed, and the entire iliac crest can be repaired with wire sutures. This repair provides a good appearance and prevents herniation.

Another method is the so-called trap-door method of harvesting bone graft (Fig. 5) (1). In this method, the crest of the ilium is elevated along with the attached abdominal muscles and fascial attachments. The crest is then hinged in place as a trapdoor, and the underlying cancellous bone is removed. The fascial attachments of the crest and of the gluteal muscles are used to repair the trapdoor and close the defect.

Bicortical grafts occasionally are harvested from the anterior ilium. If the amount of bone needed is small, three techniques exist. One is to remove the bone between the anterior superior and anterior inferior iliac spines, as one harvests bone graft for a Salter innominate osteotomy (Fig. 3C). This procedure is less cosmetically acceptable, because it changes the contour of the pelvis. An alternatively is to obtain bicortical graft just posterior

to the anterior superior spine. Such defects should be no more than 2 to 3 cm to prevent herniation through the defect (Fig. 3E). These grafts often are used in anterior interbody fusion, in the filling of defects, or in anterior cervical fusion. The third technique is to remove a bicortical window just inferior to the crest. In this technique the iliac crest is not disturbed, so all the attachments are left in place.

Smith (28) reported a case in which a patient had appendicitis in the postoperative period after an iliac bone graft. Because of the usual bone graft pain, the appendicitis was not diagnosed until the appendix had ruptured. Smith cited this as a reason for obtaining the graft from only the left side.

Posterior Iliac Crest Technique

The posterior iliac crest provides the greatest volume of bone, is the most accessible in posterior spinal exposures, and is the

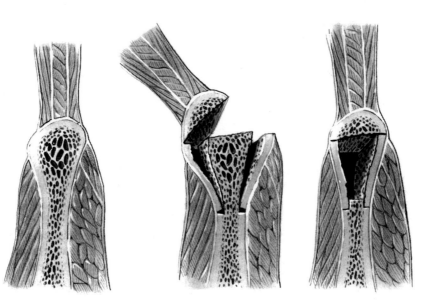

FIGURE 5. Trap-door method of harvesting bone graft allows harvesting of cancellous bone while preserving the fascial attachments of the crest and gluteal muscles.

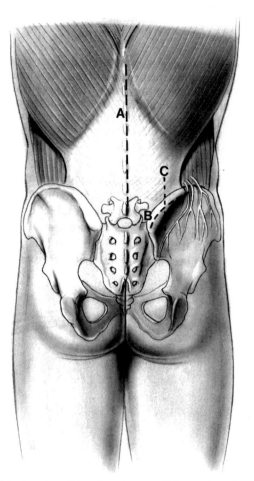

FIGURE 6. Location of the cluneal nerves. Points *A, B,* and *C* indicate the three incisions to be used to harvest graft.

narrow osteotome; then a curved osteotome is used to elevate the corticocancellous piece off the outer table. This can be removed as a single large piece, which can be cut into a variety of shapes or into strips or matchsticks (Fig. 7). As an alternative, some surgeons prefer to place linear, parallel cuts 2 to 3 mm wide in the outer table graft before harvesting it to produce strips of bone that can be removed with a wide, curved osteotome.

After the bone of the outer table is removed, a medium-sized, curved gouge is used to remove additional strips of cancellous bone from the medullary cavity, from the area immediately under the crest, and from the posterior recess toward the sacroiliac crest. A 3 to 4 mm spoon or ring curette can be used to remove additional bone. Care should be taken not to penetrate the inner table, the sacroiliac joint, or the ligaments of the sacroiliac joint. The cortex and ligaments of the sacroiliac joint should be preserved.

The inner cortex or inner table occasionally is violated. The iliacus muscle, with it overlying femoral nerve, and the ilioinguinal nerve are in proximity and can be damaged through penetration of the inner table. A sheet of gelatin foam (Gelfoam) can be placed over the defect at the end of the procedure. I have never encountered a hernia due to a full-thickness defect either

most frequently used source of iliac bone in these procedures. The posterior iliac crest can be approached in one of three ways (Fig. 6). In a midline approach in which the level of incision extends to L4 or L5, the skin and subcutaneous tissues can be undermined and the posterior crest approached through the same incision. When the crest cannot be approached in this manner, a separate incision can be made along the crest of the ilium. This incision should not be extended more than 8 cm anterior to the posterior superior iliac spine to avoid endangering the cluneal nerves. The third alternative is a longitudinal incision centered approximately 4 cm from the posterior superior iliac spine.

In any of these three methods, once the subcutaneous tissues have been incised, the posterior superior spine is identified and the periosteum incised. In operations on patients with mature skeletons, the periosteum is incised directly over the crest of the ilium. In operations on patients with immature skeletons, it is incised just inferior to the iliac apophysis. The periosteum is elevated inferiorly toward the sciatic notch, and a Taylor retractor is placed in the depths of the wound under direct vision. The Taylor retractor should not be placed in the sciatic notch. The periosteum is elevated posteriorly and toward the sacroiliac joint. The extent of the cortical graft is outlined with a sharp,

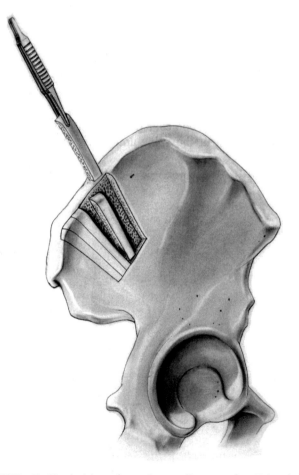

FIGURE 7. Matchsticks of corticocancellous graft. Unicortical matchsticks of corticocancellous graft are harvested from the posterior outer iliac crest.

during the immediately operative period or as a postoperative complication. In all cases the iliac crest was intact.

Bleeding can be controlled by means of placing bone wax at the bleeding points or placing hemostatic agents on the bleeding surface. These include sheets of gelatin foam; gelatin foam soaked in thrombin, or collagen hemostat (Avitene). In one study, the use of collagen hemostat was found to be slightly more effective than other methods but was also more expensive (7). A variety of power instruments are available that can be used to harvest iliac bone. These include ultrasound-powered gouges, compressed air–powered gouges, and devices that cut out a dowel of bone graft.

Strut Grafts

Strut grafts often are used in operations on patients with kyphosis. Most often they are made from ribs or the fibula. Free vascularized bone grafts are useful in a variety of orthopaedic surgical situations. In the spine, vascularized fibular grafts have not been used, or at least have not yet been described in the literature. Nonvascularized fibular grafts often have been used as a strut in anterior spinal operations, such as in the management of spinal tuberculosis and other types of vertebral body collapse. Nonvascularized fibular grafts also have been used in reconstruction after surgical management of bone tumors. Rib osteoperiosteal grafts have been harvested for use in the management of long-bone fractures and nonunions (12); they have not been

used in spinal surgery except when they are removed as part of the exposure.

Rib or fibula placed anterior to the spine takes as long as 2 years to replace living bone. The graft is at its weakest point 6 months postoperatively (4,5). Bradford (4) found a fracture incidence of 50% during bone consolidation when healing grafts were placed more than 4 cm anterior to the apical vertebra.

The fibula is a strong tubular bone that provides greater strength in supporting the spine anteriorly than do comparable rib grafts. Morbidity associated with fibular grafts includes potential damage to the peroneal nerve, hematoma, and weakness. There is less morbidity than that associated with comparable grafts from the tibia. A graft of up to 26 cm can be harvested from the fibula of an adult (Fig. 8) (33). Figure 9 shows use of a fibular strut graft in the management of Pott's paraplegia. After drainage of the anterior tuberculous abscess and resection of necrotic vertebral bodies, a fibular graft was harvested and used to strut the spine anteriorly. Postoperative magnetic resonance images show decompression of the spinal cord and the fibular strut keyed in place in the vertebral body.

Anterior spinal surgery often involves thoracotomy or a thoracoabdominal approach in which a rib is harvested as part of the approach. Such grafts can be used either as morselized bone chips or as an intact strut, but the rib is a weak strut. Such strut grafts usually are nonvascularized free grafts. As such, they are subject to the process of replacement through creeping substitution and are weakest 6 months after surgery (4,5). Bradford (4)

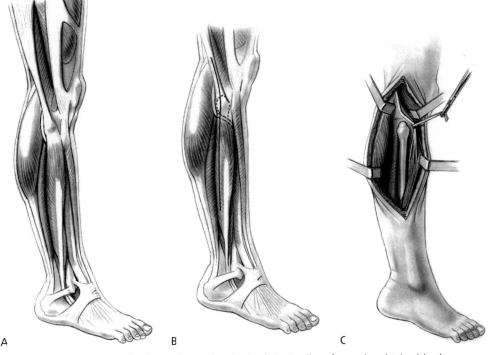

A   B   C

FIGURE 8. A variety of fibular grafts can be obtained. **A:** Small grafts can be obtained in the area between the extensor digitorum and the peroneus longus muscles. The fibula can be exposed by means of the Henry method for the harvest of intact or long pieces of fibula. **B, C:** Line of incision for the Henry method of displacing the peroneal nerve and peroneal muscle.

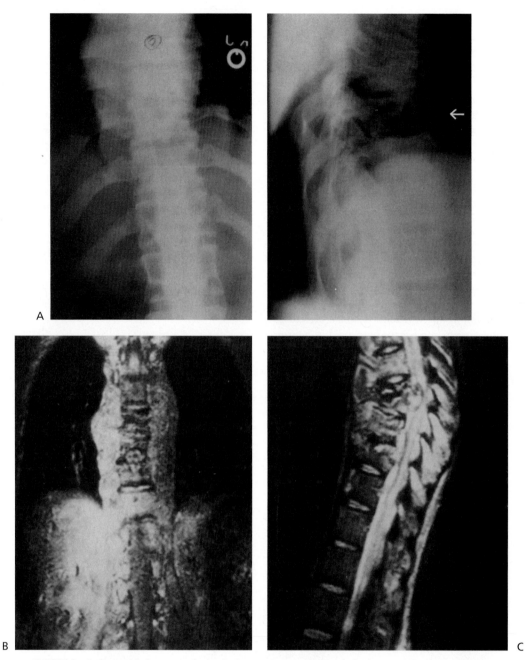

FIGURE 9. Patient with Pott paraplegia. **A:** Anteroposterior radiograph shows mediastinal widening *(left)*. Lateral radiograph shows vertebral collapse *(right)*. **B:** Magnetic resonance (MR) image shows massive paraspinous widening. **C:** Lateral MR image further delineates vertebral collapse and spinal cord compression. *(Figure continues.)*

described a technique of using a rib with a vascular pedicle to form a strut for the kyphotic thoracic spine. The thoracotomy level is chosen to comply with the level to be strutted. For kyphosis with apices between T2 and T5, a rib two or three segments below the apex of the kyphosis should be removed. The distal end of the rib is rotated to the superior vertebra to be strutted. If the apex of the kyphosis is at T6 or below, a rib two to three segments more proximal to the apex is used. The distal side is rotated to the distal vertebra of the body to be fused. A cuff of

intercostal muscle is left with the rib (Fig. 10). Electrocautery is avoided. The rib is divided at the costochondral junction. This procedure requires meticulous technique. Great care must be taken to identify the appropriate level and to preserve the vascular supply.

McBride and Bradford (23) described another technique in which a vascularized rib graft is used. In this technique a femoral head allograft is used to replace a vertebral body. A thoracoabdominal approach is made through the tenth rib. The rib is

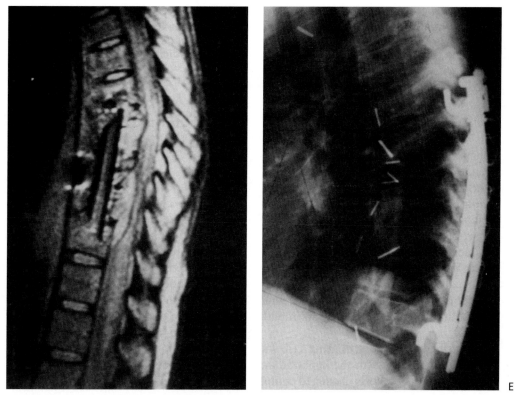

FIGURE 9. *Continued.* **D:** Postoperative MR image shows relief of spinal cord compression with the fibular strut graft in place. **E:** Lateral radiograph after second-stage posterior spinal fusion.

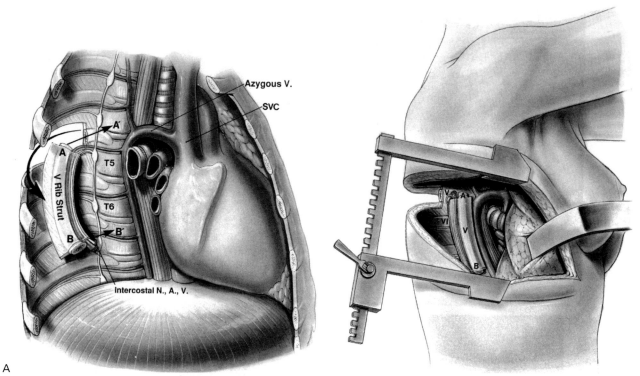

FIGURE 10. Vascularized rib grafting technique. **A:** The rib must have a wide margin of intercostal muscle. There should be minimal periosteal stripping of the ends of the graft. **B:** The graft is keyed into position. Care is taken not to kink the vascular pedicle.

harvested as a vascularized pedicle. After corpectomy, a femoral head allograft is shaped to replace the body. A burr is used to make a trough in the femoral head and adjacent bodies. The vascularized rib is then keyed into the trough. Tomograms showed bridging bone between the rib and allograft at 7 weeks. The advantage of this technique is that the femoral head provides structural support and the vascularized graft may enhance incorporation.

Local Salvage

Bone removed during exposure and decortication of the spine should be salvaged. In limited or short fusion this is a small amount, but in more extensive fusion this bone can add to the volume grafted. The surgeon should clean the spinous processes of all soft tissue and remove the cartilaginous cap. In a large patient, a half-inch (1.25 cm) straight osteotome can be used to split the spinous processes and remove them to provide two pieces of bone graft. Any decorticated fragments of spine are left in place. Any bits of bone removed during preparation of the facet joints, laminectomy, or laminotomy for hook insertion are salvaged. If for any reason a portion of the vertebral body is removed, this too can be salvaged. The bone is thoroughly cleaned of soft tissue and cut into small bits of bone for grafting. An additional rib or ribs also may be harvested. Patients undergoing thoracoplasty by means of rib resection have abundant bone available.

Patients also can autodonate their bone. In severe neuromuscular diseases such as cerebral palsy, a painful dislocated hip can be resected and used during spinal fusion. Such bone can be banked under proper banking conditions to be used at a later time (see Chapter 7). Although it is unusual, bone from amputation or resection in the management of severe neuromuscular conditions can be used for graft material.

COMPLICATIONS

As with all surgical procedures, bone-graft harvesting must be done with great care. Most complications are minor, but some may have severe disabling consequences.

Herniation

Cowley and Anderson (9) reviewed 18 cases of herniation through the ilium, 15 of which were associated with previous harvest of full-thickness graft. In all 18 cases, the graft was obtained from the midportion of the ilium, and the iliac crest was not left intact (3,6,9,14,20,22,24–26). They and others recommend that if it is necessary, a full-thickness graft should be obtained either anteriorly or posteriorly and the fascial insertion reinserted so that there is no defect (3,25). Harvest of an anterior full-thickness graft is cosmetically less acceptable because it changes the contour of the pelvis. A sizable graft can be obtained from between the two tables with the technique of Wolfe and Kawamoto (32) or with the trap-door technique (Figs. 4, 5).

Nerve Injury

Nerves that can be injured in the course of obtaining iliac bone graft include the lateral femoral cutaneous nerve, the superior cluneal nerves, and the ilioinguinal nerves (Fig. 11). Damage to the lateral femoral cutaneous nerves has been reported in as many as 10% of cases (30). The lateral femoral cutaneous nerve emerges from the lateral border of the psoas muscle and runs downward and laterally across the anterior surface of the iliacus (18) (Fig. 2B). It gains access to the thigh slightly medially and inferiorly to the anterior superior iliac spine, passing just behind the inguinal ligament. It is most often isolated or identified by means of incision of the fascia over the upper medial origin of the sartorius muscle. It supplies skin sensation over the lateral aspect of the thigh from the level of the greater trochanter to the knee. Pain caused by damage to this nerve is called *meralgia paresthetica* (15,31). The nerve can be damaged during surgical exposure to obtain a graft when it is cut it with a knife or electrocautery or when pressure is applied during retraction. The nerve has an anomalous course in as many as 10% of cases (15). It can exist over the anterior crest, making it more to injury when the iliac crest is incised. The nerve also can be injured by means of direct pressure incurred while the patient is lying prone on special pads or frames used for posterior spinal procedures.

The ilioinguinal nerve emerges through the lateral border of the psoas muscle and runs obliquely downward and laterally across the quadratus lumborum on the posterior abdominal wall (18) (Fig. 12). It enters the transverse abdominis muscle just above the iliac crest. It penetrates the internal oblique muscle to reach the superficial inguinal ring. Its sensory distribution is

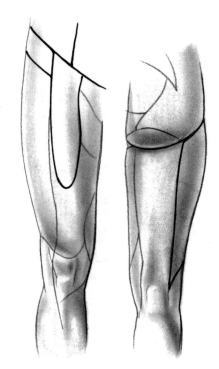

FIGURE 11. Anatomic distribution of nerves at risk during the harvest of anterior iliac crest bone grafts.

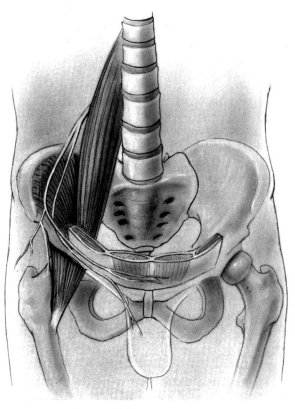

FIGURE 12. Anterior view of the inner pelvis, shows the course of the iliohypogastric and ilioinguinal nerves.

to the skin on the base of the penis and scrotum in male patients and the mons pubis and labium majus in female patients. It usually is damaged by neurapraxia during the course of exposure of the inner table during stripping or retraction of the iliac and abdominal wall muscles. When the ilioinguinal nerve is injured, it causes pain, paresthesia, and numbness in the distribution of the nerve (29).

Most of the sensation of the midportion of the skin of the buttocks is supplied by the superior cluneal nerves, typically three in number (18). These are the cutaneous continuation of the lateral branches of the dorsal rami of the upper three lumbar nerves. The lateral branches of the dorsal rami of the first three sacral nerves supply the medial aspect of the buttocks and form the three middle cluneal nerves. As it leaves the cover of the gluteus maximus muscle, the posterior femoral cutaneous nerve gives off the inferior cluneal nerves around the lateral border of this muscle to supply the skin over the lower part of the buttocks. Damage to these nerves can decrease sensation in the skin of the buttocks and cause postoperative paresthetic pain.

Infection

Infection in donor sites was reported among 2.4% and 2.7% of patients in two respective studies (27,31). Some surgeons emphasize the importance of preventing cross-contamination by means of using separate instruments, gowns, and gloves for the harvesting and grafting procedures. Suction drainage and the use of topical hemostatic agents also have been recommended. I have never routinely changes gown, gloves, or instruments during an operation except when the patient has had a tumor. Donor site infections are uncommon. Most donor site wound infections respond to standard treatment, including drainage, wound management, and intravenous antibiotics.

Hematoma

Hematoma has been reported among 4% to 10% of patients (10,27,30). Anterior donor sites are said to have a higher incidence of hematoma (10,11,19). Kurz et al. (19) reported that suction drainage for 24 to 48 hours is useful and clearly decreases the incidence of serious wound hematoma to less than 1%. I prefer not to routinely use suction drainage at iliac donor sites. I place hemostatic agents such as gelatin foam or bone wax on the donor site of the ilium, and the close the wound in layers. I also do not place drains in posterior spinal fusion wounds. Patients are nursed supine for 6 to 8 hours postoperatively in the hope that direct pressure will aid hemostasis. Aspiration of a liquefied hematoma on the fifth or sixth postoperative day rarely is necessary.

Heterotopic Bone Formation

Heterotopic bone rarely may form in an area of the iliac bone graft. This is more common anteriorly than posteriorly and tends to occur among adults rather than among children.

Peritoneal Perforation and Herniation

Kurz et al. (19) reported two cases of peritoneal perforation during anterior approaches to the inner table of the ilium. Herniation is known to occur after removal of iliac bone graft has been documented frequently. In all reported cases of herniation, harvest of a bicortical graft, including the crest of the ilium, was involved (3,5,6,9,14,20–22,24,25). It does not occur when the crest of the ilium is preserved. It is important to repair the abdominal muscles and suture the gluteal muscles securely to the crest of the ilium after an iliac graft is obtained.

Vascular Complications

Escalas and DeWald (13) reported a case of arteriovenous fistula as a result of iliac bone grafting. The case involved a 15-year-old girl with a mature skeleton being treated for idiopathic lumbar scoliosis. A traumatic injury to the superior gluteal artery caused an arteriovenous fistula and a ureteral injury. The bone graft had been removed from the posterior aspect of the ilium. A Taylor retractor used for exposure accidentally dislodged and penetrated into the sciatic notch. The ureter and iliac vessels are in proximity to the sciatic notch in the female pelvis (Fig. 13). The bleeding was controlled by means of electrocauterization. During the postoperative period, an arteriovenous fistula in the proximal portion of the right superior gluteal artery was found when an arteriogram showed no right renal function. The fistula cleared spontaneously. No obvious cause of the ureteral obstruction that caused the renal malfunction was demonstrated.

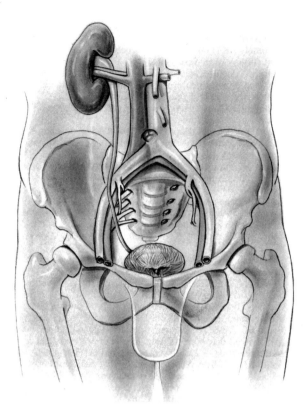

FIGURE 13. View of the inner table of the iliac wings and pelvic contents shows the relation of the kidneys, ureters, and common iliac vessels to the posterior aspect of the pelvis in the sacroiliac joint.

Sacroiliac Joint Instability

The integrity of the sacroiliac joint can be disturbed during harvesting of a posterior iliac crest graft (8,21) (Fig. 14). The posterior sacroiliac ligaments can be damaged during removal of the bone, and the articular cartilage can be breached from the subchondral iliac side of the joint. If the exposure is too generous, the iliac side of the joint can be removed. Patients can have postoperative pain and pelvic instability. Because the pelvis is a closed ring, loss of integrity of the sacroiliac joint can place stress on the symphysis pubis. Spurring and cystic degenerative changes in the pubis may become apparent on radiographs after a long time (8).

Coventry and Topper (8) reported six cases in which patients experienced pelvic instability after removal of iliac bone for bone grafting. The authors believed that this persistent disability was caused by instability of the sacroiliac joint, the symphysis, or both. The patients had pain in the sacroiliac joint during stress tests and pain in the pubic symphysis and medial aspect of the thighs. Special techniques of imaging the pelvis were necessary to see the instability. In these cases the posterior superior supporting ligaments of the sacroiliac joint were compromised at removal of the bone graft (Fig. 12). Management of this condition is fusion of the sacroiliac joint.

Other Complications

Other complications associated with graft harvest have been reported but are infrequent. Persistent pain can occur at the donor

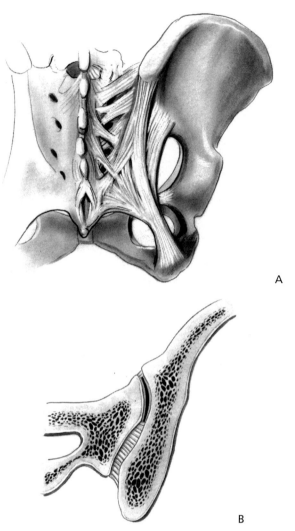

FIGURE 14. **A:** Posterior view shows the sacroiliac ligaments. **B:** Horizontal cross-section of the sacroiliac joint.

site (10,31). A mild limp may develop but is usually not persistent. In one series of 86 patients who underwent reconstructive procedures of the facial skeleton with autologous bone graft, 2.3% had disturbance of motor function, usually a slight limp. Reduced sensibility occurred among a small percentage of patients, and infection developed in 2.4% of cases (31). Seventy-five of the 86 patients had no subjective symptoms.

A stress fracture of the iliac spine and wing of the ilium has been reported (17). In this case a large bicortical graft was obtained from the left ilium, and a portion of the anterior iliac crest was left intact. Ten days postoperatively, the patient experienced the onset of weakness in the left lower extremity over a 24-hour period. Femoral neuropathy due to pressure by hematoma beneath the iliac fascia was suspected, and a large hematoma was evacuated. A fracture was found at the base of the remaining 4-cm iliac strut.

REFERENCES

1. Abbott LC (1947): The evaluation of cortical and cancellous bone as grafting material: a clinical and experimental study. *J Bone Joint Surg* 29:381–414.

2. Albee FH (1944): The evolution of bone graft surgery. *Am J Surg* 63: 421–421.
3. Bosworth D (1955): Repair of herniae through iliac crest defects. *J Bone Joint Surg* 37:1069–1073.
4. Bradford DS (1980): Anterior vascular pedicle bone grafting for the treatment of kyphosis. *Spine* 5:318–323.
5. Bradford DS (1987). *Moe's textbook of scoliosis and other spinal deformities,* 2nd ed. Philadelphia: WB Saunders.
6. Challis JH (1975): Strangulated lumbar hernia and volvulus following removal of iliac crest bone graft. *Acta Orthop Scand* 46:230–233.
7. Cobden RJ (1976): Topical hemostatic agents to reduce bleeding from cancellous bone. *J Bone Joint Surg* 58:70–70.
8. Coventry MB, Topper E (1972): Pelvic instability: a consequence of removing iliac bone for grafting. *J Bone Joint Surg* 54:83–101.
9. Cowley SP, Anderson L (1983): Hernias through donor sites for iliac bone grafts. *J Bone Joint Surg* 65:1023–1025.
10. DePalma A (1972): Anterior interbody fusion for severe cervical disk degeneration. *Surg Gynecol Obstet* 134:755–758.
11. Dick IL (1999): Iliac-bone transplantation. *J Bone Joint Surg* 28:1–14.
12. Dineen JR (1962): Rib osteoperiosteal grafts: a preliminary report of their use in the treatment of fresh and ununited fractures of the long bones. *J Bone Joint Surg* 44:1653–1653.
13. Escalas F, DeWald R (1977): Combined traumatic arteriovenous fistula and ureteral injury: a complication of iliac bone grafting. *J Bone Joint Surg* 59:270–271.
14. Froimson AI (1971): Iliac hernia following hip arthrodesis. *Clin Orthop* 80:89–91.
15. Ghent WR (1961): Further studies on meralgia paresthetic. *Can Med Assoc J* 85:871–875.
16. Ghormely RK (1942): Choice of bone graft methods in bone and joint surgery. *Ann Surg* 115:427.
17. Guha SC (1983): Stress fracture of the iliac bone with subfacial femoral neuropathy: unusual complications at bone graft donor site. *Br J Plast Surg* 36:305–306.
18. Hollingshead WH (1969): *Anatomy for surgeons,* vol 3. New York: Harper & Row.
19. Kurz LT (1989): Harvesting autogenous iliac bone grafts: a review of complications and techniques. *Spine* 14:1324–1331.
20. Lewin ML (1949): Traumatic iliac hernia with extensive soft tissue loss. *Surgery* 26:601–607.
21. Lichtblau S (1962): Dislocation of the sacroiliac joint: a complication of bone grafting. *J Bone Joint Surg* 44:193–198.
22. Lotem M (1971): Lumbar hernia at an iliac bone graft donor site. *Clin Orthop* 80:130–132.
23. McBride GG, Bradford DS (1983): Vertebral body replacement with femoral head allograft and vascularized rib strut graft: a technique for treating post-traumatic kyphosis with neurologic deficit. *Spine* 8:406–415.
24. Oldfield MC (1945): Iliac hernia after bone grafting. *Lancet* 248:810–812.
25. Pytek LJ (1960): Management of herniation through large iliac bone defects. *Ann Surg* 152:998–1003.
26. Reid RL (1968): Hernia through an iliac bone graft donor site. *J Bone Joint Surg* 50:757–760.
27. Sacks S (1965): Anterior interbody fusion of the lumbar spine. *J Bone Joint Surg Br* 47:211–223.
28. Smith RB (1973): A reason for taking iliac bone grafts from the left side in young patients. *Plast Reconstr Surg* 52:425.
29. Smith SE DeLee JC, Ramamurthy S (1984): Ilioinguinal neuralgia following iliac bone grafting. *J Bone Joint Surg* 66:1306–1308.
30. Stauffer RN (1972): Posterolateral lumbar spine fusion: analysis at the Mayo Clinic series. *J Bone Joint Surg* 54:1195–1204.
31. Stoll P SW (1981): Long term follow-up of donor and recipient site after autologous bone graft for reconstruction for the facial skeleton. *J Oral Surg* 39:676–677.
32. Wolfe SA, Kawamoto H (1978): Taking the iliac-bone graft: a new technique. *J Bone Joint Surg* 60:411.
33. Wright PE (1987): Microsurgery. In: Canale ST, ed. *Campbell's operative orthopaedics,* 7th ed. St. Louis: Mosby.

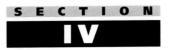

SECTION

IV

SURGICAL APPROACHES AND TECHNIQUES

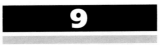

SURGICAL APPROACHES TO THE CRANIOCERVICAL JUNCTION

ARNOLD H. MENEZES

The first anatomic description of craniocervical junction abnormalities was reported in the early part of the nineteenth century (47). These autopsy examinations stimulated clinical interest, but confirmation of a diagnosis was lacking until the patient's death. The advent of roentgenographic studies in the early part of the twentieth century shed new light on the craniocervical abnormalities and on trauma to this region. However, it was only after Chamberlain's classic radiographic study of basilar invagination in 1939 that lesions in and around the craniocervical junction emerged from the realm of anatomic and pathologic curiosity to the practical, clinical field of neuroscience (46). Postmortem reports were replaced by clinical and radiographic studies of abnormalities in this region.

Recent advances in neurodiagnostic imaging, microsurgical instrumentation, and the understanding of craniocervical biomechanics have increased our surgical armamentarium and given us a better understanding of the needs of stability. Up until the early 1970s, anteriorly placed lesions of the craniocervical border were approached by means of posterior decompression and sometimes associated fusion. The morbidity and mortality for such ventrally situated lesions were extremely high (40). In 1977, I proposed surgical physiologic management of abnormalities of the craniocervical junction based on an understanding of the dynamics and stability of the craniocervical region as well as the site of encroachment and associated neural abnormalities. Since then, I have evaluated more than 3,700 patients with neurologic symptoms and signs of abnormalities of the craniocervical junction at the University of Iowa Hospitals and Clinics. This chapter describes the commonly used procedures for decompression and fusion at the craniocervical junction.

METHOD OF APPROACH

The following factors influence specific treatment (47):

1. Reducibility—whether the bony abnormality can be "reduced" to normal position to relieve compression on the cervicomedullary junction. This also implies restoration of anatomic relations of the craniospinal axis.

2. The cause of the lesion—bony or soft tissue. Vascular abnormalities, syrinx, tumors, and Chiari malformation fall into this category.

3. The presence of ossification centers and epiphyseal growth plates in congenital conditions such as fetal warfarin syndrome, Down syndrome, Goldenhar syndrome, and spondyloepiphyseal dysplasia.

4. The mechanics of compression and the direction of encroachment.

The primary goal governing treatment is to relieve compression at the cervicomedullary junction (Fig. 1). If a lesion is reducible, stabilization is essential to maintain neural decompression. Irreducible lesions necessitate decompression at the site at which encroachment has occurred. This treatment is further subdivided into ventral and dorsal compression categories. In the former, the operative approach is transpalatopharyngeal decompression and less often, a Le Fort dropdown maxillotomy or the lateral extrapharyngeal route (43). For lesions that have lateral or dorsal compression, posterolateral decompression or a dorsal decompression is needed. If instability is present after any form of decompression, posterior fixation is mandated.

A particularly interesting and difficult problem arises in the care of very young infants with an unstable craniocervical junction and conditions such as spondyloepiphyseal dysplasia, mucopolysaccharidosis, Goldenhar syndrome, bone-softening states such as osteogenesis imperfecta, and allied situations (43). In such instances it is essential for the treating physician to identify the potential for osseous development by recognizing the epiphyseal growth plates that can be seen only with thin-section computed tomography (CT) and three-dimensional reconstructions. When there is an absence of growth plates, my colleagues and I have allowed growth to take place by supporting the occipitocervical region with custom-built cervical orthoses which are changed every few months. The toddler or young child is reevaluated periodically with diagnostic procedures aimed at identifying the status of the developing craniocervical junction and neural compromise. Once the child is 3 to 4 years of age, when all the components of the craniocervical junction should be present, surgical therapy may be advanced if the situation remains unchanged. The operative procedure selected is described in this chapter.

A. H. Menezes: Division of Neurosurgery, University of Iowa Hospitals and Clinics, Iowa City, Iowa 52242.

TREATMENT OF CRANIOVERTEBRAL ABNORMALITIES

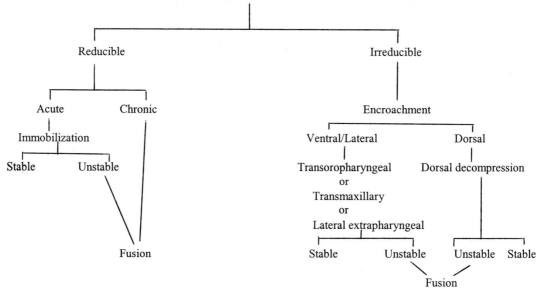

FIGURE 1. Decision tree for management of craniovertebral abnormalities.

NEURORADIOLOGIC INVESTIGATIONS

The initial investigation consists of plain radiography, which must include the lateral view of the skull showing the cervical spine, anteroposterior and open-mouth views to define the odontoid process, and oblique views of the cervical spine (42,47). Supplemental views, such as the Towne view in the anteroposterior projection of the foramen magnum, are obtained as necessary. Radiography should be followed by magnetic resonance imaging (MRI) of the head and upper cervical spine in the sagittal, coronal, and axial planes. At my institution, MRI is performed both in the T1-weighted and T2-weighted modes. Dynamic flexion-extension views are obtained in the T2-weighted mode (Fig. 2). This helps identify reducible lesions and the mechanics of compression. Associated neural abnormalities such as hindbrain herniation syndromes, intradural tumors,

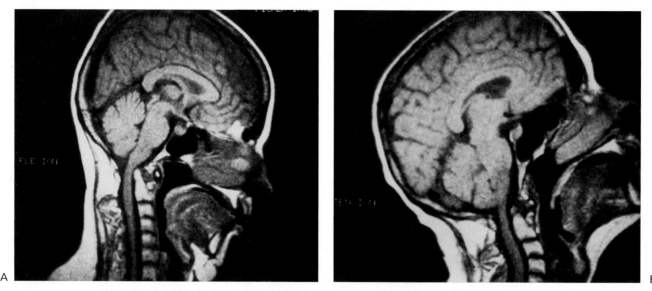

FIGURE 2. A: Midsagittal T1-weighted magnetic resonance (MR) image of the head and cervical spine with flexion at the craniovertebral junction. Atlantoaxial dislocation is present and the odontoid process impinges on the ventral cervicomedullary junction. B: Midsagittal T1-weighted MR image with extension at the craniocervical junction. The atlantoaxial dislocation is reduced, and cervicomedullary compression has been relieved.

cerebrospinal fluid abnormalities, syringohydromyelia, and vascular abnormalities are easily detected. Magnetic resonance angiography is used in selected cases, as is CT angiography. Cervical traction when used is followed by plain lateral radiography and MRI to document the reducibility and confirm the restoration of alignment and relief of neural compromise.

Rapid-acquisition spiral CT is commonly used to obtain three-dimensional images of the craniocervical junction. In all investigation techniques at my institution, dynamic stress views of the craniocervical region are necessary to assess stability and angular-osseous relations to the neural structures. This provides information regarding the optimal position of fixation if fixation is needed. CT examination of toddlers and young children is necessary to recognize the presence or the absence of epiphyseal growth plates and the extent of fusion, "missing" osseous components, and segmentation defects.

Angiography is used to identify obstruction and potential occlusion with dynamic changes of the craniocervical junction. Because of its morbidity, angiography has been relegated to evaluations of the few patients who have unexplained neurologic symptoms or signs. However, with magnetic resonance angiography and CT angiography, a better understanding of the unexplained pathologic processes is possible without morbidity.

SURGICAL APPROACHES TO DECOMPRESSION OF THE CRANIOCERVICAL JUNCTION

Common to most craniocervical procedures is the ability to stabilize the craniocervical junction with an external orthosis or temporary craniocervical traction. Skeletal traction with an MRI-compatible halo device is used in the care of young children. I prefer a crown rather than a complete ring. The youngest infant to tolerate a crown halo for traction has been 10 months of age. However, I would not recommend this routinely. For children younger than 2 years, I have used 8- to 10-point pin fixation. The pin pressure is maintained with thumb and forefinger pressure, which usually does not generate more than 1 to 1.5 lb (450 to 680 g) torque pressure. At 5 years of age the maximum pin pressure used is 4 lb (1.8 kg). Traction is initiated at a low starting rate of 3 to 4 lb (1.4 to 1.8 kg) for a 5-year-old child and does not exceed 7 lb (3.2 kg).

Reducible lesions caused by inflammation or recent trauma respond to conservative treatment with external immobilization once reduction is achieved. Healing is usually ligamentous and at times may include bony reconstitution. If this does not occur, or if the condition is not caused by trauma or infection, bony fixation is mandated. For young children, the traction device is placed in the operating room with the patient under general anesthesia. A cervical collar is used for protection during intubation. General mask anesthesia is used first. Fiberoptic intubation then is accomplished through a mask, the mask is removed, and the halo ring is put in place. It is important that the halo vest be placed with fluoroscopy to achieve the ideal reduced state. However, if an operative procedure is to be performed, the halo vest is not be placed until at least 48 hours after the completion of the operative procedure and extubation.

Older children who can tolerate cervical traction have the

crown halo ring placed with intravenous sedation and are subsequently nursed in an intensive care setting to try to achieve bony reduction. In a grossly unstable but reducible state, the crown halo ring with the halo vest is placed under general anesthesia and the child is turned prone onto the operating table. The posterior struts are removed to allow operative intervention with the ventral struts in place to provide immobilization. Once the procedure is completed, the halo vest is reapplied. The patient is then left intubated until fully awake.

For most conditions, the halo vest is not completed in the operating room, and the definitive operation is performed with cervical traction maintained dynamically over a pulley bar. At the end of the operative procedure, a cervical collar is placed around the neck, and the halo vest is finally placed 48 hours after extubation has been accomplished.

The surgical approaches to the craniocervical junction for decompression can be divided into ventral, lateral and dorsal routes (Table 1) (2,4–7,9,12,13,15,19,21). The aim of therapy for osseous pathologic conditions differs from that of therapy for neoplastic process, in which complete excision should be attempted. Likewise, degenerative diseases differ from congenital disorders and the developmental abnormalities that occur among children. The ability to work through the oral cavity into the ventral and ventrolateral aspects of the craniocervical junction has made access to this region safe and effective. However, this avenue of approach carries potential risk to the cranial nerves, the vertebral and the carotid systems, and the eustachian tubes. Primary neoplastic lesions of the craniocervical region tend to spread into the prevertebral space. Such spread often occurs among the pediatric population, a common example being chordoma of the clivus. The only limitations to tumor expansion then become the temporal fossae and expansion into the sphenomaxillary and pterygopalatine regions. In this situation lateral approaches that allow entrance into this space give a better chance for resection.

Several surgical limitations and considerations must be given attention in designing an approach to the craniocervical junction

TABLE 1. SURGICAL APPROACHES TO DECOMPRESSION OF THE CRANIOCERVICAL JUNCTION

Ventral
  Midline
    Transoral transpalatopharyngeal
    Sublabial Le Fort I maxillary osteotomy with maxillary down fracture
    Transsphenoethmoid
    Lateral rhinotomy
    Median labiomandibular glossotomy
  Anterolateral
    Transcervical extrapharyngeal
    Preauricular infratemporal
Lateral
  Infratemporal fossa transzygomatic
  Translabyrinthine and retrosigmoid
  Far lateral transcondylar
Dorsal
  Posterior lateral 'transcondylar' with rerouting of vertebral artery
  Dorsal decompression of posterior fossa and upper cervical

TABLE 2. SURGICAL APPROACHES TO THE FORAMEN MAGNUM AND UPPER CERVICAL SPINAL CANAL

Approach	Indications	Extent of Exposure	Advantages	Disadvantages	Complications
Transsphenoethmoidal	Extradural clivus and sellar abnormalities	Ventral clivus and opposite side of transethmoid route	Short midline approach	Limited to midline and opposite side. Foramen magnum not reached.	Injury to cavernous sinus and optic nerves.
Transfacial Le Fort I dropdown maxillotomy	Angiofibroma, fibrous dysplasia, extradural chordoma	Paranasal sinuses, clivus, and anterior skull base	Wide anterior base exposure. Can be combined with transoral.	Poor dural coverage if arachnoid violated. Needs miniplate fixation.	Needs tracheostomy. Dural coverage poor.
Transoral transpalatopharyngeal	Extradural lower clivus and C1–2 abnormalities	30 mm width of lower clivus, C1–2 and C3 vertebrae	Procedure done in extension. May be combined with transpalatal and mandibulotomy.	Pterygoid plates limit lateral extension as hypoglossal nerves, eustachian tube, and vertebral artery.	CSF leakage. Retropharyngeal abscess. Instability requiring occipitocervical fusion.
Lateral extrapharyngeal	Chordoma, metastasis, some bony malformations and fusions	Clivus to petrous apex and to C3 if the facial nerve is released in parotid	No oropharyngeal contamination. Ventral CVJ fusion possible.	May cause CN IX, X and XII palsies. Difficulty swallowing. Narrow field.	Limited exposure. Lower CV dysfunction.
Median mandibulotomy with glossotomy	Extradural disease, including oropharyngeal malignant tumor	Wide exposure if combined with palatal split-clivus to C4	May be combined with all ventral procedures.	May lose a central incisor, tracheostomy, miniplate fixation.	Same as transoral. Mandibular infection, malocclusion, tracheostomy.
Far lateral transcondylar	Meningioma, neurinoma, chordoma	Lower clivus and jugular bulb to C3 and below	No oropharyngeal contamination. Good vertebral artery control. May be combined with posterior fossa and infratemporal procedures.	Sigmoid and venous sinuses.	CSF leakage. Vascular injury. Potential instability.
Infratemporal fossa approaches	Intradural tumors of clivus, middle and posterior fossa and skull base	Petrous bone, upper clivus, foramen magnum	No brain stem or cerebellar retraction. Good control of carotid artery. Good muscle pedicle flaps possible.	Needs combined approaches to access lower clivus. Sacrifice of condyle of mandible and eustachian tube.	Problems chewing. Hearing loss and facial palsy.
Posterolateral lateral cerebellar	Extradural and intradural of CVJ abnormality	90–120 degree arc from lateral condyles to past midline	No brain stem retraction with good vertebral artery control. Fusion possible.	Limited by sigmoid sinus, basilar artery, and occipitocervical joints.	CSF collection. Vascular injury.
Posterior midline decompression and upper cervical laminectomy	Dorsal and lateral tumor. Bony decompression of foramen magnum.	Covers 120 degrees of dorsal foramen magnum	Can easily be combined with fusions.	Not indicated for ventral and lateral lesions.	Very few disadvantages if indicated.

CSF, cerebrospinal fluid; CVJ, craniovertebral junction; CN, Cranial nerve.

(Tables 1, 2). It is important that one recognize violation of the orodigestive tract, the need to cross the midline, the ability to look around the corner, and limitations of a narrow circumference ringed by vascular structures and neural tissue and mobile joints. Thus attention to appearance and stability have a part to play in the surgical management of lesions in this region. Table 2 enumerates the advantages, limitations, and indications for each approach. The extent of exposure is illustrated in Fig. 3.

Transoral-Transpalatopharyngeal Approach

The main indication for the anterior transoral approach is an extradural lesion located within an area extending from the mid-clivus down to the level of the C3 vertebral body and laterally for 2 cm to either side of the midline (Fig. 4) (19,42,46). The youngest child for whom my colleagues and I have had to proceed with anterior decompression of the cervicomedullary junc-

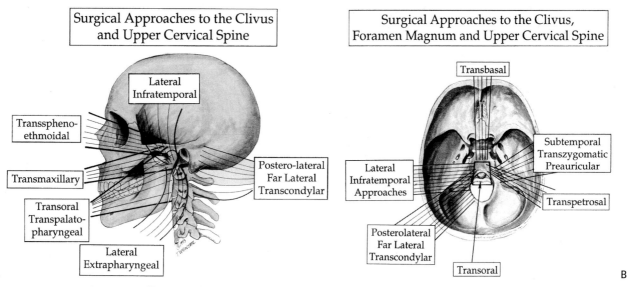

FIGURE 3. A: Illustration shows extent of surgical exposures obtained by the different routes to the clivus and upper cervical spine in lateral projection. B: Illustration in basal view shows the extent of surgical exposure to the clivus, foramen magnum, and upper cervical spine.

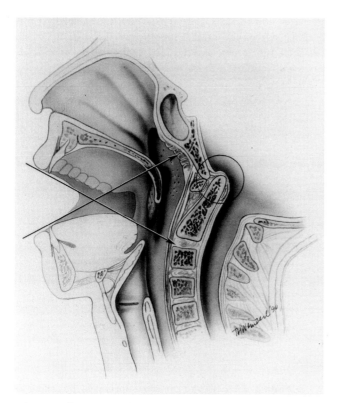

FIGURE 4. Illustration in lateral projection shows the extent of exposure obtained with a transoral-transpalatopharyngeal approach.

tion was 2 years of age, and the extent of exposure was quite satisfactory. Further inferior access may be gained by means of median labial mandibular glossotomy in operations on patients older than 12 years (2,4,5,28,48). Rostral extension of the exposure may be obtained with limited resection of the caudal hard palate or sublabial Le Fort I maxillotomy with maxillary dropdown fracture (4,6,12,34,44). Another option is lateral rhinotomy combined with the transoral procedure for a child older than 12 years. This is because the growth center for forward expansion of the midface is situated in the midline anteriorly, above the hard palate. My colleagues and I prefer not to violate this area with a rhinoseptal approach (44).

The indications for resection of craniocervical lesions by the transoral route include irreducible osseous lesions, extradural osseous and infectious lesions, and neoplasms. Intradural pathologic conditions arising from the extradural space, such as clivus chordoma, also may be approached in this manner. However, only a rare case of intradural schwannoma or meningioma would require a primary ventral transoral approach. As a rule, intraarachnoid disease is best approached by an anterolateral, lateral, or posterolateral route unless these avenues have proved ineffective.

A transoral procedure for removal of a ventrally situated bony abnormality causing cervicomedullary compression has the following advantages: (a) direct safe route with access to either side of the midline, (b) no retraction of neural structures, and the head is usually positioned in an extended position that avoids increasing the bony abnormality invaginating into the cervicomedullary junction, and (c) abnormal cerebrospinal fluid dynamics can be restored, thereby relieving the craniospinal-cerebrospinal fluid dissociation and allowing resolution of syringohydromyelia. The disadvantages of a transoral procedure are greater potential for infection and the fact that ventral fusion between the skull and the upper cervical spine has proved difficult and does necessitate dorsal fixation to overcome the biomechanical forces on this region.

Preoperative Assessment

The nutritional status of children with symptoms must be evaluated. Young children and those with juvenile rheumatoid arthritis may have limited ability to open the mouth. In such circumstances, the surgeon should assess the width of exposure between the upper and the lower incisors. A working distance of 25 to 30 mm is considered satisfactory. If this is not possible, a median mandibular split with midline glossotomy may be essential for the transoral operation, or an alternative route must be sought. Before the operation, the surgeon must assess the patient's nutritional condition, ability to swallow, and respiratory function. Preoperative compromise of the lower cranial nerves may necessitate tracheostomy (42,46).

Operative Procedure

The patient is transported to the operating theater on a fracture bed. Skeletal traction applied to older children with an MRI-compatible halo. For children who cannot tolerate preoperative traction because of age or other circumstances, a cervical collar is placed around the neck before intubation. This is done through mask induction and followed by fiberoptic intubation through the mask. Once this is accomplished, the patient is positioned supine on the operating table in mild extension on a padded horseshoe headrest. Traction is maintained over a pulley bar. My colleagues and I desist from use of head clamps because of potential instability during the operative procedure. Nasal endotracheal intubation has been avoided because this tends to disrupt the integrity of the high nasopharyngeal mucosa, which is the avenue of approach to the craniocervical region.

Somatosensory evoked potentials with particular attention to brain stem latencies were used initially but were later found to be impractical (62). In rare instances, tracheostomy is needed when the operation involves the lower clivus and structures rostral to the foramen magnum that cause brain stem compromise.

The laryngopharynx is occluded with a throat pack, and cleaning of the circumoral area and oral cavity is begun with 10% povidone-iodine followed by hydrogen peroxide and a saline rinse. A modified Dingman self-retaining mouth retractor is inserted. Over the past 4 years my colleagues and I have moved the nonarmored endotracheal tube to the side of the mouth, where it is secured to the skin of the chin. This reduces postoperative tongue swelling without compromising exposure of the oral cavity and pharynx. The soft palate is infiltrated with 0.5% lidocaine solution with 1:200,000 epinephrine in the median raphe.

A midline incision is made in the soft palate. The incision extends from the hard palate to the base of the uvula and deviates to one side. The stay sutures applied to the soft palate in the midline incision hold apart the leaves of the palate to expose the high nasopharynx (Fig. 5A). The nasopharyngeal mucosa is anesthetized with topical 2.5% cocaine supplemented with 0.5% lidocaine solution with 1:200,000 epinephrine injected into the median raphe. The posterior pharyngeal midline incision is made, and the pharyngeal flaps are retracted to either side (Fig. 5B). This exposes the lower clivus and the longus capitis and longus colli muscles over the ventral aspect of the anterior arch of the atlas and axis. The prevertebral fascia and longus capitis and longus colli muscles are dissected free of the osseous and ligamentous attachments to expose the caudal clivus, the anterior atlas arch, and the axis. Lateral exposure is limited to 15 mm to either side of the midline to preserve the integrity of the eustachian tube orifice and to prevent injury to the hypoglossal nerves and vertebral arteries.

The anterior arch of the atlas is removed with a high-speed

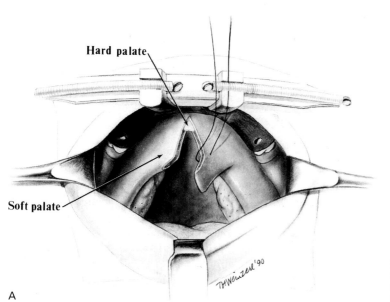

Hard palate

Soft palate

FIGURE 5. A: Illustration shows operative procedure of transoral craniocervical decompression. Self-retaining mouth retractor is in position, and the soft palate incision is made. *(Figure continues.)*

A

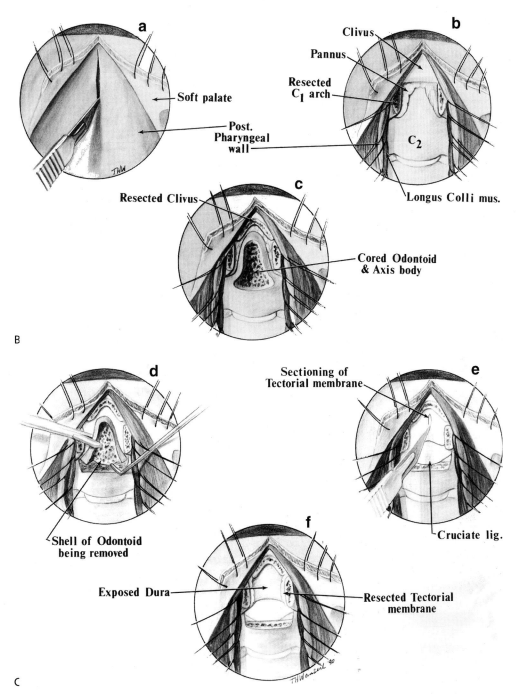

FIGURE 5. *Continued.* **B:** Views through an operating microscope during transpharyngeal craniovertebral exposure. *a,* Incision of the posterior pharyngeal wall. *b,* Resection of the anterior arch of the atlas and caudal clivus brings invaginated odontoid process into view. *c,* Odontoid process is cored out. **C:** View through an operating microscope shows transpharyngeal exposure of the craniocervical junction. *d,* Odontoid shell is being removed. *e,* Tectorial membrane is incised. *f,* Dural decompression.

drill, as is the caudal clivus. The soft tissue ventral to the odontoid process is resected with rongeurs. Removal of the odontoid process is performed in a rostral-caudal dimension with a high-speed drill with a cutting burr first and then with a diamond burr (Fig. 5C). Pannus indicates chronic instability and has to be resected. Division of the odontoid process at its base and downward traction have been advocated by some surgeons, but this maneuver endangers the patient and is fraught with difficulty. This is especially so if the pannus is tough and the odontoid process has achieved a subarachnoid location.

After removal of portions of the tectorial membrane, the surgeon is assured of adequate bony decompression when the pulsatile dura protrudes into the decompression site. It is wise to leave the transverse portion of the cruciate ligament intact for partial stability of the atlas. The extent of bone resection is governed by analysis of diagnostic images, which must be available during the surgical procedure. Extradural neoplasms such as chordoma and the like necessitate careful correlation of the diagnostic procedures to locate the position of intraarachnoid vessels.

An extension of the transoral procedure is a transpalatal approach. The soft-palate incision is extended into the hard palate in the midline for a distance of 3 cm. The mucosa is swept laterally toward the alveolar margins to preserve the greater palatine vessels. The hard palate is then removed for a distance of up to 2 cm. The lateral extent of this removal is approximately 1.0 cm to either side. The vomer is then identified and removed in the posterior aspect. Should the operative procedure require clival exposure, the vomer is excised, as is the midline septum of the sphenoid sinus. This extent of basisphenoid exposure is necessary for dealing with clivus chordoma in children.

Should an intraarachnoid lesion be present and the surgical procedure be performed into the subarachnoid spaces, careful closure of the dura is imperative. The external oblique fascia or fascia lata is harvested and laid against the dura. The fascial closure is reinforced with tissue glue and carefully covered with a fat pad. The wound is approximated in a layered manner. If the surgeon anticipates that the dura will be violated, a lumbar subarachnoid drain usually is installed preoperatively, and cerebrospinal fluid drainage is maintained for 5 to 10 days postoperatively.

The longus colli and longus capitis muscles are approximated in the midline, and the posterior pharyngeal muscles are closed subsequently. The layered closure is accomplished with 3-0 polyglycolic acid sutures in interrupted manner. The posterior pharyngeal mucosa is likewise approximated with simple sutures of similar strength. The soft palate is approximated in two layers: the nasal mucosa is brought together with simple interrupted technique, and the muscular layer together with the oral mucosa approximated with vertical mattress sutures of 3-0 polyglycolic acid. Before closure of the soft palate, a feeding tube is installed into the stomach by the nasal route under direct vision.

In the event that the dura is violated during the operative procedure, intravenous administration of cefotaxime, metronidazole, and nafcillin is begun and continued for 5 days. In the absence of cerebrospinal fluid leakage or infection, cefotaxime is discontinued after 5 days. Nafcillin and metronidazole are continued for another 5 days for a total of 10 days of antibiotic therapy. A lumboperitoneal shunt was required by only 1 of 42 patients in whom an intraarachnoid lesion was removed by the transoral route among 460 patients who underwent transpalatopharyngeal surgery at the craniocervical junction.

Postoperative Care

No oral intake is permitted postoperatively, and the head of the bed is elevated to 30 degrees. Cervical traction is discontinued, and a cervical collar placed around the neck. The endotracheal tube is left in place for the first 2 to 3 days after the transoral procedure until lingual swelling has abated. Nasogastric tube feedings are initiated once chest and abdominal radiographs confirm the position of the endotracheal tube and the nasogastric feeding tube in the stomach or transpyloric location.

In most circumstances, the transpalatopharyngeal procedure is immediately supplemented with a craniocervical stabilization fusion procedure. Cervical traction is discontinued in the postoperative phase, and a cervical collar is used for immobilization until 48 hours after extubation. At that time the halo vest is placed.

Oral intake is permitted with a clear liquid diet at the end of 5 days. After this, the patient is advanced at 5-day intervals to a full liquid diet and then to a pureed diet. Postoperative intravenous antibiotics are maintained only for the first 24 hours in an uncomplicated situation. Surgical fusion has been accomplished in all children who have undergone ventral craniocervical decompression (Fig. 6).

Complications

The most feared complication of the transoral operative procedure is cerebrospinal fluid leakage (40). If intradural disease is recognized during diagnostic studies, preoperative subarachnoid drainage is installed; otherwise it is placed postoperatively. Intraoperative closure of the wound is described earlier. Delayed cerebrospinal fluid infection occurred in two individuals in the series of 460 patients described earlier. However, this complication never occurred among the pediatric population.

The occurrence of meningitis should signify cerebrospinal fluid leakage, which must be controlled after intravenous administration has been instituted (19,30,42,63). The ventral aspect of the operative site is imaged by means of the direct nasopharyngeal fiberoptic approach and by CT and MRI.

A child with Down syndrome may have severe tongue swelling. This complication occurs mainly among older patients with rheumatoid arthritis. In these circumstances, intravenous administration of dexamethasone in the postoperative period has been found helpful to reduce swelling.

Bleeding during the transoral operation at the level of the circular sinus must be controlled by means of clipping both leaves of the venous sinuses. Careful packing with microfibrillar collagen and oxidized cellulose may be helpful. Bleeding from the vertebral artery branches may occur, especially during tumor resection. If this happens, hemostasis is secured by the use of bipolar cauterization and at times the use of aneurysm clips. This does not spell disaster because the opposite vertebral artery supplies the posterior circulation in approximately 90% of patients. Nonetheless, if the surgeon suspects that the vertebral artery may be destroyed, a preoperative angiogram should be obtained to confirm that the contralateral vessel is patent.

Palatal dehiscence necessitate immediate reclosure. Pharyngeal wound dehiscence that occurs within the first week implies improper closure and must be redone. However, pharyngeal wound dehiscence after 2 weeks indicates the presence of a retropharyngeal abscess.

The most commonly unrecognized complication is postoperative craniovertebral instability (12,42). It is thus essential that this be addressed in the care of every patient who undergoes surgical fusion, especially those in whom it is believed that the region is stable.

Seven percent of children may have velopalatine incompetence. My colleagues and I have seen it more commonly among

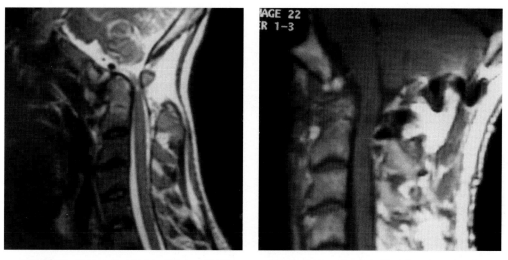

FIGURE 6. Composite of midsagittal magnetic resonance image of craniocervical junction shows irreducible atlantoaxial dislocation with gross cervicomedullary compression by the invaginated odontoid process (*left*) and shows spinal cord contusion. Ventral compression is relieved (*right*) after transoral-transpalatopharyngeal resection of the caudal clivus, anterior atlas arch, and odontoid process. Dorsal occipitocervical fusion has been accomplished. The cervicomedullary decompression is complete and craniocervical alignment satisfactory.

children with preoperative brain stem dysfunction (40). This usually signifies inadequate closure of the pharynx and the soft palate. However, if this has been properly attended to, velopalatine incompetence in children manifests itself between the third and the fourth month after the operation. This complication is caused by fibrosis in the soft palate and initially manifests as nasal regurgitation and a peculiar voice. The situation necessitates formal evaluation of the nasopharynx, including video endoscopy. Should the situation not correct itself, a palatal prosthesis or a nasopharyngeal flap may be needed.

Results

Neurologic improvement has been the rule among all 146 children who have undergone a transoral-transpalatopharyngeal procedure. There have been no deaths or major complications. Retropharyngeal infection occurred as a result of wound dehiscence, iatrogenic in origin caused by a patient's injudicious use of Yankow suction postoperatively. The youngest patient to undergo a transoral procedure was 2 years of age, and the oldest was 82 years. Patients ventilator dependent from previous posterior fossa decompression had resolution of their neurologic symptoms and signs. More important, children with Chiari malformations and basilar invagination who underwent primary ventral decompression had resolution of the symptoms and regression of the syrinx visualized at MRI (Fig. 7).

Lateral Transcervical Extrapharyngeal Approach to the Ventral Foramen Magnum

The anterior retropharyngeal approach to the upper cervical spine has been described by several authors (14,39,42,56,61). The lateral transcervical extrapharyngeal approach provides ex-

posure of the midline foramen magnum, the lower clivus, and the anterior surfaces of the upper cervical vertebrae. This route is indicated in the management of tumors, such as chordoma, that affect the ventral aspect of the craniovertebral junction and extend laterally, predominantly to one side. It has been used for ventral decompression of rheumatoid basilar invagination and ventral fusion. The exposure is pyramidal with the apex at the site of surgical interest. A wider exposure can be gained by rerouting the facial nerve and the hypoglossal nerves (44). This approach has the advantage of being extracavitary from the oropharynx and allows for ventral craniovertebral fusion.

Operative Technique

The awake patient undergoes fiberoptic intubation by the nasoendotracheal route. The oral cavity is kept free of any tubes. The same precautions are taken regarding intubation and anesthesia as with the transoral route. The patient is positioned supine with the head maintained in traction and resting on a padded headrest. The head is then turned to the left for a right-handed surgeon. The cervical incision starts behind the ear over the mastoid process and extends approximately two fingerbreadths below the angle of the mandible and the proceeds anteriorly to the midline just above the hyoid bone (Fig. 8A). An inferior extension converts the transverse incision into a *T*.

The dissection is made through the subcutaneous tissue and platysma muscle. The platysma is elevated, and the skin flaps are defined. The inferior branch of the facial nerve is identified and dissected to allow later elevation of the facial nerve and the parotid gland. Superficial veins draining into the common facial vein are sacrificed. The fascia of the parotid gland and the facial nerve are identified, and the dissection proceeds into the deep cervical triangle to elevate the parotid fascia with the facial nerve. The deep fascia at the anterior border of the sternomastoid mus-

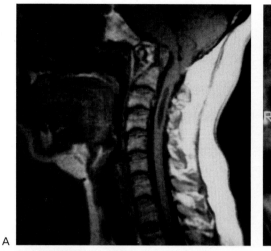

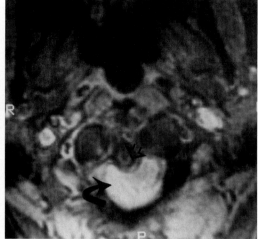

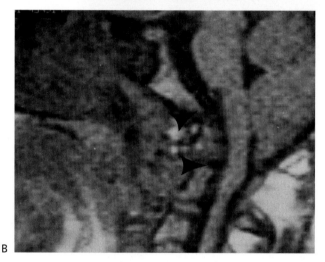

FIGURE 7. A: Composite of preoperative magnetic resonance (MR) image of a 12-year-old boy with lower cranial nerve palsy and spastic quadriparesis. Midsagittal T1-weighted MR image (*left*) shows atlas assimilation, odontoid basilar invagination indenting into the medulla, Chiari I malformation, and syringohydromyelia. Axial T2-weighted MR image (*right*) through the lower medulla (*arrow*) shows invagination into the ventral medulla oblongata. **B:** Midsagittal T1-weighted MR image through the craniocervical junction of same patient as in **A** 3 days after ventral transoral clivus-odontoid resection (between *arrowheads*). Medullary decompression is evident, and high cervical cord syringohydromyelia has disappeared.

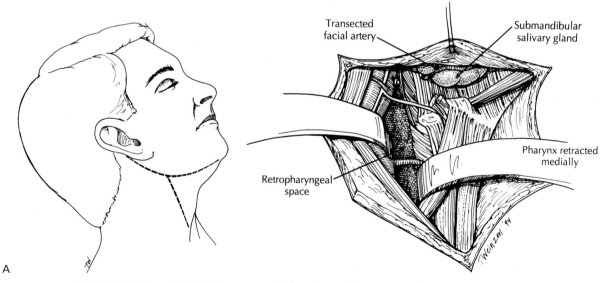

FIGURE 8. A: Line of skin incision necessary for lateral extrapharyngeal exposure of the ventral craniocervical junction. **B:** Operative procedure during lateral extrapharyngeal exposure to the lower clivus and the upper cervical spine. The vascular sheath including the carotid artery, internal jugular vein, and neurovascular bundle is retracted laterally. The tendon of the posterior belly of the digastric muscle and the stylohyoid muscle is detached at the greater cornu of the hyoid bone. The hypoglossal nerve is elevated superiorly. The pharynx is retracted medially to gain exposure of the retropharyngeal space.

cle is incised to allow a view of the carotid sheath. The blood vessels are retracted laterally.

The submandibular salivary gland is retracted anteriorly and is elevated. If it is enlarged and obstructs the view, this gland can be resected without any consequences if the duct is transected and ligated to prevent a salivary fistula. It is important to identify the posterior belly of the digastric muscle and its tendon as it comes toward the greater cornu of the hyoid bone. Here it must be transected as should the stylohyoid muscle to allow elevation and forward location of the pharynx (Fig. 8B). The hypoglossal nerve is identified and mobilized superiorly. Great care is taken to preserve the descendens hypoglossi branches. The retropharyngeal space is opened by means of blunt dissection. Any veins crossing the operative field into the jugular vein are transected after being ligated and cauterized.

The prevertebral fascia is incised in a vertical manner, and the longus colli muscles and the longus capitis are dissected free of the osseous-ligamentous attachments. The exposure provides visualization of the anterior arch of the atlas, and blunt dissection is performed. It is important to have orientation of the midline at all times with the anterior tubercle of the atlas and tubercle on the lower aspect of the clivus. This provides a midline reference. The anterior decompression is accomplished as described for a transoral procedure.

It is possible to make a tricorticate iliac crest or a fibular strut graft to be interposed between the caudal clivus and the inferior aspect of the axis. The anchorage is accomplished with a tongue-in-groove technique that provides stability. It is important not to violate the mucosa of the high nasopharynx overlying the midclivus. The wound is closed in an anatomic manner with interrupted 3-0 polyglycolic acid sutures.

Postoperative nutrition should be maintained with intravenous and nasogastric tube feedings. The procedure is not as well tolerated as a transoral operation owing to early pharyngeal dysfunction. There is a high risk of injury to the hypoglossal and glossopharyngeal nerves and difficulty in seeing the midline structures of the true craniovertebral junction. However, the approach can be ideal for extradural lesions below the level of the atlas. The dissection along the carotid sheath with posterior displacement of the structure is necessary. Therefore an important complication is embolization from carotid artery plaques and seventh nerve damage during the operative procedure.

The advantage of this procedure is that the vertebral artery can be bared during excision of the tumor and can be satisfactorily covered with a vascularized sternomastoid muscle pedicle graft. This prevents vertebral artery blowout.

Transcondylar Posterolateral Approach to the Lower Clivus, Foramen Magnum, and Upper Cervical Spinal Canal

The posterolateral transcondylar approach has been labeled the *transjugular approach,* the *extreme lateral transcondylar approach,* the *lateral suboccipital approach,* and the *extreme lateral and dorsal lateral suboccipital condylar approach.* These variants of the technique have a common denominator in that they all represent an attempt to provide exposure of the lower clivus, the foramen magnum and craniocervical border, and the upper cervical spine

without retraction of the cerebellum or spinal cord (3,9, 13,17,26,53,60). Thus this exposure requires fairly extensive posterior and lateral bony resection, which includes removal of the posterolateral squamous-occipital bone, including the rim of the foramen magnum and the medial posterior aspect of the occipital condyle. Hence, the term *transcondylar.* This exposure may be approached by a straight lateral or a posterolateral route. In any case, the posterior arch of the atlas and the posterior aspect of foramen transversarium of the atlas and the lateral atlantal mass are resected. The advantage is complete control of the extracranial and intracranial vertebral artery. A surgeon using this route can work in front of the brain stem and the cervical spinal cord and thus gain the anterior aspect of the foramen magnum. The advantage of a fusion construct with the same incision and approach enhances the use of this procedure.

Indications

The transcondylar posterolateral approach is indicated for operations on patients with intradural neoplasms situated entirely anterior to the brain stem and cervical cord and on patients with vascular abnormalities of the vertebrobasilar system. Extradural lesions of the clivus and the cervical canal can be approached with relative freedom. Lesions that affect the posterolateral and ventral foramen magnum that extends into the cervical canal can be approached by means of retrosigmoid craniotomy. Thus this route provides access for several combinations of operative intervention (2,4,13,21,22,38,44,52).

Operative Technique

I prefer to perform the procedure with the patient in the neutral prone position with the head turned slightly to the side of the exposure and fixed in a multipinned, multipurpose headrest secured to the operating table. The patient is secured to the operating table to allow rotation up to 45 degrees during the operation. This approach has been performed in a sitting position, a lateral position, and a modified decubitus or park bench position.

An inverted hockey stick incision starts at the mastoid process and ascends upward to just above the superior nuchal line. It follows the horizontal plane to just past the midline and comes down the median axis of the cervical canal to the C5 level (Fig. 9A). A cuff of muscle and fascia is maintained at the insertion into the superior nuchal line for later reapproximation and to prevent cerebrospinal fluid leakage. The paraspinous muscles are split along the spinous processes, and the resection is performed laterally to the site of the lesion. The paraspinous muscles are retracted with hooks and weights.

The lateral mass of the atlas is carefully dissected free from the vertebral artery to allow removal of the venous plexus that accompanies the vertebral artery. The ipsilateral occipital bone is removed to include the condylar fossa, the posterior rim of the occipital condyle, and the dorsal rim of foramen magnum (Fig. 9B). The posterior arch of the atlas including the transverse process and the lamina of C2 are exposed. The bony exposure is carried to the jugular bulb. Mastoidectomy may be necessary to expand the exposure.

The vertebral artery is elevated from its groove in the atlas and is dissected free from the foramen transversarium laterally

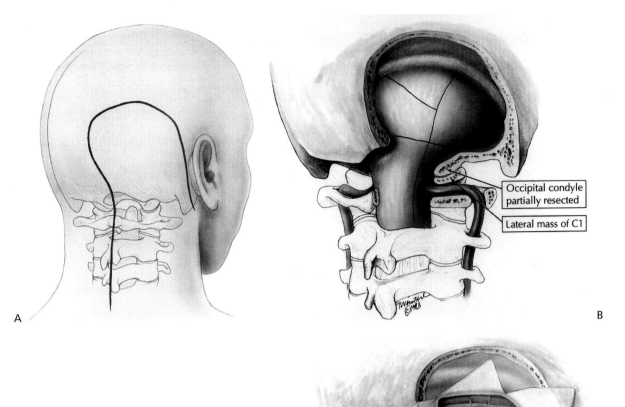

Occipital condyle partially resected

Lateral mass of C1

FIGURE 9. **A:** Skin incision for posterolateral-transcondylar exposure of the craniocervical junction and the ventral brain stem. **B:** Extent of bony removal for posterior fossa, foramen magnum, and upper cervical canal exposure to visualize the ventral craniocervical border. Illustration shows partial occipital condyle resection and resection of the lateral atlantal mass. The vertebral artery is mobilized out of the foramen transversarium. The dural incision is as marked. **C:** Extent of intradural exposure by the posterolateral-transcondylar route.

to the point of penetration into the atlantooccipital membrane medially. The lateral exposure into the posterior fossa and the upper cervical canal is better obtained when the vertebral artery is transposed. To do this the posterior aspect of foramen transversarium is removed. The vertebral artery is unroofed and dissected free down to the axis. The operating microscope is essential for this procedure. The dural opening starts at the superolateral quadrant in the posterior fossa and extends vertically downward into the cervical canal as needed. Lateral extensions from this vertical incision hold apart the leaves of the dura (Fig. 9C). The dentate ligament must be sectioned, and the cervicomedullary junction rotated upward and away from a ventrally placed lesion. In rare instances, the intradural dorsal rootlets of C1 may be sacrificed.

Removal of one third to one half of the medial aspect of the occipital condyle does not cause instability. However, if a large portion of the lateral atlantal mass and the occipital condyle have been resected, and C2 facetectomy accomplished, postoperative instability occurs (2,38,44). For this reason, fusion must be performed on the opposite side. This also can be performed on the same side to span the operative defect and go to a vertebral level below. The instrumentation used may be an angled conforming titanium loop or an angled plate. This may be secured to the occiput and the upper cervical spine wherever possible and at times may be supplemented with lateral mass pedicle screw fixation from the axis to the atlas.

The far lateral approach and the transcondylar approach carry risk of complications due to lower cranial nerve paralysis and cerebrospinal fluid leakage (2,4,52). However, at my institution these complications have not occurred, and the procedure is believed to be extremely effective and safe. A sitting position during the operation is to be avoided, if possible, to prevent air embolism.

Posterior Fossa Midline Craniectomy and Upper Cervical Laminectomy

The midline dorsal approach to the posterior fossa and upper cervical spine is indicated for decompression of the bony foramen magnum in conditions such as achondroplasia and for tumor and osseous disease in the dorsal and dorsolateral compartments of the foramen magnum and spine (Fig. 10A, B) (7,43). The advantage of this procedure is that it may be combined with a posterolateral transcondylar approach and craniospinal fixation.

Technique

Intubation must be accomplished with the patient awake in the presence of foramen magnum tumor or abnormalities at the craniocervical border. Preoperatively it is imperative that the surgeon check the patient's tolerance of the operative position

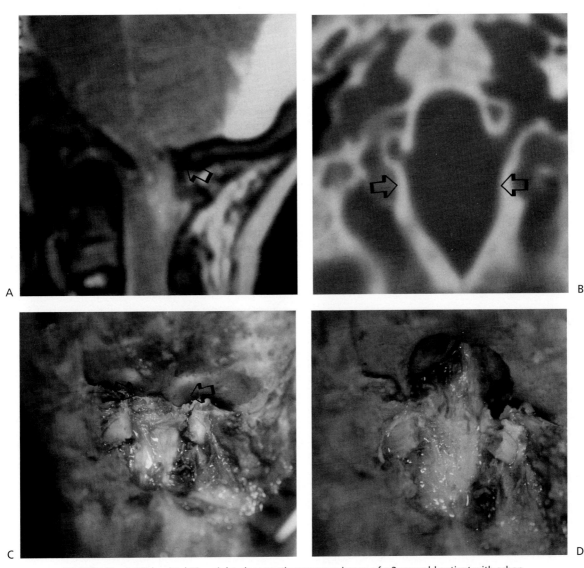

FIGURE 10. A: Midsagittal T2-weighted magnetic resonance image of a 3-year-old patient with achondroplasia, dorsal invagination of the cervicomedullary junction (*arrowhead*), and sleep apnea. **B:** Axial computed tomographic scan through the foramen magnum with bone windows (same patient as in **A**). Marked narrowing of foramen magnum is evident between the two open arrows. **C:** Photograph through operating microscope (same patient as in **A** and **B**). The foramen magnum and posterior arch of the atlas have been exposed. Posterior atlantal decompression was essential before exposure of the posterior rim of the foramen magnum and the mesially approximated occipital condyles (*arrows*). **D:** Operative photograph shows extent of dorsal decompression of foramen magnum and the posterior atlantal arch.

by mimicking the head in flexion and mild lateral rotation while the patient is awake. This is done to make sure that the patient can tolerate the position in which the head is to be maintained during the operation. Too often, vascular or neural compromise can occur with untoward results. After intubation, the awake patient should be placed in the prone position, and neurologic status should be checked. If there is no change in neurologic status, general endotracheal and intravenous anesthesia are provided.

The incision starts at the external occipital protuberance and extends to the spinous process of C6. Sharp dissection is used for subperiosteal exposure of the squamous-occipital bone and the posterior bony elements of the upper cervical spine. I prefer use of an electrocutting cautery apparatus. Dissection of the small rotator muscles from the squamous-occipital bone and the region of the foramen magnum must be accomplished by means of sharp dissection. If the patient has a condition such as osteogenesis imperfecta or achondroplasia, the posterior rim of the foramen magnum is invaginated far ahead of the dorsal laminae of C1 and C2. Hence, the foramen magnum can be reached only after laminectomy is accomplished at C1 and only by means of removal of the lower portion of the squamous-occipital bone (Fig. 10C, D). In other circumstances, posterior fossa craniectomy and upper cervical laminectomy can be performed with a high-speed drill. Bone removal is dictated by the pathologic condition. Craniectomy can be performed by means of outlining the area of bone for removal and placing two trephines at the superior lateral extent in the squamous-occipital bone. The bone incision is made with a high-speed drill powered by a footplate, and cranial bone is removed. An alternative is to use a large drill. When there is considerable compression, the footplate should not be used with the drill or with Kerrison punches. A burr should be used, and the bone should be gradually thinned.

FUSION OF THE CRANIOCERVICAL JUNCTION

The occipitoatlantoaxial articulation is complex because of the highly specialized anatomic features that provide a large range of motion between the head and the trunk. The geometric features of the articular surfaces provide mobility. Stability is provided by the muscular and ligamentous attachments that span the skull and the cervical spine (27). This versatile function necessitates numerous synovial joints and with the complex mobility of the region makes the occipitoatlantoaxial complex vulnerable to traumatic injuries among children and to diseases that affect the synovial joints and ligaments, such as Down syndrome, juvenile rheumatoid arthritis, and various other inflammatory conditions (20,23,33,50,51,54,58). In function, the craniocervical junction is a stable, interlocking unit that allows flexion-extension and lateral rotation of the head. The osseous-ligamentous elements and the muscles exert important controls over translation and limit rotation and extent of motion. The cervical spinal column functions as a series of ball and socket joints that require muscular action to prevent buckling collapse.

The muscle bulk in the neck is much more visible posteriorly and is related to the tendency of the head to be positioned in such a way that the center of gravity is positioned anterior to

TABLE 3. FUSIONS OF THE CRANIOVERTEBRAL JUNCTION

Anterior
  Occipitocervical fusion
    Bone baffle between clivus and the anterior axis body (e.g., after transoral surgery)
    Wire fixation of clivus to C1 anterior arch and C2 body and buried in methyl methacrylate
    Plate instrumentation between clivus-C1 and C2
  Atlantoaxial
    Lateral mass screws between C2 and C1
    Odontoid screw fixation for type II isolated fractures
    Plate and screw fixation
Posterior
  Occipitocervical
    Bone grafts attached to occiput and C1 and C2; spinous processes or interlaminar or facet
    Instrumentation
      Contoured loop
      Plate and screw fixation to occiput and into C2 pedicle
  Atlantoaxial
    Bone with cable fixation
    Instrumentation
      Transarticular screws C2 to C1
      Clamps between C1 and C2 laminae

the vertical support provided by the spinal column. Thus it can be seen that occipitocervical fusion is best served with a dorsal fusion mass. Fusion of the region should be capable of withstanding the forces of compression, axial loading, flexion and extension, lateral rotation, and lateral bending (1,11,16,41,57).

Occipitoatlantoaxial arthrodesis in any form must theoretically be done to act as a spacer and allow growth of children without lordosis or iatrogenic subaxial instability (36,41). The final goal of this construct is osseous integration. There is no doubt that the initial strength of the construct is greatest at surgery and subsequently is reduced in the process of the host response until the final fusion mass is achieved.

Craniocervical junction fusion can be divided into anterior and posterior types (Table 3). In the anterior variety, occipitoatlantal fusions have been performed with a baffle between the clivus and the anterior axis body, wire fixation between the clivus and the upper cervical spine buried in methyl methacrylate, and plate instrumentation. Anterior atlantoaxial arthrodesis has been accomplished with similar types of material, including lateral mass screws between C2 and C1 and plate and screw fixation. The more commonly used posterior route consists of a combination of bone and instrumentation. The commonly used fusions are described.

Dorsal Occipitocervical Fusion

The main indications for dorsal occipitocervical fusion are congenital bifid anterior and posterior arches of the atlas that cause gross instability (29,33,41). A similar situation arises with reducible basilar invagination and an unstable dystopic os odontoideum. Unilateral atlas assimilation with chronic rotary occiput-C1 and C1–2 luxation necessitates occipitocervical stabilization. This is a primary procedure in occipitocervical dislocation. Complex fractures of the craniovertebral junction that cause gross instability necessitate occipitocervical fusion, as does transoral decompression of the craniovertebral junction. Primary malignant tumors that affect the craniovertebral junction in the pediatric population, such as chordoma of the clivus and osteoblastoma, necessitate dorsal fixation. Incorporation of the occiput in craniocervical fusion has serious implications because of loss of motion segments. Occipitoatlantoaxial dorsal fixation eliminates 30 degrees of flexion and extension and the first 35 to 40 degrees of lateral rotation that normally occurs at the atlantoaxial articulation. This limitation occurs to a much lesser degree among children who adapt to the fusion mass.

Technique

The maneuvers for intubation are as described for the surgical approaches to decompression. In an operation on a young child who has not been placed in halo cervical traction, traction is applied after intubation. The patient then is turned to a prone position on the operating table, and traction is maintained. The face and halo ring rest on a padded Mayfield-Kees horseshoe headrest. The head and neck are placed in the position that shows the least neural compromise on preoperative imaging studies. Lateral radiographs document the optimal position for reduction, and this can be guided by preoperative dynamic views. Cervical traction is maintained over a pulley bar to allow dynamic changes during the operation (Fig. 11A). Paralyzing agents are prohibited during this portion of the anesthesia. A fixed-head position with a pinned headrest or halo vest allows changes in alignment between the prone and supine positions and during a prone position and hence may allow us a snaking situation. This is obviated by the use of a constantly mobile traction device that adapts to the patient's position.

The posterior scalp and cervical region are prepared, as is the area for harvesting donor bone. I prefer to use rib grafts over iliac crest grafts. Just before induction of anesthesia, the patient begins to receive intravenous cephalothin sodium, administered every 6 hours and continued for 48 hours after the operation.

A midline incision is made from the external occipital protuberance to the spinous process of C5. Subperiosteal exposure is obtained of the squamous-occipital bone and the posterior arches of the upper three cervical vertebrae by means of sharp dissection. A towel clip is passed through the spinous process of the axis, if gross instability is present. This must be maintained with muscle dissection to expose the atlas. Stabilization of the operative exposure is further obtained by means of placing angled D'Errico or Miskimmon retractors at 90-degree angles to each other. This stretches and fixes the muscle-bone relation so as to prevent movement at the craniocervical articulations.

The posterior rim of the foramen magnum is excised with Kerrison punches, and the bone is preserved for later use in the osseous construct. Craniectomy is performed to excise the posterior rim of the foramen magnum for 1 cm to either side of the midline and 1.5 to 2 cm up from foramen magnum. This is essential to remove the exoccipital inner bony ridge to facilitate passage of soft cable from laterally positioned trephines toward the midline (18). The trephines are made 1.5 cm to either side

of the midline and 3 cm above foramen magnum. A second set is made 2 cm away from the midline and 1 cm above the foramen magnum. Epidural cable is passed from the trephine to the midline craniectomy to gain purchase of the occipital bone. Sublaminar cables are passed under the posterior bony elements of C1, C2, and at times C3. I prefer to use full-thickness rib grafts placed between the occiput and the posterior arch of C1 and C2. The grafts are transfixed with the cables and thus individually anchored to the recipient surfaces of bone at the occiput, C1, and C2 respectively. The excess bone is made into matchstick slivers that are packed into the remaining crevices of the donor-recipient interface.

In operations on patients older than 8 years, I have used instrumentation for occipitocervical fusion, especially in situations such as Down syndrome and spondyloepiphyseal dysplasia (41,49). The placement of instrumentation serves only for the immediately postoperative period until osseous fusion has occurred. Custom-contoured loop instrumentation spanning the occiput and upper cervical vertebrae allows for postoperative MRI and has improved the treatment of these children (12,29). The exposure is as described for the rib graft fusion (51). However, the titanium loop instrumentation is first placed against the dorsal occipitocervical articulation and the contour of the loop is customized to the individual occipitocervical angulation (Fig. 11B). The cables secure the loop at the point of fixation to the occiput and to the lamina of C1 and C2. It is important that the transverse fixation of the inferior ends of the loop be made if the posterior arch of the inferiormost vertebra to be secured is not fully stable or strong enough. In an average 10- to 12-year-old patient, the cables are cinched down at 30 lb (13.5 kg) torque pressure at the axis and the occiput (Fig. 11C). At C1, this usually is reduced to 15 lb (6.8 kg). My colleagues and I prefer not to use ferromagnetic instrumentation. The rib grafts are placed laterally to the bony instrumentation to obtain contact with the recipient surface of the occiput and the dorsal aspect of the laminae of the cervical spine. This is secured with cerclage sutures of 2-0 polyglycolic acid to maintain them in this position (Fig. 11D).

Should midline decompression of the occiput and upper cervical spine be needed, purchase for the cables can be obtained through the inferior facet of the cervical vertebrae (Figs. 12, 13). In grossly unstable situations, transarticular screw fixation between C2 and C1 is made. The screw either is incorporated with a hook and clamp to the occipitocervical loop or is free-standing.

Atlantoaxial Arthrodesis

Dorsal atlantoaxial arthrodesis is performed in the same manner as the occipitocervical fusion except that the grafts do not extend to the occiput. Modified Gallie fusion is performed for older children for whom a satisfactory tricorticate iliac crest graft is made to fit between the undersurface of the dorsal arch of C1 and the superior aspect of the posterior arch of C2. A notch is made for the spinous process (8,16,24,46). This is maintained by means of placement of Gallie-type cable wiring that goes under the lamina of C1 and hooks beneath the spinous process

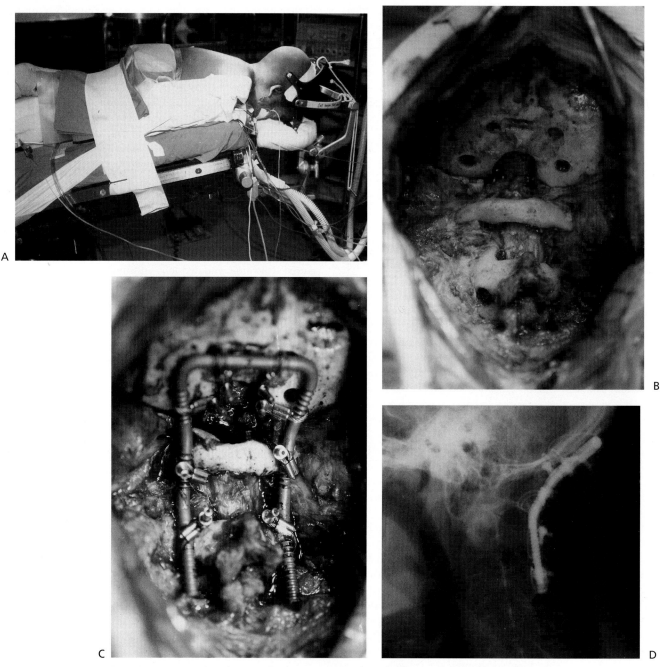

FIGURE 11. A: Operative photograph of 6-year-old child positioned prone for dorsal craniocervical fusion. The crown halo rests on a padded headrest and continuous cervical traction. **B:** Operative photograph shows exposure of the squamous-occipital bone (posterior fossa), foramen magnum, and upper cervical spine. Midline craniectomy has been performed to remove the rim of the foramen magnum. Trephines are visible in the occiput for passage of extradural cable to secure the occipital bones. **C:** Operative photograph of the same patient as in **B** shows custom-contoured threaded titanium loop instrumentation anchored to the occiput and the posterior atlantal arch and the C2 lamina. **D:** Postoperative lateral craniocervical radiograph obtained 6 months after completed dorsal occipitocervical fusion. Image shows titanium loop instrumentation and completed rib graft fusion.

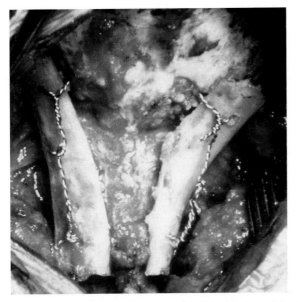

FIGURE 12. Operative view of occipitocervical dorsal rib graft fusion in the face of posterior fossa decompression. The grafts are secured to the lateral portion of the available squamous-occipital bone and to the axis facets.

of C2 (Fig. 14). The anterior portion of the cable passes around the wedge graft to be tied behind it and anchored in this position.

The severe shortcoming of this procedure is the toggling that seems to occur with any amount of graft resorption. The toggling causes failure of the fusion unless halo immobilization is provided postoperatively. I use rib graft fusion with interlaminar bridging between C1 and C2 and at times C3 (Fig. 15) (43,46). The success rate of atlantoaxial arthrodesis is 98.4% with satisfactory postoperative immobilization (51). Rib grafts have had a high incidence of fusion in my series, possibly owing to the

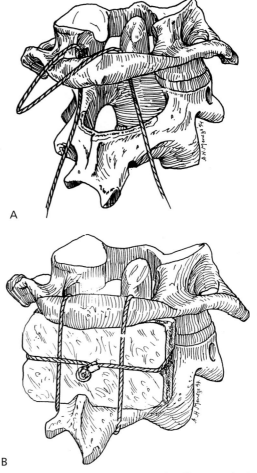

A

B

FIGURE 14. A: Cable passage for modified Gallie-type atlantoaxial fusion. The superior aspect of the lamina and spinous process has been prepared to accommodate a tricortical iliac crest bone graft. **B:** Completed dorsal atlantoaxial arthrodesis in the manner of Gallie with iliac crest graft.

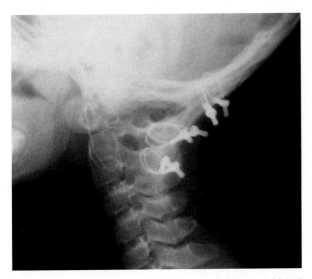

FIGURE 13. Lateral craniocervical radiograph of an 8-year-old patient with dorsal occipital–C1-2 fusion with rib graft. The extent of bone incorporation with the dorsal bony elements described is evident.

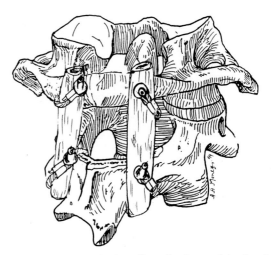

FIGURE 15. Dorsal interlaminar rib graft atlantoaxial arthrodesis.

increased amount of bone morphogenic protein present from the marrow of the rib graft. In this situation, the patient is maintained in a halo vest for 3 months, as for patients with Down syndrome (31). Otherwise a Miami J collar can be used. Occipitocervical arthrodesis requires 5 to 6 months of immobilization. Shorter immobilization has resulted in nonunion or union in an abnormal position (45). Additional cranial settling with subsequent increased neurologic deficit has occurred.

Posterior Transarticular-Atlantoaxial Screw Fixation

Indications

The maximum amount of immobilization across the atlantoaxial joint under laboratory testing is obtained with transarticular screw fixation between the axis and the atlas (16,35). This is the result of fixation at the extremes within a circle. This procedure is not indicated for every patient for whom atlantoaxial arthrodesis is being considered (55). One contraindication to this procedure is age younger than 8 to 10 years when the vertebral artery groove is so high riding it causes a marked decrease in the amount of space available at the pars interarticularis of the axis. The other contraindication is inability to reduce the atlantoaxial alignment. This eliminates approximately 30% of patients for whom the procedure is being considered. Preoperative assessment with CT must be made for this reason. Frameless stereotaxic guidance can be used to provide direction for the screw placement.

Atlantoaxial instability has traditionally been managed by means of posterior arthrodesis with wiring and bone grafts. However, the appropriate choice of operative technique and failure to provide satisfactory postoperative bracing has resulted in high failure rates. The initial development of posterior atlantoaxial screw fixation by Margrel was a way to achieve rigid internal fixation of C2–1 and thus promote arthrodesis (35). This technique is particularly useful in conditions in which postoperative immobilization is not possible and when the posterior arch of C1 is absent. My colleagues and I have used this with satisfactory results after failed attempts at atlantoaxial arthrodesis. The procedure is contraindicated when there is destruction of the lateral masses of the atlas, as in osteoporosis, osteopenia, and inflammatory states such as rheumatoid disease. Patients with atlas assimilation and occipitalization may have a meandering course to the vertebral artery, making it vulnerable to transarticular screw fixation (32,41,59). Similarly, if the anatomic landmarks of the anterior tubercle of the atlas are absent, as in patients who have undergone transoral resection of the ventral craniocervical abnormality, this procedure may be hazardous (55).

Preoperative assessment for transarticular screw fixation between the axis and the atlas demands flexion-extension radiographs to evaluate the reducibility of the lesion. CT of the craniocervical region with parasagittal reconstructions through the region of the axis pars interarticularis is mandated (Fig. 16). An aberrant position of the vertebral artery makes the procedure impossible.

The patient is positioned in crown halo traction prone on the operating table with mild neck flexion. A fluoroscope is positioned laterally for monitoring throughout the procedure (25,37,56). The precautions for intubation and exposure have been previously described. The region of the foramen magnum and the upper four cervical vertebrae has to be exposed beyond

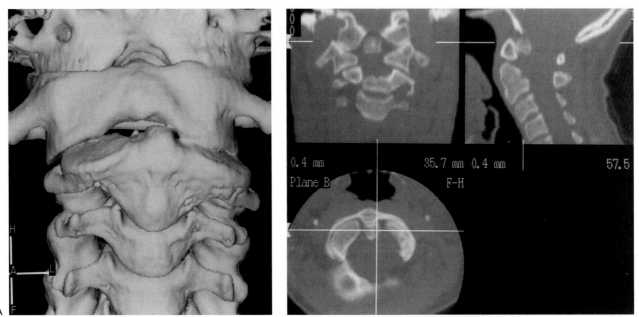

FIGURE 16. A: Frontal view three-dimensional computed tomographic (CT) scan of the craniocervical junction of a 14-year-old patient with dystopic os odontoideum and gross atlantoaxial dislocation. **B:** Two-dimensional CT scan with frontal, midsagittal, and axial reconstructions shows the dystopic os odontoideum, the integrity of the lateral atlantal masses, which is necessary for transarticular screw fixation, and atlantoaxial lateral dislocation.

the lateral facets. The skin must be prepared up to the upper thoracic region. This is to allow for the angle of drilling and may be circumvented by use of a percutaneous technique (43). The spinous processes and the lamina and the facets from C1 to C3 are exposed. The ligamentum flavum must be removed between C1 and C2, and the C2 nerve root is exposed and elevated. The facet joint between C1 and C2 is identified, and an instrument is placed there. Venous bleeding from the venous plexus around C2 is controlled with judicious bipolar cauterization and packing with oxidized cellulose cotton. Identification of the C2 pars interarticularis is important. Satisfactory alignment of the atlas and the axis must be obtained. If needed, manual reduction can be performed with somatosensory evoked control. I prefer a cannulated screw technique because of the safety of placing a K-wire before a screw and being able to identify vascular injury.

A bone awl or a drill is used to penetrate the posterior cortical bone of C2 at the inferior facet 3 to 4 mm from the medial edge of the facet joint (Fig. 17A). The trajectory is marked out toward the dorsal cortical aspect of the anterior arch of C1 (Fig.

17B). The drill is placed 10 degrees to the vertical pointing medially to come through the C2 pars interarticularis. In the sagittal orientation, the trajectory is slightly medial to the vertical. The length of the screw should be measured before the procedure with CT reconstructions; the screw pathway also should be measured. The guidewire is followed with real time fluoroscopy and must past through the C1–2 facet joint. As the wire traverses the joint space, the atlantoaxial articulation becomes rigid and fixed. A new stiffness is felt in the guidewire and the tap that follows. If angulation is not possible for guidewire placement with the extent of exposure, a percutaneous technique is used whereby the carrying portion of the insertion cannula enters the skin 2 cm to either side of the midline at about the T2 level. Under fluoroscopy the cannula is guided to the space described earlier. Drilling is performed through the shaft of this cannula. The advantage is that the guidewire can be secured with a clamp at the C2 facet once it has reached its ideal position and the pneumatic drill has been disconnected.

The cannulated drill is passed over the guidewire and advanced over the guidewire with the pneumatic drill. The guide-

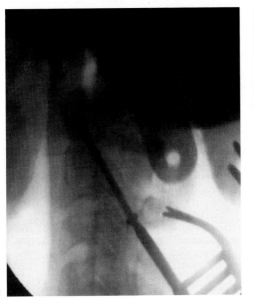

A

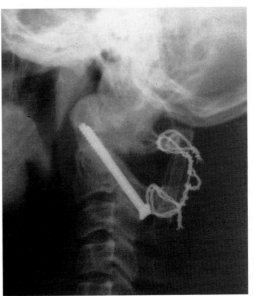

B   C

FIGURE 17. A: Extent of exposure for transarticular C1–2 screw fixation. Illustration shows the position of the vertebral arteries and the point of entry of the screw in the facet and pars of the axis and its point of traversal of the atlantoaxial joint. **B:** Radiograph of the same patient as in **A** obtained during real-time fluoroscopy and transarticular atlantoaxial C2–1 screw fixation shows crown halo traction, atlantoaxial reduction, fixation of the C2 spinous process by a towel clip, and the cannulated screw tightened over a guidewire. **C:** Lateral radiograph of same patient as in **A** and **B** obtained after transarticular C1–2 screw fixation and bilateral dorsal interlaminar rib-graft fusion.

wire is secured beyond the pneumatic drill to prevent advancement into the parapharyngeal soft tissues with the drilling technique. The drill is followed by the tap. The length of the screw is measured with preoperative CT and by means of passing a guidewire of similar length into the cannula and measuring the difference between the inserted primary guidewire and the secondary one for measurement of depth. This allows identification of ideal screw length.

The opposite side drilling is performed. This is done before placement of the screw to be able to identify each individual guidewire with lateral fluoroscopy. The screw is advanced over the guidewire and its purchases obtained into the lateral mass of the atlas. The screw head should be positioned flush against the bone. Overtightening of the screw causes shearing to the cortex of the pars interarticularis and the facet and destroys the purchase on bone.

Interlaminar bone fusion must be performed after placement of the bilateral or unilateral screw (Fig. 17C). If the vertebral artery or vein has been injured, drilling must not be performed on the opposite side. Injury to one vertebral artery will probably not cause neurologic deficit. It is therefore important not to proceed on the opposite side if injury has occurred (10,43).

Percutaneous drilling and screw insertion tools are convenient and require long drill bits and tissue sheets. My colleagues and I prefer to use 3.5-mm diameter titanium screws to allow subsequent imaging of the region. However, the widest possible screw diameter ideally should be used because of the inner diameter of the screw is the primary determinant of bending strength.

Transarticular atlantoaxial screw fixation must always be followed by interlaminar or interspinous bone fusion. The technique requires considerable expertise and has a steep learning curve.

REFERENCES

1. Abumi K, Takada T, Shono Y, et al. (1999): Posterior occipitocervical reconstruction using cervical pedicle screws and plate-rod systems. *Spine* 24:1425–1434.
2. Al-Mefty O, Borba LAB (1997): Skull base chordomas: a management challenge. *J Neurosurg* 86:182–189.
3. Al-Mefty O, Borba LA, Aoki N, et al. (1996): The transcondylar approach to extradural non-neoplastic lesions of the craniovertebral junction. *J Neurosurg* 84:1–6.
4. Ammirati M, Bernardo A (1998): Analytical evaluation of complex anterior approaches to the cranial base: an anatomic study. *Neurosurgery* 43:1398–1408.
5. Arbit E, Patterson RH Jr (1981): Combined transoral and median labiomandibular glossotomy approach to the upper cervical spine. *Neurosurgery* 8:672–674.
6. Archer DJ, Young S, Uttley D (1987): Basilar aneurysms: a new transclival approach via maxillotomy. *J Neurosurg* 67:54–58.
7. Aryanpur J, Hurko O, Francomano C, et al. (1990): Craniocervical decompression for cervicomedullary compression in pediatric patients with achondroplasia. *J Neurosurg* 73:375.
8. Brooks AL, Jenkins EB (1978): Atlanto-axial arthrodesis by the wedge compression method. *J Bone Joint Surg Am* 60:279–284.
9. Canalis RF, Martin N, Black K, et al. (1993): Lateral approach to tumors of the craniovertebral junction. *Laryngoscope* 103:343–349.
10. Coric D, Branch CL Jr, Wilson JA, et al. (1996): Arteriovenous fistula as a complication of C1–C2 transarticular screw fixation: long-term evaluation of results and efficacy. *J Neurosurg* 85:340–343.
11. Coyne TJ, Fehlings MG, Wallace MC, et al. (1995): C1–C2 posterior cervical fusion: long-term evaluation of results and efficacy. *Neurosurgery* 37:688–693.
12. Crockard HA, Pozo JL, Ransford AO, et al. (1986): Transoral decompression and posterior fusion for rheumatoid atlanto-axial subluxation. *J Bone Joint Surg Br* 68:350–356.
13. Day JD, Fukushima T, Giannotta S (1997): Cranial base approaches to posterior circulation aneurysms. *J Neurosurg* 87:544–554.
14. DeAndrade JR, MacNab I (1969): Anterior occipito-cervical fusion using an extra-pharyngeal exposure. *J Bone Joint Surg Am* 51:1621–1626.
15. Derome PJ (1977): The transbasal approach to tumors invading the base of the skull. In: Schmidek HH, Sweet WH, eds. *Current techniques in neurosurgery*. New York: Grune & Stratton, pp. 223–245.
16. Dickman CA, Crawford NP, Paramore CG (1996): Biomechanical characteristics of C1–C2 articulation: a biomechanical study comparing simple midline wiring and the Gallie and Brooks procedures. *J Neurosurg* 85:316–322.
17. Dowd GC, Zeiller S, Awasthi D (1999): Far lateral transcondylar approach: Dimensional anatomy. *Neurosurgery* 45:95–100.
18. Ebraheim NA, Lu J, Biyani A, et al. (1996): An anatomic study of the thickness of the occipital bone. *Spine* 21:1725–1730.
19. Fang HSY, Ong GB (1962): Direct anterior approach to the upper cervical spine. *J Bone Joint Surg Am* 44:1588–1604.
20. Fielding WJ, Hawkins RJ, Ratzan SA (1976): Spine fusion for atlantoaxial instability. *J Bone Joint Surg Am* 58:400–407.
21. Fisch U, Matton D (1988): Infratemporal fossa approach. In: Fisch U, Matton D, eds. *Microsurgery of the skull base*. New York: Thieme Medical Publishers, pp. 136–281.
22. Fisch U, Pillsbury HC (1979): Infratemporal fossa approach to lesions in the temporal bone and base of the skull. *Arch Otolaryngol* 105:99–107.
23. Flint GA, Hockley AD (1987): Internal fixation for atlanto-axial instability in children. *Childs Nerv Syst* 3:368–370.
24. Gallie WE (1939): Fractures and dislocations of the cervical spine. *J Bone Joint Surg Am* 46:495–499.
25. Gebhard JS, Schimmer RC, Jeanneret B (1998): Safety and accuracy of transarticular screw fixation C1–C2 using an aiming device: an anatomic study. *Spine* 23:2185–2189.
26. George B, DeMatons C, Cophignon J (1988): Lateral approach to the anterior portion of the foramen magnum. *Surg Neurol* 29:484–490.
27. Goel VK, Clark CR, Gallaes K, et al. (1988): Movement rotational relationships of the ligamentous occipito-atlantoaxial complex. *J Biomech* 21:673–680.
28. Hall JE, Denis F, Murray J (1977): Exposure of the upper cervical spine for spinal decompression by a mandible and tongue-splitting approach. *J Bone Joint Surg Am* 59:121–123.
29. Hamblen DL (1967): Occipitocervical fusion: indications, technique and results. *J Bone Joint Surg Br* 49:33–45.
30. Hayakawa T, Kamakawa, Ohnishi T, et al. (1981): Prevention of postoperative complications after a transoral transclival approach to basilar aneurysms. *J Neurosurg* 54:699–703.
31. Johnson RM, Hart DL, Simmons EF, et al. (1977): Cervical orthoses: a study comparing their effectiveness in restricting cervical motion in normal subjects. *J Bone Joint Surg Am* 59:332–339.
32. Kawaguchi T, Fujita S, Hosoda K, et al. (1997): Rotational occlusion of the vertebral artery caused by transverse process hyperrotation and unilateral apophyseal joint subluxation. *J Neurosurg* 86:1031–1035.
33. Koop SE, Winter RB, Lonstein JE (1984): The surgical treatment of instability of the upper part of the cervical spine in children and adolescents. *J Bone Joint Surg Am* 66:403–411.
34. Krespi YP, Har-El G (1988): Surgery of the clivus and anterior cervical spine. *Arch Otolaryngol Head Neck Surg* 114:73–78.
35. Magerl F, Seemans PS (1987): Stable posterior fusion of the atlas and axis by transarticular screw fixation. In: Kehr P, Weidner A, eds. *Cervical spine*. New York: Springer-Verlag, pp. 322–327.
36. Malcolm GP, Ransford AO, Crockard HA (1994): Treatment of nonrheumatoid occipitocervical instability. *J Bone Joint Surg Br* 76:357–366.
37. Marcotte P, Dickman CA, Sonntag VKH, et al. (1993): Posterior atlantoaxial facet screw fixation. *J Neurosurg* 79:234–237.

38. Matsushima T, Natori Y, Katsuta T, et al. (1998): Microsurgical anatomy for lateral approaches to the foramen magnum with special reference to transcondylar fossa (supracondylar transjugular tubercle) approach. *Skull Base Surg* 8:119–125.

39. McAfee PC, Bohlman HH. Riley LH, et al. (1987): The anterior retropharyngeal approach to the upper part of the cervical spine. *J Bone Joint Surg Am* 69:1371–1373.

40. Menezes AH (1992): Complications of surgery at the craniovertebral junction: avoidance and management. *Pediatr Neurosurg* 17:254–266.

41. Menezes AH (1995): Posterior occipitocervical fixation. *Tech Neurosurg* 1:72–81.

42. Menezes AH (1997): Indications and techniques for transoral and foramen magnum decompression. In: Bridwell KH, DeWald RL, ed. *Textbook of spinal surgery*. Philadelphia: Lippincott-Raven, pp. 1011–1026.

43. Menezes AH (2000): Craniocervical junction congenital abnormalities. In: Kaye AH, Black PM, eds. *Operative neurosurgery*. London: Churchill Livingstone, pp. 1755–1770.

44. Menezes AH, Gantz BJ, Traynelis VC, et al. (1996): Cranial base chordomas. *Clin Neurosurg* 44:491–509.

45. Menezes AH, Ryken TC (1992): Craniovertebral abnormalities in Down's syndrome. *Pediatr Neurosurgery* 18:24–33.

46. Menezes AH, VanGilder JC (1990): Abnormalities of the craniovertebral junction. In: Youmans J, ed. *Neurological surgery,* 3rd ed. Philadelphia: WB Saunders, pp. 1421–1459.

47. Menezes AH, VanGilder JC, Graf CJ, et al. (1980): Craniocervical abnormalities: a comprehensive surgical approach. *J Neurosurg* 53:444–455.

48. Moore LJ, Schwartz HC (1985): Median labiomandibular glossotomy for access to the cervical spine. *J Oral Maxillofac Surg* 43:909–912.

49. Ransford AO, Crockard HA, Pozo JL, et al. (1986): Craniocervical instability treated by contoured loop fixation. *J Bone Joint Surg Br* 68:173–177.

50. Ryken TC, Menezes AH (1994): Cervicomedullary compression in achondroplasia. *J Neurosurg* 81:43–48.

51. Sawin P, Menezes AH (1987): Basilar invagination in osteogenesis imperfecta and related osteochondrodystrophies: medical and surgical management. *J Neurosurg* 86:950–960.

52. Sekhar LN, Schramm VL Jr, Jones NF (1987): Subtemporal preauricular infratemporal fossa approach to large lateral and posterior cranial base neoplasms. *J Neurosurg* 67:488–499.

53. Sen C, Sekhar LN (1990): An extreme lateral approach to intradural lesions of the cervical spine and foramen magnum. *Neurosurgery* 27:197–204.

54. Smith MD, Phillips WA, Hensinger RN (1991): Fusion of the upper cervical spine in children and adolescents: an analysis of 17 patients. *Spine* 16:695–701.

55. Solanki GA, Crockard HA (1999): Peroperative determination of safe superior transarticular screw trajectory through the lateral mass. *Spine* 24:1477–1482.

56. Stevenson GC, Stoney RJ, Perkins RK, et al. (1966): A transcervical transclival approach to the ventral surface of the brain stem for removal of a clivus chordoma. *J Neurosurg* 24:544–551.

57. Stillerman CB, Wilson JA (1993): Atlanto-axial stabilization with posterior transarticular screw fixation: technical description and report of 22 cases. *Neurosurgery* 32:948–955.

58. Taggard DA, Menezes AH, Ryken TC (1999): Instability of the craniovertebral junction and treatment outcomes in patients with Down's syndrome. *Neurosurg Focus* 6:3.

59. Taitz C, Arensburg B (1991): Vertebral artery tortuosity with concomitant erosion of the foramen of the transverse process of the axis: possible clinical implications. *Acta Anat (Basel)* 141:104–108.

60. Wen HT, Rhoton AL Jr, Katsuta T, et al. (1997): Microsurgical anatomy of the transcondylar, supracondylar, and paracondylar extensions of the far-lateral approach. *J Neurosurg* 87:555–585.

61. Whitesides TE Jr (1983): Lateral retropharyngeal approach to the upper cervical spine. In: Cervical Spine Research Society, ed. *The cervical spine*. Philadelphia: JB Lippincott, pp. 517–527.

62. Yamada T, Ishida T, Kudo Y, et al. (1986): Clinical correlates of abnormal P14 in median SEP's. *Neurology* 36:765–771.

63. Yamaura A, Makino H, Isobe K, et al. (1979): Repair of cerebrospinal fluid fistula following transoral transclival approach to a basilar aneurysm: technical note. *J Neurosurg* 50:834–838.

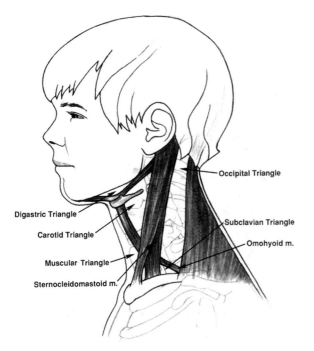

FIGURE 3. Triangles of the neck.

the four components of the deep cervical fascia. It surrounds the neck and encloses the sternocleidomastoid and trapezius muscles. The next three layers of deep fascia are considered to be the middle layers of the deep fascia. The first of these layers encloses the strap muscles and the omohyoid muscle in the anterior cervical region then extends laterally to the scapula.

The deepest component of the middle layer is the visceral fascia, which surrounds the larynx, trachea, esophagus, and thyroid gland. The recurrent laryngeal nerve also is enclosed within the visceral fascia. Care should be taken to avoid entering this fascial plane so that the enclosed structures will not be injured. The fourth portion of the deep fascia is the alar fascia, which spreads like wings (hence its name) behind the esophagus and surrounds the carotid sheath structures laterally.

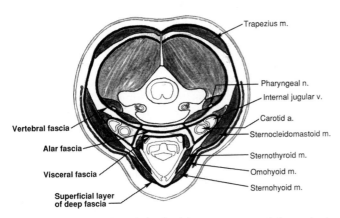

FIGURE 4. Cross-section of the fascial compartments of the neck at the level of the thyroid cartilage.

The deepest layer of fascia in the neck is the prevertebral fascia, which surrounds the vertebral bodies in the paraspinous muscles. Also enclosed in this layer are the phrenic nerve and the scalene muscles. It is continuous with the lumbodorsal fascia in its caudalmost extent. The prevertebral fascia and alar fascia are both considered portions of the deepest layer of the deep fascia. The alar fascia blends with the prevertebral fascia at the level of the transverse processes but generally does not have connections with the prevertebral fascia in the midportions of the neck. In a standard anteromedial approach to the cervical spine, the fascial layers are transected as follows: The superficial fascia is transected in conjunction with the platysma muscle. The superficial layer of the deep fascia is transected sharply at the medial border of the sternocleidomastoid muscle. The middle layer of the deep fascia is transected just anteriorly to the anterior border of the carotid artery, generally by means of finger dissection. The alar fascia and prevertebral fascia are transected sharply directly in the midline to obtain access to the vertebral bodies and discs of the anterior cervical spine (Fig. 5).

Anteromedial Approach to the Vertebral Bodies and Intervertebral Discs from C3 through C7

This approach was described by Robinson, Southwick, and Riley (11,12,14) and is the standard approach to the anterior cervical spine from C3 through C7. This approach allows the discs between C2–3 and C7–T1 and all intervening discs to be exposed in a relatively easy manner.

There has been considerable discussion of whether the approach is more advantageous on the right or left side of the midline. The rationale for approaching on the left side of the midline is that the recurrent laryngeal nerve ascends in the neck on the left side between the trachea and the esophagus, having branched off from its parent nerve, the vagus, at the level of the arch of the aorta. The right recurrent laryngeal nerve travels alongside the trachea in the neck after passing beneath the right subclavian artery. In the lower part of the neck, the right recurrent laryngeal nerve is vulnerable to damage as it crosses from the subclavian artery to the tracheoesophageal groove. Its course in relation to the groove is more variable on the right than on the left. Therefore the right recurrent laryngeal nerve is slightly more vulnerable to injury than the left. An approach from the left side can injure the thoracic duct, which enters the jugular vein–subclavian vein junction at the base of the neck on the left. However, many surgeons prefer to make the incision and approach to the right of the midline if they are right-handed, believing that this facilitates both orientation and technical performance of the procedure. Still others believe that the incision should be made on the side of the predominant lesion. Because generous exposure of the anterior cervical spine can be obtained from either side, the surgical approach should be made on the side that is most comfortable to the surgeon.

The operation can be performed through a transverse or a longitudinal skin incision. In general, the transverse skin incision is sufficient to expose three consecutive vertebral bodies and two consecutive intervertebral discs. If more than two intervertebral discs must be exposed and a prolonged segment of the cervical

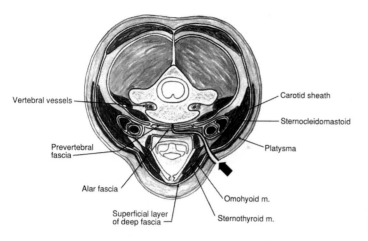

FIGURE 5. Order of transection of layers of cervical fascial in the anteromedial approach to C3–7.

spine has to be accessed, as in multiple vertebrectomy and strut grafting, an oblique incision should be made to parallel the anterior border of the sternocleidomastoid muscle. A transverse skin incision should extend to the midline and be centered over the anterior border of the sternocleidomastoid muscle over the segment of the spine to be exposed (Fig. 6). The fifth, sixth, and seventh cervical segments in general should be approached through a transverse incision placed two to three fingerbreadths superior to the clavicle. The third, fourth, and fifth cervical segments should be approached through a transverse skin incision placed three to four fingerbreadths superior to the clavicle. A lateral radiograph obtained before the incision is made helps ensure proper placement of the incision. A longitudinal or oblique incision should be made over the medial border of the sternocleidomastoid muscle and can extend from the tip of the

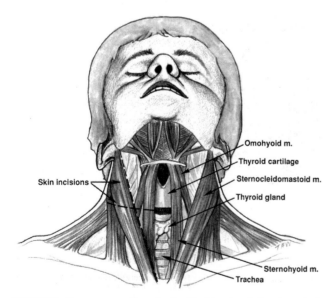

FIGURE 6. Transverse and longitudinal incision in relation to underlying muscles of the neck. The head should be placed in neutral position before a transverse incision is made. We prefer to make both types of incisions on the right side.

mastoid process to the suprasternal notch if this degree of exposure is necessary.

Once the skin incision is made, the platysma muscle is sharply incised at the level of the lateral limb of the transverse incision or at the caudal limb of the longitudinal or oblique incision. It can be bluntly separated from the underlying structures with an instrument passed deep to the muscle. This step is important to prevent unintentional incision of the underlying structures, which would include the sternocleidomastoid muscle at the lateralmost extent of the transverse incision or at the caudal extent of an oblique incision. On the medial aspect of the incision, the thyroid gland may be vulnerable to injury during the course of transection of the platysma muscle. The anterior border of the sternocleidomastoid muscle is clearly identified once the platysma muscle has been transected. The fascia investing the sternocleidomastoid muscle should be sharply incised at the medial border of the sternocleidomastoid muscle so that it can be retracted laterally. The middle layer of the cervical fascia is now well demonstrated, and the omohyoid muscle is seen to cross the field in the midportion of the neck, generally just above the level of the vertebral body of C6. This muscle may be mobilized and retracted inferiorly or superiorly or divided and retracted to provide adequate exposure. The external jugular vein may be encountered deep to the sternocleidomastoid muscle, and both the external jugular vein and the anterior jugular vein may have to be divided and cut if they interfere with adequate exposure.

The vessels and nerves coursing from lateral to medial generally are located in the layer of the middle portion of the deep cervical fascia. Palpation beneath the sternocleidomastoid muscle for the carotid pulse identifies the contents of the carotid sheath. The sternocleidomastoid muscle and the carotid sheath should be retracted together laterally, and the middle cervical fascia should be transected by means of finger dissection during lateral retraction of these structures. The following structures should be identified in the middle layer of the deep cervical fascia: The digastric muscle, hypoglossal nerve, and glossopharyngeal nerve are found in the superiormost portion of this exposure. These should be retracted superiorly. The superior thyroid artery and vein and the superior laryngeal nerve are the next structures encountered inferiorly. These should be identified and retracted as necessary. The middle thyroid vein courses from lateral to medial below the thyroid vessels and can be transected and ligated if necessary. The inferior thyroid vein and artery are the inferiormost vascular structures during this approach and can be retracted inferiorly or superiorly, according to the level being exposed.

Once the deep layer of the middle cervical fascia is traversed with blunt dissection and the appropriate structures are retracted, palpation of the anterior surface of the cervical spine usually is possible. At this point, the viscera and the midline should be inspected. The esophagus may be seen just posteriorly to the trachea; more superiorly, it lies posterior to the larynx. The esophagus is often thin and ribbonlike and should be retracted with care to avoid perforation. A blunt retractor such as a Cloward retractor is ideal for medial retraction of the esophagus, trachea, and thyroid gland (Fig. 7).

The prevertebral fascia is incised longitudinally in the midline of the neck and retracted to either side. This fascia must be incised as closely to the midline of the cervical spine as possible to avoid injury to the other structures in the neck (Fig. 8). It has been emphasized that the surgeon must not mistake the palpable anterior tubercles of the transverse processes for the vertebral bodies. Otherwise, an incision that was intended to be made through the prevertebral fascia in the midline of the cervical spine may be made instead through the longus colli muscle, which lies immediately lateral to the midline of the cervical spine. Incising the longus colli can damage the cervical sympathetic chain or the vertebral artery, which is deep in the longus colli muscle, and cause excessive bleeding. Once the prevertebral fascia is incised in the midline, the longus colli muscles are sharply elevated from the intervertebral disc and the vertebral bodies. They are then retracted laterally to allow more complete exposure of the entire segment of the vertebral bodies and intervertebral disc. Before the longus colli muscle is elevated, its medial edge should be coagulated to prevent unnecessary bleeding. At this point, there should be adequate exposure of the vertebral bodies and disc spaces to perform a variety of procedures, including discectomy, corpectomy, biopsy, or fusion.

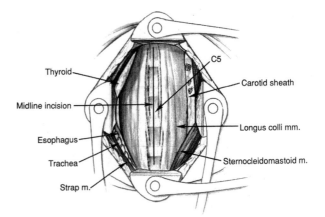

FIGURE 8. Once the prevertebral fascia is visualized by means of appropriate retraction of medial and lateral structures, it should be incised as closely to the midline as possible to minimize damage to contiguous structures.

Consequences of Injury to the Neurovascular Structures during the Anterior Approach

The vertebral artery is at risk of injury during the anterior approach. This can occur during excision of a cervical disc when the dissection is carried posteriorly to a position lateral to the joints of Luschka. The vertebral arteries pass through the transverse foramen at each cervical level from C6 cephalad to C1. Once it reaches C1, the vertebral artery curves posteriorly immediately over the lateral masses between C1 and C2 and then follows a groove in the posterior arch of the atlas to pass into the foramen magnum. The vulnerability of these vessels at this location is discussed in the section on posterior approaches. At each level, the cervical nerve root passes directly behind the vertebral artery. Therefore the roots are in jeopardy if the vertebral artery is tied blindly when surgical injury occurs. If it is injured and bleeding cannot be controlled with tamponade, the artery must be exposed in the region of the transverse foramen and controlled proximally and distally before ligation. In operations on young patients, it usually is safe to ligate one vertebral artery, but this may cause cerebral or cerebellar ischemia among older patients. This complication occurs when one vertebral artery is compromised by spurring around the foramen or when traumatic disruption or occlusion of one vertebral vessel occurs. In these circumstances, surgical compromise of the contralateral vessel produces marked ischemia.

Injury to neural structures during the approach can include damage to the cervical sympathetic chain, which is a deep structure located near the longus colli muscles. The sympathetic chain lies deeply in a reflection of the carotid sheath along the anterior surface of the lateral masses and prevertebral muscles. It extends from C2 downward and exhibits three gangliotic enlargements: the superior ganglion in front of C2 and C3, the middle ganglion in front of C5, and the inferior ganglion, frequently fused with the first thoracic ganglion just below C7 and called the *stellate ganglion.* Injury to the cervical sympathetic chain can cause Horner syndrome.

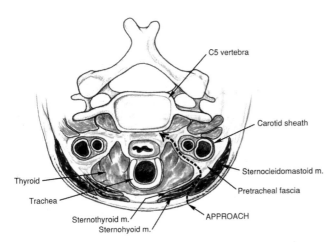

FIGURE 7. The midline musculovisceral column can be bluntly retracted medially as a unit. The lateral structures include the sternocleidomastoid muscle and the contents of the carotid sheath.

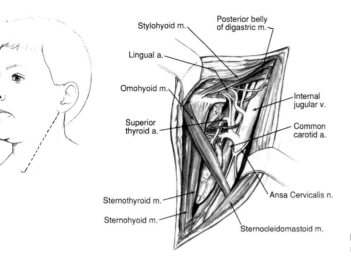

FIGURE 9. Neurovascular structures encountered in the anteromedial approach.

Other neural structures vulnerable to injury include the pharyngeal and superior laryngeal branches of the vagus nerve, which are deep to the carotid and superior thyroid arteries. These supply the tracheal muscles of the back of the pharynx and sensory innervation to the larynx and the cricothyroid. These are generally retracted with the viscera, and because they run in a longitudinal oblique course, they are not damaged as part of usual exposures.

The recurrent laryngeal nerve arises from the vagus nerve at the level of the subclavian artery on the right, recurs below the subclavian artery, and ascends between the trachea and esophagus, protected by the visceral fascia. The left recurrent laryngeal nerve arises at the level of the aortic arch and passes around the arch to ascend in a manner similar to that on the right. Retraction may cause temporary paralysis of the recurrent laryngeal nerve during the anterior approach, but this is less likely to happen with a left-sided approach because the recurrent laryngeal nerve is more frequently situated in the tracheoesophageal groove on the left than on the right. The nerve branches to all muscles of the larynx except the cricothyroid. It communicates with the internal laryngeal nerve and supplies sensory filaments to the mucous membrane of the larynx below the level of the vocal cords. It also carries afferent fibers from the stretch receptors in the larynx. Injury to both recurrent laryngeal nerves causes the vocal folds to be motionless in the same position they normally assume in tranquil respiration. When only one recurrent laryngeal nerve is injured, the vocal fold of the same side is motionless. The function in the fold of the opposite side allows phonation, but the voice is altered and weak in timbre. Injury to the superior laryngeal nerve causes anesthesia of the mucous membrane in the upper part of the larynx so that foreign bodies can readily enter the cavity. Because the nerve supplies the cricothyroid muscle, the vocal folds cannot be made tense, and the voice is deep and hoarse (19) (Fig. 9).

Anterior Approach to C1 and C2

The anterior approach to C1 and C2 is attributed to Crowe and Johnson by Robinson and Southwick (12,14). However, Riley (11) attributed this approach to Fang. This approach historically has been used primarily for drainage of retropharyngeal abscess and biopsy of the anterior arch of C1 and the body of C2. A midline longitudinal incision is carried through the pharyngeal membrane and fascial planes directly to the mass or to the bone. The midpharynx usually is avascular, and the small number of vessels cut can be ligated with absorbable sutures. Partial closure with interrupted catgut sutures usually is used. When used to drain abscesses, this incision should not be closed. The transoral approaches have the obvious limitations of being small exposures with small spaces in which to work. However, with the use of an operating microscope, it is possible to perform transorally procedures such as odontoid resection. The reported rate of infection with these exposures is high. For more extensive work on the upper cervical spine, alternative exposures should be considered (Figs. 10, 11).

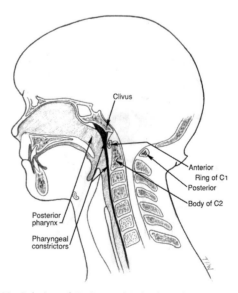

FIGURE 10. Relation of C1 ring and C2 body to the posterior pharynx. The relation of the hard and soft palates to the atlantoaxial junction is evident.

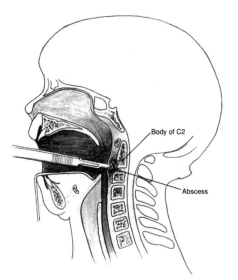

FIGURE 11. Transoral pharyngeal approach to drainage of retropharyngeal abscess.

Anterior Extrapharyngeal Approaches to the Upper Cervical Spine

Three extrapharyngeal approaches to the upper cervical spine have been used as alternatives to transpharyngeal approaches. These include approaches described by De Andrade and Macnab (4) and the approach described by Riley (11), which requires anterior dislocation of the mandible on the side of the approach along with resection of the submaxillary gland with an extensive dissection of the anatomic structures in this area. Both of these approaches are medial to the carotid sheath. The lateral retropharyngeal approach to the upper cervical spine described by Whitesides et al. (17,18) is a modification of Henry's (8) approach to the vertebral artery and is carried anterior to the reflected sternocleidomastoid muscle but posterior to the carotid sheath. The approach can be extended medially into the retropharyngeal space to expose all the vertebral bodies of C1 through C7.

Extrapharyngeal approaches can be used in the management of a variety of problems in the cervical spine in which upper cervical spine exposure is needed. These include os odontoideum, fracture, nonunion or malunion, and postlaminectomy deformity. These also may be undertaken for stabilization in the management of problems relating to inflammatory and collagen diseases, such as rheumatoid arthritis, ankylosing spondylitis, scleroderma, and lupus erythematosus. Biopsy and management of tumors of the upper cervical spine are common reasons for use of this approach. Although infection can be managed with this approach, the transoral retropharyngeal approach may be more common in this situation.

Lateral Retropharyngeal Approach to the Upper Cervical Spine

Whitesides originally described the use of this approach for anterior cervical fusion in a patient with neurofibromatosis who needed extensive anterior fusion for a recurrent deformity (17,18). The procedure can be performed with the neck in halo traction in slight extension and rotation to the contralateral side the approach. However, neither rotation nor extension is needed to successfully approach the anterior cervical spine with this method. Because of risk of respiratory problems due to swelling after extensive retropharyngeal dissection, elective tracheostomy can be performed before the procedure is begun. If respiratory problems are not anticipated, nasotracheal intubation is performed to allow the mandible to be unobstructed during the procedure.

It is helpful to prepare the ipsilateral ear inside and out and to sew the earlobe anteriorly to the cheek to facilitate exposure of the sternocleidomastoid insertion through the posterior limb of the hockey stick incision. The hockey stick incision is the initial horizontal portion of the incision, which begins just posterior to the tip of the mastoid process and is carried across the tip of the mastoid process anteriorly until the anterior border of the sternocleidomastoid muscle is reached. The incision is turned inferiorly in an oblique manner along the anterior border of the sternocleidomastoid muscle (Fig. 12). Once the skin is incised, the great auricular nerve should be identified and is retracted cephalad. If retraction is not possible and it impedes further exposure, this structure can be divided and ligated. This produces a minor sensory deficit in the distribution of the terminal portion of the greater auricular nerve.

The platysma muscle is divided along the oblique portion of the incision just anterior to the sternocleidomastoid muscle, and the deep fascia along the medial border of the sternocleidomastoid muscle is divided sharply. The interval between the sternocleidomastoid muscle and the contents of the carotid sheath are developed by means of finger dissection in the cephalic portion of the wound (Fig. 13). If only the upper portion of the cervical spine is being approached, the sternocleidomastoid muscle is retracted posterolaterally, the carotid sheath contents are retracted anteromedially, and the dissection is continued in this

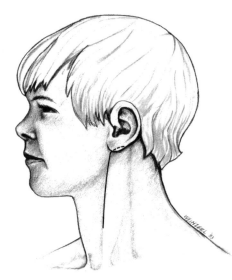

FIGURE 12. Incision for lateral retropharyngeal approach (Whitesides technique).

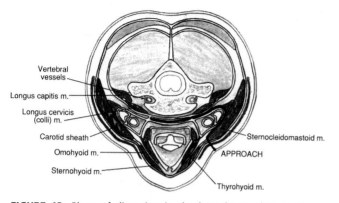

FIGURE 13. Plane of dissection in the lateral retropharyngeal approach is anterior to the sternocleidomastoid muscle and posterior to the carotid sheath.

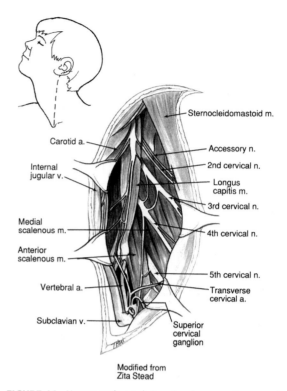

FIGURE 14. Nerves and vessels in retropharyngeal approach.

area. However, if the sternocleidomastoid muscle is well developed, or if exposure of both the upper and lower cervical spine is needed for the procedure, the sternocleidomastoid muscle can be divided at its insertion along the mastoid process.

Before the sternocleidomastoid muscle is divided at its insertion, the entrance of the spinal accessory nerve into the sternocleidomastoid muscle should be visualized. The spinal accessory nerve generally enters the sternocleidomastoid muscle 2 to 3 cm caudad to the tip of the mastoid process. Care should be exercised in posterolateral retraction of the sternocleidomastoid muscle after division of its insertion so that excessive traction is not placed on the spinal accessory nerve. It may be necessary to dissect the spinal accessory nerve from the jugular vein toward the jugular foramen to effect safe lateral retraction of the sternocleidomastoid muscle. After reflection of the sternocleidomastoid muscle, the interval just posterior to the carotid sheath contents is developed by means of finger dissection, and the prominent transverse process of C1 is palpated. If the patient's head is turned toward the contralateral side of the body, the transverse process of C1 will be rotated away from the transverse process of C2.

Henry's original description of this approach involved access to the vertebral artery for ligation (8). A portion of the vertebral artery extending between the transverse foramen of C2 and the transverse foramen of C1 was the cephalic extent of Henry's second stage of the vertebral artery. Because the interval between the C2 transverse foramen and the C1 transverse foramen is larger than the other contiguous transverse foramina of the cervical spine, this site is accessible for ligation of the vertebral artery (Figs. 14, 15).

As the dissection is carried medially from the transverse processes of the upper cervical vertebral bodies, the sagittal fascial band, which binds the midline viscera to the prevertebral fascia (the fibers of Charpey), is divided so that the anterior musculovisceral column can be retracted anteromedially. Thus the retropharyngeal space is entered with the prevertebral fascia visible along the anterior cervical vertebral bodies and the longus colli and longus capitis muscles evident in the more anterolateral aspect of these vertebral bodies. Sharp transection of the prevertebral fascia may be performed after coagulation of the edges of

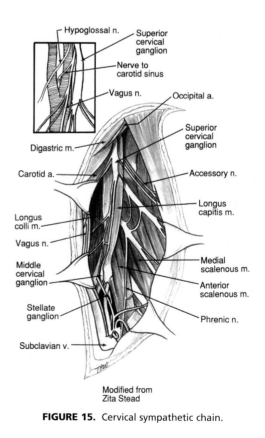

FIGURE 15. Cervical sympathetic chain.

the muscle fibers in the area. Subperiosteal dissection then is performed to expose the anterior cervical vertebral bodies and their intervening disc spaces. The anterior cervical muscles down to the level of the upper thoracic region can be removed during the course of this anterior subperiosteal exposure if such exposure is required.

This approach may be used for simultaneous exposure of the right and left lateral C1–2 articulations for procedures such as screw fixation, as described by Barbour (1,5,13). Other uses of this exposure include vertebrectomy and incision of the odontoid process, biopsy of lesions in all areas of the anterior cervical spine, fusion of C1 to T1, and exposure of a small amount of the basiocciput for fusion to that area when necessary. Once the procedure is concluded, the sternocleidomastoid muscle is reapproximated to its origin at the mastoid tip with absorbable suture. A drain should be left deep within the wound. The platysma muscle is closed with absorbable suture and the skin approximated with a subcutaneous stitch. External immobilization with a halo vest may be needed for some types of fusion in this area.

Complications associated with the approach include facial nerve palsy, which may be caused by retraction of the digastric muscle and subsequent injury to the seventh cranial nerve. There also is risk of injury to the spinal accessory nerve, which would denervate the sternocleidomastoid muscle. It is important to identify the jugular vein in the course of dissection posterior to the contents of the carotid sheath so that this structure is not injured. The infection rate has been acceptably low, especially in relation to that for the transoral approach. Whitesides and McDonald (18) reported a 2.5% incidence of infection. In general, this approach is a safe, effective means of exposing both the upper cervical spine and the upper and lower cervical spine combined.

Anteromedial Retropharyngeal Approach to the Upper Cervical Spine and Basiocciput

The anteromedial retropharyngeal approach to the upper cervical spine and basiocciput to gain access to the basiocciput for occipitocervical fusion was described by De Andrade and Macnab (4). It is a cranial extension of the approach made popular by Smith and Robinson and Bailey and Badgley. It involves extending the oblique incision along the medial border of the sternocleidomastoid muscle as used in the anteromedial approach cephalad to the angle of the mandible.

The platysma muscle and deep cervical fascia are divided sharply, and the lower cervical spine is approached with the dissection used in the anteromedial approach. The branches of the external carotid artery, which prevent access to the retropharyngeal space in the upper cervical spine, are divided and ligated to facilitate this portion of the exposure. These include the superior thyroid, lingual, and facial arteries. The other structures that hinder access to the retropharyngeal space in the upper cervical and craniocervical junction are the digastric muscle, hypoglossal nerve, and pharyngeal and laryngeal branches of the vagus nerve, which are retracted during the procedure. Traction on the pharyngeal and laryngeal branches of the vagus nerve may cause

temporary or permanent hoarseness and other problems related to the timbre of the voice (Fig. 16).

Anteromedial Retropharyngeal Approach to the Upper Cervical Spine (Riley Technique)

The Riley technique (11) is essentially an alternative means of extending the standard anteromedial approach cephalad to the C1–2 vertebral bodies. The major differences involve use of a modified Schoebringer incision, excision of the submaxillary gland, and anterior dislocation of the temporomandibular joint to improve access to the upper cervical spine. The incision is begun in the submandibular area, just inferior to the edge of the mandible, and carried posteriorly in a horizontal manner to the angle of the mandible. The incision is then carried inferiorly in an oblique manner just at the posterior edge of the sternocleidomastoid muscle. At the lower third of the sternocleidomastoid muscle, the incision is gently curved anteriorly and inferiorly to cross the clavicle and terminate near the suprasternal space (Figs. 17, 18). The deeper part of the incision involves transection of the subcutaneous tissue and platysma muscle in the same line as the incision and medial retraction of skin, subcutaneous tissue, and platysma as a single flap. This exposes the underlying sternocleidomastoid muscle at the lateral border of the dissection and the musculoviseral column medially. The mandible and submaxillary fascia are visible in the superiorly aspect. The mandibular branch of the facial nerve is just inferior to the angle of the mandible. It should be identified and protected throughout the dissection.

The sternocleidomastoid muscle is freed along its medial and lateral borders and retracted laterally. The omohyoid muscle is divided in the portion just deep to the sternocleidomastoid muscle and then is retracted superiorly and inferiorly. Blunt dissection through the middle layer of the cervical fascia is carried medially to the carotid sheath toward the prevertebral fascia. The medial musculoviseral column is retracted medially, and the contents of the carotid sheath are retracted laterally with the sternocleidomastoid muscle. This step provides access to the vertebral bodies from the C2–3 disc space to the C7–T1 disc space.

Superior development of the dissection to access C1 and C2 involves identifying the superior thyroid artery, which crosses the field horizontally from lateral to medial as it exits the external carotid artery en route to the thyroid gland. The superior thyroid artery is divided and ligated for the dissection to proceed superiorly to the superior laryngeal neurovascular bundle and the hypoglossal nerve. Both of these structures should be identified and protected during the course of superior dissection. The stylohyoid muscle and digastric muscle are identified, divided, and retracted.

As the larynx and pharynx are retracted medially and the external carotid artery is retracted laterally, the floor of the submaxillary triangle becomes visible. This is retracted superiorly to reveal the base of the skull and anterior arch of C1. The exposure is improved by means of excision of the submaxillary gland and manual anterior dislocation of the temporomandibular joint (Fig. 19). The mandible is rotated out of the field of dissection to improve superior retraction of the floor of the

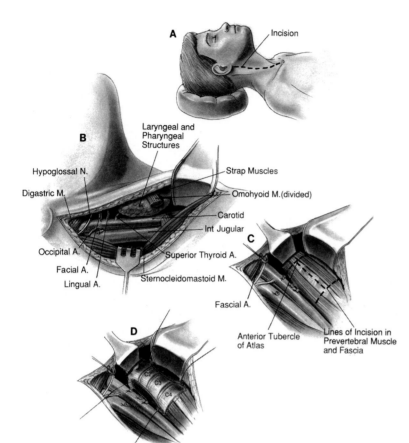

A — Incision

B

Laryngeal and
Pharyngeal
Structures

Hypoglossal N.

Digastric M.

Strap Muscles

Omohyoid M.(divided)

Carotid

Int Jugular

Occipital A.

Superior Thyroid A.

Facial A.

Sternocleidomastoid M.

Lingual A.

Fascial A.

C

Anterior Tubercle
of Atlas

Lines of Incision in
Prevertebral Muscle
and Fascia

D

FIGURE 16. Anteromedial retropharyngeal approach described by De Andrade and Macnab (4).

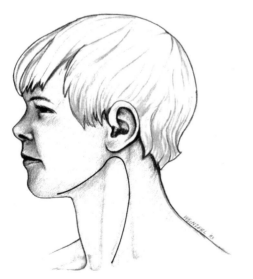

FIGURE 17. Neck incision in Riley anteromedial retropharyngeal approach.

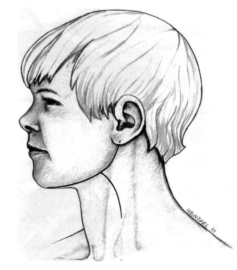

FIGURE 18. Modified Shoebringer incision, which may be used in the Riley extrapharyngeal approach to the upper cervical spine.

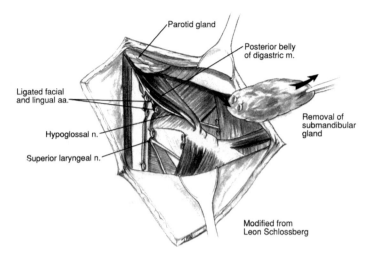

Parotid gland

Posterior belly
of digastric m.

Ligated facial
and lingual aa.

Removal of
submandibular
gland

Hypoglossal n.

Superior laryngeal n.

Modified from
Leon Schlossberg

FIGURE 19. Excision of the submaxillary gland to improve exposure.

submaxillary triangle to expose the base of the skull and the entire anterior aspect of C1. This allows adequate access to C1–2, and the vertebral arteries can be seen and controlled as necessary. Subperiosteal dissection of the longus colli muscle in a lateral direction exposes the transverse processes and the vertebral artery.

Closure is accomplished by means of relocating the dislocated temporomandibular joint and repairing the digastric and stylohyoid tendons. A suction drain is placed deep within the wound, and the platysma muscle is reapproximated throughout the incision. Subcuticular absorbable suture is used to close the skin (Fig. 20).

The disadvantages of this approach involve not only the need to excise the submaxillary gland and the potential problems with dislocation of the temporomandibular joint but also the same risk as the approach described by De Andrade and Macnab (4). The hypoglossal nerve and superior laryngeal nerve remain vulnerable to injury during this procedure, because they must be retracted as work is performed in this area.

Hodges et al. (10) reviewed complications in operations on 12 patients who underwent the anterior retropharyngeal approach to the upper cervical spine. No cases of infection occurred among these patients. Nor did permanent nerve damage or voice changes occur. Several patients had dysphasia, one had postoperative pneumonia, and one had airway obstruction that necessitated emergency tracheotomy. Hodges et al. (10) cited a previous review of the cases of 85 patients by Heeneman (9), who documented an incidence of postoperative voice changes among 11% of the patients and permanent vocal cord paralysis among 3.5%. Heeneman (9) also mentioned that a left-sided approach did not lower the incidence of injury to the recurrent laryngeal nerve in the upper cervical spine. Hodges et al. (10) concluded that the anterior retropharyngeal approach is superior to other approaches because of a low incidence of complications and the ability to gain exposure to both the upper and lower cervical spine. Before the operation patients need to be counseled regarding the complications of dysphasia, transient voice changes, and nerve damage.

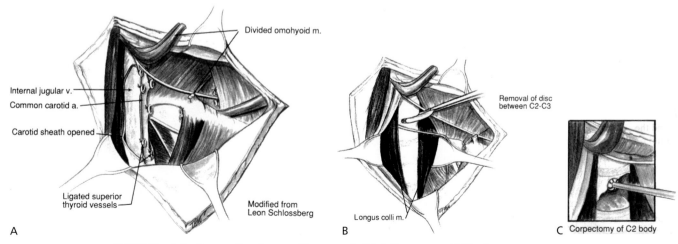

Divided omohyoid m.

Internal jugular v.

Common carotid a.

Carotid sheath opened

Ligated superior
thyroid vessels

Modified from
Leon Schlossberg

Removal of disc
between C2-C3

Longus colli m.

Corpectomy of C2 body

A   B   C

FIGURE 20. A–C: Deeper dissection provides access to C2–3 disc space and C2 body.

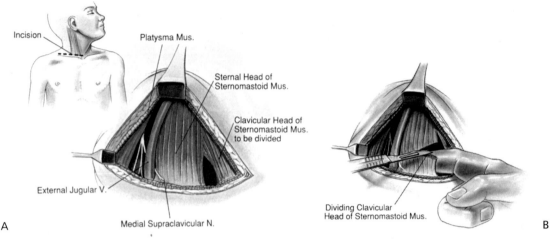

Incision

Platysma Mus.

Sternal Head of
Sternomastoid Mus.

Clavicular Head of
Sternomastoid Mus.
to be divided

External Jugular V.

Medial Supraclavicular N.

Dividing Clavicular
Head of Sternomastoid Mus.

A

B

FIGURE 21. **A, B:** Incision for supraclavicular approach.

Supraclavicular Approach to the Lower Cervical Spine

The supraclavicular approach to the lower cervical spine was described by Riley as a means of accessing the lower cervical spine through an anterolateral approach (11). It provides excellent access to the transverse processes, pedicles, and vertebral artery.

A transverse incision is placed one fingerbreadth above the clavicle. The incision extends from the midline of the neck to just beyond the posterior border of the sternocleidomastoid muscle (Fig. 21). Transection of the platysma muscle is performed in line with the skin incision, and the medial and lateral borders of the sternocleidomastoid muscle are defined by means of blunt and sharp dissection. The sternocleidomastoid muscle is separated from its underlying structures by blunt means of dissection, and the anterior jugular vein and external jugular vein are identified and ligated if necessary. The sternocleidomastoid muscle is divided by means of incision from its lateral border to its medial border. Care is taken to avoid the internal jugular vein. The muscle is retracted superiorly and inferiorly to provide access to the area of the middle cervical fascia. The omohyoid and sternohyoid muscles then can be seen. The middle cervical fascia is bluntly dissected laterally to the carotid sheath to provide access to the surface of the anterior scalene muscle (Fig. 22).

The omohyoid muscle is divided and retracted as the sternocleidomastoid muscle was to improve access to this area. The phrenic nerve is identified on the surface of the anterior scalene muscle. It crosses from the lateral to the medial aspect in its superior to inferior course. The phrenic nerve is retracted medially after it is gently freed from the surface of the anterior scalene muscle. The cords of the brachial plexus emerge from beneath the lateral border of the anterior scalene muscle. These cords should be visualized and protected throughout the dissection. The anterior scalene muscle is sharply divided approximately 1 inch (2.5 cm) inferior to the side of the desired exposure. The entire superior portion of the muscle is excised; however, the slips of origin of the anterior scalene muscle emanate from the anterior tubercles of the cervical transverse processes, so the ver-

tebral arteries are vulnerable to injury as they pass between the bony foramen and the transverse processes of the cervical vertebrae when these slips are being resected (Fig. 23).

The standard approach involves lateral retraction of the carotid sheath; however, if possible, the internal jugular vein and carotid sheath can be retracted medially. The anterior scalene muscle also can be retracted laterally rather than resected. The close relation between the anterior scalene muscle and the parietal pleura should be ascertained. The deep surface of the anterior scalene muscle is covered by a continuation of the prevertebral fascia known as the Sibson fascia, and the deep surface of the Sibson fascia is formed by the apex of the parietal pleura and lung. Care should be taken not to violate this fascial plane, because this would involve entering the thoracic cavity. The Sibson fascia is followed medially toward the transverse processes of the cervical vertebrae, where it is incised and bluntly retracted inferiorly (Fig. 24).

The recurrent laryngeal nerve is retracted medially with the carotid sheath and the medial musculovisceral column. The prevertebral fascia is sharply transected in the midline, and subperiosteal dissection of the fascial attachment and longus colli muscle is performed. The dissection can be carried superiorly to expose

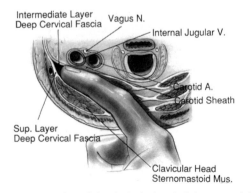

Intermediate Layer
Deep Cervical Fascia   Vagus N.

Internal Jugular V.

Carotid A.
Carotid Sheath

Sup. Layer
Deep Cervical Fascia

Clavicular Head
Sternomastoid Mus.

FIGURE 22. Transection of the clavicular head of the sternocleidomastoid muscle and the plane of dissection.

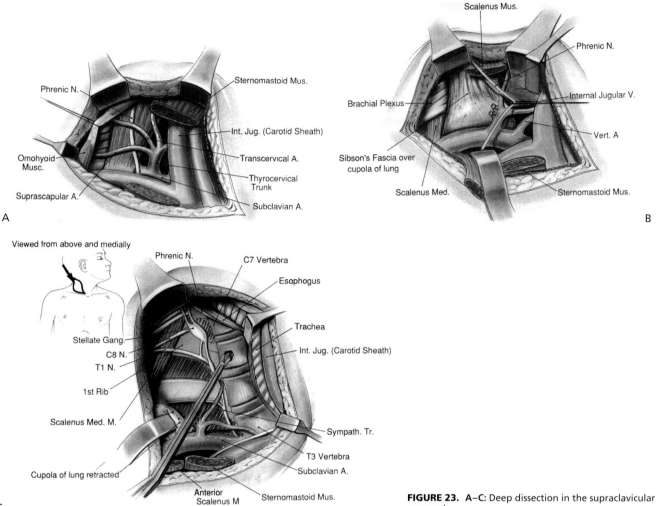

FIGURE 23. A–C: Deep dissection in the supraclavicular approach.

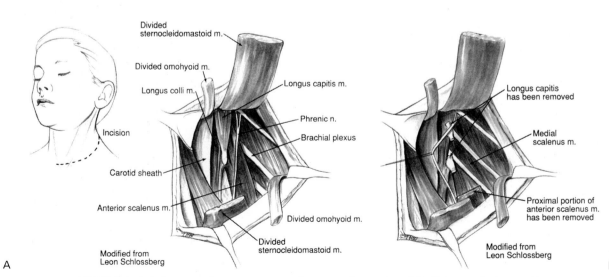

FIGURE 24. A, B: Exposure of transverse process by means of retraction of divided sternocleidomastoid muscle and resection of the cephalic portion of anterior scalene muscle.

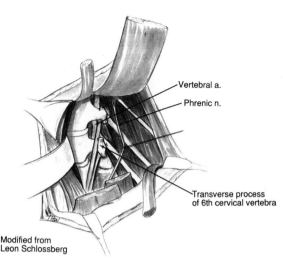

FIGURE 25. Reflection of longus colli muscle improves access to vertebral bodies, neural foramina, and vertebral artery.

vertebral bodies up to the C2–3 disc space. If the transverse processes, pedicles, or neural foramina are to be exposed, the longus colli muscle can be reflected medially (Fig. 25).

A left-sided approach makes the thoracic duct vulnerable to injury. During this approach, if it is performed from the left side, the thoracic duct should be carefully sought at its junction with the internal jugular–subclavian vein complex. If it is injured during dissection, the thoracic duct is tied proximally and distally to prevent formation of chylothorax. The other complications are pneumothorax and injury to the cervical sympathetic chain as it ascends along the longus colli muscle.

Transclavicular Approach to the Cervicothoracic Spine

A variation of the transclavicular approach to the cervicothoracic spine was described by Birch et al. (2). This approach allows mobilization of the medial portion of the clavicle and a portion of the lateral manubrium of the sternum but allows the sternocleidomastoid muscle to remain attached to the clavicle. It is a modification of the procedure described by Charles and Govender, which involved excision of a portion of the clavicle and manubrium. This approach allows access to the cervicothoracic spine from C3 to T4.

The approach usually is made from the left side. The patient is placed in semisitting position, and the head is turned slightly away from the side of the approach. A *T*-shaped incision is made with the transverse limb in the skin crease 2 cm above the clavicle and the vertical limb in the midline extending midway down the sternal body (Fig. 26A). Flaps are raised deep to the platysma and extend cephalad to the hyoid bone and caudad to the clavicle. The flaps are retained with suture. The supraclavicular nerves are protected, but sometimes the medial branches are sacrificed. The accessory nerve is on the side of the upper flap and should be protected.

The sternocleidomastoid muscle is separated from deeper

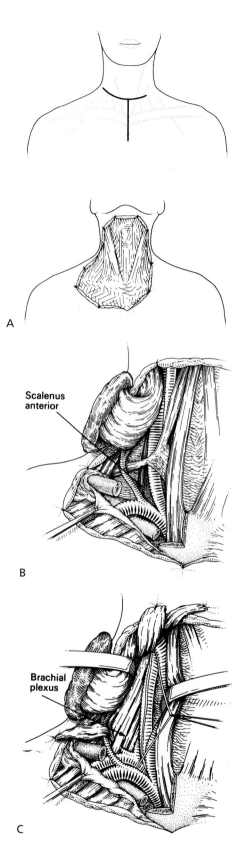

FIGURE 26. A: Skin incision and superficial structure for transclavicular approach to the cervicothoracic spine. **B:** Reflection of medial clavicle with sternocleidomastoid muscle. **C:** Deeper dissection in transclavicular approach. (From Birch R, Bonney G, Marshall RW [1990]: A surgical approach to the cervico-thoracic spine. *J Bone Joint Surg Br* 72:904–907, with permission.)

structures. The clavicle is dissected as far medially as the sterno-clavicular joint. The omohyoid muscle is divided, and the anterior portion of the internal jugular vein and the common carotid artery are defined. The upper part of the manubrium is cleared and the upper part of the sternal head of the pectoralis major muscle is detached. A saw is used to resect the cephalic lateral corner of the manubrium, and the first costal cartilage is divided. The clavicle is divided at its midpoint with a drill and a saw. The clavicle with the manubrial corner is elevated and retracted superiorly on a pedicle of sternocleidomastoid muscle (Fig. 26B).

The infrahyoid muscles, trachea, innominate veins, innominate artery, subclavian artery, common carotid artery, scalenus anterior muscle, phrenic nerve, brachial plexus, and a portion of the first rib are visible. This allows access to the brachial plexus. To access the cervicothoracic spine, the dissection is carried medially to the carotid sheath. The recurrent laryngeal nerve is identified. The anterior portion of the spine is bluntly dissected away from the prevertebral fascia from C3 through T4 (Fig. 26C).

The wound is closed by means of replacing the osseomuscular flap and reattaching the manubrium with wires and the clavicle with a plate and screws. The soft-tissues structures are restored, and the skin is closed. If the pleura has been opened, a chest tube is inserted. The primary problems encountered in the approach are airway obstruction from edema or external pressure. Tracheostomy usually is not necessary.

POSTERIOR APPROACHES

Posterior Approach to C1–2

The posterior approach to C1–2 is used for fusion involving both the C1–2 articulations and the occipitocervical articulations. The exposure can be extended cephalad to include the occiput and caudad to include the lower cervical spine.

The patient is prone on the operating table, and the head may be supported with either a headrest or a self-retaining head fixation device attached to the table. The standard incision for C1–2 posterior fusion is a midline incision from the caudal aspect of the occiput to the C3 spinous process. This is carried through the skin with a scalpel blade. Deeper dissection is performed with either a scalpel blade or an electrocautery. The midline avascular structure, the median raphe or the ligamentum nuchae, follows a tortuous course. This generally prevents dissection in a straight line from posterior to anterior if this plane is to be followed. Care should be taken to remain within this raphe; straying into the paraspinous muscle masses causes unnecessary bleeding. The dissection can be carried down to the occiput in the cephalic extent and into the spinous processes in the caudal portion of the exposure.

In operations on children, exposure of unnecessary levels should be avoided so that spontaneous fusion at levels adjacent to those necessary for the procedure does not occur. The ligamentous attachments to C2 are most prominent in this area, and dissection can begin at the C2 spinous process with either an electrocautery or a subperiosteal elevator. The dissection then proceeds from the C2 spinous process to the lamina of C2 in

a lateral direction. The dissection often is carried caudal to the C2 level to provide adequate exposure. The exposure of the C2 and C3 laminae should extend to the medial one third of the facet joint at the base of the laminae but should not extend beyond the facet joints during the lateral exposure. The occiput is exposed subperiosteally in a similar manner. The intervening area contains the ring of C1, which may be very deep with respect to C2. The posterior tubercle of C1 usually is palpable in the midline, and subperiosteal dissection with a small subperiosteal elevator proceeds from the posterior tubercle of C1 laterally.

Care must be taken during this dissection to avoid excessive pressure on the C1 ring, because it may be thin and easily fractured. Slipping of the C1 ring in a cephalic direction during subperiosteal dissection can cause penetration of the atlantooccipital membrane and injury to the underlying structures. In the case of atlantoaxial instability, direct pressure of the C1 ring against the dura can leave the dura vulnerable to injury during dissection. The dura can be penetrated on both the superior and inferior edges of the ring of C1, so care must be taken during this portion of the dissection. The pathologic condition involved must be taken into account.

The lateral extent of exposure at C1 is approximately 1.5 cm. The lateral landmark at the ring of C1 is the second cervical ganglion, which is on the lamina of C1 in the area of the groove for the vertebral artery. The medial aspect of the groove for the vertebral artery must be carefully identified on the superior border of the C1 ring. The vertebral vein usually is visualized because of its bluish color. Care must be taken in this area to avoid damage to the vertebral artery as it courses from the slightly posterior foramen transversarium of C1 in a posteromedial direction to enter the foramen magnum just above the ring of C1. The vertebral artery and vein are vulnerable in the groove at C1 and as the artery passes from the foramen transversarium of C2 to the foramen transversarium of C1, where it is in lateral and posterior proximity to the joint (Fig. 27).

The vertebral vein is encountered first as the dissection is carried from medial to lateral along the lamina. Penetration of the atlantooccipital membrane just off the superior border of the ring of C1, more medial than the usually safe 1.5-cm margin from the midline, can damage the vertebral artery. It is therefore imperative that these relations be known in exposure of the C1, C2, and occipital portions of the upper cervical spine. Self-retaining retractors are useful for maintaining retraction of the cervical paraspinous muscles during procedures on the upper and lower cervical spine. If a more lateral approach to the C1–2 facet joint is desired, the vertebral artery between the C1 and C2 articulation must be identified. In rotatory dislocations of the C1–2 articulation, the artery is stretched tightly across the joint on the side where C1 is anterior to C2 and is easily damaged.

The position of the head is important during all posterior procedures on the cervical spine. The head usually is held as close as possible to neutral alignment. Flexion often aids in the exposure by means of bringing the occiput away from the C1–2 articulations in a cephalic direction. However, the pathologic condition for which the patient is being treated must be consid-

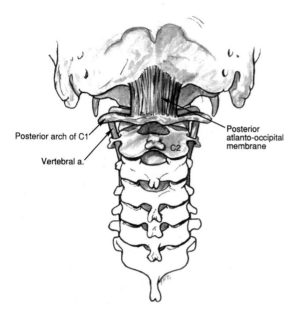

FIGURE 27. The relation between the C1 ring, C2 posterior elements, atlantooccipital membrane, and vertebral artery.

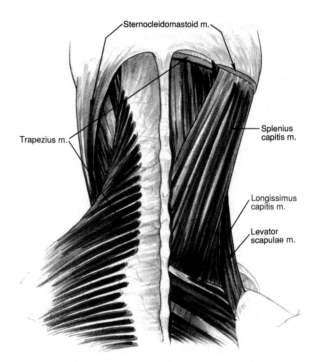

FIGURE 28. Posterior cervical muscles. Superficial layer.

ered, in that flexion of the occiput may not be possible to retain reduction of the C1–2 articulation. The ultimate position of the cervical spine must be evaluated on a lateral radiograph before any surgical incision is made. This should be assessed for both position of the neck with respect to the procedure to be performed and radiographic accessibility to the areas being operated upon, so that radiographic evaluation can be performed during the procedure.

Posterior Exposure of the Lower Cervical Spine

In exposure of the lower cervical spine, the prominent C7 spinous process should be palpated to determine the level and strength of the midline posterior cervical incision. It is important to remain within the ligamentum nuchae during the procedure to keep bleeding from the paraspinous muscles to a minimum. Once the skin and subcutaneous tissues are transected with a scalpel blade, the trapezius fascia is incised, and the muscle mass on the side of the lesion is retracted. Subperiosteal dissection of the cervical paraspinous muscles then is performed. These muscles include the splenius, the semispinalis capita, the lower semispinalis cervicis, and the multifidus. Dissection of these muscles can be performed with Bovie electrocautery, which is the method preferred by some. If removal is not indicated, the extensor muscular insertions at C2 should be retained to preserve both function and stability. Exposure of the laminae in the lower cervical spine is therefore performed with relative impunity and may be carried laterally to expose the medial two thirds of the zygapophyseal joints. Dissection beyond the zygapophyseal joints may denervate the paraspinous muscles. It also can make the vertebral artery vulnerable to injury should the dissection be carried beyond the joint and slightly

anterior to the crossing of the vertebral artery between the foramen transversarium of two adjacent bodies (Fig. 28). Just as in exposure of the upper cervical spine, a lateral radiograph obtained before surgical preparation is extremely important (Figs. 29, 30).

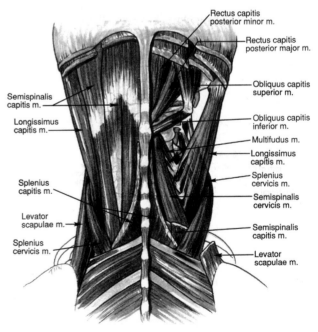

FIGURE 29. Posterior cervical muscles. Deep layer.

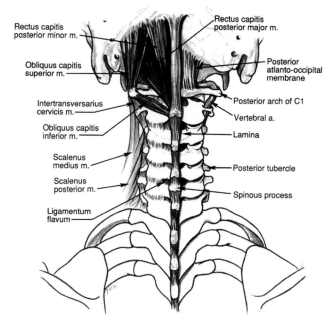

FIGURE 30. Muscle attachments of upper cervical spine.

Rectus capitis posterior minor m.

Rectus capitis posterior major m.

Obliquus capitis superior m.

Posterior atlanto-occipital membrane

Intertransversarius cervicis m.

Posterior arch of C1

Vertebral a.

Obliquus capitis inferior m.

Lamina

Scalenus medius m.

Posterior tubercle

Scalenus posterior m.

Spinous process

Ligamentum flavum

REFERENCES

1. Barbour JR (1971): Screw fixation in fractures of the odontoid process. *S Aust Clin* 5:20–24.
2. Birch R, Bonney G, Marshall RW (1990): A surgical approach to the cervico-thoracic spine. *J Bone Joint Surg Br* 72:904–907.
3. Cervical Spine Research Society Editorial Committee (1989): *The cervical spine,* 2nd ed. Philadelphia: JB Lippincott, pp. 805–807.
4. De Andrade JR, Macnab I (1969): Anterior occipito-cervical fusion using an extra-pharyngeal exposure. *J Bone Joint Surg Am* 51: 1621–1626.
5. Du Toit G (1976): Lateral atlantoaxial arthrodesis: a screw fixation technique. *S Afr J Surg* 14:9–12.
6. Frymoyer JW (1991): *The adult spine.* New York: Raven Press.
7. Grodinsky M, Holyoke EA (1938): Fascial and fascial spaces of the head, neck and adjacent regions. *Am J Anat* 63:367.
8. Henry AK (1973): *Extensile exposure.* New York: Churchill Livingstone.
9. Heeneman H (1973): Vocal cord paralysis following approaches to the anterior cervical spine. *Laryngoscope* 83:17–21.
10. Hodges DS, et al. (1998): Complications of the anterior retropharyngeal approach in cervical spine surgery: a technique and outcomes review. Presented at the 26th Annual Meeting of the Cervical Spine Research Society, December.
11. Riley LH (1973): Surgical approaches to the anterior structures of the cervical spine. *Clin Orthop* 91:16–20.
12. Robinson RA, Southwick WO (1978): Surgical approaches to the cervical spine. *Instr Course Lect* 17:299–330.
13. Simmons EH, du Toit G (1978): Lateral atlantoaxial arthrodesis. *Orthop Clin North Am* 9:1101–1113.
14. Southwick WO, Robinson RA (1976): Surgical approaches to the vertebral bodies in the cervical and lumbar regions. *J Bone Joint Surg Am* 39:631–644.
15. Watkins RG (1983): *Surgical approaches to the spine.* New York: Springer-Verlag.
16. Whitecloud TS, LaRocca H (1976): Fibular strut graft in reconstructive surgery of the cervical spine. *Spine* 1:33–43.
17. Whitesides TE Jr, Kelly RP (1966): Lateral approaches to the upper cervical spine for anterior fusion. *South Med J* 59:879–883.
18. Whitesides TE Jr, McDonald AP (1978): Lateral retropharyngeal approach to the upper cervical spine. *Orthop Clin North Am* 9: 1115–1127.
19. Williams PL, Warwick R, eds. (1980): *Gray's anatomy,* 36th ed. Philadelphia: WB Saunders.

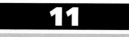

SURGICAL APPROACHES TO THE THORACIC AND THORACOLUMBAR SPINE

KIYOSHI KANEDA

The aim of spinal surgery is to reconstruct spinal function by means of the following procedures: resection of the pathologic lesions in the spinal column or the spinal nervous tissue, neural decompression, correction and stabilization of the spinal deformity, and restoration of spinal stability. Surgical approaches must attain these aims without causing additional damage to the surrounding tissues. The surgical approach is determined by the purpose of the operative procedure, anatomic features of the spinal, and the location, size, level, and pathologic features of the primary lesion to be controlled. As a rule, several concerns must be addressed. The patient must be on a stable positioning frame or table to ensure patient safety. The size of the incision must allow adequate visibility, wound illumination must be adequate, and there must be enough room to work with spinal implants if they are to be used. The surgeon must bear in mind that poor positioning or draping of the patient may make an operation difficult or even dangerous. Surgical approaches to the thoracic and thoracolumbar spine are principally divided into anterior, posterior, and combined approaches.

ANTERIOR APPROACHES

Cervicothoracic Junction and Upper Thoracic Spine

If the lesion involves the cervicothoracic junction (lower cervical and upper thoracic vertebral bodies), the following approaches can be used.

Standard Anterior Approach to the Cervical Spine

T1, the C7–T1 disc, and sometimes the T1–2 disc can be reached with a standard anterior approach to the cervical spine. When resection of the T2 vertebral body or correction of kyphotic deformity, including the T1–2 portion, is needed, the anterior approach is not recommended. The costotrans-

K. Kaneda: Department of Orthopaedic Surgery, Hokkaido University School of Medicine, Sapporo 060, Japan.

versectomy approach to or thoracotomy (anterolateral approach) to the upper thoracic spine should be used instead.

For exposure of the C7 to T2 vertebral bodies, the patient is positioned supine without skeletal traction, except in the presence of fresh traumatic instability. A pillow is placed between the shoulder blades and beneath the cervical spine. The neck is slightly extended, and the head is turned toward the right (Fig. 1). An oblique skin incision along the anterior border of the sternocleidomastoid muscle should be made from the left side to avoid damage to the recurrent laryngeal nerve. An approach to the T1–2 vertebrae sometimes requires considerable retraction, which can damage the great vessels, particularly the innominate brachiocephalic vein. Retraction of the esophagus and the trachea with displacement to the right exposes the C7, T1, and T2 vertebral bodies.

Cervical Sternum-Splitting Approach (Cervical Sternotomy)

Cervical sternotomy is used for resection of lesions from the lower cervical to the T1, T2, or T3 vertebral bodies and for anterior fusion. It is difficult to reach below the T4 body.

The patient is positioned supine with the neck slightly extended and rotated to the right. A skin incision is made obliquely along the anterior border of the left sternocleidomastoid muscle and is extended distally and vertically on the midsternum toward the jugular notch and the xiphoid process (Fig. 2). After the anterior side of the lower cervical spine is exposed by means of blunt dissection, the retrosternal adipose tissue and thymus residues are retracted from the manubrium craniad to caudad with cotton applicators. The tip of the xiphoid process is detached from the muscular aponeuroses, and the retrosternal fatty tissue is bluntly dissected in a superior to inferior direction. A narrow malleable retractor is inserted for security at the sternotomy under the sternum (between the sternum and the detached fatty tissue), as shown in Fig. 2. Median sternotomy is performed with a sternotomy saw. Hemostasis must be maintained in the region of the divided sternal edge with an electric coagulator and bone wax. Injury to the pleura should be avoided. The muscles of the sternohyoid, sternothyroid, and omohyoid are ligated and transected. The left brachiocephalic vein is ex-

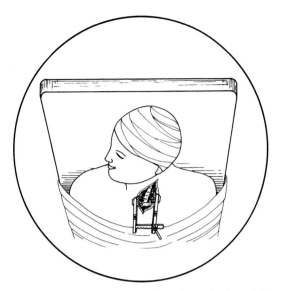

FIGURE 1. Standard anterior approach to the cervicothoracic junction.

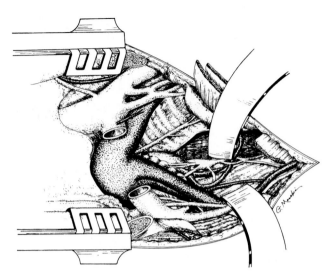

FIGURE 3. Anatomic features of the cervicothoracic junction. The left brachiocephalic vein is cut. The aortic arch and left and right common carotid arteries are shown. The anterior aspect of the cervicothoracic junction will be exposed with narrow malleable retractors.

posed and doubly ligated bilaterally; it is transected if it hinders access to the vertebrae (Fig. 3).

Exposure of the vertebrae is accomplished by means of ligating and transecting the inferior thyroid artery. The esophagus, trachea, and cervical fascia are cautiously retracted medially while the thoracic duct and vessels are retracted laterally. The pretracheal fascia is split in the middle and retracted. The anterior aspect of the lower cervical and upper thoracic vertebral bodies

is exposed (Fig. 4). Caution must be exercised not to traumatize the pleura, the recurrent laryngeal nerve, and the thoracic duct with excessive retractor pressure. After the necessary procedures, the sternotomy is closed with transosseous wire sutures. The omohyoid, sternohyoid, and sternocleidomastoid muscles are rejoined with the retained sutures, and the ordinary anterior cervical closures are performed. Use of a drain is recommended.

One disadvantage of this approach is the amount of work required. In addition, transection of the brachiocephalic vein can cause postoperative venous reflux in the left upper extremity.

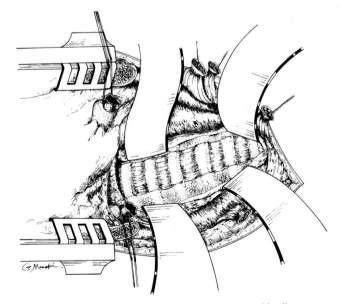

FIGURE 2. Cervical sternum-splitting approach (cervical sternotomy).

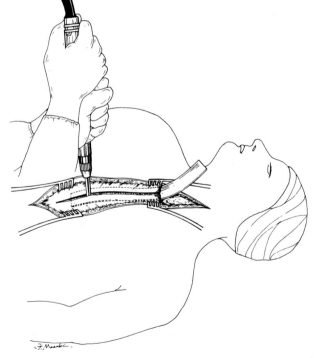

FIGURE 4. Exposure of C6–7 to T1–3 vertebral bodies.

Combination Anterior Cervical and Thoracotomy Approach

In the case of a swan-neck deformity (postlaminectomy kyphosis or tuberculosus spondylitis with severe kyphosis) of the cervicothoracic junction, it is necessary to expose a wide portion of the spine from C6 or C7 to T4, T5, or T7 for anterior correction and stabilization with fibular strut grafts. For anatomic reasons, this large portion of the lower cervical and upper thoracic spine cannot be exposed with a single approach. Therefore the combination of a right anterior cervical approach and right high thoracotomy is recommended.

The patient is positioned on his or her left side because the thoracotomy approach is conducted from the right side if there is no special reason to see the section with anterolateral thoracotomy. The right arm is placed free to expose both the cervical and the thoracic vertebrae. The right upper thoracotomy and the anterior cervical exposure are connected under a tunnel through the chest wall and the clavicle. The vertebrae are exposed in the same way as for either approach.

Thoracic Spine

Costotransversectomy (Extrapleural or Thoracotomy)

This posterolateral approach provides access to both the lateral aspect of the vertebral bodies and the posterior elements from the upper thoracic to the middle thoracic spine. It is especially useful in the upper thoracic spine because other approaches to this area provide only limited exposure. For example, it is impossible to reach the spine below T3 with the cervicosternal approach, and the anterolateral approach exposes the anterolateral elements only.

The patient is placed in the prone or semilateral position. I recommend a semilateral or lateral position with axillary padding under the contralateral side to avoid compression of the axial neurovascular structures. The upper arm of the approach side should be elevated and fixed superiorly and anteriorly so that the scapula does not disturb the exposure. This approach exposes both the posterolateral and anterior aspects of the upper thoracic spine. A prone position also can be used, but a direct view of the anterior portion is difficult in this position.

The skin incision for exposure of the upper thoracic to T7 vertebral bodies is made posteriorly in a straight line midway between the medial margin of the scapula and the spinous processes. If there is severe kyphosis, the skin incision should be changed according to the curvature. For operations on the upper thoracic vertebrae, the scapula may have to be moved anteriorly and superiorly with a scapula retractor. During retraction of the scapula, the trapezius and rhomboid muscles are divided, and the medial border of the latissimus dorsi may have to be cut. The ribs should come into view. The paravertebral muscles are retracted posteriorly to expose the costotransverse joints and the transverse processes; these muscles are divided if necessary. The ribs to be resected are stripped subperiosteally and cut 6 to 10 cm from the costotransverse joint. The ligaments of the costotransverse joint are cut. At this time, the pleura is detached from the chest wall and pushed away for extrapleural exposure. The pleura can be detached easily from the lateral and anterior aspects of the vertebrae if there is no severe adhesion. The costovertebral joint is exposed, the radiate ligaments of the costovertebral joint are cut, and the rib is completely removed (Fig. 5). If a wider exposure is necessary, the adjacent ribs are removed in the same way. Next, the transverse processes are removed. Two or three costotransversectomies provide sufficient access to three or four vertebrae. The intercostal vessels are ligated if necessary. The pleura and lung should be protected with a sponge and malleable retractors (Fig. 6). At this stage, access to the anterolateral aspect of the vertebrae can be achieved for resection of the vertebral bodies.

In an approach below T7, the proximal longitudinal part of the skin incision is made at the lateral quarter of the vertebral muscles, and the distal oblique part of the skin incision is made on the rib to be resected for costotransversectomy. Resection of the rib and exposure of the vertebrae are almost the same as the procedures described for the approach to the upper thoracic vertebrae.

The costotransversectomy approach seems to have been supplanted by thoracotomy, which provides better exposure. But costotransversectomy is extremely useful for exposing the upper

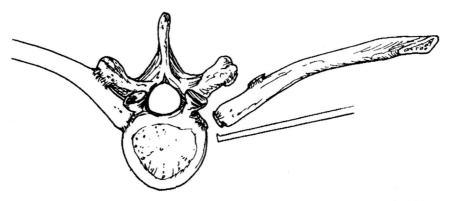

FIGURE 5. Costotransversectomy. The ligaments of the costotransverse and costovertebral joints are divided.

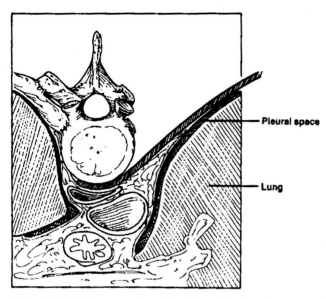

FIGURE 6. Costotransversectomy. Resection of the rib and exposure of the anterolateral spine. The parietal pleura is pushed away from the chest wall and the vertebra.

thoracic vertebrae and is indicated when tumor or infection that involves both the posterior elements and the vertebral body has to be resected in one operation.

Transthoracic Approach: Anterolateral Thoracotomy (Transpleural or Extrapleural)

The thoracic vertebral bodies from T2 to T12 can be exposed with the transthoracic approach (anterolateral thoracotomy). The thoracotomy can be performed extrapleurally or transpleurally. An extrapleural exposure is recommended in cases of infection or tumor, but it is sometimes difficult in operations on aged patients because the pleura is thin and easily torn. These approaches are used for a variety of reasons, including anterior spinal cord decompression and reconstruction with or without instrumentation, resection of vertebral bodies with lesions such as tumors or infection, reconstruction, spinal osteotomy, and correction of spinal deformity.

Upper Thoracic Spine (T1 to T4)

Approaching the upper thoracic vertebral bodies is difficult. If the vertebrae to be accessed are above T4 or the cervicothoracic junction has to be exposed, the approaches described above can be used. The upper thoracic spine is generally approached from the right because of the location of the aortic arch. The patient is positioned on the left side, with the right arm placed as far craniad as possible. This is important for pulling the scapula anteriorly and superiorly.

The skin incision is made around the medial and inferior angle of the scapula (Fig. 7). The trapezius muscle is dissected along the skin incision. The latissimus dorsi muscle is divided as far caudally as possible. The greater rhomboid muscle is di-

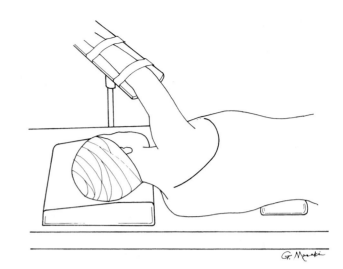

FIGURE 7. Position and skin incision for high thoracotomy.

vided near the scapula, but the serratus anterior muscle is divided as far caudally as possible to avoid damage to the long thoracic nerve (Fig. 8). After these procedures, the scapula can be retracted with a scapula hook. The rib to be resected is easily counted from the first rib to the caudal ribs. When approaching T1–4 vertebral bodies, the third or fourth rib usually is resected. Then the thoracic retractor is applied, and the upper thoracic vertebrae are exposed extrapleurally or transpleurally (Fig. 9).

In cases of infection or tumor, the extrapleural exposure is recommended. If there is a risk of spinal fluid leakage due to anterior spinal cord decompression, the extrapleural exposure is

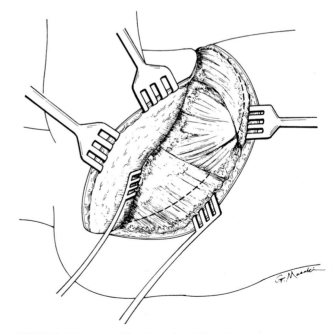

FIGURE 8. Exposure of the trapezius, infraspinatus, teres major, and latissimus dorsi muscles. *Dotted line,* transection of the muscles.

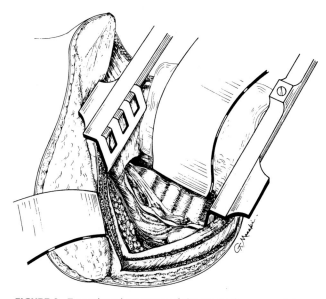

FIGURE 9. Transpleural exposure of the upper thoracic vertebrae.

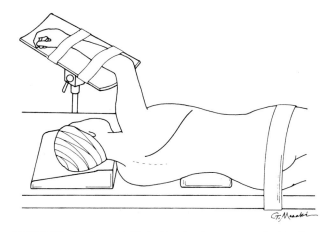

FIGURE 10. Position and skin incision for thoracotomy of mid to lower thoracic spine.

strongly recommended. In the extrapleural approach, the rib is exposed subperiosteally and resected. The parietal pleura is separated from the chest wall (the rib and muscle layers) with fingers and gauze. This separation should be started from the posterior mediastinum because the parietal pleura adheres loosely to the chest wall but is more firmly attached at the lateral part of the thoracic wall. If the pleura is torn, it has to be closed; extrapleural separation can continue, or a transpleural approach can be performed. After the necessary procedures, the integrity of the pleura must be checked by means of pouring tepid water into the extrapleural cavity. If the pleura is ruptured, it must be sutured, which is sometimes difficult. In such a case, a suction drain must be inserted into the intrapleural cavity. Wound closure is conducted as usual with insertion of a thoracic drain. Chest cage closure is performed with a rib approximator. The transected muscles are sutured as described for the transpleural approach (see later).

Mid to Lower Thoracic Spine (T3–4 to T10–11)

The anterior portion of the mid to lower thoracic spine can be approached from either the right or the left side, but the right side is preferable because of the location of the aorta. Anterior procedures for the management of scoliosis always are performed on the convex side.

The patient is positioned with the approach side up and the spinal column parallel to the operating table. The rib chosen to be resected usually is the one above the uppermost level of the spinal lesion. If the ribs have a sharply descending course (far from horizontal) on a chest radiograph, the rib chosen to be resected should be two or three levels above the vertebra to be approached. It is sometimes necessary to resect two ribs (but not contiguous ones) in a severe scoliotic deformity. The skin incision is made over the selected rib. The latissimus dorsi muscle is cut completely through along the skin incision, but this must

be done as far caudally as possible to avoid damaging the thoracodorsal nerve (Fig. 10).

The vertebrae to be approached are exposed transpleurally or extrapleurally. When the vertebral lesion is infectious or tumorous or if there is risk of spinal fluid leakage due to anterior spinal cord decompression, extrapleural exposure is recommended. The technique is the same as the extrapleural approach to the upper thoracic spine. The segmental vessels are exposed, ligated, and transected at the midline.

In exposing the thoracic vertebrae with the anterior approach, the critical supply zone of the spinal cord—the watershed—should be kept in mind. The watershed generally lies between T4 and T9. The segmental arteries on the vertebrae in this area should be transected as far as possible in the anterior direction. Coagulation of the segmental vessels near the intervertebral foramen should be avoided to prevent damage to the blood supply to the spinal cord, particularly in the watershed area.

After a thoracic drain is inserted, a rib approximator is applied to close the rib resection gap. The pleura and the intercostal muscles are sutured continuously. The transected muscles of the lateral serratus and the latissimus dorsi are sutured.

Intercostal Thoracotomy without Rib Resection

Intercostal thoracotomy without rib resection is useful in operations on children and adolescents with a mobile thorax, especially if only two or three vertebrae have to be exposed and no rib grafting is scheduled. Patient positioning is the same as for conventional thoracotomy. After transection of the latissimus dorsi muscle and the anterior serratus muscle, the selected intercostal space is entered. Then the usual exposure is accomplished.

Extended Posterior Approach (Bilateral Costotransversectomy and Pedicular Resection)

The extended posterior approach is designed primarily for resection of vertebral tumors. It allows access to all levels of the thoracic and lumbar spine, provides exposure of the posterior and anterior structures of the spine, and can be used unilaterally or bilaterally. Total vertebrectomy in the thoracic spine can be performed in a single procedure with this approach. It is important to understand, however, that because the approach is extensive, the risk of neurologic complications is high from direct damage to the spinal cord or interruption of the blood supply in the watershed area of the thoracic spinal cord.

The patient is placed prone on a frame to prevent compression of the thoracic and abdominal contents. A usual midline posterior incision is made on the spinous processes and must be three to four levels cranial and caudal to the area of resection to give sufficient retraction. Transverse division of the paravertebral muscles sometimes is necessary to provide a wide enough exposure to remove the vertebral bodies safely. When total vertebrectomy is being done, complete laminectomy of the vertebral levels to be resected is performed. At this point, the spinal canal and its contents are visible. The ribs are divided 3 to 5 cm lateral to the costotransverse joints. Rib resection is performed extrapleurally if possible. The particular processes and pedicles are resected. The posterior mediastinal structures are pushed away by hand with gauze by means of detaching the pleura from the chest wall and from the vertebral bodies. The segmental vessels must be ligated and divided to mobilize the vascular structures from the anterior aspect of the vertebral bodies (Fig. 11A–C).

After the posterior mediastinum is mobilized, malleable retractors are inserted bilaterally (Fig. 11D). The vertebral bodies are excised, usually through the disc spaces above and below the lesion. The vertebral bodies above and below the lesion can be sectioned with a Gigli saw starting anteriorly and extending through the anterior two thirds of the vertebral bodies from anterior to posterior (Fig. 11E). The posterior third of the vertebral body still in place is cut with a thin, sharp osteotome. The posterior longitudinal ligament should be cut with a knife (Fig. 11F). Before anterior resection, posterior stabilization with posterior instrumentation should be applied (a pedicular screw and plate or a rod system is suitable for rigid stabilization). Then resection of the vertebral bodies is performed. The gap of the vertebrectomy is replaced with a strut graft consisting of femur or tibia allograft or with a ceramic vertebral prosthesis. Posterior stabilization is performed by means of bone grafting (Fig. 11G). The extended posterior approach to resection of vertebral bodies is extensive in both surgical time and invasiveness. Therefore this type of surgery must be conducted with great care.

Anterolateral Approach to the Thoracolumbar Spine

The bodies of T10, T11, T12, L1, and L2 are exposed by the extrapleural-retroperitoneal approach or the transpleural-retroperitoneal (thoracoabdominal) approach. I use the former approach to expose the thoracolumbar vertebral bodies if there are no special contraindications. The extrapleural approach is less invasive, and the postoperative care is easier (no chest tube). The extrapleural-retroperitoneal approach is especially useful in operations on patients with an infectious disease or a tumor. In the extrapleural exposure, the procedure of detaching the pleura from the chest wall should be performed with care, because the pleura can be ruptured easily. Because the pleura is relatively

thick and strong in children and adolescents, this approach is a good choice for pediatric patients.

Extrapleural-Retroperitoneal Approach

The extrapleural-retroperitoneal approach is used below T10 to the lumbar spine. I use this approach to manage thoracolumbar scoliosis with anterior instrumentation. However, in operations on patients with severe thoracolumbar scoliosis (Cobb angle greater than 70 to 80 degrees with severe vertebral rotation), the transpleural approach is easier than the extrapleural approach because the route to the vertebral bodies is much shorter.

The extrapleural-retroperitoneal approach can be made from the right or the left side, depending on the location of the lesions. If there are no special considerations, the left-sided approach is preferable for the following reasons. The liver is larger on the right side. The vena cava is on the right and is easily torn, and bleeding from the vena cava can be difficult to control. Although the spleen on the left is fragile, it is smaller than the liver and more easily retractable. The aorta is easier to locate than the vena cava owing to its pulsation (even among infectious or scar tissue), it is less susceptible to damage than the vena cava, and bleeding from the aorta is much easier to control.

The patient is placed on the operating table with the side to be operated on facing up (thus the patient most frequently lies on the right side for a left-sided approach). An axillary pad is used to prevent circulatory disturbance of the right upper extremity. Pressure on the peroneal nerve of the right side should be eliminated to avoid nerve palsy. The skull is kept on a pillow with the cervical spine straight. The chest cage is supported on the sternum and the back with pads and adhesive tape. The pelvis is fixed with a gluteal pad and adhesive tape on the greater trochanter. The patient should remain stable in this position even when the table is tilted during the operation (Fig. 12).

The rib one level above the uppermost level of the lesion is resected—usually the tenth or eleventh rib. This allows exposure below T10 or T11 to the lower lumbar spine. After a skin incision is made over the tenth or eleventh rib, the latissimus dorsi and external oblique muscles are cut along the course of the rib with a diathermal knife. The periosteum of the rib is transected with a diathermal knife along its entire length, and the rib is stripped subperiosteally (Fig. 13). The rib is dissected with a knife at the costochondral junction, elevated dorsally, and transected with a rib cutter at the exposed proximal end. After the rib is removed, the abdominal muscle layers (external and internal oblique and transverse) are transected along the skin incision line. After the costochondral cartilage is divided longitudinally with a knife, the peritoneum is forced apart bluntly from the abdominal wall, the quadratus lumborum and iliopsoas muscles, and the vertebral bodies. The parietal pleura is carefully detached with a wide-blade nerve root retractor or the fingers and is pushed away from the abdominal wall (Fig. 14). The extrapleural space should be widened carefully to avoid damage to the pleura. The diaphragm is detached from the chest wall, and an edge is left for resuturing. Several marking sutures are made in the dissected edges of the diaphragm.

The most important part of this approach is detaching the

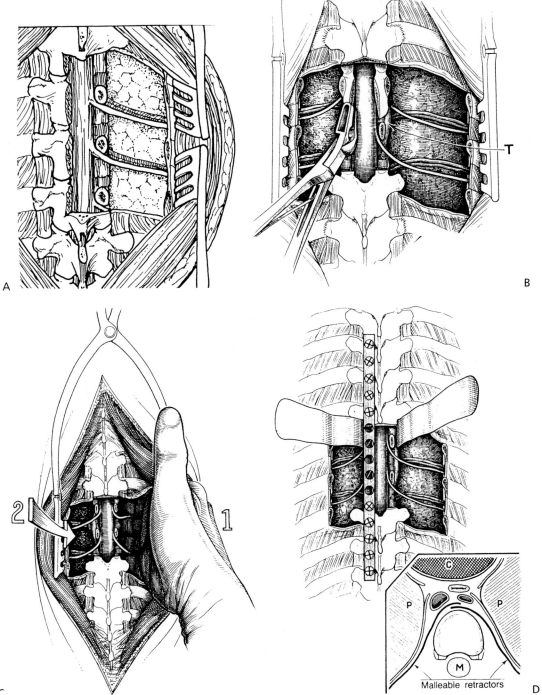

FIGURE 11. Extended posterior approach to resection of the vertebral bodies. **A:** Unilateral costotransversectomy and pedicular resection. **B:** Bilateral costotransversectomy and pedicular resection. **C:** Pleural detachment from the chest wall and the vertebral bodies with fingers. **D:** Insertion of two malleable retractors to protect the posterior mediastinum. The transpedicular screw and plate system is applied unilaterally. *(Figure continues.)*

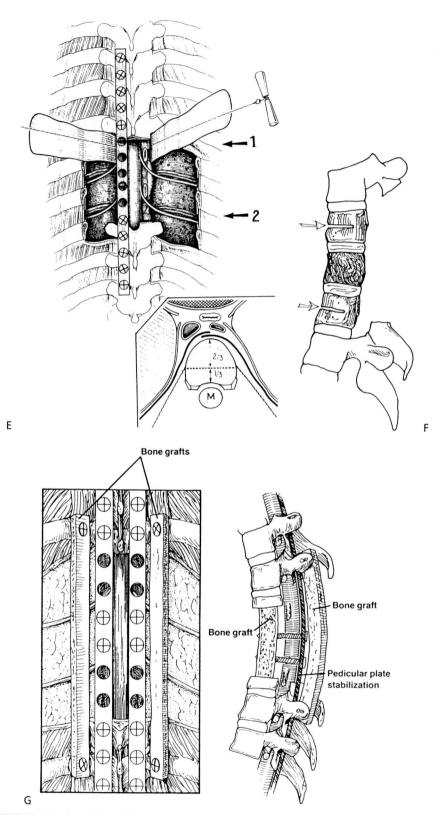

E

F

Bone grafts

G

FIGURE 11. *Continued.* **E:** Partial anterior vertebral body resection with Gigli saw. **F:** Lateral view shows partial anterior vertebral body resection. **G:** Anterior reconstruction and posterior stabilization. (From Kostuik JP [1991]: Surgical approaches to the thoracic and thoracolumbar spine. In: Frymoyer JW, ed. *The adult spine: principles and practice.* New York: Raven Press, pp. 1243–1266 and Roy-Camille R, Benazet JP [1989]: Extradural tumors of the spine. In: Laurin CA, Riley LH Jr, Roy-Camille R, eds. *Atlas of orthopaedic surgery,* vol 1. Masson, pp. 273–293, with permission.)

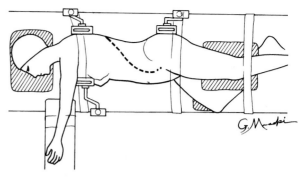

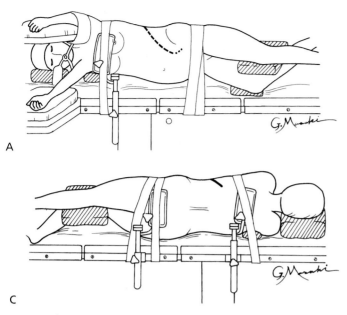

FIGURE 12. Positioning and skin incision for the anterolateral approach to the thoracolumbar and lumbar spine. **A:** From front. **B:** From top. **C:** From back.

pleura and the diaphragm from the chest wall to connect the extrapleural cavity and retroperitoneal space. Even if the pleura is ruptured during the procedure, the extrapleural part of the operation can be continued. The rupture can be repaired at closure. If a large rupture is made at the beginning of the operation, the transpleural approach is used.

After the intended procedures are finished, it is necessary to check the integrity of the pleura by means of pouring tepid water into the extrapleural cavity and looking for bubbles. When a small pleural rupture is found, the hole is closed and the lung fully expanded without a chest tube. The diaphragm is resutured with the marking sutures. Closure is the same as for the transpleural approach from this point.

Transpleural-Retroperitoneal Approach

The transpleural-retroperitoneal approach usually is used in operations on the thoracolumbar spine. The patient positioning, rib selection, skin incision, rib removal, and exposure of the retroperitoneal space are the same as for the extrapleural-retroperitoneal approach. After these steps, the thorax is opened by means of longitudinal division of the parietal pleura in the bed of the resected rib. The thoracotomy is widened with a rib spreader or chest opener. The peritoneum has already been stripped from the dome of the diaphragm, so the diaphragm can be transected circumferentially. An edge is left about 2 to

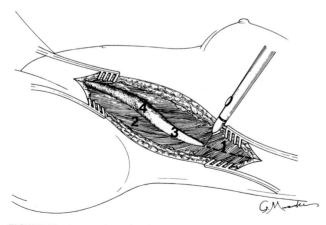

FIGURE 13. Approach to the thoracolumbar spine. Transection of the external abdominal oblique and latissimus dorsi muscles on the tenth rib. *1,* latissimus dorsi muscle; *2,* external oblique muscle; *3,* tenth rib; *4,* cartilage of the tenth rib.

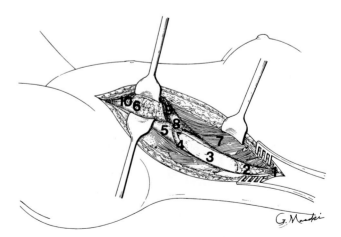

FIGURE 14. Resection of the tenth rib for the extra- or transpleural and retroperitoneal approaches to the thoracolumbar spine. *1,* stump of tenth rib; *2,* parietal pleura; *3,* diaphragm; *4,* periosteum of tenth rib; *5 and 9,* internal oblique muscle; *6,* peritoneum; *7,* external oblique muscle; *8,* cartilage of tenth rib; *10,* transversus abdominis muscle.

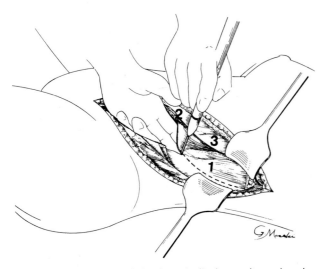

FIGURE 15. Transection of the thoracic diaphragm (transpleural approach). *1,* thoracic diaphragm; *2,* divided costal cartilage; *3,* external oblique muscle.

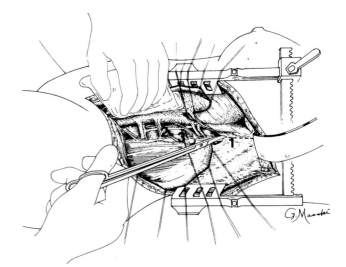

FIGURE 17. Exposure of vertebrae by means of splitting parietal pleura and retroperitoneal tissue. *1,* parietal pleura; *2,* lumbar segmental vessels; *3,* left medial crus.

2.5 cm away from the chest wall (the attachment of the diaphragm) for resuturing (Fig. 15).

It is convenient to leave bilateral marking sutures at the site of transection of the diaphragm (Fig. 16). The parietal pleura on the vertebrae to be accessed is cut with a scissors along the axis of the vertebral column. The segmental vessels running transversely on the vertebral bodies are ligated and cut (Fig. 17). Dissection is started over the intervertebral disc, which is always prominent and has no segmental vessels. The surfaces of the vertebral bodies and discs are exposed with Cobb elevators or cotton applicators. The origin of the psoas major muscle is detached from the intervertebral discs and retracted posteriorly to expose the base of the transverse processes as far as the interverte-

bral foramen (Fig. 18). This approach provides access to the promontory of the sacrum if a sufficiently long incision is made.

After the necessary procedures on the vertebrae, the psoas major muscle and parietal pleura are reinserted or closed to restore the original position. The diaphragm is closed from the medial dorsal direction to the lateral ventral. Finally, the cartilage of the rib is resutured (Fig. 19). Two drains are inserted: one

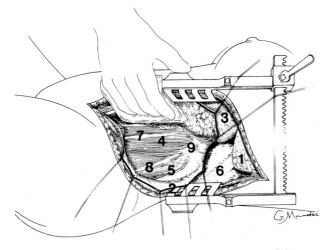

FIGURE 16. Transection of the diaphragm and exposure of the retroperitoneal space. *1,* lung; *2 and 3,* diaphragm; *4,* psoas major muscle; *5,* quadratus lumborum muscle; *6,* eleventh rib; *7,* ilioinguinal nerve; *8,* iliohypogastric nerve; *9,* medial arcuate ligament.

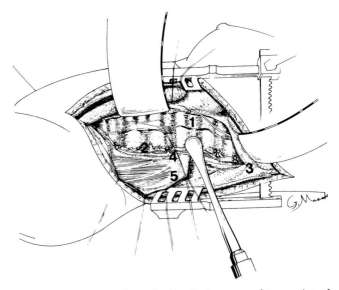

FIGURE 18. Exposure of vertebral bodies by means of transection of segmental vessels and retraction of the psoas major muscle and parietal pleura. *1,* anterior longitudinal ligament; *2,* lumbar segmental vessels (ligated and dissected); *3,* parietal pleura; *4,* medial arcuate ligament; *5,* lateral arcuate ligament.

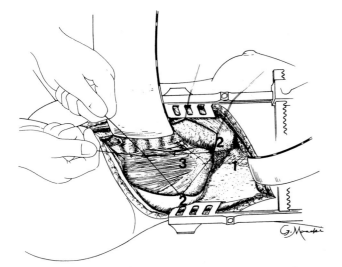

FIGURE 19. Suture of diaphragm. *1,* parietal pleura; *2,* thoracic diaphragm; *3,* psoas major muscle.

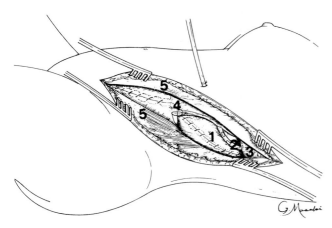

FIGURE 20. Closure of thoracic and abdominal walls. *1,* sutured thoracic diaphragm; *2,* drain (chest tube); *3,* lung; *4,* sutured costal cartilage; *5,* external oblique muscle.

into the thoracic cavity and one into the retroperitoneal space. The rib resection gap is closed with a rib approximator, and the thoracic wall muscles, latissimus dorsi, anterior serratus, and abdominal muscles are sutured (Fig. 20).

POSTERIOR APPROACH

The indications for a posterior approach are fusion for fractures and spinal deformities such as scoliosis and kyphosis and laminectomy for tumors or degenerative diseases in the spinal canal. The patient is placed prone on a supporting frame, such as a Relton-Hall frame, and supported on four parts of the supporting pillow, which are placed in a *V*-shaped arrangement. The pelvis should be supported bilaterally on the pillows between the iliac crest and the trochanteric area. The anterior aspect of

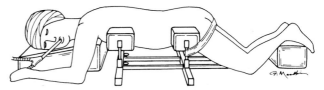

FIGURE 21. Prone position on a modified Relton-Hall frame.

the iliac crest is carefully protected because the lateral cutaneous femoral nerve is vulnerable. The hips are flexed to maintain normal lumbar lordosis (Fig. 21). Care should be taken not to compress the abdomen. Compression increases pressure on the inferior vena cava and causes high pressure on the Batson venous plexus and increases venous hemorrhage during the operation. For operation on the cervicothoracic junction or the high thoracic area, the cervicothoracic spine should be kept in a neutral position. The headrest (face support) of a horseshoe frame usually is used in combination with a chest (sternum) supporter and modified Relton-Hall frame.

A straight midline skin incision is made, even in operations on patients with scoliosis. When posterior spinal instrumentation is to be used, the skin incision should be one or two seg-

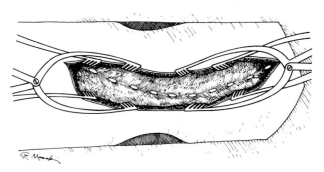

FIGURE 22. Skin incision and exposure of the subcutaneous tissue.

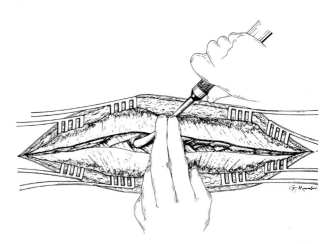

FIGURE 23. Subperiosteal stripping of the spinous processes and laminae.

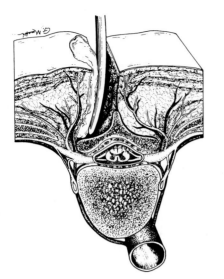

FIGURE 24. Cross section of the thoracic spine and posterior subperiosteal exposure.

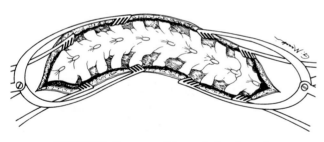

FIGURE 25. Exposure of the posterior elements.

ments longer than the intended fusion area. The subcutaneous tissue is dissected as far as the fascia (Fig. 22). In operations on children and adolescents, the cartilaginous cap apophyses of the spinous processes are split in the midline in a longitudinal direction together with the interspinous ligaments. The apophyses and the adhering periosteum can be detached easily with Cobb elevators from the spinous processes and the laminae (Fig. 23). Subperiosteal stripping is easy in operations on children and adolescents. In operations on adults, however, the fascia and semispinalis and multifidus muscles have to be detached with a diathermal knife or an ordinary knife and Cobb elevators, because there is no cartilaginous apophysis. Subperiosteal stripping should be done carefully so that the neurovascular supply of the musculature and the muscle itself are not damaged (Fig. 24). Subperiosteal dissection is continued laterally as far as the bases or ends of the transverse processes (Fig. 25). From this point, the posterior elements are removed as necessary to meet the surgical purposes.

REFERENCES

1. Bauer R, Kerschbaumer F, Poisel S (1987): Spine, anterior approaches; spine, posterior approaches. In: *Operative approaches in orthopedic surgery and traumatology.* New York: Georg Thieme Verlag, pp. 1–87.
2. Kaneda K (1990): Anterior surgical approach to the thoracolumbar and lumbosacral spine. In: Weinstein JN, Wiesel SW, eds. *The lumbar spine.* Philadelphia: WB Saunders, pp. 975–986.
3. Kostuik JP (1991): Surgical approaches to the thoracic and thoracolumbar spine. In: Frymoyer JW, ed. *The adult spine: principles and practice.* New York: Raven Press, pp. 1243–1266.
4. Louis R (1983): *Surgery of the spine: surgical anatomy and operative approaches.* New York: Springer-Verlag, pp. 232–261, 292–313.
5. Roy-Camille R, Benazet JP (1989): Extradural tumors of the spine. In: Laurin CA, Riley LH Jr, Roy-Camille R, eds. *Atlas of orthopaedic surgery,* vol 1. Masson, pp. 273–293.

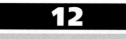

EXTRACAVITARY APPROACHES TO THE THORACOLUMBAR SPINE

ROBERT F. MCLAIN

With a sound understanding of the three-dimensional anatomic configuration of the lumbar spine and a well-considered surgical plan, a spine surgeon can safely gain access to any lesion in any region of the spinal column. Because many spinal disorders affect the anterior vertebral column, calling for an anterior or combined anterior-posterior surgical approach, the surgeon must be well prepared to use the proper anterior exposure in the appropriate situation (2,9). Traditional transthoracic or retroperitoneal approaches have proved versatile and useful in the management of a variety of disorders and are well described elsewhere in this text. The standard thoracoabdominal approach gives wide exposure of the entire thoracolumbar spine and is the most widely used exposure for thoracolumbar fractures, tumors, and anterior instrumentation for deformity. The extracavitary approach to the thoracic and thoracolumbar spine is not as well known but has proved useful in a variety of conditions requiring anterior surgical exposure.

The extracavitary approach is extensile, provides a true anterior exposure, and simplifies management of the diaphragm in thoracolumbar approaches. It may reduce the incidence of some complications of transthoracic procedures, including intrapleural migration of bone graft and formation of pleural adhesions. The principles for success with this approach remain the same as for any other: careful assessment of the patient, fundamental knowledge of the three-dimensional anatomic configuration of the spinal, recognition of complicating factors and hazards, and skillful and meticulous surgical technique.

PREOPERATIVE PLANNING

Preoperative assessment of the patient parallels that for any anterior exposure. The surgeon must consider the patients ability to tolerate the anterior approach, the risk of life-threatening complications, and the patient's medical and surgical history. Although an anterior approach may be the best, or even the only, reasonable approach to a given lumbar lesion, a history of infection, local irradiation, or previous operation through the

same region considerably increases the likelihood of complications. Furthermore, previous surgery, irradiation, or extensive infection or tumor may make an extracavitary approach impossible, leaving the traditional transthoracic thoracoabdominal approach the best option.

Patient preparation and positioning play a key role in the success of any anterior exposure. Spinal cord monitoring and cell saver equipment should be routinely arranged in advance, and radiographic or fluoroscopic imaging should be available. The appropriate operating table and positioning frame should be arranged in advance, and the operating room staff should be familiar with the use of the equipment.

THE SURGICAL APPROACHES

Some pathologic processes that affect the spine can be reached only through a direct anterior approach. Infection or neoplasm of the vertebral body, anterior compressive lesions due to fracture or focal kyphosis, and structurally rigid scoliotic curves frequently necessitate use of an anterior approach as either the primary procedure or part of a combined anterior-posterior operation. The type of anterior approach chosen is determined by the level of the pathologic process, but most thoracic and thoracolumbar lesions can be adequately and safely exposed through an extracavitary approach.

Extrapleural Thoracotomy

The thoracic spine can be accessed from T4 to T10 by means of extrapleural thoracotomy. The patient can be intubated with a double-lumen endotracheal tube to allow selective deflation of the ipsilateral lung, but this step is not necessary. The patient is placed in a full lateral decubitus position, usually with the right side down, on a standard operating room table. An axillary roll is placed under the right chest wall, and a bean bag is used to keep the patient from rolling backward or forward. The flank is centered over the central hinge of the table. After the table is broken to expose the left flank, the kidney rests are elevated and the bean bag is deflated to maintain a true decubitus position. The table can then be rolled side to side to facilitate exposure without confusing the surgeon's orientation during the surgical

R. F. McLain: Section of Spine Surgery, Department of Orthopaedic Surgery, The Cleveland Clinic Foundation, Cleveland, Ohio 44195.

approach. The top leg is flexed in a figure-of-four over the bottom leg to relax the psoas muscle and prevent pressure between bony prominences. All bony prominences should be well padded. The arms usually are positioned over a biplane arm board, but the top arm can be draped out separately for upper thoracic exposures.

The level of the incision is determined by the most rostral extent of the anterior procedure, but the proximal extent of the incision is kept at least 2 cm caudal to the tip of the scapula. The skin incision is carried from the posterior angle of the rib to the costochondral junction and is centered over the rib itself. If the third or fourth ribs must be exposed, the scapula is retracted out of the way before the incision is carried down to the underlying rib. The subcutaneous tissues are divided by means of cauterization down to the rib, and the latissimus dorsi and serratus anterior muscles are divided in line with the skin incision. The erector spinae muscles are elevated and retracted medially but do not have to be divided. The periosteum of the rib is elevated, and the full length of the rib is exposed. After the inner periosteum is stripped with a Doyen elevator, the rib is cut posteriorly and disarticulated from the chondral junction anteriorly. The rib bed is carefully incised to expose the parietal pleura (Fig. 1).

After the periosteum is incised, a blunt dissector is introduced to gently separate the periosteum from the loosely adherent parietal pleura. Once an initial separation is made the dissection is continued with a sponge stick or finger to separate the layers cranially and caudally.

The periosteal incision is extended as the dissection is carried anteriorly to the costochondral junction and posteriorly to the rib head and the anterior vertebral column. Moist sponges are packed over the exposed surface of the parietal pleura, and the pleura, visceral pleura, and underlying lung are retracted to the midline with fans or a malleable retractor. The vertebral bodies, discs, and segmental vessels are easily seen at the depth of the wound (Fig. 2).

An incision through a single rib bed generally gives access to four or even five contiguous disc spaces. If the curve is severe, full discectomy may not be possible at the extremes of the exposure, and only three or four discs may be adequately removed. If additional disc spaces must be accessed, either the subjacent rib can be osteotomized and retracted distally or a second rib can be incised distally or proximally to give access to additional disc spaces. This is necessary only in the management of large-magnitude curves that have proved extremely rigid. A second rib incision facilitates application of anterior spinal instrumentation such as rod and screw constructs. This second rib incision is performed through the same skin incision by means of simple distal or proximal retraction of the skin over the bed of the selected rib two or three levels above or below the initial resection. The second periosteal incision is made through the bed of the rib, but the rib is not resected.

Once the surgical procedure is completed, the parietal pleura is allowed to fall back over the anterior vertebral body and segmental vessels to contain any graft that is placed and seal the extracavitary space. A chest tube connected to a water seal is placed in the extrapleural space and positioned to exit through an uninjured intercostal space in the midaxillary line. The chest

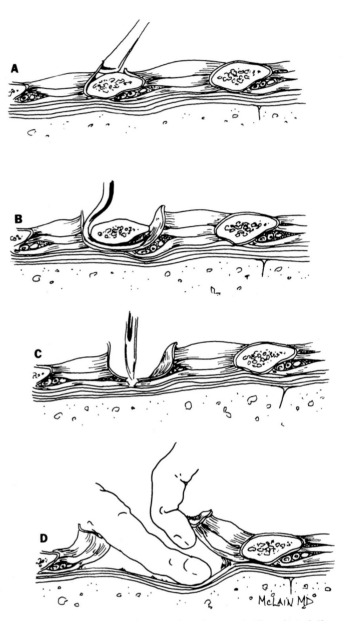

FIGURE 1. Entrance into the extrapleural space. **A:** The selected rib is exposed as in standard thoracotomy with an elevator to raise the periosteum. **B:** A pigtail or Doyen elevator is used to separate the rib from its inner periosteal bed. The rib can be retained or removed at the surgeon's discretion. **C:** The periosteal rib bed is carefully incised to expose the potential space between the intercostal muscles and the parietal pleura. **D:** Sponge-stick or digital dissection is used to sweep the parietal pleura away from the chest wall.

tube is left in place until drainage is minimized and there is no evidence of pneumothorax. Once the tube is removed, an adhesive dressing is placed over the incision with occlusive gauze to prevent pneumothorax. A second, intrapleural chest tube may be needed to drain a persistent pleural effusion, but this tube is not typically inserted during the operation.

The surgical closure is simple. The incision is closed by means of repairing the periosteal bed of the rib with interrupted sutures. A second set of sutures is used to approximate adjacent ribs by

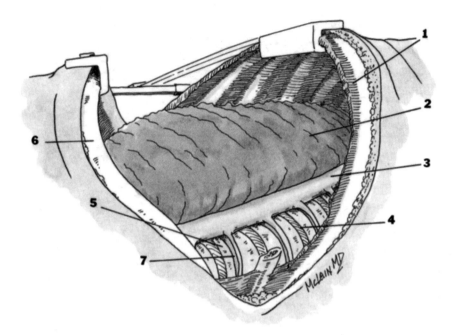

FIGURE 2. Exposure of the spinal column. Once the chest wall is opened, the lung tends to collapse out of the way to expose the great vessels and the spinal column. *1,* intercostal muscles; *2,* parietal pleura, overlying visceral pleura and lung; *3,* aorta; *4,* thoracic disc; *5,* vertebral body; *6,* subjacent rib; *7,* segmental artery and vein.

means of passing the suture over the top of the supraadjacent rib and through a hole made in the lower rib so that the lower intercostal nerve is not compressed (Fig. 3). The chest wall is closed in the usual manner. Tears in the pleura can be repaired with small, absorbable sutures, or they can be left alone.

Thoracoabdominal Exposures

The extracavitary approach can be used to provide thoracoabdominal exposure when the thoracolumbar spine is involved in the spinal abnormality. The thoracic cavity is opened through the tenth rib bed. The incision crosses the costochondral junction before turning obliquely across the abdominal wall toward the lateral border of the rectus abdominis sheath. The parietal pleura is dissected away from the inner thoracic wall as described earlier. The rib is disarticulated from the costochondral junction, and the costal cartilage is split longitudinally to enter the abdominal cavity. The external oblique muscle is split along the line of its fibers, and the internal oblique muscle is divided with an electrocautery. The transversus abdominis fascia is entered near

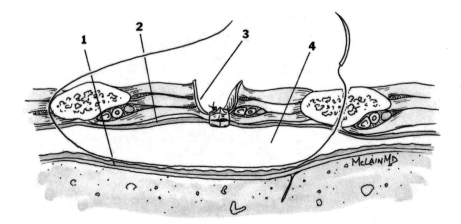

FIGURE 3. Wound closure. If the rib has been excised, the rib bed is closed, and the two adjacent ribs are approximate with suture. If the rib was not removed, the exposed rib is reapproximated directly to its neighbor. *1,* parietal and visceral pleura; *2,* intercostal surface of chest wall; *3,* periosteum of resected rib; *4,* extrapleural space.

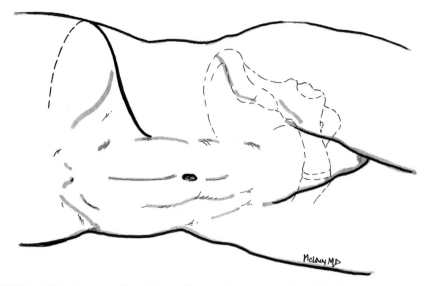

FIGURE 4. Incision for a combined thoracoabdominal approach. The incision is based over the tenth rib and runs from the anterior rectus sheath to the head of the rib.

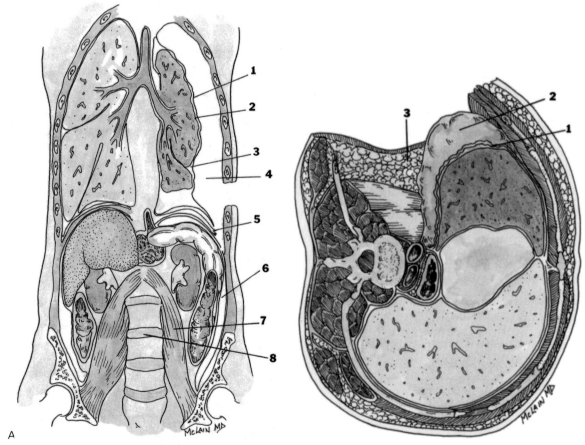

A

B

FIGURE 5. **A:** Coronal section shows the extracavitary and retroperitoneal approaches to the thoracolumbar spine. *1,* parietal pleura; *2,* visceral pleura; *3,* pleural cavity; *4,* extrapleural cavity; *5,* diaphragm; *6,* retroperitoneal space; *7,* psoas muscle; *8,* intervertebral disc. (Adapted from Moskovich R, Benson DR, Zhang ZH, et al. [1993]: Extracoelomic approach to the spine. *J Bone Joint Surg Br* 75:886–898, with permission.) **B:** Thoracoabdominal approach. Axial section at the level of the diaphragm shows confluent extracavitary and retroperitoneal spaces. *1,* parietal and visceral pleurae; *2,* diaphragm detached from chest wall; *3,* retroperitoneal space.

the rectus sheath where it is thinnest. After the area between the fascia and the peritoneum is developed, blunt dissection continues along the abdominal wall while the fascia is split with an electrocautery. If there is scarring in the retroperitoneum, the surgeon must take particular care to identify the ureter before introducing the electrocautery. The ureter usually follows the parietal peritoneum and is easily dissected out of the plane. The psoas muscle must be identified, and dissection must stay anterior to it (8).

By means of proximal and distal dissection through the retroperitoneal and the extrapleural spaces, the attachment of the diaphragm is identified along the insertion into the chest wall. The diaphragm is bluntly detached from the chest wall, and dissection is carried posteriorly to the crus. Wet sponges are used to retract the lung, diaphragm, and peritoneal contents anteriorly away from the spine to allow exposure from the midlumbar to the midthoracic spine through a single incision (Figs. 4, 5).

When the spinal procedure is completed, the pleural and peritoneal tissues are allowed to fall back into their normal positions. The diaphragm is not directly reattached to the chest wall but is allowed to reapproximate to the wall through adhesion of peritoneal and pleural tissues. A large intercostal chest tube is placed in the extrapleural space, and the costal cartilages are reapproximated to initiate closure of the abdominal incision. Rapid readhesion of the parietal pleura to the entire chest and abdominal walls provides fixation of the diaphragm and early restoration of normal diaphragmatic and pulmonary function.

CLINICAL RESULTS

Moskovich et al. (7) presented their results with 65 consecutive operations performed with either the extracavitary or the traditional transthoracic–transthoracic-retroperitoneal approach. Most of the patients were treated for scoliosis, but several were treated for burst fracture, and two were treated for infection. Excluding patients with particularly complex spinal procedures, there was no difference in blood loss between the extracavitary and the traditional transthoracic approaches. There also were no differences in length of chest tube placement, length of hospital stay, operative time, or postoperative complications. Among patients who underwent a thoracoabdominal approach, reconstruction of the costophrenic junction was considerably simplified. Another purported advantage was that multilevel discectomy could be performed through this approach without ligation of the segmental vessels. This, theoretically at least, reduces the risk of ischemic injury to the spinal cord through unintentional disruption of the segmental blood supply (3). If spinal instrumentation is applied anteriorly, the vessels usually need to be ligated. In this case, however, the extracavitary approach provides parietal covering of the implants once the procedure is concluded and provides a barrier between the metal edges and the great vessels and surrounding visceral tissues.

COMPLICATIONS

Performed skillfully, an anterior spinal approach to an uncomplicated operation can provide excellent exposure with little blood loss. The risk of severe and even catastrophic complications increases considerably among patients who have undergone previous operation or irradiation or have had an infection or those undergoing radical resection of tumors, infection, or correction of severe kyphosis. Adhesions and scar obscure the tissue planes and margins that lead to the great vessels and can even invest the vessel walls themselves. Tumor tissue can adhere directly to the great vessels, making dissection around the aorta and vena cava most challenging. Previous irradiation or infection can render vessels friable and easily damaged, and even blunt trauma during dissection can cause severe hemorrhage. In such situations, vascular injury can prove difficult to control and repair.

Avulsion of segmental vessels at the base requires careful closure of the vessel wall. This is particularly difficult on the vena caval side. For this reason, the left-sided approach to either the thoracic or the lumbar spine is preferred whenever possible.

Injury to abdominal organs, particularly the liver or spleen, can occur through excessive retraction or direct penetration with a surgical instrument. Gentle retraction under the diaphragm minimizes these risks. The spleen occasionally is damaged during left-sided exposure, and the liver is at somewhat greater risk when right-sided exposure is used (5). The risk of injury decreases when the surgeon frequently checks and rechecks the position of the retractors and takes care to make sure the assistant does not apply excessive pressure to the underlying viscera.

The spinal cord, cauda equina, individual nerve roots, and the sympathetic chain and plexus all are at risk during an anterior approach. Injuries to the cauda equina and spinal cord can occur during exposure and bony decompression, and injuries to the sympathetic neural plexus can occur during exposure of the lower lumbar spine and lumbosacral junction. Risk of injury to the cord and cauda equina can be reduced when care is taken during positioning of the patient. The surgeon must carefully maintain orientation during vertebrectomy and discectomy to avoid penetrating the canal. If the patient is placed in a position other than the straight decubitus, it is always crucial to recognize the oblique orientation of the posterior vertebral body to prevent unintentional penetration of the canal.

In operations on patients with tumors or fractures, simply positioning the patient on the table introduces some risks. Great care should be taken in transferring the patient with an unstable spine. Somatosensory evoked potential monitoring should be done before and after positioning the patient and throughout the surgical procedure.

A rare complication of anterior operations on the thoracolumbar region is anterior spinal cord ischemia. Ischemic cord injury can occur in aortic trauma or repair of an aortic aneurysm and in procedures that require prolonged cross-clamping above the renal arteries or ligation of several segmental vessels (6). Spinal artery ischemia is a rare complication associated with scoliosis surgery or osteotomy (3,4,6). Cord injury due to ligation of a single unilateral segmental vessel has not been reported. For multilevel procedures, Apel et al. (1) have recommended evaluating the contribution of segmental vessels by means of monitoring changes in somatosensory evoked potentials during temporary occlusion of prominent segmental vessels with a small vascular clip.

SUMMARY

The extracavitary approach to the thoracic and thoracolumbar spine is a useful option. The extracavitary approach carries no increased risk of hemorrhage or complications but simplifies repair of the diaphragm in thoracoabdominal approaches and maintains a tissue barrier between bone graft or instrumentation and the pleural cavity.

REFERENCES

1. Apel DM, Marrero G, King J, et al. (1991): Avoiding paraplegia during anterior spinal surgery: the role of somatosensory evoked potential monitoring with temporary occlusion of segmental spinal arteries. *Spine* 16: S365–S370.
2. Cauthen JC (1988): *Lumbar spine surgery.* Baltimore: Williams & Wilkins.
3. Dommisse GF (1974): The blood supply of the spinal cord: a critical vascular zone in spinal surgery. *J Bone Joint Surg Br* 56:225–235.
4. Dommisse GF, Enslin TE (1970): Hodgson's circumferential osteotomy in the correction of spinal deformity. *J Bone Joint Surg Br* 52:778 (Abstract).
5. Hodge WA, DeWald RL (1983): Splenic injury complicating the anterior thoracoabdominal approach for scoliosis: a report of two cases. *J Bone Joint Surg Am* 65:396–397.
6. Kiem HA, Sadek KH (1971): Spinal angiography in scoliosis patients. *J Bone Joint Surg Am* 53:904–912.
7. Moskovich R, Benson DR, Zhang ZH, et al. (1993): Extracoelomic approach to the spine. *J Bone Joint Surg Br* 75:886–893.
8. Southwick WO, Robinson RA (1957): Surgical approaches to the vertebral bodies in the cervical and lumbar regions. *J Bone Joint Surg Am* 39: 631–635.
9. White AH, Rothman RH, Day CD (1987): *Lumbar spine surgery: techniques and complications.* St Louis: Mosby.

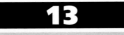

SURGICAL APPROACHES TO
THE LUMBAR SPINE

JAMES N. WEINSTEIN
WILLIAM A. ABDU

Surgical approaches to the lumbar spine should allow complete exposure and visualization of all portions of that structure as well as the contents within the spinal canal. Choice of approach is dictated by the site of the primary pathologic condition. If the disease or deformity primarily involves the vertebral bodies, then it is usually best to approach them anteriorly through the abdomen or flank. On the other hand, the posterior elements of the lumbar spine are best approached directly through a vertically oriented posterior midline incision. This allows direct access to the spinous processes, laminae, and facets. By extending the dissection more laterally through the posterior approach, adequate exposure to the transverse processes and pedicles can be attained without difficulty. As an alternative, the posterolateral muscle-splitting approach provides direct access to the transverse processes and pedicles but more limited exposure of the vertebral bodies themselves.

As in any surgical procedure, the anatomic features of the proposed operative site have to be reviewed and understood before surgery. The surgeon should carefully study a skeletal model in conjunction with plain radiographs, computed tomography scans, magnetic resonance images and other images to produce a mental three-dimensional image of the structures that will be treated surgically. Particularly for anterior procedures around the lumbar spine, the approach should be planned so that it can be extended if necessary during the operation. The principles of any surgical procedure must be strictly observed during operations on the lumbar spine. These considerations include appropriate patient positioning, comfort, visibility related to the size of the incision, illumination, visualization, and maneuverability of instrumentation. The surgeon should never be constrained by poor positioning or draping.

POSTERIOR APPROACH

The posterior approach to the lumbar spine is by far the most common and widely used. It usually is made through a longitu-

dinal midline incision to gain direct access to the spinous processes, laminae, and facets of all levels of the lumbar spine. Through the direct posterior approach, the surgeon can remove some or all of the posterior osseous structures (laminotomy or laminectomy) and gain access to the posterior aspect of the cauda equina, conus medullaris, lumbar vertebral disc, pedicles, and vertebral body. With this approach, removal of an extruded portion of herniated disc and exploration of the thecal sac and nerve roots usually can be performed. With further dissection and retraction of the paraspinous muscles laterally, the facet joints and full extent of the transverse processes can be easily seen.

After satisfactory induction of anesthesia, the patient is gently log rolled and positioned prone on a spinal frame. Proper positioning allows the abdomen to hang free to reduce abdominal pressure and diminish venous engorgement and intraoperative bleeding at the operative site. With a midline posterior approach (Fig. 1), an incision is made longitudinally over the palpable spinous processes. Before the incision is made, skin bleeders can be controlled in part with subdermal injection of a 1:500,000 dilution of epinephrine. The addition of local anesthetic to this injection and at wound closure as preemptive analgesia may greatly diminish postoperative pain (10).

Sharp dissection with a scalpel or electrocautery is carried through subcutaneous tissue in line with the midline skin incision, and hemostasis is obtained with electrocoagulation. The thoracolumbar fascia (thoracodorsal fascia) is identified in the midline as it merges with the supraspinous ligaments. All efforts should be made to maintain the integrity of the supraspinous and interspinous ligaments. The thoracolumbar fascia can be incised just laterally to the supraspinous ligament. The paraspinous muscles incised subperiosteally can be elevated laterally off the spinous processes, laminae, and facet joints with a Cobb elevator and gauze packing.

The tip of the spinous processes has a bulbous configuration (Fig. 2). The interspinous plane lies directly in the midline between the two paraspinous (sacrospinalis) muscles, each of which receives its segmental nerve supply from the posterior primary rami of the lumbar nerves of its corresponding side. The bony exposure can continue laterally to expose the capsule of the facet joint, which should be protected if fusion is not planned. In preparation of the posterior elements for fusion, the lateral aspect

J. N. Weinstein: Dartmouth Medical School, Hanover, NH 03155.
W. A. Abdu: Department of Orthopaedics, Dartmouth-Hitchcock Medical Center, Lebanon, NH 03756.

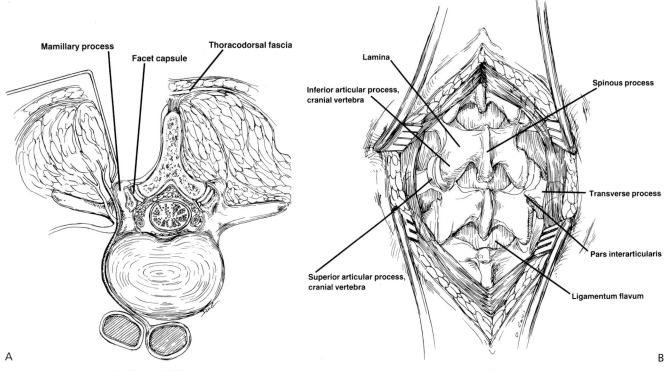

FIGURE 1. Midline posterior approach in axial plane. Posterior osseous exposure of the lumbosacral spine. (Redrawn from Hoppenfeld S. *Surgical exposures in orthopaedics.* Philadelphia: J.B. Lippincott, 1984, with permission.)

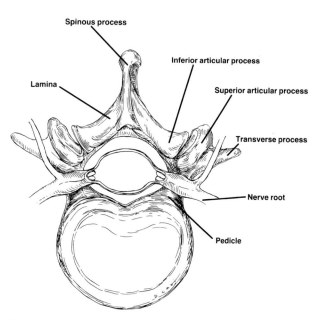

FIGURE 2. Transverse (axial) plane section of a lumbar segment emphasizes orientation of the bulbous tip of the spinous process, facet articular processes, pedicle, and neuromotor elements. (Redrawn from Watkins R, *Surgical approaches to the spine.* New York: Springer-Verlag, 1983, with permission.)

of the superior articular facet should be cleared and the dissection continued laterally to expose the transverse processes by means of dissection down the lateral side of the superior facet and onto the transverse process itself.

The ligamentum flavum (yellow ligament), which fans between the lumbar laminae, originates cranially approximately midway under the cephalad laminae and inserts under the cephalic edge of the caudal laminae (Fig. 3). The ligamentum flavum has a superficial portion and a deep portion and is thinnest in the midline. The ligamentum flavum extends down anteriorly to form the anterior capsule of the facet joint (Fig. 4). Variable portions of the laminae can be removed (laminotomy or laminectomy) to expose the underlying thecal sac, nerve roots, and surrounding soft-tissue structures. Removal of bone can continue laterally to involve the medial aspect of the pedicle or the medial aspect of the facet joint (hemifacetectomy) (Fig. 5), or the facet joint can be completely removed (total facetectomy).

The anatomic key to lumbar spine surgery is the pedicle. Three-dimensional thinking is essential for accurate spinal surgery and necessitates an ability to orient intracanal anatomic structures from visualization of the posterior elements. The center of the pedicle is generally at a point formed by the intersection of three lines: the axes of the transverse process, superior facet, and pars interarticularis (Fig. 6). With identification of the pedicle, the cephalic disc and caudal nerve root can be accurately located. Immediately cephalic to the pedicle is the intervertebral disc; immediately caudal to the pedicle is the exiting nerve root. Meticulous probing is mandatory in the pedicular portion of

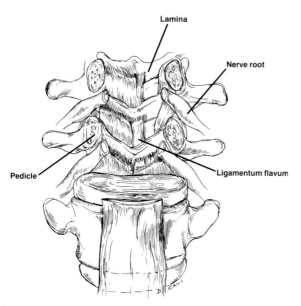

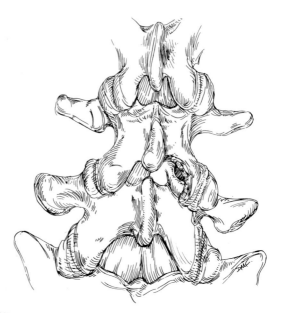

FIGURE 3. View from inside the canal and facing posteriorly shows the anatomic features of the ligamentum flavum. The ligamentum flavum inserts approximately midway under the cephalic lamina and inserts into the cephalic edge of the caudal lamina below. The ligamentum flavum is thinnest in the midline, providing the easiest point of entrance into the spinal canal. (Redrawn from Watkins R, *Surgical approaches to the spine*. New York: Springer-Verlag, 1983, with permission.)

FIGURE 5. Laminotomy with partial (hemi) facetectomy on the right side to expose underlying nerve root and disc lesion. The medial portion of the L4 inferior facet and the medial portion of the L5 superior facet are removed to expose the nerve root.

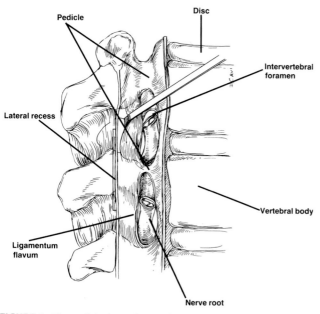

FIGURE 4. View of the boundaries of the neural foramen from inside the spinal canal facing out. (Redrawn from Watkins R, *Surgical approaches to the spine*. New York: Springer-Verlag, 1983, with permission.)

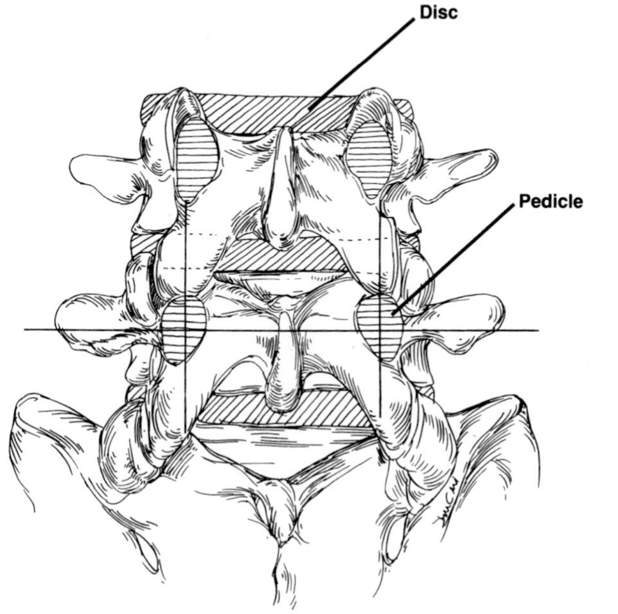

FIGURE 6. View of the pedicle with posterior elements intact. (Redrawn from Watkins R, *Surgical approaches to the spine*. New York: Springer-Verlag, 1983, with permission.)

the canal, because the pedicular vascular plexus in this region can be a source of troublesome bleeding. In surgical maneuvers within the spinal canal, the epidural venous system must be appreciated. Bipolar electrocauterization is essential in dealing with the epidural venous plexus.

As the dissection progresses cephalad, it is important to remember the location of the nerve root above and its relation to the interlaminar space. The L5–S1 disc is located approximately at the level of the interlaminar space between L5–S1, whereas the L2–3 disc space is well cephalic under the laminae of L2 rather than directly at the level of the interlaminar space between L2–3. It is also critical to identify the location of the pars interarticularis during any decompression. The interpedicular distance narrows from L5 to L1; this anatomic feature places the pars at risk of iatrogenic injury and instability from unintended facetectomy.

Decompressive laminectomy and foraminotomy are performed through the posterior approach. The neural foramen is a canal in which the nerve root and its accompanying vascular structures are located. The margins of the canal are formed anteriorly by the disc and vertebral body, posteriorly by the facet joint, inferiorly by the pedicle of the level below, and superiorly by the pedicle of the level above (Figs. 4, 7). A neural foramen by definition is a canal or tunnel with three dimensions (height, width, depth); it is more than than a simple open hole or foramen. The blood supply around the facet joints and pars interarticularis is rich with multiple muscular branches (Fig. 8). The arterial supply has been found to be remarkably constant in its anatomic distribution (8). Knowledge of the anatomic location of these articular and muscular branches allows the surgeon to identify and cauterize these vessels to minimize intraoperative bleeding.

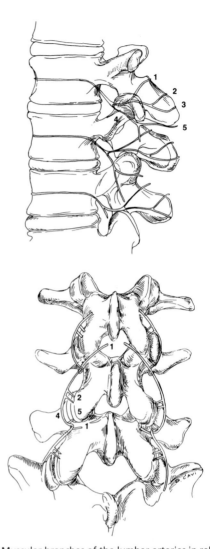

FIGURE 8. Muscular branches of the lumbar arteries in relation to the operative exposure. Rich and abundant blood supply is present around the facet joint, pars interarticularis, and transverse process. The interarticular artery is immediately lateral to the pars interarticularis. *2, 3,* The two superior articular arteries are immediately lateral to the tip of the superior articular facet. The communicating artery is a large vessel immediately lateral to the superior articular facet that extends onto the dorsum of the transverse process. The inferior articular artery is in the angle formed by the transverse process and superior articular facet (Redrawn from Macnab I, Dall D [1971]: The blood supply of the lumbar spine and its application to the technique of intertransverse lumbar fusion. *J Bone Joint Surg Br* 53:628–638, with permission.)

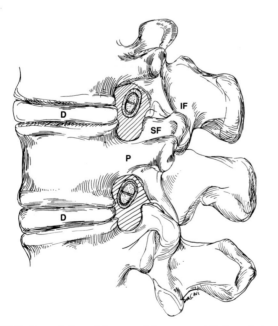

FIGURE 7. Lateral view of the neural foramen and its boundaries: superior facet, inferior facet, facet joint, pedicle, disc.

POSTEROLATERAL APPROACH

The posterolateral approach is popular for posterolateral lumbosacral fusion (10). This approach can provide direct access to the transverse processes and to the mammillary processes of the facets. Through this approach the transverse process can be removed to expose the nerve root from the level above. This approach also provides access to the pedicle. The lateral aspects of the vertebral body may be exposed in a limited manner. Two types of skin incisions can be used. A midline incision can be made with elevation of a subcutaneous tissue flap to expose the

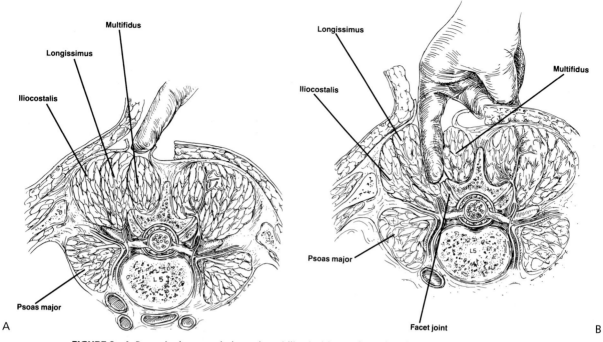

FIGURE 9. **A:** Paraspinal approach through a midline incision and muscle-splitting exposure of facets and transverse processes (Wiltse LL, Batemen JG, Hutchinson RH, et al. [1968]: Paraspinal sacrospinalis-splitting approach to the lumbar spine. *J Bone Joint Surg Am* 50:919–926; Wiltse LL, Spencer CW [1988]: New uses and refinements of the paraspinal approach to the lumbar spine. *Spine* 13:696–706.) A space is made between the multifidus and longissimus muscle groups. **B:** Further digital dissection places the surgeon's finger easily into the facet joint. The multifidus, longissimus, and iliocostalis muscles often are collectively called the *sacrospinalis group.* (Redrawn from Wiltse LL, Spencer CW [1988]: New uses and refinements of the paraspinal approach to the lumbar spine. *Spine* 13:696–706, with permission.)

thoracodorsal fascia. Then bilateral paraspinous incision can be made through the thoracodorsal fascia to expose the sacrospinalis muscle groups.

Muscle splitting between the multifidus and longissimus muscles provides direct access to the facet joint and transverse processes (Fig. 9). An alternative is to make bilateral paraspinous skin incisions (Fig. 10) approximately 1.75 inches (4.4 cm) lateral to the midline followed by a muscle-splitting division of the sacrospinalis group. This allows a direct approach to the facet joint and transverse processes. This approach has been popular-

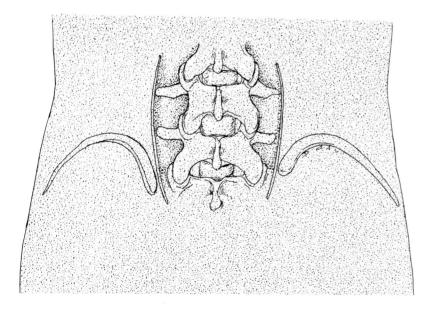

FIGURE 10. Skin incisions for bilateral paraspinous approach to lower lumbar spine, followed by muscle splitting to visualize facet joints, transverse processes, and ala of sacrum. (Redrawn from Watkins R, *Surgical approaches to the spine.* New York: Springer-Verlag, 1983, with permission.)

ized by Wiltse et al. (8,9) who consider it advantageous because it provides less muscle mass retraction medially and may decrease operative bleeding. Additional advantages of this approach are access to far lateral disc herniations, some intraforaminal discs, decompressions of the "far out syndrome" and access to the iliac crest for harvesting bone graft.

ANTERIOR APPROACHES

Although most operative procedures on the lumbar spine are performed by means of classic posterior approaches, selective indications arise for anterior approaches at one or several levels (Fig. 11). The anterolateral retroperitoneal flank approach usually allows visualization of all lumbar vertebrae. However, the exposure that it provides at its cranial and caudal extents is limited. For full access and exposure to L1, a thoracoabdominal approach is recommended. For satisfactory anterior exposure of L5 and S1, the transperitoneal approach often is needed.

ANTEROLATERAL RETROPERITONEAL APPROACH TO THE LUMBAR VERTEBRAE

The anterolateral approach to the lumbar vertebrae is an extension of the standard flank incision used for years by general surgeons for lumbar sympathectomy (Fig. 11). It provides excellent exposure for complete débridement or reconstructive bone grafting, which can include L2, L3, and L4. The access is more limited to L5. By dividing portions of the insertion of the arcuate ligament of the diaphragm on the first lumbar transverse process, this approach can provide limited access as high as T12. However, if an extensive reconstructive procedure or grafting is planned for L1 or T12, it is recommended that consideration be given to the thoracoabdominal T10 retroperitoneal approach.

The lumbar vertebrae are approached retroperitoneally from the left side if all other considerations are equal and the lesion can be resected from this side. The liver, located on the right side, is large and difficult to retract without injury. The inferior vena cava and its associated veins often are difficult to locate and are more fragile than the left-sided arterial system. Vena caval hemorrhage can be difficult to control. The spleen, on the left, is fragile but is much smaller than the liver, more mobile, and easily retracted; it can be sacrificed in an emergency. Hodge and DeWald (6) described a splenic injury with an anterior approach from the left side.

The patient is placed on the operating room table in the right lateral decubitus position. The kidney rest or inflatable roll is elevated and the table flexed to open the left flank. The left hip should be slightly flexed to relax the psoas muscle, an important landmark in the retroperitoneal approach. The level of incision varies according to the level of the lumbar spine requiring treatment (Fig. 12). This approach entails muscle-splitting dissec-

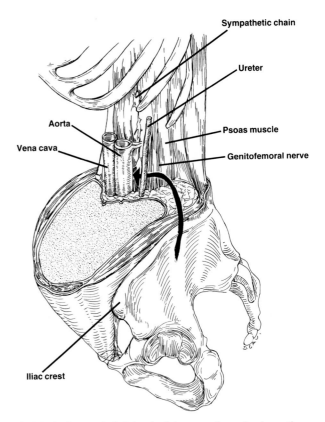

FIGURE 11. Removal of abdominal viscera and muscles shows the anatomic features of the flank. *Arrow* directs the surgical route to approach the anterolateral portion of the lumbar spine between the peritoneum anteriorly and the retroperitoneal structures posteriorly. (Redrawn from Hoppenfeld S. *Surgical exposures in orthopaedics.* Philadelphia: JB Lippincott, 1984, with permission.)

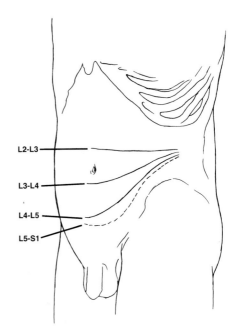

FIGURE 12. Patient in lateral decubitus position, right side down. Levels of incision for anterior retroperitoneal approach according to the level of the spine to be approached. (Redrawn from Watkins R, *Surgical approaches to the spine.* New York: Springer-Verlag, 1983, with permission.)

tion. It starts with electrocautery transection of the external oblique muscle and fascia and then the internal oblique muscle and fascia (Fig. 13A). The transversus abdominis muscle often is very thin or absent. Deep to the transversus abdominis muscle is the transversalis fascia. The transversalis fascia in the midline is adherent to the underlying peritoneum. For safe entrance into the retroperitoneal space, the transversalis fascia should be opened in the posterior aspect of the wound (Fig. 13B).

The peritoneum is thickest laterally and easiest to separate from the transversalis fascia laterally. The peritoneum thins toward the midline. If it is unintentionally entered, the peritoneum should be closed before the operation proceeds. The retroperito-

neal fat and retroperitoneal contents, including the ureter, are gently elevated off the quadratus lumborum muscle and psoas muscle, the key to the retroperitoneal space. The surgeon must avoid entering the retropsoas space, which is a blind pouch between the psoas and the quadratus lumborum muscles. The genitofemoral nerve must be identified and protected as it exits through the iliopsoas muscle belly, variably at approximately L3. The lumbar spine is immediately medial to the psoas and often is partially obscured by the psoas muscle. The paravertebral sympathetic chain is just medial to that muscle (Fig. 11). The ureter is reflected medially with the under surface of the peritoneum within the contents of the retroperitoneal fat. Digital palpation

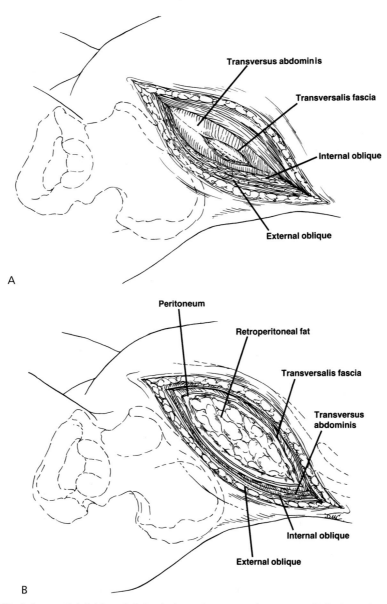

FIGURE 13. **A:** Sequential division of abdominal muscles exposes the transversalis fascia. **B:** The retroperitoneal cavity with its retroperitoneal fat, especially in posterior aspect of wound, is entered. *(Figure continues.)*

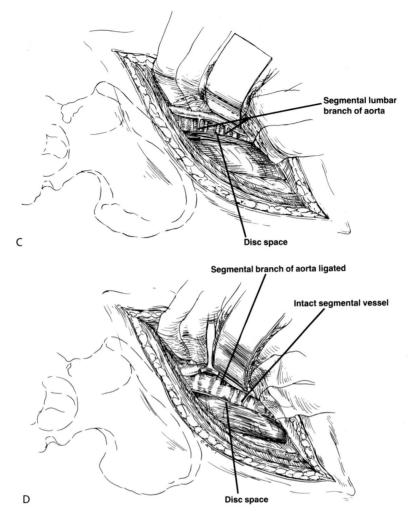

FIGURE 13. *Continued.* **C:** Psoas muscle exposed. **D:** Ligation of segmental vessels, aorta mobilized medially to reach the anterior and anterolateral positions of the vertebral body. (Redrawn from Watkins R, *Surgical approaches to the spine.* New York: Springer-Verlag, 1983, with permission.)

medial to the psoas leads directly to the vertebral bodies, and the raised white soft discs can be palpated directly.

An intraoperative radiograph should be obtained to identify the appropriate level. The psoas muscle is retracted laterally to expose the anterolateral aspect of the vertebral bodies (Fig. 13C). At the midlevel of each lumbar vertebra are the segmental vessels, which must be identified. When necessary, these vessels should be ligated to control bleeding. Injury to these vessels can cause profuse bleeding. After satisfactory control of the segmental vessels, the aorta can be mobilized more medially to fully expose the anterior aspect of the lumbar vertebrae (Fig. 13D). At the L4–5 level, the ascending iliolumbar vein crosses the left L4–5 disc level and must be identified and ligated for satisfactory exposure of the L4–5 disc space and L5 vertebral body. The anterior longitudinal ligament can be elevated or resected from the midportion of the vertebral body as desired for the indicated reconstructive surgery around the vertebral body. The retroperitoneal approach described can be combined with the transtho-

racic retroperitoneal approach for complete anterior exposure from L5 to the upper thoracic level as required.

ANTERIOR APPROACH TO THE LUMBOSACRAL SPINE THROUGH A PARAMEDIAN INCISION

In some cases, L4, L5, and the sacrum can best be approached anteriorly through the anterior abdominal wall in the midline. This approach is particularly advantageous for procedures around L5–S1, but it can be used for L4–5, although it involves a great deal of mobilization of the great vessels. This approach may require the assistance of a general or vascular surgeon, a urologist, or a colleague more familiar with the area to be exposed. The patient is placed supine on the operating table and positioned in slight hyperextension. A paramedian incision is made (Fig. 14) over the abdomen that extends from the umbilicus to the pubis. The rectus fascia beneath is identified and

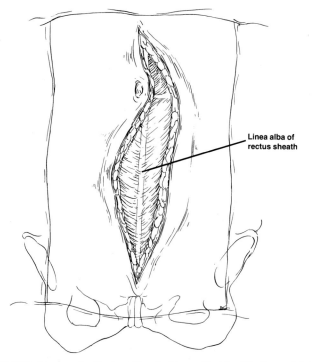

FIGURE 14. Longitudinal midline incision with identification of the rectus sheath. (Redrawn from Hoppenfeld S. *Surgical exposures in orthopaedics*. Philadelphia: JB Lippincott, 1984, with permission.)

opened longitudinally in line with the incision. The rectus abdominis muscle is mobilized laterally to expose the underlying posterior rectus fascia. The peritoneum is encountered and a decision is made to proceed transperitoneally (2,4) or retroperitoneally (9).

Transperitoneal Approach

The peritoneum is opened longitudinally in line with the skin incision; care is taken to protect the intestine beneath from injury. The intraabdominal contents are then packed cranially to expose the posterior peritoneum over the great vessels and vertebral body (Fig. 15). The posterior peritoneum is incised longitudinally in the midline over the sacral promontory. Presacral and parasympathetic nerve fibers should be preserved.

The deep surgical dissection consists of freeing the distal ends of the aorta and vena cava from the vertebrae in the L4–5 vertebral area. The aorta divides on the anterior surface of the L4 vertebra into the two common iliac arteries. The common iliac vessels then generally divide at approximately the S1 level into the internal and external iliac vessels (Fig. 16). The left common iliac vein lies below the left common iliac artery, whereas the right common iliac artery is below and medial to the right common iliac vein. The parasympathetic nerves in the presacral area exist as a diffuse plexus of nerves that course around the aorta and head inferiorly from the bifurcation along the anterior surface of the sacrum beneath the posterior peritoneum. This plexus should be protected if at all possible to preserve adequate sexual function and prevent retrograde ejaculation (1). The middle sac-

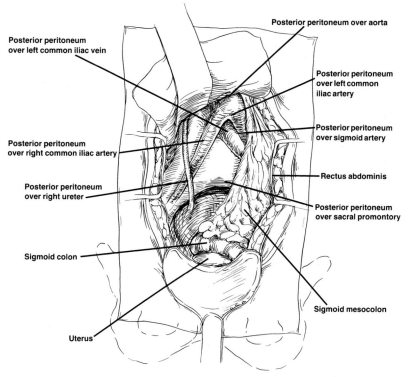

FIGURE 15. The posterior peritoneum is incised to reveal the bifurcation of the aorta and vena cava, parasympathetic nerve fibers, anterior longitudinal ligament, and sacral promontory. (Redrawn from Hoppenfeld S. *Surgical exposures in orthopaedics*. Philadelphia: JB Lippincott, 1984, with permission.)

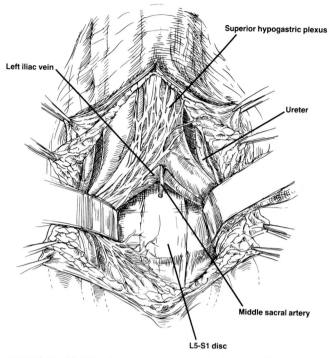

Left iliac vein

Superior hypogastric plexus

Ureter

Middle sacral artery

L5-S1 disc

FIGURE 16. Mobilization of the great vessels, ligation of the middle sacral artery, and gentle retraction of the hypogastric plexus for adequate exposure of L5–S1 or L4–5. (Redrawn from Watkins R, *Surgical approaches to the spine.* New York: Springer-Verlag, 1983, with permission.)

ral artery (Fig. 16) often is adherent to the vertebral bodies, and some difficulties may be encountered in mobilization of this vessel. In this situation, the artery can be ligated with vascular clips. In difficult procedures preoperative angiography can be helpful to define the vascular anatomic features.

Retroperitoneal Approach

Once exposure through the anterior abdominal wall is complete, the spine still can be approached with a retroperitoneal plane

of dissection rather than a transperitoneal plane. The left side is again preferred; dissection stays posterior on the renal fascia plane posterior to the ureter. Retroperitoneal dissection provides a less direct route to the spine, but if the tissue planes are well developed with blunt dissection and the abdominal contents are packed away, satisfactory exposure is obtained with less risk to the viscera and hypogastric plexus. The midline anterior approaches often are used in operations for spondylolisthesis, tumors, pseudarthrosis, or failures of previous posterior operations, for which anterior interbody fusion is indicated. Complications among male patients include impotence or sterility, although the incidence is reported to be less than 1% (3). Care must be taken not to extend the dissection well below the pelvic brim, where the parasympathetic or pudendal nerves can be injured.

REFERENCES

1. Flynn JC, Price CT (1984): Sexual complications of anterior fusion of the lumbar spine. *Spine* 9:489–492.
2. Freebody D, Bendall R, Taylor RD (1971): Anterior transperitoneal lumbar fusion. *J Bone Joint Surg Br* 53:617–627.
3. Hodge WA, DeWald RL (1983): Splenic injury complicating the anterior thoracoabdominal surgical approach for scoliosis: a report of two cases. *J Bone Joint Surg Am* 65:396–397.
4. Lane JD Jr, Moore ES Jr (1948): Transperitoneal approach to the intervertebral disc in the lumbar area. *Ann Surg* 127:537–551.
5. Macnab I, Dall D (1971): The blood supply of the lumbar spine and its application to the technique of intertransverse lumbar fusion. *J Bone Joint Surg Br* 53:628–638.
6. Southwick WO, Robinson RA (1957): Surgical approaches to the vertebral bodies in the cervical and lumbar regions. *J Bone Joint Surg Am* 39:631–635.
7. Watkins MB (1953): Posterolateral fusion of the lumbar and lumbosacral spine. *J Bone Joint Surg Am* 35:1014–1018.
8. Wiltse LL, Bateman JG, Hutchinson RH, et al. (1968): Paraspinal sacrospinalis-splitting approach to the lumbar spine. *J Bone Joint Surg Am* 50:919–926.
9. Wiltse LL, Spencer CW (1988): New uses and refinements of the paraspinal approach to the lumbar spine. *Spine* 13:696–706.
10. Woolfe CJ, Chong MS (1993): Preemptive analgesia: treating postoperative pain by preventing the establishment of central sensitization. *Anesth Analg* 77:362–79.

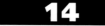

14

ANTERIOR AND POSTERIOR APPROACHES TO THE LUMBOSACRAL JUNCTION AND SACRUM

JACK C. Y. CHENG
K. Y. FUNG

The choice of surgical approach to the lumbosacral junction and the sacrum should primarily be dictated by the underlying pathology that needs to be treated surgically. For pathology localized primarily to the vertebral body, an anterior approach is preferred. This can be done transperitoneally or retroperitoneally. For pathology localized primarily to the posterior elements of the spine, a posterior or posterolateral approach is preferred. The other important considerations that affect the choice of approach are the need for nerve root decompression, the need for reduction of deformity, the need for instrumentation and pedicle screw placement, the need for spinal fusion, the presence of previous surgical procedures or complications, the need for extension of the surgical exposure, and last but not least, the experience and expertise of the surgeon or team of surgeons.

Alternative approaches to the lumbosacral spine using minimal invasive surgery through a laparoscopic anterior approach or an arthroscopic-spinoscopic posterior approach are discussed in other chapters. This chapter covers the following topics:

Indications for surgery at the lumbosacral junction and sacrum
Special surgical anatomy of the lumbosacral junction and sacrum
Techniques of anterior approach, posterior approach, and combined approach
Advantages, disadvantages, and pitfalls of the different surgical approaches
Complications specific to the approaches

INDICATIONS FOR SURGERY AT THE LUMBOSACRAL JUNCTION AND SACRUM

The most common indications for surgery at the lumbosacral junction and sacrum are degenerative conditions, including de-

generative disc problems, spinal stenosis, spinal instability, and spondylotic changes. The other common indications are for spondylolisthesis and other deformities, such as congenital hemivertebrae and neuromuscular scoliosis (1,5,23,24,28,37,42, 44,47,48,52,56,60). Rare pyogenic and tuberculous infections affecting L5 and the sacrum may require surgical decompression and fusion (6). Some fractures involving the sacrum, ilium, and sacroiliac joint may need surgical stabilization and instrumentation. A number of tumors have been reported to occur in the sacrum than can be treated with en bloc excision. These includes the more common chordomas and others, such as schwannomas, Ewing sarcoma, teratomas, presacral tumors, chondrosarcomas, osteosarcomas, giant cell tumors, and others (21,57,58,62,62). A growing number of salvage reconstructions are being done for pseudarthrosis resulting from failed scoliosis or kyphosis procedures, L5 listhesis below the level of the previous fusion, sagittal plane malalignment with clinical symptoms, significant residual and unacceptable deformity, oblique take-off at the lumbosacral junction, and progressive curve deterioration as a result of the crankshaft phenomenon or excessively short fusion of previous scoliosis deformity (38,45,46).

SPECIAL SURGICAL ANATOMY OF THE LUMBOSACRAL JUNCTION AND SACRUM

In approaching this region, the surgeon must be aware of a number of special anatomic facts. The sacral vertebral body is relatively small and difficult to access anteriorly. The anterior column is relatively insufficient. The cortical bone, is thin and the body is made mostly of trabecular bone that can be very osteoporotic in elderly patients. Therefore, for any implant fixation, the purchase could be more difficult. Only properly positioned bicortical S1 or S2 screws can have a reliable purchase and fixation. These facts, together with the large moment arm occurring at the slanting and mobile lumbosacral junction, can account for the higher rate of postsurgical pseudarthrosis. This can also explain why there are so many different fixation systems designed to improve purchase and fixation: alar hooks and screws, promontory screws, iliac screws, iliosacral screws, intrailiac rods, Galveston technique, sacral blocks, intrasacral rods,

J. C. Y. Cheng and K. Y. Fung: Department of Orthopaedics and Traumatology, Chinese University of Hong Kong, Prince of Wales Hospital, Hong Kong SAR.

sacral bars, sacral plates, and so forth (26,30–34,41,49–51, 53–55,59,65,66).

The surgical anatomy of the lumbosacral junction demands special attention whether one is approaching anteriorly or posteriorly. The bifurcation of the aorta anteriorly and the main branches of arteries and veins, common iliac vessels, internal iliac vessels, lumbosacral vein, and midsacral vessels are the most important structures that can be injured during the exposure or instrumentation. The spinal canal with the dural sac and the emerging lumbosacral trunk and sacral nerves anteriorly and spinal nerve roots posteriorly can easily be damaged. The presacral plexus is particularly prone to injury by cautery during the anterior transperitoneal approach (2,11,29). The visceral and pelvic organs are not far away from the anterior vertebral body. Thorough understanding of the anatomy and preoperative detailed imaging workup and planning are absolutely necessary for the surgeon operating in the lumbosacral area.

ANTERIOR APPROACHES

Hodgson and colleagues popularized the anterior approach to the lumbar spine through their extensive experience in treating tuberculous infection of the spine (6). In the lumbosacral junction, the anterior approach has the distinct advantages of restoration of the natural height of the anterior column and re-creation of natural lordosis that cannot be achieved through a posterior approach. In patients requiring fusion, the compressed bone graft can provide additional mechanical stability. Exposure of the lumbosacral junction can be accomplished through one of the following approaches: anterolateral retroperitoneal, paramedian retroperitoneal, and transperitoneal (3,4,7–9,12–16, 25,27,36).

Anterolateral Retroperitoneal Approach

The spine is commonly approached from the left side because the left common iliac vessels are longer than those of the right side and thus can be better retracted across to the right without undue tension. The patient is placed in the right lateral position with 40 degrees off to the back using either the vacuum beanbag or simply proper positioning of sandbags underneath the left buttock and the left shoulder. The right knee is flexed to 90 degrees, and a pillow is placed beneath the left leg to flex the left hip slightly and thereby relax the psoas muscle (Fig. 1). In this position, the visceral organs fall away from the spine, and little retraction is required. This is especially important when operating on obese patients with pendulous abdomen. The patient is positioned so that the lumbosacral junction is right over the bridge of the operating table, which is raised to open up the disc space. At the end of the operation, lowering the bridge allows impaction of interbody bone grafts. Insertion of a Foley catheter decompresses the bladder and is recommended in all anterior approaches.

The surgeon stands on the right side of the patient because this provides a direct anterior view of the spine after exposure. As a general guideline, the skin incision is placed in a more anterior and inferior position in the abdomen for lower lumbar

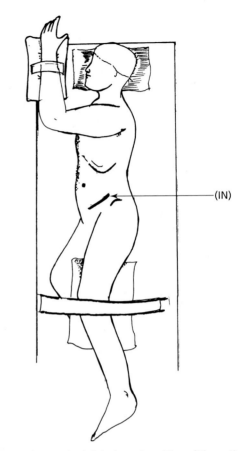

FIGURE 1. The standard right lateral position of the patient with 40 degrees tilt to the back showing the incision (IN) for the anterolateral approach to the lumbosacral spine.

and lumbosacral spine. An oblique incision is made from a point slightly caudal to midway between the iliac crest and the lowest rib to the lateral border of rectus abdominis muscle midway between the umbilicus and pubis on the left side (7–9, 13–16,27). Palpation of the sacral promontory helps to identify the level of incision accurately. Electric cautery is used to incise successively the subcutaneous fat, superficial and deep fascia, external oblique, internal oblique, and transversus abdominis muscle in the line of the skin incision. Often, the external oblique muscle can be split along its fibers.

The transversalis fascia is then stripped from the peritoneum. It is best to start stripping the peritoneum laterally. This part of the peritoneum is thicker and often covered by a good layer of extraperitoneal fat that can provide a good plane of dissection (8). The fat can be separated from the peritoneum by the surgeon's finger or a blunt instrument, such as a Deaver retractor. After defining the plane, the peritoneum can be slowly dissected off of the anterior overlying rectus muscle over the medial side of the incision. Here, the peritoneum is thin and adherent, especially in multipara. A sponge stick is then used to sweep the peritoneum further from the undersurface of the muscles both proximally and distally to facilitate the retraction of the peritoneum to the midline. Further medially, part of the anterior and the posterior rectus sheaths are divided with Metzenbaum scissors, leaving the rectus muscle and the inferior epigastric vessels intact. This releases the tension of the incision and allows better retraction. The peritoneum is then carefully stripped medially starting from anterior to the psoas muscle, followed by the abdominal aorta and common iliac vessels along a loose areola tissue plane.

To avoid unnecessary bleeding, it is important not to work too far and too deep laterally in the interval between the psoas and quadratus lumborum muscles. The ureter can be identified as a whitish wriggling structure adherent to the peritoneum and is retracted together with the peritoneum medially. If the peritoneal cavity is inadvertently opened, it can be closed with 3-0 atraumatic sutures immediately, although some surgeons do not always repair it if the hole is small (36). The sympathetic chain, found between the vertebral bodies and the psoas, is preserved and retracted laterally together with the psoas muscle. The genitofemoral nerve lying on the anterior surface of the psoas is protected.

The vertebral bodies can be palpated well at this stage. The segmental vessels lying on the midportion of L4 vertebral body can be ligated and divided to allow better retraction and mobilization of the surrounding structures. Using the Deaver retractor, the peritoneum is further retracted toward the midline to bring the main vessels into view. The left common iliac artery is identified and mobilized carefully. Small sympathetic fibers passing over the artery can be divided. Proximally along the vessels, the paraaortic lymph glands encountered can be dissected off with patience. Working caudally along the left common iliac artery, the left common iliac vein can be seen in a deeper plane. The left common iliac vein and its continuation, the external iliac vein, are carefully freed, and the iliolumbar vein running upward laterally and then posterior to the medial border of the psoas muscle should be identified. The iliolumbar vein can be single or double; when occurring as a single branch, it is often short and bifurcates immediately. To avoid damage to the vein, which can lead to troublesome bleeding, a good length of the iliolumbar vein must be freed before it is ligated and divided (Fig. 2).

The soft tissue over the anterior aspect of the vertebra is gradually stripped toward the right side with a Cobb elevator and dental swab held by artery forceps. Small vessels running into the anterior longitudinal ligament from the vena cava are cauterized and divided. To facilitate the exposure, the psoas muscle can be retracted laterally by means of a positioning Steinmann pin with protective rubber tubing. The common iliac vessels, together with all the retroperitoneal tissue, which contains the fibers of hypogastric plexus, can be safely displaced and retracted toward the right side by a shoehorn retractor, thus exposing the whole of lumbosacral disc, L5 body, and upper part of the sacrum (Fig. 3).

Paramedian Retroperitoneal Approach

The retroperitoneal approach to the lumbar and lumbosacral spine can be achieved through a paramedian incision (5). The patient is placed in the supine position with the lumbar spine extended. This can be done by putting a sandbag behind the lower back or by raising the bridge of the operating table at that level. A left paramedian incision is made from umbilicus to the

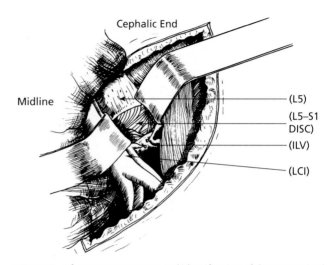

FIGURE 2. After proper exposure and identification of the L5 vertebral body, L5 to S1 disc, and sacral promontory, the left common iliac vessels (LCI) are retracted toward the midline. The left iliolumbar vein (ILV) is then carefully exposed on its whole length before it is ligated and divided.

pubis (Fig. 4). The anterior rectus sheath is opened longitudinally in line with the skin incision. Note that the rectus abdominis muscle receives its nerve supply from the lower six thoracic nerves that lie between the internal oblique and transversus abdominis muscles before they finally pierce the posterior part of rectus sheath to reach the rectus muscle. To preserve its nerve supply, the rectus is retracted laterally to expose the posterior rectus sheath.

The arcuate line that marks the lower end of the posterior rectus sheath is identified. The preperitoneal space can be entered here (Fig. 5). The peritoneum is carefully stripped off directly from the posterior rectus sheath before incising the sheath. Great caution is taken to preserve the inferior epigastric

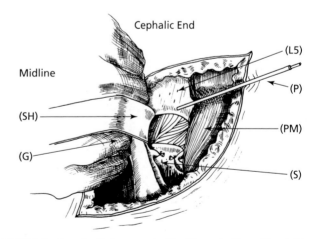

FIGURE 3. Use of a Steinmann pin (P) with protective rubber tubing to retract the psoas muscle (PM) laterally, and use of loose gauze packing (G) beneath the large blunt shoehorn retractor (SH) to protect the great vessels and hypogastric plexus medially. The whole lumbosacral disc, L5 body, and upper sacrum (S) can be exposed.

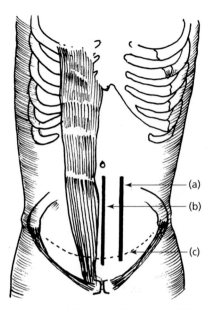

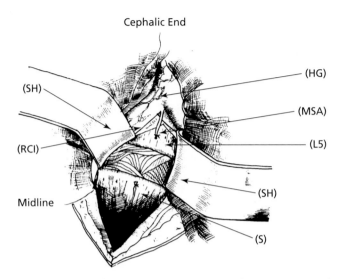

FIGURE 4. Shown are the left paramedian incision (*A*) from the umbilicus to the pubis for a paramedian retroperitoneal approach an the vertical (*B*) versus transverse (*C*) skin incisions for the transperitoneal approach.

FIGURE 6. At the final exposure in the paramedian retroperitoneal approach, two large shoehorn retractors (SH) are placed to protect the great vessels. The middle sacral artery (MSA) is ligated and divided. This artery is often adherent to the disc and L5 body and needs to be mobilized before ligation. The hypogastric plexus (HG) is retracted together with the right common iliac vessels (RCI).

vessels while cutting the sheath. The peritoneum is often very thin and adherent here. As the peritoneum is mobilized from medial to lateral, extraperitoneal fat is encountered. The peritoneum can be separated from the fat and the posterior abdominal wall with the hand or a blunt instrument, such as a Deaver retractor. While doing this, the psoas muscle can be felt and the peritoneum stripped off from the anterior surface in the same

manner as described in the section for the anterolateral retroperitoneal approach.

For exposure of the L5 to S1 disc, dissection is made just medial to the left common iliac artery and vein. The soft tissue, together with the hypogastric plexus, which lies in the retroperitoneal tissue overlying the aortic bifurcation, is mobilized from left to right. The middle sacral artery is then identified on the middle of the L5 to S1 disc. The artery may be adherent to the disc and L5 vertebral body, and it must be carefully mobilized before it is ligated and divided. The anterior wall of the sacrum can then be dissected from the rectum easily. The iliac vein, which lies within the aortic bifurcation in front of the L5 body, can be retracted proximally and protected by a shoehorn retractor to allow better exposure of the L5 vertebral body (Fig. 6).

If cautery is used in this area, the bipolar type is recommended to minimize the chance of damage to the hypogastric plexus. With careful attention, this retroperitoneal procedure is safe and causes minimal injury to the hypogastric plexus (3,5). If necessary, it allows placement of a suction drain after the operation.

Transperitoneal Approach

The transperitoneal approach provides excellent exposure of the lumbosacral junction (4,12,14,15,27). This can be achieved through either a vertical midline skin incision or a transverse skin incision (Fig. 4). The transverse incision is cosmetically superior but requires transection of the rectus abdominis muscle and the sheath. The patient is placed in the supine position with the lumbosacral spine extended. A vertical midline infraumbilical incision is sufficient for lumbosacral interbody fusion. The linea alba, the conjoined layer of the rectus sheath, is divided and dissected to expose the peritoneum, which is then opened longitudinally in line with the skin incision, with protection of the underlying bowel.

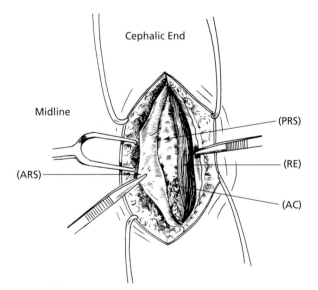

FIGURE 5. In the paramedian approach, after opening the anterior rectus sheath (ARS), the rectus abdominis (RE) is retracted laterally, and the posterior rectus sheath (PRS) and the arcuate line (AC) at its lower end are identified.

The operating table is inclined with the cranial side tilted downward about 10 to 15 degrees. The bowel contents fall away from the aorta and iliac vessels and are packed away and protected with a moist towel. The aortic bifurcation at the L4 to L5 region and the sacral promontory can be identified by palpation. The softer texture of the L5 to S1 disc can easily be recognized. Saline infiltration of the loose connective tissues just anterior to the L5 to S1 disc elevates the posterior peritoneum and helps the subsequent dissection. The posterior peritoneum is picked up, and a longitudinal incision is made in the midline. Blunt dissection with a dental swab held with an artery forceps in the region exposes the L5 to S1 disc. The middle sacral artery, which runs down the midline along the anterior aspect of the sacrum, is dissected free and then ligated and divided for further exposure. Great caution should be taken to protect the left iliac vein that runs across the L5 vertebral body and is found just below the aortic bifurcation. The left common iliac vessels are retracted to the left and the hypogastric plexus and the right iliac vessels are retracted to the right. Care must be taken not to injure the left ureter, which crosses the left common iliac vessel over the sacroiliac joint during the dissection. Cautery should be avoided as far as possible to prevent damage to the hypogastric plexus. If diathermy is necessary, the bipolar type is preferred. Shoehorn retractors are then used to protect the vessels on both sides to allow for further procedures on the L5 to S1 disc or the lumbosacral junction.

POSTERIOR APPROACHES

Standard Posterior Approach

The midline posterior approach is the most commonly used approach in posterior spinal surgery. It allows excellent exposure of the lumbosacral area from the midline extending laterally to the pedicle and transverse processes. By removing the posterior spinous process and lamina partially or completely, a direct approach to the spinal canal, thecal sac, cauda equina, nerve roots, and the L5 to S1 disc, and through the disc to expose part of the L5 and S1 vertebral body, is possible. By extending the midline incision upward and downward, a thorough exposure of the whole spine and sacrum can be achieved readily in cases of long fusion for spinal deformities.

After being anesthetized in the supine position, the patient is carefully turned into the prone position. Different types of frames can be used to support and position the patient, including a radiolucent spinal frame, four-post frame, or knee-chest frame, depending on the requirement of the operation. It is important to take into consideration the sagittal alignment of the lumbosacral area. In cases in which no instrumentation is required, the knee-chest or kneeling position with the lumbar spine flexed would allow better exposure of the lumbosacral area and the spinal canal posteriorly. In cases in which posterior instrumentation is anticipated, however, the lumbar lordosis must be maintained as near to the anatomic sagittal plane as possible (i.e., with the hips flexed to about 30 degrees to avoid iatrogenic flattening of the normal lumbar lordosis). The abdomen must hang loose and free from pressure to minimize venous engorgement and intraoperative bleeding, which can be troublesome.

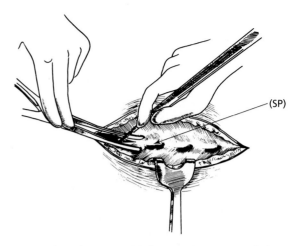

FIGURE 7. A large hemostat with downward pressure can help to stabilize the soft tissue over the spinous process (SP) and allows the incision and exposure of the spinous process to proceed in the midline.

Additional bolsters beneath the shoulder and anterior superior iliac spine may help to relieve the pressure further. In female patients, care should also be made to shift the breasts away from direct pressure. Headlight visualization can be helpful to the surgeon.

A standard midline skin incision is done with or without prior subdermal diluted epinephrine infiltration. After controlling bleedings from the skin edges with cautery, the spinous processes of the L4, L5, and S1 discs are identified. Depending on the nature of the surgery, exposure can be extended upward or downward accordingly. To prevent slipping of the knife during the midline incision, a large hemostat can be used to mark and stabilize the midline structures on both sides of the spinous process (Fig. 7). The midline cut is then done with cautery directly through the thoracolumbar fascia down to the spinous process. The hemostat is then slowly released to allow time for the cautery to catch up the bleeding vessels from the edges of the supraspinous ligaments. A true subperiosteal approach is done with the Cobb elevator, with the assistant tensing up the paraspinal muscle on the side to be stripped with another Cobb elevator. Using this double-Cobb technique, the muscles can be stripped nicely subperiosteally, which prevents muscle tearing and unnecessary bleeding. If the Cobb elevators are positioned on each of the adjacent lamina synchronously, the interlaminar structures can be stripped and cut with cautery easily from the midline laterally (Fig. 8). Sequential stripping can then proceed laterally, and if the exposure of the pedicle and transverse process is necessary, the capsule of the facet joints can be opened by cautery. Bleeding encountered during the procedure can usually be controlled by proper gauze-packing technique. Occasionally, bleeding comes from nutrient vessels at the lamina or near the facet, which can only be controlled by plugging with bone wax over a small dental swab over a small hemostat. If fusion is not planned, the capsule of the facet joints should be protected and kept intact.

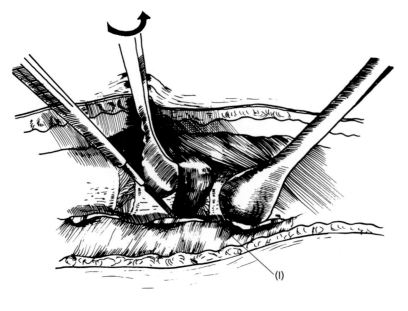

FIGURE 8. Double Cobb technique: After the initial subperiosteal stripping of adjacent lamina, with the upper Cobb elevator acting as a retractor, the lower Cobb is rotated to tense up the interlaminar structures (I) and to allow a clean cautery stripping from the midline laterally at the plane just above the ligamentum flavum.

In the L5 to S1 area, the paraspinal muscles are usually tight. After adequate initial exposure of both sides of L5 to S1, strong adjustable self-retaining retractors with proper depth and width help to keep the area clear. Intelligent use of Meyerding retractors of different sizes by the assistant can offer additional help. Careful use of periosteal elevators and sharp bone curettes can then help to clean the area and prepare for further procedure. When approaching the lateral side of the pedicle on the way to the transverse process, it is common to encounter significant bleeding. The anatomy of the blood supply in this region should be remembered clearly. In the interspinous plane, the pedicle of the segmental neurovascular bundle from the posterior primary rami of the lumbar nerves of its corresponding side appears and should be protected and not inadvertently damaged. The arterial supply has been found to be relatively constant in its anatomic distribution (13). This consists of the interarticular artery lying lateral to the pars interarticularis. The superior articular artery lies immediately lateral to the tip of superior articular facet. The communicating artery appears as a large vessel immediately lateral to the superior articular facet and extending onto the dorsum of the transverse process. The inferior articular artery can be found at the angle formed by transverse process and superior articular facet (Fig. 9).

With proper retraction, blunt dissection with the help of cautery sculpturing can be done along the lateral side of the superior articular process down to the transverse process subperiosteally. Identification of the mammillary process and the transverse process with the blunt Cobb elevator can help to define the anatomic landmarks more precisely. Care must be taken to avoid cutting into the adjacent muscles, which can lead to profuse bleeding, which can be difficult to control in the depth of the wound.

Note that with proper identification of the pedicle, the cephalad disc and caudal nerve root can be accurately located. Immediately cephalad to the pedicle is the intervertebral disc; immedi-

ately caudal to the pedicle is the exiting nerve root. The L5 to S1 disc is near the level of the interlaminar space between L5 and S1, in contrast to the L2–3 disc space, which is well cephalad under the laminae of L2 rather than directly at the level of the interlaminar space between L2–3 (Fig. 10).

For additional exposure of the spinal canal, the ligamentum flavum can be removed with or without additional laminotomy, laminectomy, facetectomy, or foraminotomy, depending on the nature of the procedure. The ligamentum flavum fanning between the lumbar laminae originates cranially about midway under the cephalad laminae and inserts under the cephalad edge of the caudal laminae. The ligamentum flavum is thinnest in

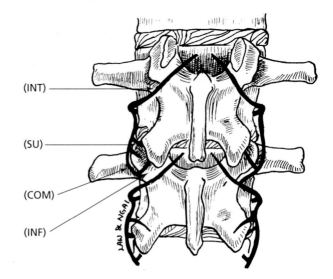

FIGURE 9. Blood supply of the pedicles posteriorly showing the interarticular artery (INT), the superior articular artery (SU), the inferior articular artery (INF), and the communicating artery (COM).

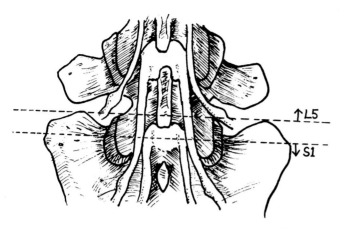

FIGURE 10. Surface landmark of the lumbosacral disc.

the midline and extends down anteriorly to form the anterior capsule of the facet joint. Variable portions of the laminae can be removed to expose the underlying thecal sac, nerve roots, and surrounding soft tissue structure. Epidural venous plexus bleeding can be controlled by packing or with bipolar cautery.

For placement of instrumentation or pedicle screws in the lumbar sacral area, one of the prerequisites is that the exposure must be adequate from the midline to near the tip of the transverse process so that the anatomic landmarks for preparation of pedicle screw insertion can be clearly localized. The most reliable procedure is to have the transverse process, pedicles, and lamina on both sides clearly exposed.

For exposure of the sacrum, the midline exposure is relatively easy, whereas the pedicles and lateral dense bone are more difficult to identify. The S1 pedicle location is halfway between the lumbosacral facet and the first posterior sacral neural foramen,

medial from and about one third the distance of the neural foramen to the midline. For pedicle screw insertion, the sacral ala exposure should extend 1 cm laterally and about 2 cm superiorly and inferiorly.

Posterolateral Approach

As an alternative to the standard posterior approach, the spine can be approached through a bilateral posterolateral approach (17–19,40). This is particularly useful in patients with midline scarring from previous operations and with defects in the posterior elements of the spine or when pedicle screw placement is planned without the necessity of exploring the spinal canal. It allows direct access to the transverse processes and facet joints of the lumbosacral area. Decompression of lateral disc herniation or "far-out syndrome" is possible. The exposure also allows posterolateral bone fusion, with simultaneous bone graft harvesting from the iliac crest. The posterolateral approach can be achieved by one of three different skin incisions (Fig. 11): the midline longitudinal skin incision and bilateral paraspinal approach, the transverse skin incision and bilateral paraspinal approach, or the paraspinal skin incision approach. After the skin incision, there are two different methods of approaching the spine: the lateral paraspinal approach and the paraspinal muscle-splitting approach of Wiltse.

Lateral Paraspinal Approach

This approach is useful for wide exposure from L4 down to the sacrum and for procedures requiring good posterolateral fusion with or without instrumentation. A longitudinal incision is made along the outer border of the paraspinal muscles and curves slightly medially near the caudal end as the incision crosses the

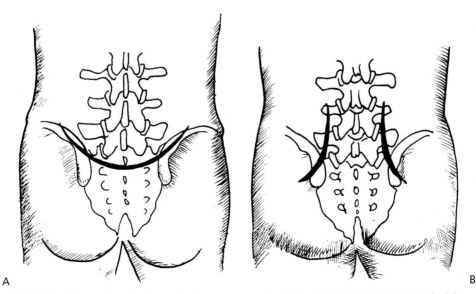

A   B

FIGURE 11. Skin incisions for the posterolateral approach. **A:** One transverse skin incision. **B:** The bilateral paraspinal incision approach.

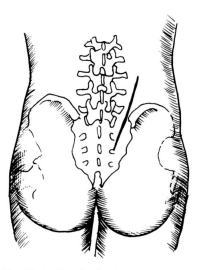

FIGURE 12. Skin incision for the lateral paraspinal approach.

is retracted laterally to allow an incision along the posterior third of the iliac crest and subperiosteal exposure of the posterior portion of the ilium. The exposure is then carried medially from the tips of the transverse processes, clearing the tissues off the superior articular process. The joint capsule is excised, and the exposure is carried medially, exposing the lamina to the base of the spinous process, except in patients with laminar defects. The exposure is continued distally to uncover the first two sacral segments.

If the patient has a spondylolisthesis at the lumbosacral level, the defect in the pars interarticularis can be visualized. For fusion from L4 to the sacrum, the transverse process of L4 and L5 are decorticated along with the pars interarticularis and the lateral aspects of the superior articular process of L4 and L5. After decortication and grafting, the retractors are removed, and the soft tissues are allowed to fall into place. The gluteal muscle and fascia are securely approximated with interrupted sutures through drill holes made in the intact medial crest of the posterior ilium.

posterosuperior iliac spine (Fig. 12). The thoracolumbar fascia is incised, and dissection is done in the plane between the paraspinal muscles medially and the fascia overlying the transversus abdominis muscle laterally. The tip of the transverse processes of L5 can be palpated in the depth of the wound. About 3 cm of the posterior iliac crest, including the posterosuperior iliac spine, can be osteotomized superficially and retracted medially, along with the reflected sacrospinalis muscle, thus exposing the ala of the sacrum (Fig. 13).

For obtaining iliac bone grafts for fusion, the lateral skin flap

Muscle-splitting Approach of Wiltse

The Wiltse approach is similar to the lateral paraspinal approach. Instead of keeping lateral to the sacrospinalis, the thoracodorsal fascia is incised and the muscle plane between the multifidus and longissimus muscles developed with the help of finger palpation (20,64). The approach is directly over the facet joint and transverse processes. The posterior elements are then subperiosteally exposed from the base of the spinous process to the tip of the transverse process. Wiltse believes that this approach is better than the midline incision because the spinous processes with their ligaments and blood supply are not disturbed, thus maintaining the stability (Fig. 14).

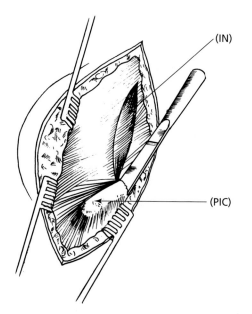

FIGURE 13. Incision over the lateral part of the paraspinal muscle (IN), followed by osteotomy of the posterior iliac crest (PIC) to expose the ala of the sacrum.

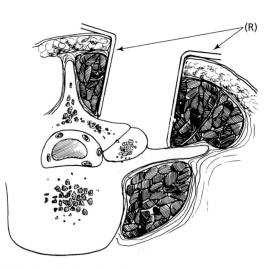

FIGURE 14. Paraspinal muscle-splitting approach of Wiltse: The interval is developed between the multifidus and longissimus muscle and retracted with deep retractors (R) to expose directly the facet joint and adjacent structure.

COMBINED ANTERIOR AND POSTERIOR APPROACH

The combined anterior and posterior approach may be indicated in situations in which difficult circumferential fusion of the lumbosacral area is required after salvage reconstruction of failed fusion after deformity surgery, degenerative spine, or spondylolisthesis (24,38,45). This may be done in single stage or in two stages. One of the most important indications is for en bloc excision of malignant tumor in the sacrum (21,57,58,62,63). Among all the tumors described in this area, sacral chordoma is the most common (Fig. 15). The anterior approach is required for control of the neurovascular elements and exposure of the anterior aspects of the tumor. The posterior incision allows control of the nerve roots and excision of the tumor. The detailed steps depend primarily on the nature and pathology of the sacral tumor. Detailed preoperative imaging study of the pathoanatomy and preoperative planning are vital. This often means a combination of radiographs, computed tomography scans, magnetic resonance imaging studies, arteriograms, and other investigations.

Some surgeons prefer approaching the posterior side first, followed by the anterior approach. Others believe that the anterior should be approached first, followed by the posterior surgery. If one uses the anterior approach first, a retroperitoneal approach is preferred for unilateral lesions, whereas a midline transperitoneal approach is better indicated for bilateral lesions that cross the midline. Through the anterior approach, the lumbosacral trunk can first be controlled at the medial edge of the iliopsoas muscle. The anterior sacral osteotomy is done between the sacral foramina corresponding to the roots that are to be preserved. Profuse bleeding may occur at this stage, which requires proper packing. After wound closure, the patient is turned over for the posterior incision. A laminectomy is performed on L5 and the sacrum, allowing identification of the roots that were marked from within the pelvis. The osteotomy is then completed posteriorly. If the rectum must be included in the resected specimen, the procedure is begun anteriorly, continued posteriorly, and completed finally from the front. After the anterior resection, the rectum is removed en bloc with the sacrum through the posterior exposure. After this posterior incision is closed, the patient is replaced in the supine position, and the abdominal incision is reopened to perform a colostomy.

When the posterior approach is done first, after the laminectomy, the dura are opened and the L4, L5, and S1 nerve roots in intervertebral foramina are exposed and protected. This is followed by a separate anterior incision or anterolateral incision extending horizontally to join the posterior incision.

ADVANTAGES AND DISADVANTAGES OF THE DIFFERENT APPROACHES

Posterior Approach

Advantages

The posterior approach allows direct access to most of the posterior osseous structures—the spinous process, laminae, facets, and transverse processes of L5 and S1. It also allows direct access to the posterior aspects of the cauda equina, thecal sac, nerve roots, lumbar disc, pedicles, and even the vertebral body.

Disadvantages

The paraspinal muscle is usually tight, making retraction difficult and traumatizing. The approach to the lateral side of the

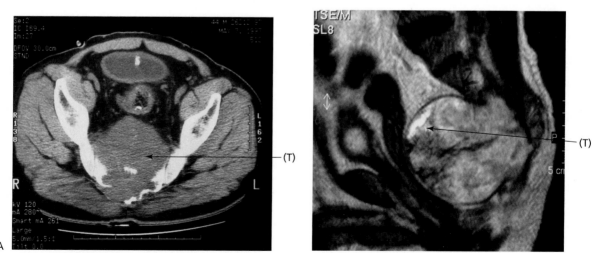

FIGURE 15. A: A typical case of sacral chordoma arising anteriorly from the sacrum. The anteroposterior and lateral computed tomography scan illustrates the extension of the tumor (T) anteriorly compressing on the rectum and posterior into the sacral spinal canal. **B:** A combined anterior and posterior approach is necessary to excise the chordoma.

pedicle and transverse process can be difficult, and exposure may not be adequate for decortication and posterolateral fusion or insertion of pedicle screws.

Posterolateral Approach

Advantages

The posterolateral approach allows direct access to the transverse processes, facets and mammillary processes of the facets, pedicles, far lateral disc herniations, intraforaminal discs, and iliac crest for bone graft with less retraction.

Disadvantages

Simultaneous approach to the spinal canal and decompression would be difficult. The approach may cause scarring of the paraspinal muscles and skin, which may affect subsequent surgery that requires more extensive exploration of spinal canal.

Anterolateral Retroperitoneal Approach

Advantages

This method permits an extensive retroperitoneal approach to the lumbar spine. With extension of the incision, the L3 to L4 and L4 to L5 discs and the lumbosacral junction can be exposed simultaneously. With distal retraction of the wound, the left ilium can be reached for harvesting bone graft without an additional skin incision.

Disadvantages

This is a muscle-cutting approach, and the patient may experience pain with postoperative deep breathing exercise. Retraction of the rectus muscle to the medial side may denervate part of the muscle. There is a potential risk for damage to the hypogastric plexus.

Anterior Paramedian Retroperitoneal Approach

Advantages

This approach avoids cutting of abdominal muscles and provides direct anterior access to the lower lumbar and lumbosacral junction simultaneously. Mild grades of L5 to S1 spondylolisthesis (grades I and II) can be reduced easily after discectomy and with the patient in the supine position with the back hyperextend.

Disadvantages

A vertical incision is not as cosmetically pleasing as an oblique incision. The same approach can be used with a transverse incision, but it requires transection of the rectus abdominis muscle and the sheath. Previous abdominal surgeries can make the approach difficult. A separate incision is needed for harvesting the bone graft from the ilium. The hypogastric plexus, which is the direct extension of the aortic plexus overlying the common iliac

vessels and the L5 body, has to be mobilized, and this can introduce potential urogenital complication of retrograde ejaculation in male patients.

Anterior Transperitoneal Approach

Advantages

This approach is the shortest route to the lumbosacral region and is particularly useful in patients who underwent previous retroperitoneal surgery. Because of its direct access, this method can be used for anterior fusion of all grades of spondylolisthesis.

Disadvantages

The great vessels and the hypogastric plexus have to be mobilize through the retroperitoneal tissue. There is a greater risk for damaging this plexus as compared with the other retroperitoneal approaches. This method is limited to the lumbosacral junction. Upward extension and exposure cannot be accomplished without generous mobilization of the wound, thus increasing the chance of damaging the hypogastric plexus. The approach is particularly difficult in obese patients.

COMMON PITFALLS OF DIFFERENT APPROACHES
Posterior Approach

Pitfalls of the posterior approach include the following:

- Failure to keep to midline during the initial exposure, thus cutting into muscle and causing unnecessary damage and bleeding
- Exposure of the lamina and spinous process that is not subperiosteal
- Mistaking L4 for L5
- Inadvertent damage to a facet joint not intended to be included in the fusion
- Trauma to paraspinal muscles with excessive retraction
- Damage to neurovascular pedicle at the L5 and sacral foramen

Many other pitfalls may occur when exposing the spinal canal, including failure of adequate decompression and bony fusion.

Anterolateral Retroperitoneal Approach

The techniques of handling and ligation of the vessels are vital in this operation. Failure to use long-handled instruments significantly affects the surgeon's operative view while dissecting the soft tissue. Vascular complications are not uncommon, and most of them are minor tears of the vein. Panic and failure to control the bleeding when encountering a tear in the iliac vein and iliolumbar vein can be disastrous. If a hole is made in the big vein, a finger is put on the bleeding spot to control the bleeding temporarily. Two shoehorn retractors are placed in a V manner to press the vein firmly against the spine to block off the bleeding and expose the bleeding point. Atraumatic Prolene suture of 5-0 or 6-0 can then be used to repair the hole properly.

In cases of L5 to S1 spondylolisthesis with instability, the dissection can be tedious because of the fibrous adhesion between the spine and the big vessels. Normally, the lumbosacral angle is easily defined. In L4 to L5 spondylolisthesis, however, the disc can be prominent and mistaken for the lumbosacral angle.

Anterior Paramedian Retroperitoneal Approach

In the anterior paramedian retroperitoneal approach, damage may be done to the inferior epigastric vessel during the cutting of the rectus sheath. Tearing of the peritoneum under the posterior rectus sheath may also occur at the site where it is often very thin and adherent. In the later part of the operation, part of the medial wall of the left common iliac vein within the aortic bifurcation may slip out underneath the retractor and become entrapped during impaction of the bone graft. Cautery in the region of the bifurcation can cause damage to the hypogastric plexus inadvertently.

Anterior Transperitoneal Approach

Failure to mobilize adequately before ligating the middle sacral artery can often lead to unnecessary bleeding. Cautery in the region of the aortic bifurcation is more likely to cause damage to the hypogastric plexus than the other anterior approaches. Other common pitfalls are similar to those of the other anterior approaches.

COMPLICATIONS SPECIFIC TO DIFFERENT APPROACHES

Posterior Approaches

Complications from posterior approaches are not common because this is the most familiar approach to most surgeons. Some of the more likely potential complications are injury to the nerve roots and dural tears during exposure of the spinal canal. Bleeding from epidural veins can sometimes be troublesome. Injury to major vessels in front of the vertebral body has been reported as a result of perforation of the anterior longitudinal ligaments during discectomy or posterior interbody fusion (61). Transient paralytic ileus and urinary retention are not uncommon after posterior surgery.

Anterior Approaches

Apart from a few specific complications, most complications are similar among the different anterior approaches as they are discussed here. For retroperitoneal approaches, denervation of the rectus abdominis can occur. Visceral injuries to the intestine, spleen, kidney, and in particular the ureter may occur (39,43). Peritoneum perforation is not uncommon. Injury to the sympathetic chain and the genitofemoral nerve over the psoas muscle frequently occurs. Vascular injury is the most serious complication that can include injury to the inferior epigastic vessels, mid-

dle sacral vessels, iliolumbar veins, ascending lumbar veins, and external or common iliac veins (22,61). Excessive trauma and cautery in the bifurcation of the aorta can injure the hypogastric plexus and lead to retrograde ejaculation in male patients (10,35,43). The actual incidence, however, is not as common as often described.

The transperitoneal approach can be complicated by injury to the viscera, including the intestines, bladder, and other pelvic structures. The middle sacral artery and the left iliac vein lying just in the aortic bifurcation can be damaged as a result of improper mobilization and retraction during the exposure of the L5 to S1 disc. This approach also carries additional risk for damaging the hypogastic plexus and sacral nerves with potential possibility of retrograde ejaculation and problems of penile erection in male patients.

Other Complications

Other complications can be related to complications of the implant fixation, specific instrumentation techniques, and of the specific spinal disorders. Failure of bone purchase or bone fusion and breakage of implants, instruments, and the linkage system have been reported regularly. Instrument and implant malposition can lead to neurovascular and visceral organ damage.

ACKNOWLEDGMENTS

We wish to thank Dr. K. S. Leung for helping to write part of this chapter and Drs. S. W. Law and Y. H. Ngai for their great support in drawing all the illustrations in this chapter.

REFERENCES
Classic References

1. Cummine JL, Lonstein JE, Moe JH, et al. (1979): Reconstructive surgery in the adult for failed scoliosis fusion. *J Bone Joint Surg Am* 71: 1151–1161.
2. Elaut L (1932): The surgical anatomy of the so called presacral nerve. *Surg Gynecol Obstet* 53:581–589.
3. Flynn JC, Hoque MA (1979): Anterior fusion of the lumbar spine: end-result study with long-term follow up. *J Bone Joint Surg Am* 61: 1143–1150.
4. Freebody D, Bendall R, Taylor RD (1971): Anterior transperitoneal lumbar fusion. *J Bone Joint Surg Br* 53:617–627.
5. Harmon PH (1963): Anterior excision and vertebral body fusion operation for intervertebral disc syndromes of the lower lumbar spine: three to five year results in 244 cases. *Clin Orthop* 26:107–27.
6. Hodgson AR, Stock FE, Fang HSY, et al. (1960): Anterior spinal fusion: the operative approach and pathologic findings in 412 patients with Pott's disease of the spine. *Br J Surg* 48:172–178.
7. Hodgson MB, Wong SK (1968): A description of a technique and evaluation of results in anterior spinal fusion for deranged intervertebral disc and spondylolisthesis. *Clin Orthop* 56:133–162.
8. Hodgson AR, Yau AMC (1969): Anterior surgical approaches to the spinal column. In: Graham A, ed. *Recent advances in orthopaedics.* London: J and A Churchill, pp. 314–323.
9. Humphries AW, Hawk WA, Berndt AL (1961): Anterior interbody fusion of lumbar vertebrae: surgical technique. *Surg Clin North Am* 41:1685–700.
10. Kedia KR, Markland C, Fraley EE (1975): Sexual function following high retroperitoneal lymphadenectomy. *J Urol* 114:237–241.

11. LaBate JS (1938): The surgical anatomy of the superior hypogastric plexus: "presacral nerve." *Surg Gynecol Obstet* 67:199–211.
12. Lane JD Jr, Moore ES Jr (1948): Transperitoneal approach to the intervertebral disc in the lumbar area. *Ann Surg* 127:537–551.
13. Macnab I, Dall D (1971): The blood supply of the lumbar spine and its application to the technique of intertransverse lumbar fusion. *J Bone Joint Surg Br* 53:628–638.
14. Sacks S (1966): Anterior interbody fusion of the lumbar spine: indications and results in 200 cases. *Clin Orthop* 44:163–170.
15. Southwick WO, Robinson RA (1957): Surgical approaches to the vertebral bodies in the cervical and lumbar regions. *J Bone Joint Surg Am* 39:631–635.
16. Stauffer RN, Coventry MB (1972): Anterior interbody lumbar spine fusion: analysis of Mayo Clinic series. *J Bone Joint Surg Am* 54:756–768.
17. Stauffer RN, Coventry MB (1972): Posterolateral lumbar-spine fusion: analysis of Mayo Clinic series. *J Bone Joint Surg Am* 54:1195–1204.
18. Watkins MB (1959): Posterolateral bone grafting for fusion of the lumbar and lumbosacral spine. *J Bone Joint Surg Am* 41:388–396.
19. Watkins MB (1953): Posterolateral fusion of the lumbar and lumbosacral spine. *J Bone Joint Surg Am* 35:1014–1018.
20. Wiltse LL, Bateman JG, Hutchinson RH, et al. (1968): Paraspinal sacrospinalis splitting approach to the lumbar spine. *J Bone Joint Surg Am* 50:919–926.

General References

21. Anson KM, Byrne PO, Robertson ID, et al. (1994): Radical excision of sacrococcygeal tumours. *Br J Surg* 81:460–461.
22. Baker JK, Reardon PR, Reardon MJ, et al. (1993): Vascular injury in anterior lumbar surgery. *Spine* 18:2227–2230.
23. Balderston RA, Winter RB, Moe JH, et al. (1986): Fusion to the sacrum for nonparalytic scoliosis in the adult. *Spine* 11:824–828.
24. Boachie-Adjei O, Dendrinos GK, Ogilvie JW, et al. (1991): Management of adult spinal deformity with combined anterior-posterior arthrodesis and Luque-Galveston instrumentation. *J Spinal Disord* 4:131–41.
25. Burrington JD, Brown C, Wayne ER, et al. (1976): Anterior approach to the thoracolumbar spine: technical consideration. *Arch Surg* 111:456–463.
26. Carlson GD, Abitbol JJ, Anderson DR, et al. (1992): Screw fixation in the human sacrum: an in vitro study of the biomechanics of fixation. *Spine* 17[Suppl]:S196–S203.
27. Crock HV (1993): *A short practice of spinal surgery,* 2nd revised ed. New York: Springer Verlag Wien, pp. 79–98.
28. Dubousset J (1997): Treatment of spondylolysis and spondylolisthesis in children and adolescents. *Clin Orthop* 337:77–85.
29. Ebraheim NA, Lu J, Biyani A, et al. (1997): The relationship of lumbosacral plexus to the sacrum and the sacroiliac joint. *Am J Orthop* 26:105–110.
30. Ebraheim NA, Xu R, Biyani A, et al. (1997): Morphologic considerations of the first sacral pedicle for iliosacral screw placement. *Spine* 22:841–846.
31. Ebraheim NA, Xu R, Challgren E, et al. (1998): Location of the sacral pedicle, foramina, and ala on the lateral aspect of the sacrum: a radio49.-graphic study. *Orthopedics* 21:703–706.
32. Edwards CC, Curcin A (1995): *New alternatives for secure sacral screw fixation: biomechanical testing and clinical trials.* Paper No. 261 presented at the annual meeting of the American Academy of Orthopaedic Surgeons, Orlando, FL, February 16–21, 1995.
33. Esses SI, Botsford DJ, Huler RJ, et al. (1991): Surgical anatomy of the sacrum: a guide for rational screw fixation. *Spine* 16[Suppl]:S283–S288.
34. Farcy JP, Rawlins BA, Glassman SD (1992): Technique and results of fixation to the sacrum with iliosacral screws. *Spine* 17[Suppl]:S190–S195.
35. Flynn JC, Price CT (1984): Sexual complications of anterior fusion of the lumbar spine. *Spine* 9:489–492.
36. Fraser RD, Gogan WJ (1992): A modified muscle-splitting approach to the lumbosacral spine. *Spine* 17:943–948.
37. Gau YL, Lonstein JE, Winter RB, et al. (1991): Luque-Galveston procedure for correction and stabilization of neuromuscular scoliosis and pelvic obliquity: a review of 68 patients. *J Spinal Disord* 4:399–410.
38. Grob D, Scheier HJ, Dvorak J, et al. (1991): Circumferential fusion of the lumbar and lumbosacral spine. *Arch Orthop Trauma Surg* 111:20–25.
39. Hodge WA, DeWald RL (1983): Splenic injury complicating the anterior thoracoabdominal surgical approach for scoliosis: a report of two cases. *J Bone Joint Surg Am* 65:396–397.
40. Humke T, Grob D, Dvorak J, et al. (1998): Translaminar screw fixation of the lumbar and lumbosacral spine: a 5-year follow-up. *Spine* 23:1180–1184.
41. Jackson RP, McManus AC (1993): The "iliac buttress": a computed tomographic study of sacral anatomy. *Spine* 18:1318–1328.
42. Jeanneret B, Miclau T, Kuster M, et al. (1996): Posterior stabilization in L5–S1 isthmic spondylolisthesis with paralaminar screw fixation: anatomical and clinical results. *J Spinal Disord* 9:223–233.
43. Johnson RM, McGuire EJ (1981): Urogenital complications of anterior approaches to the lumbar spine. *Clin Orthop* 154:114–118.
44. Kostuik JP, Hall BB (1983): Spinal fusions to the sacrum in adults with scoliosis. *Spine* 8:489–500.
45. Kostuik JP, Maurais GR, Richardson WJ, et al. (1988): Combined single-stage anterior and posterior osteotomy for correction of iatrogenic lumbar kyphosis. *Spine* 12:259–266.
46. Lagrone MO, Bradford DS, Moe JH, et al. (1988): Treatment of symptomatic flatback after spinal fusion. *J Bone Joint Surg Am* 70:569–580.
47. Lehmer SM, Steffee AD, Gaines RW Jr (1994): Treatment of L5–S1 spondyloptosis by staged L5 resection with reduction, and fusion of L4 onto S1 (Gaines procedure). *Spine* 19:1916–1925.
48. Leong JC, Day GA, Luk KD, et al. (1993): Nine-year mean follow-up of one-stage anteroposterior excision of hemivertebrae in the lumbosacral spine. *Spine* 18:2069–2074.
49. McCord DH, Cunningham BW, Shono Y, et al. (1992): Biomechanical analysis of lumbosacral fixation. *Spine* 17:S235–S243.
50. Miladi LT, Ghanem IB, Draoui MM, et al. (1997): Iliosacral screw fixation for pelvic obliquity in neuromuscular scoliosis: a long-term follow-up study. *Spine* 22:1722–1729.
51. Mirkovic S, Abitbol JJ, Steinman J, et al. (1991): Anatomic consideration for sacral screw placement. *Spine* 16:S289–S294.
52. Muschik M, Zippel H, Perka C (1997): Surgical management of severe spondylolisthesis in children and adolescents: anterior fusion in situ versus anterior spondylodesis with posterior transpedicular instrumentation and reduction. *Spine* 22:2036–2042.
53. Pashman RS, Hu SS, Schendel MJ, et al. (1993): Sacral screw loads in lumbosacral fixation for spinal deformity. *Spine* 18:2465–2470.
54. Peretz AM, Hipp JA, Heggeness MH (1998): The internal bony architecture of the sacrum. *Spine* 23:971–974.
55. Roy-Camille R, Benazet JP, Desauge JP, et al. (1993): Lumbosacral fusion with pedicular screw plating instrumentation: a 10-year follow-up. *Acta Orthop Scand* 251[Suppl]:100–104.
56. Saer EH III, Winter RB, Lonstein JE (1990): Long scoliosis fusion to the sacrum in adults with non paralytic scoliosis: an improved method. *Spine* 15:650–653.
57. Samson IR, Springfield DS, Suit HD, et al. (1993): Operative treatment of sacrococcygeal chordoma: a review of twenty-one cases. *J Bone Joint Surg Am* 75:1476–1484.
58. Santi MD, Mitsunaga MM, Lockett JL (1993): Total sacrectomy for a giant sacral schwannoma: a case report. *Clin Orthop* 294:285–289.
59. Smith SA, Abitbol JJ, Carlson GD, et al. (1993): The effects of depth of penetration, screw orientation, and bone density on sacral screw fixation. *Spine* 18:1006–1010.
60. Steffee AD, Biscup RS, Sitkowski DJ (1986): Segmental spine plates with pedicle screw fixation: a new internal fixation device for disorders of the lumbar and thoracolumbar spine. *Clin Orthop* 203:45–53.
61. Szolar DH, Preidler KW, Steiner H, et al. (1996): Vascular complications in lumbar disk surgery: report of four cases. *Neuroradiology* 38:521–525.

62. Tomita K, Tsuchiya H (1990): Total sacrectomy and reconstruction for huge sacral tumors. *Spine* 15:1223–1227.

63. Waisman M, Kligman M, Roffman M (1997): Posterior approach for radical excision of sacral chordoma. *Int Orthop* 21:181–184.

64. Wiltse LL, Spencer CW (1988): New uses and refinements of the paraspinal approach to the lumbar spine. *Spine* 13:696–706.

65. Xu R, Ebraheim NA, Robke J, et al. (1996): Radiologic and anatomic evaluation of the anterior sacral foramens and nerve grooves. *Spine* 21:407–410.

66. Zindrick MR, Wiltse LL, Widell EH, et al. (1986): A biomechanical study of intrapedicular screw fixation in the lumbosacral spine. *Clin Orthop* 203:99–112.

Pediatric Spine Surgery, 2nd ed., edited by Stuart L. Weinstein. Lippincott Williams & Wilkins, Philadelphia © 2001.

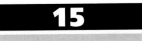

ANTERIOR AND POSTERIOR CERVICAL SPINE FUSION AND INSTRUMENTATION

VINCENT ARLET
MAX AEBI

Cervical spine fusions in children require specific knowledge of the pediatric pathology as well as an extensive expertise in spine surgery. Fusion of the pediatric cervical spine may require no or minimal instrumentation (Fig. 2, shown later) or, on the contrary, very advanced spinal instrumentation (Figs. 7 to 9 and 14, shown later). This means that one must be familiar with different surgical techniques ranging from simple decortication and bone graft to the most modern spinal implants to stabilize the cervical spine. Likewise, one must be as comfortable with a soft collar prescription in cases of stable instrumentation or with the realization of a Minerva or a halo cast to immobilize the neck postoperatively in case no or little instrumentation has been applied.

Although we have acquired extensive experience with all sorts of modern internal fixation in the adult cervical spine (1–4,6,13), we hesitate to use hardware to enhance fusion in the pediatric spine. The reasons are the following: In small children, the hardware may be too large for the vertebrae or the bone too weak, with sublaminar wires cutting out or screws pulling out or with little or no purchase. In older children, we also hesitate because in most instances fusion can be achieved with little or no hardware, provided appropriate external immobilization are used. And these are usually extremely well tolerated in the pediatric patients.

The indications for internal fixation are limited to malformations and instability, especially in the upper cervical spine, and occasionally tumors, trauma, and bone dysplasia. The operating field for the posterior approach must be more extensive whenever more than simple wire techniques for internal fixation is required. This is a disadvantage because the pediatric spine tends to spontaneously fuse where muscles have been dissected subperiosteally (10) (Fig. 16, shown later). Extension of the dissection above or below the area of interest frequently results in an unwanted creeping fusion to the adjacent laminae above and below. Therefore in most cases stabilization of the pediatric C spine is

achieved with simple means such as tension band wiring or cerclage and proper postoperative immobilization. One has to be aware that some of the techniques presented below are rarely indicated in the pediatric C spine and are reserved for extraordinary cases that cannot be treated with more conservative methods.

NONINSTRUMENTED AND INSTRUMENTED FUSION IN THE UPPER CERVICAL SPINE

The indications for fusion of the upper cervical spine are mainly malformation and instabilities secondary to trauma or bony dysplasia. In most cases, the upper cervical spine in children and adolescents is approached posteriorly.

Posterior Procedures

The craniocervical junction is often the location of a malformation or an instability. The requirement of a brain-stem decompression may necessitate a cervicooccipital posterior fusion as in Morquio syndrome after a laminectomy of C1 and a foramen magnum decompression. (As with most cases of Chiari malformation, there is no need for an occipitocervical fusion if the laminectomy did not extend below C2 and if the facets have been kept intact and the appropriate postoperative immobilization has been done.) Instability of the craniocervical junction due to trauma, malformations, skeletal dysplasias such as spondyloepiphyseal dysplasia, and odontoid anomalies (13,14) may be an indication for a C1 to C2 fusion or, rarely, an occipitocervical fusion. Rotatory subluxation of C1 to C2, caused by trauma or infection of the upper respiratory tract, may occasionally need a C1 to C2 fusion if they have not been reduced by traction (7,10).

Positioning

The head of the patient is positioned on a horseshoe rest with Gardner tongs if traction is necessary, with a Mayfield head rest, or with the help of a halo. In most cases, the head is horizontal

V. Arlet and Max Aebi: Department of Surgery, Health Center, McGill University, Montreal, Quebec, Canada.

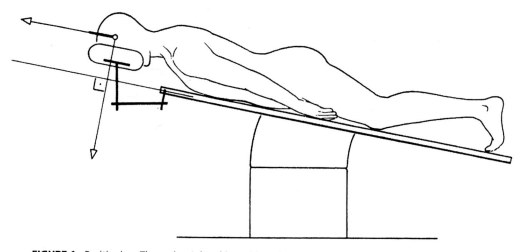

FIGURE 1. Positioning. The patient's head is positioned horizontally in relation to the table, with traction if necessary. In some cases, a flexed position is necessary to allow easier access for decompression; in others, an extended position is required for the reduction of a C1 to C2 dislocation. The position is always checked radiographically or fluoroscopically before the operation begins and before the instrumentation.

to the table (Fig. 1). In some cases, however, the neck must be flexed and the head retropulsed to facilitate the approach when, for instance, a foramen magnum decompression or a laminectomy of C1 is required. The head therefore needs to be repositioned before the fixation to avoid kyphosis. In many cases, however, the positioning of the patient (previously checked with dynamic magnetic resonance imaging, flexion extension film, or traction films) has achieved the indirect decompression. The head therefore is positioned to achieve this indirect decompression. Radiographs or the use of the image intensifier should always be used to check proper positioning before fixation.

Bone Graft Only

If only a bone graft procedure (as in very young children) is chosen, great care should be given to the harvest of the iliac bone graft, which requires corticocancellous strips of significant length (Fig. 2A) to span the whole fusion area. Thorough decortication of the posterior elements down to the bleeding cancellous bone must be done so that fusion ensues. This is best accomplished with a small and sharp rongeur rather than a burr that burns and wastes the bone. The strips must lie over the decorticated area (Fig. 2B), and the surgeon must be careful to prevent their migration in case of a posterior laminectomy. Small sutures passed around the posterior elements left intact or through the facets or burr holes can prevent such graft migration. Adequate immobilization must be done postoperatively with a posterior half cast shell (Fig. 2C), which is replaced 5 to 7 days postoperatively with a Minerva cast (Fig 2D) or with a halo cast if a halo has been applied. Total immobilization requires 3 to 4 months, usually in a position of extension of the head (Fig. 2).

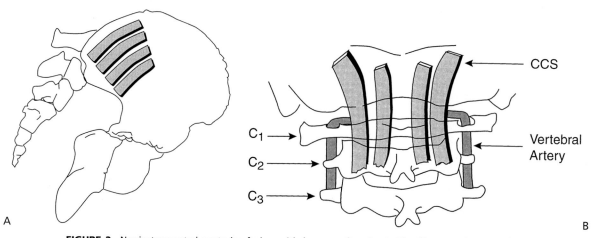

FIGURE 2. Noninstrumented posterior fusion with bone graft only. **A:** The iliac crest bone graft is harvested to obtain long corticocancellous strips, which will span the levels to be fused. **B:** The strips of bone are laid over the decorticated area. They can be sutured with nonabsorbable sutures to the posterior elements and lamina or through burr holes. (*Figure continues.*)

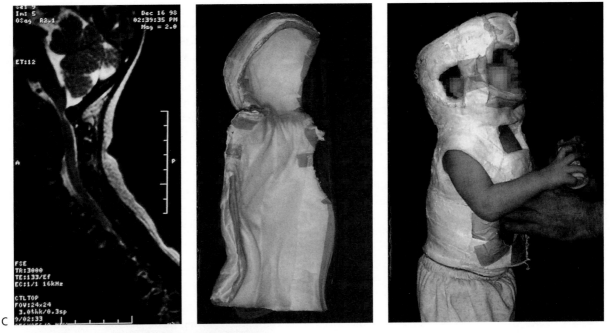

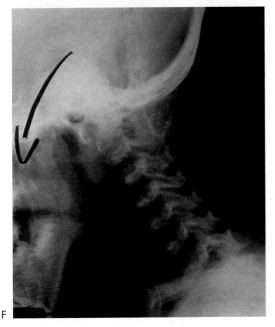

FIGURE 2. *Continued.* **C:** Three-year-old boy with Morquio syndrome and a delay in walking. The severe foramen magnum stenosis can be seen. Treatment will consist of a laminectomy of C1 with enlargement of the foramen magnum and a posterior spine fusion down to C2 with corticocancellous strips only. **D:** The patient is immobilized in a posterior minerva shell postoperatively (which was made preoperatively. **E:** A minerva cast with extension of the head is done 5 days later and kept for 15 weeks. No instrumentation at all is used. **F:** Two years later, the fusion is perfectly solid.

Wiring Technique

Most C1 to C2 instabilities in children can be treated with a C1 to C2 wiring technique. Different wiring techniques are available. We use the modified Gallie (Fig. 3) and the Brooks-Jenkins (Fig. 4) techniques. In both techniques, the central portion of the arch of C1 (2 cm) and C2 must be exposed. Care must be taken not to carry the exposure too far laterally so as not to traumatize the venous plexus around the vertebral artery or the artery itself. The artery turns medially after perforating the foramen transversarium of C1. An injury of this plexus may lead to extreme bleeding that can be stopped only by local compression with Gelfoam or with bipolar coagulation.

The Gallie fusion is illustrated in Figure 3 and the technique of Brooks and Jenkins in Figure 4. Both techniques are tension-banding systems, but the Brooks-Jenkins technique provides better rotational stability and tension strength than the Gallie technique. Both techniques have the disadvantage of requiring the passage of a wire around the C1 arch; the Brooks-Jenkins technique also requires wire passage around the C2 lamina. This

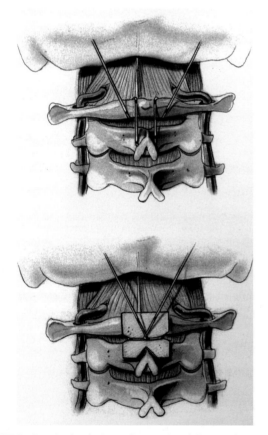

FIGURE 3. Standard technique of C1 to C2 stabilization (Gallie procedure). A 1.2-mm wire is first inserted below the spinous process of C2 through the soft tissue without cutting the ligament (to prevent a postoperative C2 to C3 kyphosis). The two free ends are each fixed to a suture previously passed around the arch of C1. The wires are then pulled with the suture and inserted from a cranial direction and looped over the superior surface of C1. The two free ends of the wire, which are laterally placed, are brought across to the midline after a cortico-cancellous graft (measuring 3 to 4 cm) has been shaped (like an "H") to match the posterior surfaces of C1 and C2.

maneuver may be the cause of intraspinal injury (e.g., dural tear, injury of the spinal cord), but we have never encountered such an injury. Neither technique can be used in cases of a fracture or a bifid C1 arch, C2 lamina, or nonfused spinous process often encountered in very young patients and in patients with a dysplastic spine. Likewise, the wiring can erode the thin posterior arch of young children (17). Because both techniques are tension-banding systems, they reduce the anterior subluxation of C1. Care must be taken not to create a posterior subluxation by tightening the wire too much in the Gallie technique. The Gallie technique should not be used in posterior dislocations of C1 on C2 (Fig. 5). The postoperative care in both techniques is simple and consists of wearing a firm collar or a Minerva cast, depending on the patient's age, the initial instability, the etiology, and the reliability of the patient.

Transarticular Screw Technique

The transarticular screw technique (3,11,12) is extremely useful in cases in which posterior element damage prevents the use of conventional wiring techniques and a high degree of instability is present. In cases in which the incidence of nonunion is high, as in Down syndrome, we recommend this technique. This technique is biomechanically superior to wiring techniques (18,21) and allows maintenance of the reduction. It is normally combined with a Gallie-Brooks fusion. The fact that screws need to be inserted into the isthmus of the very narrow and short pedicle of C2 limits the application of this technique to adolescents, in whom there is enough space to insert screws without damaging the vertebral artery lateral to the screw path. This technique is highly demanding and should not be used by surgeons who are not familiar with it and do not use it on a regular basis.

Preoperative computed tomography is helpful to identify the exact anatomy and location of the vertebral artery, especially in case of malformation. The reduction of C1 to C2 is checked using lateral image intensifier control. The neck is flexed as much as possible to facilitate insertion of the screws, and the image intensifier is used to exclude redislocation. A midline incision is made from the occiput down to C3. The arch of C1, spinous process, lamina, and inferior articular process of C2 are exposed subperiosteally. The rest of the cervical spine is not exposed in children to avoid undesired creeping fusions. Persistent anterior dislocation of C1 or C2 may be reduced by pushing on the spinous process of C2 or by pulling gently on the posterior arch of C1 with either a Kocher clamp or a sublaminar wire. Direct pressure in the mouth with a sponge on a stick may help reduce the anterior C1 dislocation. Persistent posterior dislocation requires the opposite forces (1). The insertion of the screws is best described in Figure 6.

Occipitocervical Plating

The indications for occipitocervical plating in children are the following: occipitocervical instability, cranial settling, and revision for C1 to C2 pseudoarthroses. The function of the occipitocervical plate is to act as a buttress and partially as a tension

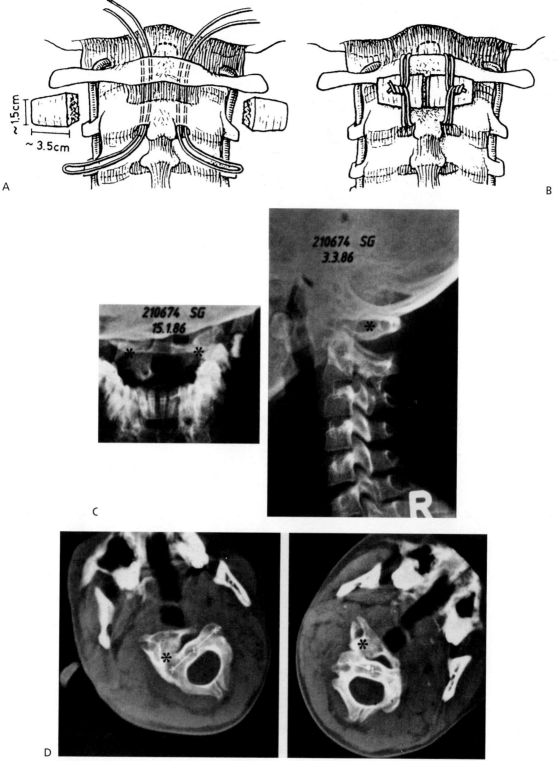

FIGURE 4. Brooks and Jenkins C1 to C2 fusion. **A:** Two wire loops (measuring 1.2 mm each) are passed from the superior aspect of C1 around the arch of C1 and further distally beneath the lamina of C2. **B:** Two corticocancellous bone grafts measuring about 1.5 by 2.5 cm are fashioned into a wedge with the cortical portion posterior. The inferior surface of C1 and the superior surface of C2 are decorticated. The two bone wedges are placed between the inferior arch of C1 and the superior arch of C2. The double wires are twisted to press the bone graft against the lateral arch. **C:** Typical C1 to C2 fixed rotatory luxation in a 9-year-old boy. Note the overlapping of the C1 and C2 lateral masses on the anteroposterior view (*asterisk*) and the obliquity of C1 on the lateral view (*asterisk*). **D:** The dynamic computed tomography scan demonstrates the locked rotational luxation (asterisk). (*Left side:* rotation to the left; *right side:* rotation to the right) (*Figure continues.*)

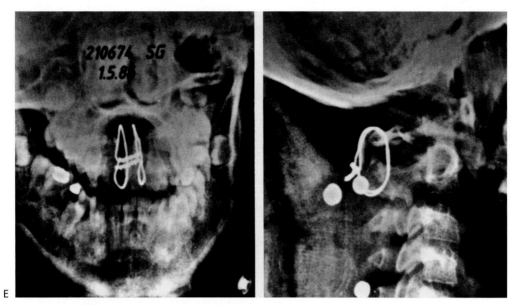

E

FIGURE 4. *Continued.* **E:** Despite conservative treatment with traction, the dislocation did not reduce a C1 to C2. Brooks fusion was therefore carried out.

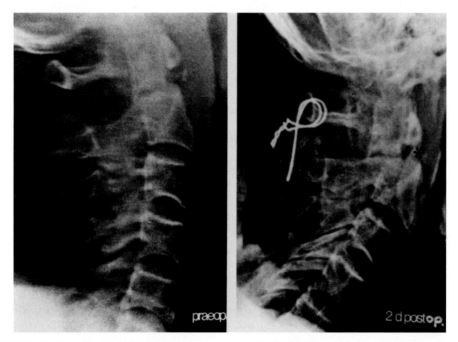

FIGURE 5. Overcorrection with Gallie fusion in a case of odontoid fixation. Note the overcorrection with posterior dislocation (*asterisk*). This problem is inherent in this technique because of the tension-banding character of the wiring technique.

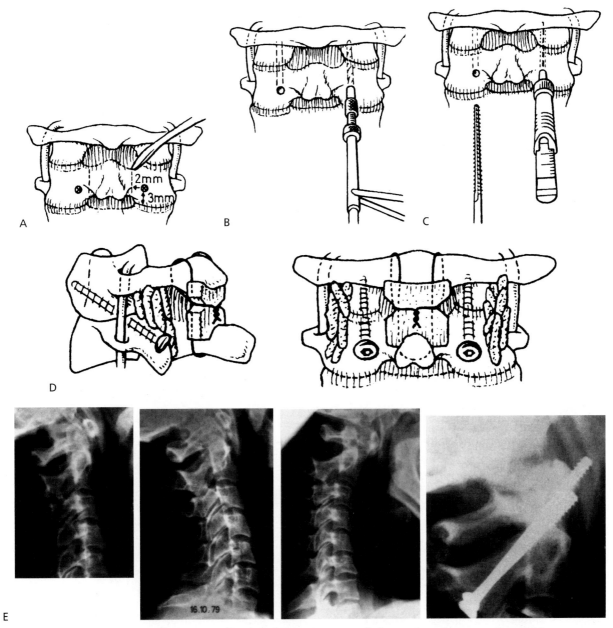

FIGURE 6. Transarticular screw fixation of C1 to C2. **A:** A small dissector is used to expose the cranial surface of the lamina and isthmus of C2 by careful subperiosteal dissection of the posterior capsule of the atlantoaxial joint. The atlantoaxial membrane is visible medial to the isthmus. **B:** Using lateral image intensifier control, a long 2.5-mm drill is inserted in a strictly sagittal direction. In such cases, we use long drill bits inserted percutaneously at the base of the neck to avoid exposing the lower cervical spine and to prevent a possible creeping fusion. The entry point of the drill is at the lower edge of the caudal articular process of C2. The drill goes through the isthmus near its posterior and medial surface. It then enters the lateral mass of the atlas close to its posteroinferior edge. Anteriorly, the drill perforates the cortex of the lateral mass of C1. The same maneuver is repeated on the opposite side. **C:** The screw length is measured and checked using the image intensifier. The screws are inserted after tapping with a 3.5-mm cortical tap. Proper caudocranial drilling is sometimes difficult because the neck muscles and the upper torso prevent the correct placement of the drill. Gently pulling the spinous process of C2 cranially with a towel clamp facilitates drilling. Drilling in a horizontal direction must be avoided because at the level of C2, the vertebral artery runs upward, anterior to the C1 to C2 joint, and could be damaged. The screw could exit C2 anteriorly and not enter the atlas. **D:** After bilateral screw fixation, Gallie posterior C1 to C2 fusion is performed to increase stability. The postoperative care consists of immobilization with a firm collar for 6 to 10 weeks, but the patient is allowed to remove the collar for daily care. If an additional Gallie-Brooks wiring technique is been used, no collar is necessary postoperatively. **E:** An example of a transarticular screw fixation of C1 to C2 combined with nonresorbable sutures instead of wires in an 18-year-old woman with instability resulting from rupture of the transverse ligament of C1.

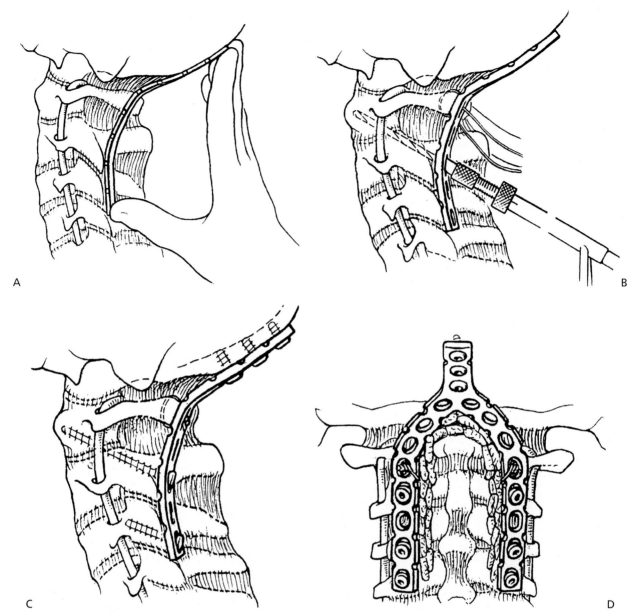

FIGURE 7. Technique for an occipitocervical plate fixation. **A:** The template is contoured to fit the occipital and cervical spine. **B:** A sublaminar wire can be placed beneath either side of the C1 arch, and a C1 to C2 transarticular screw of appropriate length is inserted through the contoured plate. **C:** The screws are inserted in the occiput in the midline (where the bone is thicker) below the inion. The screws in the lateral masses are inserted and tightened, as are the sublaminar wires. **D:** *Y*-shaped cervicooccipital plate.

band (Fig. 7). It is far superior to cerclage wires tightened to a contoured rod because it prevents settling and sliding of the occiput on the rod and subsequent loss of correction. This technique is technically demanding, however, with potential neurovascular injury. In addition, the purchase of the screw is poor away from the midline in the occiput, and the head position needs to be perfectly adjusted before fixation. In cases of basilar invagination, it is our experience that traction can reduce the vertical instability, reverse the invagination of the odontoid from the brain stem, and improve the neurologic signs.

Maintenance of the reduction is best achieved with cervicooccipital plating (Fig. 8). In cases in which the reduction cannot be achieved with traction and the odontoid is still compressing the brain stem, the fixation must be combined with a transoral resection of the dens (Fig. 9). This highly demanding fixation usually requires a transarticular screw at C1 to C2, a C1 sublaminar cerclage, screws in the thick part of the occiput, and sometimes lateral masses screws in C3 (Figs. 8 and 9). Different surgical techniques can be used: plates, *Y*-shaped plates, or the Cervifix (16).

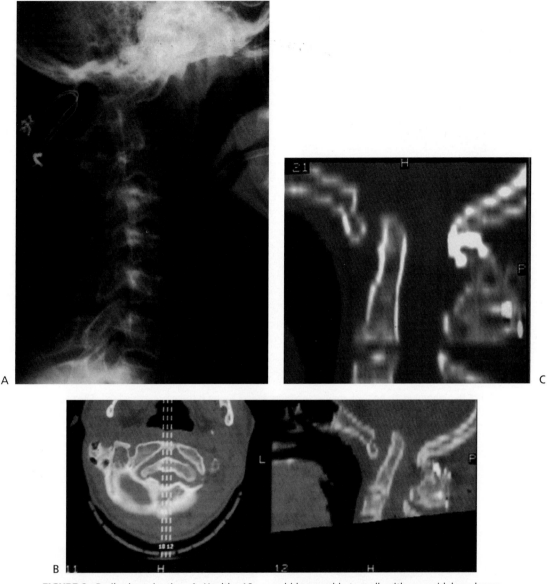

FIGURE 8. Basilar invagination. **A:** Healthy 16-year-old boy unable to walk with pyramidal syndrome. He previously had posterior surgery with an attempted O to C2 fusion. **B:** Computed tomography (CT) scan with reconstruction clearly shows the basilar invagination. **C:** A new CT is done after 15 lb of traction have been applied. One can see that the invagination of the odontoid from the skull has markedly decreased. His neurologic symptoms were much improved. (*Figure continues.*)

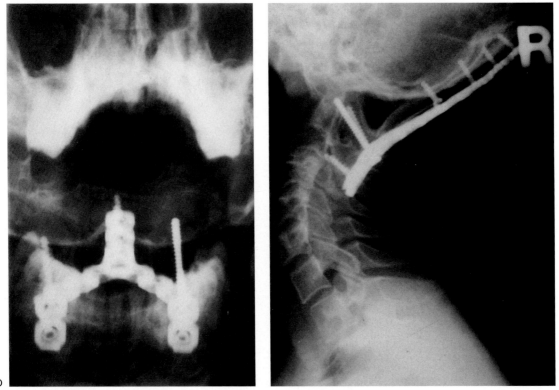

FIGURE 8. *Continued.* **D:** An instrumented occipitocervical fusion is therefore carried out. The patient will resume normal activities after the fusion becomes solid.

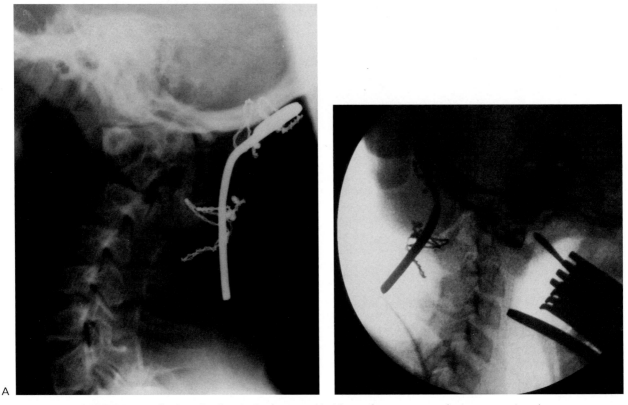

FIGURE 9. Basilar invagination. **A:** Twelve-year-old girl seen for severe neurologic compromise who had an attempted cervicooccipital fusion elsewhere. **B:** Because of the fixed deformity, a transoral dens resection is first carried out to decompress the cord. (*Figure continues.*)

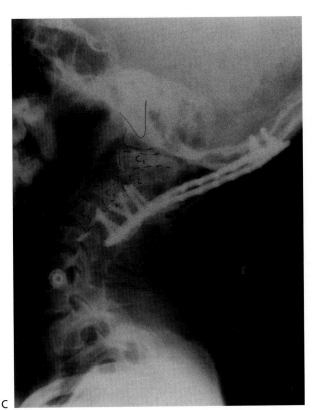

FIGURE 9. *Continued.* **C:** A cervicooccipital plate will stabilize the craniocervical junction and improve the patient's persistent neurology.

Anterior Procedures

To date, we have performed only one anterior screw fixation in a child (Fig. 10). The 16-year-old boy had a type II odontoid fracture that was unstable. Odontoid fractures in young children are traumatic epiphysiolysis and can be treated successfully with a cast. In older children, they can still be treated with appropriate casting if they are stable and reduced in extension. Therefore, use of the anterior internal fixation technique for the upper cervical spine in the case of odontoid fractures (type II) is an extremely rare occurrence and is not discussed in this chapter, as it has been described in detail elsewhere (1–3,9).

INSTRUMENTED FUSION IN THE LOWER CERVICAL SPINE

The indications for instrumented fusions in the middle and lower cervical spine are mainly malformations and trauma. In some instances, the requirement of an extensive laminectomy done for spinal cord tumors requires surgical stabilization. Fortunately, postlaminectomy kyphosis is seldom seen because of the wider use of laminoplasty techniques combined with proper postoperative immobilization. Tumors are mostly benign (22), and when surgery is indicated, it can generally be performed without fusion in cases of an osteoid osteoma or without instrumentation (Fig. 13, shown later).

Posterior Procedures

Wiring Techniques

Different wiring techniques have been developed for posterior fixation of the lower cervical spine. The most simple and least

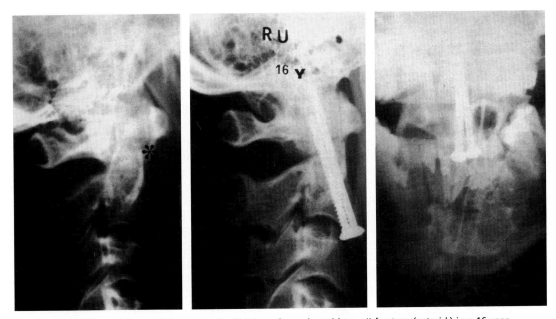

FIGURE 10. Example of direct anterior fixation of an odontoid type II fracture (*asterisk*) in a 16-year-old boy.

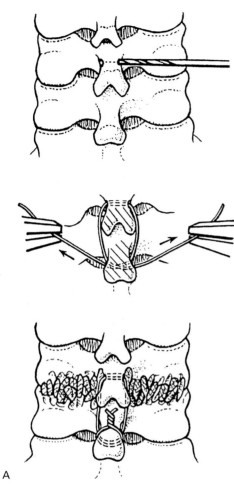

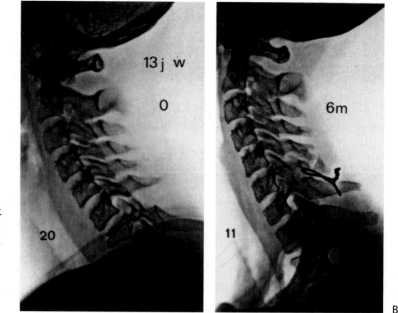

FIGURE 11. Simple wiring techniques. **A:** A hole is drilled on each side of the base of the spinous process of the upper vertebra. The entry point corresponds to the junction of the upper and middle portions of the process. An 0.8- to 1.2-mm wire is passed through the hole and then around the base of the inferior spinous process, leaving the interspinous soft tissues intact. The wire ends are curved around the inferior spinous process and twisted tight. The laminae are decorticated with a high-speed burr or curette, and cancellous bone graft is applied. **B:** A 16-year-old girl with a wedge compression fracture of C7. The result 6 months postoperatively with remodeling of the compressed C7 vertebral body.

dangerous is the tension-banding principle using interspinous wiring. It is indicated in trauma when rupture of predominantly the posterior ligament complex is present (Fig. 11). The anterior approach should be avoided in young children to prevent growth disturbances caused by destroying the growth plate during anterior fusion. If we are successful in reducing an anterior compression or wedge compression fracture by applying a tension-band fixation posteriorly, some anterior growth potential may be preserved, and a secondary deformation can be avoided. Posterior wiring techniques are relatively easy to perform and can be limited to one segment whenever possible. The hardware does not need space; hence, ample posterior bone surface is available for the fusion. The disadvantages are wire breakage and wire cutout, and the technique cannot be used in fractures of the vertebral arch including the spinous process. These techniques require an appropriate postoperative external immobilization (Fig. 11B).

Plating and Rod Techniques

Several different plates can be used: the hook plate of Magerl, the 3.5-mm one-third tubular plate, the 3.5-mm reconstruction AO/ASIF plate, the titanium reconstruction plate of Anderson (4,6), and the Cervifix of Jeanneret (16). All these plates are anchored to the spine by screws in the lateral mass according to

Magerl's technique (3,15) (Fig. 12). Because of the obliquity in two planes in Magerl's technique, a longer bone path exists, resulting in a better screw grasp than the straight direction of Roy-Camille's technique (20). The danger of injuring the vertebral artery or the nerve roots is less with Magerl's technique than with Roy-Camille's technique.

All posterior plate systems act as tension-banding systems. The primary stability achieved with plate fixations is superior to that of interbody fusions and posterior cerclage wiring technique (21). In addition, there is less danger of dural or spinal cord injuries than with sublaminar wiring because the spinal canal remains untouched. However, the plating technique is more demanding than the wiring procedures and certainly more traumatic to soft tissue. This may be important in view of the risk for spontaneous fusion above and below the originally stabilized and fused segment. For specific descriptions of each of the surgical techniques (plate, Cervifix, hook plate), refer to Aebi and colleagues (3). The hook plates are specifically useful in unisegmental posterior fixation. In bisegmental fixation or even more extensive fusion, a plate may be more appropriate. However, this indication is extremely rare in children.

As an alternative to the hook plates, 3.5-mm reconstruction plates or one-third tubular plates (hammered flat) may be used. These plates provide stable tension-band fixation in flexion, in-

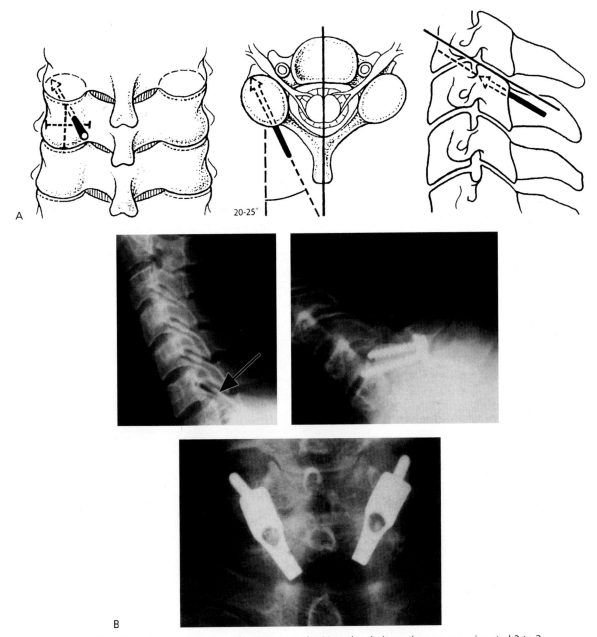

FIGURE 12. Lateral masses screw fixation. **A:** In the Magerl technique, the screws are inserted 2 to 3 mm medially and cranially from the center of the articular mass. Each screw diverges by 25 degrees anteriorly and is parallel to the facet joint. (The exception is at the axis level, where the screw goes into the pedicle of C2 according to Judet with a 25-degree medial direction.) **B:** Example of a 17-year-old patient with a hook plate stabilization performed for a traumatic ligamentous instability of C6 to C7. The divergent orientation of the screws can be seen.

creasing stability in rotation and buttressing in extension. The indications are mainly cervical spine trauma, tumor reconstruction, or malformation. The advantage of this type of fixation is that several segments can be bridged. The stability is superior to that achieved with wiring techniques, and plates can be used in the presence or absence of laminar or spinous process fractures or in cases of postlaminectomy kyphosis. No special instrumentation is required when the basic AO/ASIF plate screw set is available (4). Ideal screw placement is sometimes difficult

because of the spacing of the holes, which is why Anderson and associates (6) designed a titanium reconstruction-type plate with screw hole distances of 8 or 12 mm to fit the anatomic conditions of the cervical spine. This was further improved by Jeanneret (16) with the Cervifix, in which the screw positioning can be optimized because its placement is independent of the rod.

All these techniques require a standard posterior midline incision with subperiosteal exposure of the laminae and lateral masses of the corresponding vertebrae. The use of an image intensifier is necessary to avoid unnecessary exposure.

Anterior Procedures

Bone Graft Only

Anterior fusion without instrumentation is indicated in exceptional cases of tumor in which the spine needs to be reconstructed after the tumor excision. It is possible to use no instrumentation provided that the posterior elements of the spine are intact and only a one-level fusion is done (Fig. 13). The graft must be keyed so that intrinsic stability is maintained. Postoperative immobilization with a Minerva or halo jacket or cast is necessary in the young noncompliant patient.

Anterior Plating

Anterior fusion with instrumentation consists of anterior plating and interbody fusion. Although different plate systems exist, we use the simple H plate of the AO/ASIF group or the titanium cervical spine locking plate (CLSP) (Fig. 14), which is a more stable standardized anterior plate system introduced by Morscher and colleagues (19). Although used extensively in adults for trauma (5), anterior plating is rarely used for that purpose in children because of the reason mentioned previously. We have used this system in children only for malformation (Fig. 14B). The goal of anterior plating is to increase the stability of the anterior column after grafting. The AO/ASIF plates function as a tension band in extension and as a buttress plate in flexion. Anterior plating is indicated when support of the anterior column is needed, when instability persists, and particularly when there is loss of height of the vertebral body or after partial or total vertebrectomy for decompression of the spinal cord. Refer to Figure 12 and to Aebi and colleagues (3). The simple H plate allows more versatility regarding screw direction, an eccentric screw placement that allows the compression of the graft, and the use of either a 2.7- or 3.5-mm screw (Fig. 14B). Its disadvantages are the requirement to perforate the posterior

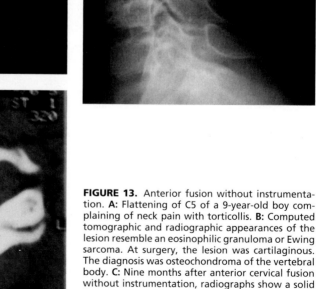

FIGURE 13. Anterior fusion without instrumentation. **A:** Flattening of C5 of a 9-year-old boy complaining of neck pain with torticollis. **B:** Computed tomographic and radiographic appearances of the lesion resemble an eosinophilic granuloma or Ewing sarcoma. At surgery, the lesion was cartilaginous. The diagnosis was osteochondroma of the vertebral body. **C:** Nine months after anterior cervical fusion without instrumentation, radiographs show a solid fusion.

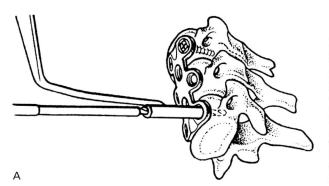

A

FIGURE 14. Anterior plating techniques. **A:** Titanium cervical spine locking plate. The screws are 14 mm long and do not perforate the posterior cortex. They are locked into the plate by means of a small conical expansion screw. **B:** Anterior H plate. *(1)* Fifteen-year-old patient with neurofibromatosis combined with hydrocephalus, syringomyelia and a huge hemangioma in the neck extending from the occiput to C7 *(arrows). (2)* This massive tumor led to a progressive subluxation of C1 to C2 and specifically C2 to C3 anteriorly. *(3)* Flexion-extension radiographs demonstrate the frank instability and the incomplete reduction. *(4)* The dislocation is reduced as much as possible with traction. *(5)* Anterior graft and plating from C2 to C4. The patient was immobilized in a Minerva brace until the fusion was solid. An anterior procedure was chosen over posterior instrumentation because of the massive hemangioma posteriorly. The patient subsequently received radiation treatment posteriorly.

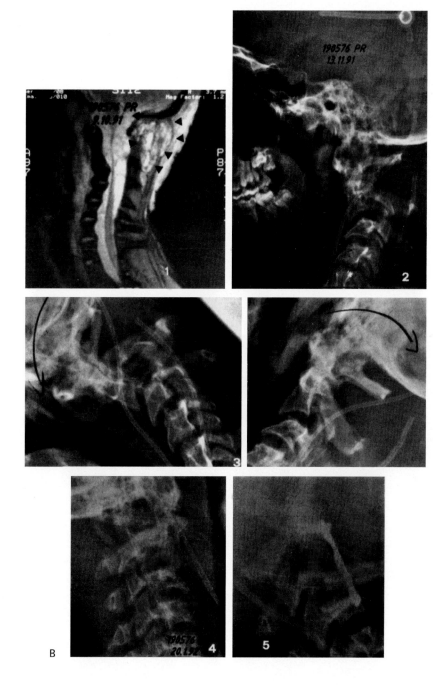

B

cortex (with potential risk to the spinal cord), the possibility of screw loosening, and the lack of intrinsic stability between the screw and the plate. The CLSP plate was made to overcome all the aforementioned disadvantages, but the lack of versatility of the screw placement and the fact that no axial compression is possible must be taken in consideration.

PITFALLS IN PEDIATRIC CERVICAL FUSION AND INSTRUMENTATION

It is impossible to enumerate all the pitfalls and complications of pediatric cervical spinal fusion and instrumentation. We chose, therefore, to mention a few classic pitfalls.

The pediatric cervical spine has some specificities. Despite the good reputation of the pediatric cervical spine to achieve a solid fusion, we have observed pseudarthroses in our practice. The pseudarthroses are usually a result of lack of adequate postoperative immobilization or surgical stabilization or lack of bone graft. We do not recommend the use of synthetic or cadaveric bone graft. This results too often in a pseudarthrosis that requires revision (Fig. 15). The morbidity of harvesting iliac crest is extremely low in children, and almost none of these patients complain of donor site pain. Therefore, we strongly recommend the use of autologous bone, classically taken from the iliac crest either as corticocancellous strips (Fig. 2) or in the shape of a H or a trapezoid wedge-shaped tricortical bone graft for anterior surgery.

Conversely, the pediatric spine may fuse where it was not expected to fuse. We have often observed creeping fusions resulting from too large subperiosteal dissection of the cervical spine (Fig. 16). To avoid such pitfalls, the use of an image intensifier or radiographic marker is essential to limit the approach to only the segments to be fused.

In trauma, ligamentous lesions may occur without any bony lesions, or a fracture may be associated with posterior disruption injuries at several levels. Failure to recognize this problem may lead to kyphosis above or below the instrumentation. Likewise, too much exposure of the cervical spine may lead to injury of the posterior structures (ligament nuchae and posterior capsules) and subsequent kyphosis above or below the instrumentation.

Another pitfall to consider is the reliability of the patient. Because the osteosynthesis required is often simple (cerclage wire, for instance), the postoperative immobilization must be adequate, especially in young turbulent children or teenagers. The surgeon may therefore choose a postoperative cast or a halo cast for the postoperative immobilization. However, complications may be observed with a halo cast (pin loosening, pin penetration, pin infection) or a Minerva cast (lack of appropriate immobilization, pressure sores). When there is no or little osteosynthesis, we believe that braces are not indicated.

Finally, some pathologies, such as Down syndrome (8), are more prone to complication such as infection and nonunion. Techniques such as placement of the C1 to C2 transarticular screw are strongly recommended in these cases and obviate the need for postoperative halo immobilization in these unreliable patients.

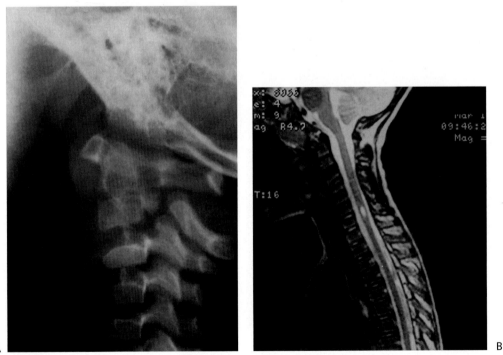

FIGURE 15. Pseudarthroses. **A:** Congenital spondylolysis of C2 in a 4-year-old boy. **B:** Magnetic resonance imaging study shows a syringomyelia and a Chiari malformation. (*Figure continues.*)

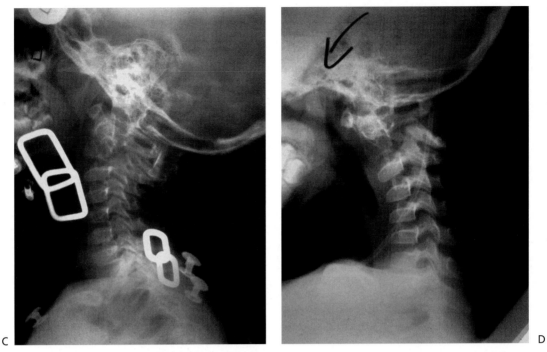

C

D

FIGURE 15. *Continued.* **C:** A Chiari decompression is performed; at the same time, a noninstrumented occipitocervical fusion is done. **D:** At 9 months' follow-up, the pseudarthrosis is evident, and the graft has melted away. This can be explained by insufficient immobilization (only a Minerva brace was used) and by the use of only artificial bone graft.

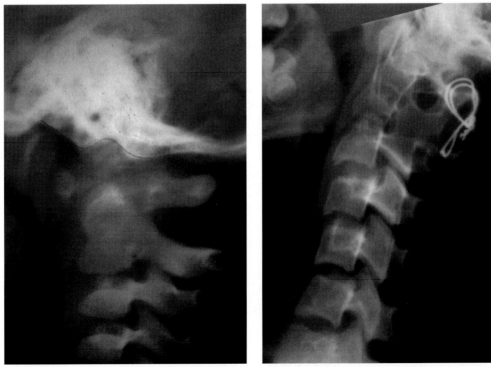

A

B

FIGURE 16. Creeping fusion. **A:** Patient with C1 to C2 instability due to a hypoplasia of the odontoid. He is operated at 8 years of age. **B:** Ten years later, the patient's C1 to C2 fusion is perfectly solid but has creeped down to C3.

REFERENCES

1. Aebi M (1991): Surgical treatment of cervical spine fractures by AO-techniques. In: Bridwell KH, de Wald RL, eds. *Textbook of spinal surgery.* Philadelphia: JB Lippincott.
2. Aebi M, Etter C, Coscia M (1989): Fractures of the odontoid process: treatment with anterior screw fixation. *Spine* 14:1065–1070.
3. Aebi M, Thalgott JS, Webb JK (1998): *AO ASIF principles in spine surgery,* Chaps 5 and 6. Berlin: Springer-Verlag, pp. 42–82.
4. Aebi M, Webb JK (1991): The spine. In: Müller ME, Allgöwer M, Schneider R, et al., eds. *Manual of internal fixation,* 3rd ed. Berlin: Springer-Verlag.
5. Aebi M, Zuber K, Marchesi D (1991): The treatment of cervical spine injuries by anterior plating. *Spine* 16:38–45.
6. Anderson PA, Hentey MB, Grady MS, et al. (1991): Posterior cervical arthrodesis with AO reconstruction plates and bone grafts. *Spine* 16: 72–79.
7. Arlet V, Rigault P, Padovani JP (1992): Instabilités et luxations reconnues ou négligées du rachis cervical supérieur de l'enfant: A propos de 20 observation. *Rev Chir Orthop* 78:300–311.
8. Arlet V, Rigault P, Padovani JP (1992): Atlantoaxial instability in children with Down syndrome: atlantoaxial arthrodesis or occipitoaxial fusion. *Rev Chir Orthop* 78:240–242.
9. Böhler J (1982): Anterior stabilization for acute fractures and non-unions of the dens. *J Bone Joint Surg Am* 64:18–27.
10. Fielding JW (1983): Cervical spine injuries in children. In: Cervical Spine Research Society, eds. *The cervical spine.* Philadelphia: JB Lippincott, pp. 268–281.
11. Grob D, Magerl F (1987): Operative Stabilisierung bei Frankturen von C1 und C2. *Orthopädie* 16:46–54.
12. Grob D, Jeanneret B, Aebi M, et al. (1991): Atlantoaxial fusion with transarticular screw fixation. *J Bone Joint Surg Br* 73:972–976.
13. Hensinger RN (1983): Congenital anomalies of the odontoid. In: Cervical Spine Research Society, ed. *The cervical spine.* Philadelphia: JB Lippincott, pp. 164–174.
14. Hensinger RN (1983): Congenital anomalies of the atlanto-axial joint. In: Cervical Spine Research Society, ed. *The cervical spine.* Philadelphia: JB Lippincott, pp. 155–160.
15. Jeanneret B, Magerl F, Ward EH, et al. (1991): Posterior stabilization of the cervical spine (C2–7) with hook plates. *Spine* 16:56–63.
16. Jeanneret B (1996): Posterior rod system of the cervical spine: a new implant allowing optimal screw insertion. *Eur Spine J* 5(5):350–356
17. Lowry DW, Pollack IF, Clyde B, et al. (1997): Upper cervical spine fusion in the pediatric population. *J Neurosurg* 87(5):671–676.
18. Montesano PX, Inach EC, Anderson PA, et al. (1991): Biomechanics of cervical spine internal fixation. *Spine* 16:10–16.
19. Morscher E, Sutter F, Jenny H, et al. (1986): Die vordere verplattung der halswirbelsäule mit dem hohlschrauben-plattensystem aus titanium. *Chirurg* 57:702–707.
20. Roy-Camille R, Saillant G, Mazel C (1989): Internal fixation of the unstable cervical spine by posterior osteosynthesis with plates and screws. In: Sherles HH, ed. *The cervical spine.* Philadelphia: JB Lippincott.
21. Ulrich C, Wörsdörfer O, Claes L, et al. (1987): Comparative study of the stability of anterior and posterior cervical spine fixation procedures. *Arch Orthop Trauma Surg* 106:226–231.
22. Verbiest H (1983): Benign tumors of the cervical spine. In: Cervical Spine Research Society, ed. *The cervical spine.* Philadelphia: JB Lippincott, pp. 430–477.

16

POSTERIOR SPINAL FUSION

JESSE H. DICKSON

According to Scott (17), Ollier described the use of an osteoperiosteal graft in an attempt to obtain a spinal fusion in 1867. However, it is generally acknowledged that Hibbs (5) and Albee (1) were the first to describe a specific technique and give end results. According to Howorth (11), Hibbs observed that in tuberculosis of the spine, bony ankylosis occurred after spinal immobilization. This fusion was often incomplete and sometimes required many years to become complete. Hibbs reasoned that if spinal ankylosis could be achieved operatively, the disease process would heal more quickly. Hibbs performed his first spinal fusion on January 5, 1911, and reported on three cases in May 1911. His original procedure was described as greensticking the spinous processes at their base, leaving the caudal portion attached to the lamina. They were then turned down into the next inferior vertebra, which had its spinous process green-sticked and turned down to the next vertebra. Thus, the spinous process of one vertebra made contact with the cancellous bed of the next inferior spinous process, which had been green-sticked.

During the next 8 years, Hibbs reported various modifications of his technique (6–9). The classic Hibbs procedure is described in his 1924 article (10). This technique included not only turning down the spinous processes, as described in his original article, but also overlapping strips of bone upward and downward from each lamina and curetting the cartilage from the facet joints. In each of his articles, Hibbs emphasized the importance of meticulous subperiosteal dissection. He did not advocate the use of a bone graft but did suggest in his original article that a bone graft from the leg may be necessary in very young patients.

Albee is also considered one of the founders of spinal fusion. In fact, he may have antedated Hibbs. In his original article, Albee described a procedure he had used in five cases; it consisted of splitting the spinous processes and turning them down to come into contact with the next adjacent spinous process. Because of the uncertainty of fusion in these cases, he believed that a bone graft was needed. In his 1911 article, Albee described his modified procedure, which was to split the spinous processes and lay a strip of the crest of the tibia between the split spinous processes longitudinally. His 1911 report gave the results of his

modified procedure in three cases, the first having been performed in June 1911. Therefore, one may surmise that at least one of Albee's original five cases must have been performed before to Hibbs' first case in January 1911. Albee arrived at his decision to attempt to fuse the spine because of the rapid disappearance of tuberculosis he had observed in other joints when a fusion was obtained—whether the fusion had occurred spontaneously or by means of an operative procedure, such as his technique for hip fusion.

Since then, many modifications have been introduced concerning decortication of the lamina, destruction of the facet joints, and the use of extra bone. Howorth's (11) 1943 article on the evolution of spinal fusion probably described the then-current state of art of spinal fusion. This included meticulous subperiosteal dissection far enough laterally to expose the facets; removal of the spinous processes, which are cut into strips and used as graft; partial removal of the ligamentum flavum; destruction of the facet and packing of the defect with a piece of bone; decortication of the lamina into strips; the interlocking of these strips with strips from the lamina above and below; and, finally, placement of the cut strips of spinous process across the interlaminal spaces.

Moe (14) in 1958 critically analyzed the results of four types of bone fusion that were all modifications of Hibbs' technique. Moe described a procedure in which the thoracic and lumbar facets were destroyed and blocks of cancellous and cortical bone were inserted into the defects, as described by McBride (12). This has become known as the Moe fusion procedure.

In 1959, Goldstein (4) described his technique of spinal fusion in which all the posterior elements from the tip of transverse process to the tip of the opposite transverse process were decorticated with a hand gouge. No attempt was made to denude the articular cartilage of the facet joints in the thoracic or lumbar regions. The strips of bone removed from the posterior elements were repositioned over the more lateral surfaces of the decorticated posterior elements. Goldstein's procedure differed from Moe's in that no attempt was made to destroy the facet, nor were the strips of bone from the posterior elements left attached to the spine.

Moe did not advocate use of autogenous bone but did use it in some cases. Goldstein strongly recommended the use of large amounts of autogenous bone and even described his technique for obtaining the graft from the ilium.

Since the late 1950s, numerous articles have appeared de-

J. H. Dickson: Department of Orthopedic Surgery, Institute of Spinal Disorders, Baylor College of Medicine, Houston, Texas 77030.

scribing various techniques of obtaining a spinal fusion. They all have in common a meticulous subperiosteal dissection and a thorough decortication of the posterior elements. The facets may or may not be destroyed, and extra bone—autogenous, homogenous, or both—may or may not be added.

POSITIONING AND PREPARATION

Positioning of the patient is important (Fig. 1). The abdomen should be fully suspended so that abdominal pressure is lessened. Pearce (15) demonstrated that any abdominal pressure that resulted in partial or complete occlusion of the inferior vena cava produced a marked increase in venous pressure below the occlusion. This increased pressure caused the blood from the lower half of the body to be shunted into the vertebral plexus around the vertebral bodies, as had been demonstrated by Batson (2). This in turn caused an increase in blood loss during posterior spinal surgery. This abdominal suspension can be obtained by supporting the pelvis and the chest wall with frames, such as the Relton-Hall frame (16), or by using chest rolls. Chest rolls are advantageous because they not only suspend the abdomen

by supporting the pelvis and the clavicle and subclavicular area but also support the entire lateral chest wall. This adds stability to the spine so that when the decortication for fusion is undertaken, less vibration of the spine occurs, and less bleeding is encountered.

In procedures in which maintaining lumbar lordosis is important, the type of suspension may be important. Tan and colleagues (18) showed that lumbar lordosis is better maintained on chest rolls than on some of the other frames.

The arms should not be raised past 90 degrees from the side of the body. If they are, there is a greater chance for the development of a brachial plexus palsy. The elbows should be padded so that there will be no compression of the ulnar nerve at the elbow.

Pads are placed beneath the knees, and a pillow is placed beneath the distal tibiae and ankles so that the feet hang free without any pressure on the toes. After the patient is positioned, the pulses at the ankles should be checked to ensure that there is no occlusion of the femoral artery at the groin by whatever device is used to support the patient on the operating table.

The skin is prepared in a sterile aseptic technique. In patients who are to have exposure of the high thoracic spine (T1 through

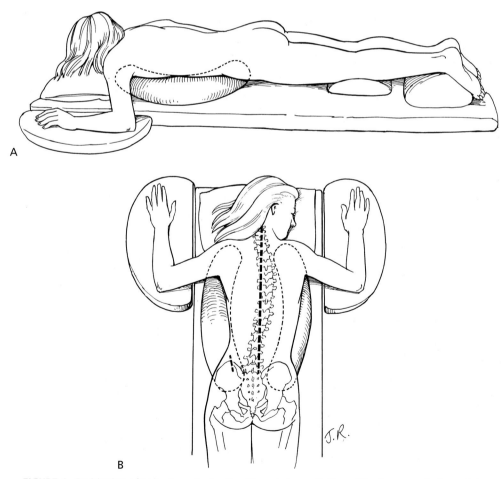

FIGURE 1. Positioning of patient on chest rolls with pads beneath the ankles, knees, and elbows (**A**). Arms are positioned with shoulders at an angle of less than 90 degrees. A small separate vertical incision is made for the graft. A straight midline incision is made for the back exposure (**B**).

T4), care is taken to ensure that the skin is prepared up to the midcervical level. If this is not accomplished, exposure of the upper thoracic spine will be difficult after drapes are applied.

BONE GRAFT

If a bone graft is to be obtained, it can be obtained through a separate incision or by dissecting laterally from a midline incision, which may or may not be curved at its caudal end toward the side from which the graft is to be taken. The author prefers a separate incision (Fig. 1) because more bone graft can be obtained through a separate incision than by dissecting subcutaneously to the iliac crest from the midline. This incision, in a young patient who is not overweight, can be 2 inches in length and is made parallel to the midline of the body. The incision is placed just lateral to the posterosuperior iliac spine and crest. The lower portion of the incision stops at the caudal level of the posterosuperior iliac spine. The skin can then be moved up, down, and sideways to expose the posterior one third of the ilium. I prefer to take the graft before starting the spinal exposure. If the spine is fully exposed while the graft is being obtained, especially in a patient with scoliosis, there will be more bleeding than would occur if the graft is obtained first. Blood can be obtained from the graft site to bathe the strips of bone graft until they are placed on the decorticated surface of the spine.

INCISION AND EXPOSURE

The extent of the incision depends on the object of the surgical procedure. The following description applies to exposure of the spine for a posterior spinal instrumentation and fusion for scoliosis. Shorter incisions are made for other surgical procedures, but the same principles apply.

A midline incision (Fig. 1) is made from one level above to one level below the superior and inferior vertebrae to be instrumentated and fused. First, the skin is partially incised as a marker for the rest of the skin incision. The skin and subdermal tissues are infiltrated with a 1:500,000 solution of adrenaline and saline. Rarely is more than 20 to 25 mL necessary. Some surgeons inject the adrenaline solution into the paravertebral muscles as well as subperiosteally around the posterior elements. If this is done, 200 to 300 mL of adrenaline solution is needed. I do not believe that this is necessary; the decrease in bleeding in these areas can be accomplished by staying in the midline and performing a meticulous subperiosteal dissection. This infiltration with adrenaline can be performed before closing the skin over the graft site, giving the adrenaline solution time to take effect while the skin over the graft site is closed.

A straight incision is made even in the presence of a markedly curved spine. When the incision is closed, the back will appear straighter with a straight incision than with a curved incision. After the skin has been infiltrated with the adrenaline solution, the deeper portions of the dermis and subcutaneous tissue are incised using cautery or a knife. I prefer cautery to help minimize blood loss. As the subcutaneous tissues are dissected, traction is applied on the skin by applying self-retaining retractors just beneath the skin. This facilitates exposing the spinous processes and the midline raphe of the back. In small curves, this is not a problem; in larger curves, the muscle on the convex side—especially in the thoracic region—sometimes overlaps the midline at the apex of the curve, which makes exposure difficult.

After the midline of the spine has been exposed, pressure is applied to both sides of the spinous processes (Fig. 2). A scalpel

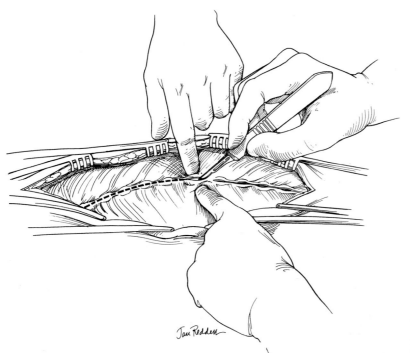

FIGURE 2. Pressure is applied to the sides of each spinous process. A scalpel is used to cut directly into the bone of the spinous process through the cartilaginous cap if present.

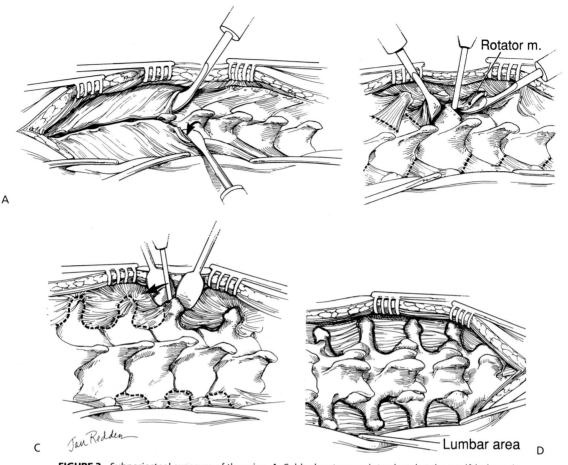

FIGURE 3. Subperiosteal exposure of the spine. **A:** Cobb elevators are introduced at the twelfth thoracic vertebra and moved upward, separating the midline. **B:** Each lamina is dissected subperiosteally, leaving the short rotator muscles attached to the inferior edge of the lamina. These muscles are then incised and the transverse process subperiosteally exposed. **C:** The soft tissue attached to the transverse processes in the intertransverse process area is incised. **D:** In the lumbar region, each lamina is dissected individually out to the tip of the transverse process.

is used to make an incision through the cartilaginous cap, if present, to the bone of the spinous process. This is performed at each level starting at the most inferior exposed spinous process. After all the spinous processes have been so incised, Cobb elevators are introduced subperiosteally at the twelfth thoracic vertebra on both sides of the spinous processes down to the level of the lamina (Fig. 3A). With the surgeon and assistant working simultaneously, the Cobbs are rotated outward starting at the base of each spinous process. During this maneuver, it is important not to bury the Cobb elevators completely beneath the paravertebral muscles. If this occurs, the elevators will pierce the periosteum and dissect into the paravertebral muscles, causing more bleeding. As the Cobbs are moved up the spine, the midline is separated, exposing the spinous processes. Because of the attachment of the muscle fibers in the lumbar region, this maneuver cannot be performed there. In the lumbar region of the spine, each individual level is exposed, first by exposing the spinous processes and then by dissecting about half the laminae subperiosteally. As one exposes the lower portion of the incision, the

upper portion, which has already been separated, is packed tightly with sponges to control bleeding.

After exposure of the spinous processes, the self-retaining retractors are repositioned on the midline raphe, and traction is applied laterally. At each individual vertebral level (Fig. 3B), the laminae are further dissected subperiosteally out to the base of the transverse process, leaving the short rotators attached to the inferior surface of the lamina above. Using a knife, cautery, or sharp Cobb, the surgeon detaches the short rotators from the lamina out to the base of the transverse process. The Cobb is then rotated, and the muscles and periosteum over the transverse process are lifted to expose the tip of the transverse process. Electric cautery is used to cauterize the bleeders and to clear the transverse process of soft tissue (Fig. 3C). The superior articular artery located at the junction of the base of the superior portion of the transverse process and the lamina is the most persistent. This exposure is performed at each level in the thoracic region. In the lumbar area, the lamina at each level is dissected free. The knife, sharp Cobb, or cautery is then used to dissect the capsule from the facet joint. The transverse process is dissected subperiosteally to completely expose the transverse process out to its tip (Fig. 3D).

MacNab and Dall (13) demonstrated the arterial vessels, which are encountered when exposing the lumbar lamina, pars interarticularis, facet, and transverse process. If one is mindful of these vessels, especially the superior and inferior articular arteries, they can be cauterized quickly on exposure, thus lessening blood loss. After the posterior elements are completely exposed, the intertransverse process soft tissues at each level that remain are cut with a cautery or knife, completing the exposure.

FUSION

The object of the fusion is to decorticate the spine completely from the tip of one transverse process to the tip of the opposite transverse process in both the thoracic and lumbar regions. If the fusion is to extend to the sacrum, the decortication is extended out onto the ala of the sacrum. Little or no bone graft is placed in the midline; all of it is placed laterally over the decorticated transverse process, the lateral surface of the superior facet and pars of the fifth lumbar vertebra, the decorticated facet between the fifth lumbar vertebra and the sacrum, and the ala of the sacrum (Fig. 4). If the fusion is to extend from the fourth lumbar vertebra to the sacrum, the decortication and bone graft include the facet between the fourth and fifth lumbar vertebrae and the pars and transverse process of the fourth lumbar vertebra.

Decortication can be achieved by the use of osteotomes, gouges, rongeurs, or power-driven instruments. The objective is

not only to decorticate the posterior elements to create a bleeding cancellous bed but also to obtain additional bone graft material. Little extra bone is obtained when a power-driven burr is used. The facets can be ignored as advocated by Goldstein or destroyed as advocated by Moe.

The following is my technique for decorticating the posterior elements. In those procedures in which the spinous processes can be removed, they are first split in half with a ½-inch osteotome (Fig. 5A). They are then removed at their base with an angled bone cutter, thus creating a relatively flat surface of the remaining posterior elements consisting of the lamina and transverse process. The spinous processes are cut in half again, creating three or four strips of corticocancellous bone graft material. In the thoracic region, each inferior facet is removed with a ¼-inch osteotome as if a distraction hook is to be inserted (Fig. 5B). The cartilage and subchondral bone of the exposed superior facet are removed. The transverse process is split in half using a ½-inch osteotome (Fig. 5B,C). Then, starting in the cancellous bone where the spinous process has been removed, the osteotome is advanced laterally and subcortically to meet with the cut in the transverse process. Thus, the entire cortex of the lamina and transverse process is removed as one unit. This is then cut lengthwise with a bone cutter to create two or more strips of bone to use as bone graft. Cancellous bone is placed over the decorticated surfaces, and the cut strips of bone removed by decortication are placed on top of the cancellous bone (Fig. 5D).

In the lumbar region, after removal of the spinous process (Fig. 6), a ½-inch osteotome is used to decorticate the posterior elements completely from the exposed cancellous surface of the removed spinous process out to the tip of the transverse process.

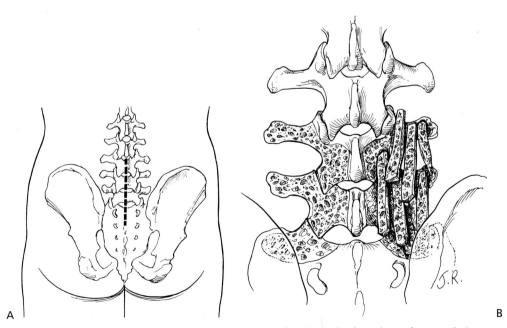

FIGURE 4. Lumbosacral fusion. **A:** Incision for exposure of the lower lumbar spine and sacrum. **B:** Area of decortication and placement of bone graft for a fusion from the fourth lumbar vertebra to the sacrum. Note that the third and fourth lumbar facets are not destroyed when the fusion includes the fourth lumbar vertebra. Also note the decortication of the ala of the sacrum.

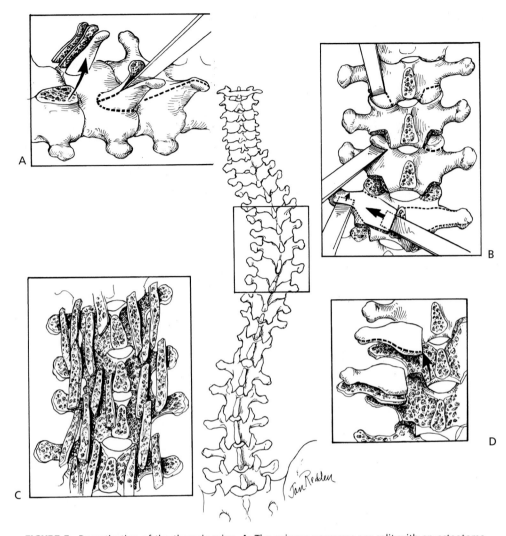

FIGURE 5. Decortication of the thoracic spine. **A:** The spinous processes are split with an osteotome and cut into strips. **B:** The inferior facet is removed with a ¼-inch osteotome. The cartilage and subchondral plate are removed from the exposed adjacent superior facet. The posterior cortex of the lamina and transverse process is removed with an osteotome. **C:** Cancellous bone graft and strips of bone removed by decortication are placed on top of the decorticated spine. **D:** The cortex that was removed from the lamina and transverse process is split in half.

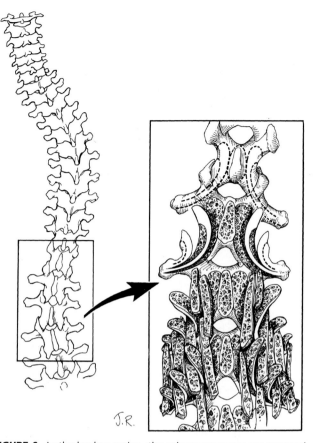

FIGURE 6. In the lumbar region, the spinous processes are removed. The posterior elements are decorticated by taking multiple cuts with a ½-inch osteotome starting at the base of the removed spinous process. Cancellous bone graft and strips of removed decorticated bone are placed over the decorticated surface.

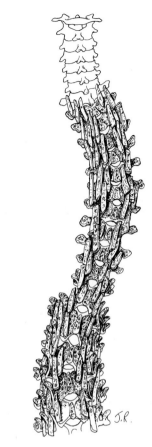

FIGURE 7. When the fusion is completed, the entire spine has been decorticated from the tip of the transverse process to the tip of the opposite transverse process. Bone graft has been inserted on top of the decorticated surfaces.

This is performed by taking multiple cuts (at least three) across the lamina through the facet out to the tip of the transverse process. About 70% to 80% of the facet is removed. This decorticated bone is lifted up, and strips of cancellous bone graft are placed on top of the lateral decorticated surfaces of the posterior elements. The bone graft should be placed from transverse process to transverse process and along the lateral aspect of the lamina and decorticated pars interarticularis region as well as over the remaining facet.

When the spinous processes are not removed, it is difficult to obtain a complete decortication with a curved osteotome. The thoracic facets are handled in the same manner as described when the spinous processes are removed. The thoracic and lumbar laminae and transverse processes are completely decorticated using a rongeur or a curved gouge. This decorticated bone is removed, saved for bone graft, and reinserted on top of the cancellous bone, which is placed as previously described.

When the fusion has been completed (Fig. 7), the entire spine, from the tip of the transverse processes to the tip of the opposite transverse processes, has been decorticated, as have the facets in the thoracic region. Cancellous bone from the graft site and the strips of bone removed by the decortication are placed on top of the decorticated spine.

CLOSURE

When the fusion is completed, there is a large surface of exposed, decorticated bone that continues to bleed. Towel clips are used to close the incision rapidly (Fig. 8). This allows pressure to begin to build up in the operative area to help control some of this bleeding.

Drains may or may not be inserted. If drains are used, they can be placed beneath the fascia of the paravertebral muscles or between the fascia and skin. They are removed within 12 to 36 hours. Flynn and colleagues (3) recommend harvesting the blood from the hemovac for the first 6 hours under sterile conditions. This blood is washed and centrifuged by the blood bank and can then be transfused back to the patient within 12 hours after preparation. I do not use a drain and prefer to close the fascia tightly with interrupted figure-of-eight sutures; the back pressure created by the developing hemotoma helps control the bleeding from the decorticated surfaces.

Methods of closing the fascia, subcutaneous tissue, and skin are the surgeon's choice. I prefer using inverted subcutaneous sutures to reapproximate the skin. Steri-Strips are then applied across the incision to approximate the skin edges accurately. When the incision heals, only a straight line is visible; there is

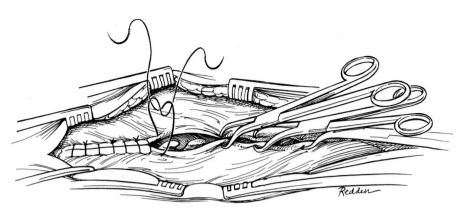

FIGURE 8. When closure is started, the incision is rapidly closed using towel clips. As the suturing progresses, the towel clips are removed.

no evidence of suture lines, as would be seen if skin sutures had been used.

A sterile, bulky dressing is applied. Patients are positioned on their backs for the first 4 to 6 hours to apply pressure to the decorticated bone surfaces to help minimize postoperative bleeding.

LATERAL APPROACH TO THE LUMBOSACRAL REGION

In 1953, Watkins (19) first described his lateral approach to the lower lumbar spine and the sacrum. His technique has subsequently been modified by Wiltse (20). The following is Wiltse's recommended procedure. This procedure is primarily used to expose the spine from the fourth lumbar vertebra to the sacrum.

A midline incision is made from the spinous process of the third lumbar vertebra to the second sacral vertebra (Fig. 9). The deep fascia is exposed two fingerbreadths lateral to the midline on either side. The deep fascia is then incised 2 cm lateral to the midline on each side for the length of the incision. There is a cleft between the multifidus and longissimus muscles (Fig. 10). A finger may be used to dissect between these two muscle planes starting at the fourth lumbar level. As the finger dissects downward, it touches the facet of fourth and fifth lumbar vertebrae. The posterior elements from the base of the spinous process to the tip of the transverse process can be exposed (Fig. 11). The posterior elements can then be decorticated, but care must be taken not to expose the lamina or facet joint of the vertebra immediately cephalad to the uppermost vertebra to be fused. Bone graft is then placed on top of the decorticated lamina, facet, and transverse process (Fig. 12). The fascia,

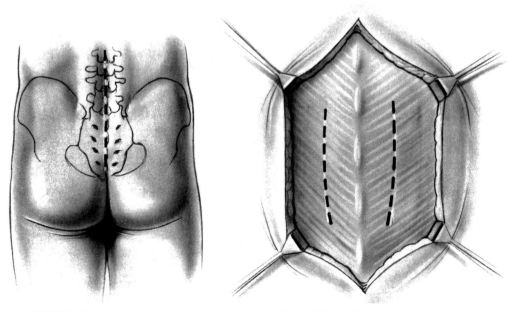

FIGURE 9. Paraspinal approach to the lumbar spine. *Left:* A midline incision is made. *Right:* The fascia is exposed two fingerbreadths on each side of the midline. (*Figure continues.*)

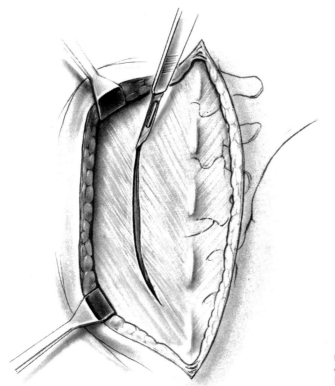

FIGURE 9. *Continued.* The fascia is incised 2 cm to each side of the midline, curving it gently toward the midline at the distal end. (Adapted from Wiltse LL, Spencer CW [1988]: New uses and refinements of the paraspinal approach to the lumbar spine. *Spine* 13:696–706, with permission.)

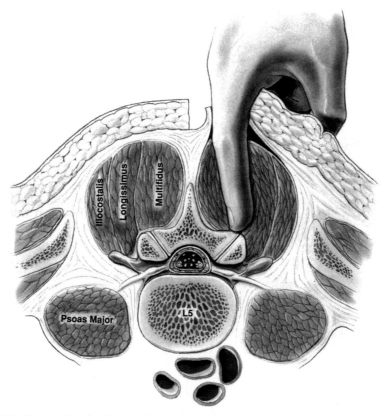

FIGURE 10. Cross-section showing the three paravertebral muscle groups and the approach between the multifidus and longissimus. (Adapted from Wiltse LL, Spencer CW [1988]: New uses and refinements of the paraspinal approach to the lumbar spine. *Spine* 13:696–706, with permission.)

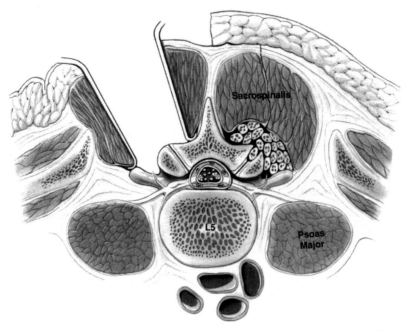

FIGURE 11. Retractors have been placed between the multifidus and longissimus muscles. The posterior elements are subperiosteally exposed from the base of the spinous process to the tip of the transverse process. (Adapted from Wiltse LL, Spencer CW [1988]: New uses and refinements of the paraspinal approach to the lumbar spine. *Spine* 13:696–706, with permission.)

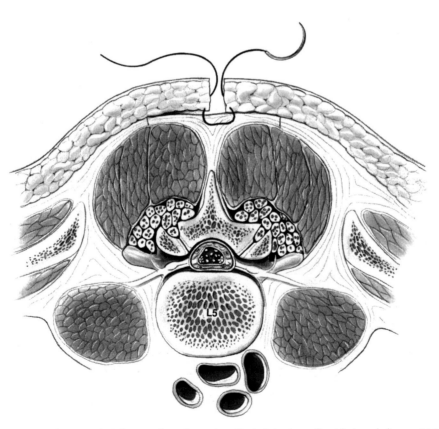

FIGURE 12. The posterior elements have been decorticated, bone graft added, and closure started. (Adapted from Wiltse LL, Spencer CW [1988]: New uses and refinements of the paraspinal approach to the lumbar spine. *Spine* 13:696–706, with permission.)

subcutaneous tissue, and skin are closed. Wiltse believes that this approach is better than the midline incision because the spinous processes with their ligaments and blood supply are not disturbed, thus maintaining stability. In addition, exposure in certain diagnoses is easier, and if care is used, less bleeding is encountered.

In this day and age of marked proliferation of hardware used in the spine, one must not forget the objective of the procedure, that is, a spinal fusion. Hardware, no matter how strong, does not permanently stabilize the spine and does not substitute for poorly performed spinal fusion.

REFERENCES

1. Albee FH (1911): Transplantation of a portion of the tibia into the spine for Pott's disease: a preliminary report. *JAMA* 57:885–886.
2. Batson OV (1940): The function of the vertebral veins and their role in the spread of metastases. *Ann Surg* 112:138–149.
3. Flynn JC, Price CT, Zink WD (1991): The third step of total autologous blood transfusion in scoliosis surgery. (Harvesting blood from the postoperative wound.) *Spine* 16:328–329.
4. Goldstein LA (1959): Results in the treatment of scoliosis with turnbuckle plaster cast correction and fusion. *J Bone Joint Surg Am* 41: 321–335.
5. Hibbs RA (1911): An operation from progressive spinal deformities. *N Y Med J* 93:1013–1016.
6. Hibbs RA (1912): An operation for Pott's disease of the spine. *JAMA* 59:433–436.
7. Hibbs RA (1912): A further consideration of an operation for Pott's disease of the spine. *Ann Surg* 55:682–688.
8. Hibbs RA (1917): Treatment of deformities of the spine caused by poliomyelitis. *JAMA* 69:787–791.
9. Hibbs RA (1918): Treatment of vertebral tuberculosis by fusion operation. *JAMA* 71:1372–1376.
10. Hibbs RA (1924): A report of fifty-nine cases of scoliosis treated by the fusion operation. *J Bone Joint Surg* 6:3–37.
11. Howorth MB (1943): Evolution of spinal fusion. *Ann Surg* 117: 278–289.
12. McBride EA (1949): A mortised transfacet bone block for lumbosacral fusion. *J Bone Joint Surg Am* 31:385–399.
13. MacNab I, Dall D (1971): The blood supply of the lumbar spine and its application to the technique of intertransverse lumbar fusion. *J Bone Joint Surg Br* 53:628–638.
14. Moe JH (1958): A critical analysis of methods of fusion for scoliosis: an evaluation in two hundred and sixty-six patients. *J Bone Joint Surg Am* 40:529–554.
15. Pearce DJ (1957): The role of posture in laminectomy (abridged). *Proc R Soc Med* (Section of Anaesthetics) 50:109–112.
16. Relton JES, Hall JE (1967): An operative frame for spinal fusion: a new apparatus designed to reduce haemorrhage during operation. *J Bone Joint Surg Br* 49:327–332.
17. Scott JC (1953): Editorial on spinal fusion. *J Bone Joint Surg Br* 35: 169–171.
18. Tan SB, Kozak JA, Dickson JH (1994): *Effect of operative position on sagittal alignment of the lumbar spine. Spine* 19(3):314–318.
19. Watkins MB (1953): Posterolateral fusion of the lumbar and lumbosacral spine. *J Bone Joint Surg Am* 35:1014–1018.
20. Wiltse LL, Spencer CW (1988): New uses and refinements of the paraspinal approach to the lumbar spine. *Spine* 13:696–706.

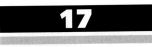

ANTERIOR SPINAL SURGERY

JOHN A. HERRING

ANTERIOR SPINAL FUSION

Indications

Anterior spinal fusion is indicated to arrest spinal growth in children with considerable spinal growth remaining, to gain flexibility when the spinal deformity is rigid, to obtain better fusion rates in neuromuscular scoliosis, to obtain a spinal fusion when posterior structures are deficient, and to stabilize spinal kyphosis. Vertebral infections, tumors, and other processes affecting the vertebral bodies are often best managed by anterior spinal surgery.

When there is a progressive scoliosis in an immature patient, an anterior fusion is often indicated in addition to a posterior fusion to arrest spinal growth. Several studies showed that a posterior fusion in immature patients is regularly followed by progressive angulation and rotation of the spine as the vertebrae continue to grow anteriorly (19,62). Dubousset and colleagues (19) termed this progression the *crankshaft phenomenon* to emphasize the rotational nature of the progressive deformity (Fig. 1). To determine the need for an anterior fusion, the physical maturity of the patient must be assessed relative to the Tanner stages of sexual maturity, the Risser grade, and the skeletal age. In addition, the maturity of the epiphysis of the elbow has a useful relationship to spinal growth. Dimeglio and Bonnel (18) showed that spinal growth follows an acceleration-deceleration pattern (Fig. 2). The deceleration phase begins at the time of closure of the physis of the capitellum, which is followed in some months by the first appearance of the Risser sign. Menarche usually occurs at Risser 1 or 2, further into the decelerated phase of spinal growth. Sanders and coworkers found that curve progression after posterior fusion was much more likely in patients with open triradiate cartilages than in those whose triradiates were closed (48). Little and coworkers showed that the most accurate predictor of growth of the spine was the estimate of the time of peak growth velocity in the adolescent (36). This measure is more accurate than either menarche or standard radiographic signs of maturity because it identifies the exact peak of the adolescent growth spurt. The average peak growth velocity is 8 cm per year in girls and 9.5 cm per year in boys.

The phase of spinal growth is an important factor in predict-

ing the outcome of a posterior fusion. Growth is rapid in the accelerated phase, which starts as the child enters puberty. A posterior fusion done during or before this period usually is complicated by unacceptable postoperative progression. In this period, a circumferential fusion of the immature spine is necessary to arrest further growth and produce permanent correction (34,52) (Fig. 3). After the patient has reached the decelerated phase of spinal growth and has passed the peak growth velocity, a posterior fusion suffices because the anterior growth is insufficient to produce significant crankshaft progression (18). If a large deformity remains, an anterior fusion may be advisable in the early decelerated phase (Risser 1) to gain better correction and to eliminate any postoperative progression. Crankshaft progression has been observed in patients with idiopathic, neuromuscular, and congenital scoliosis.

The indications for anterior fusion to prevent growth in congenital scoliosis are less clear than those for other etiologies (62). Growth patterns are variable in congenital scoliosis, and congenital deformities with anterior bar formation may have no significant anterior growth potential, in which case an anterior fusion is unnecessary. Other congenital curves with intact anterior growth centers progress after posterior fusion and should be managed with circumferential fusion. Computed tomography may be useful in identifying the intact or blocked growth centers.

An anterior fusion is also indicated in idiopathic scoliosis to gain spinal mobility when the deformity is severe and the spine is rigid. A period of halo traction after an anterior release and fusion may improve the ultimate correction obtained with posterior instrumentation. In addition, idiopathic thoracolumbar and lumbar curves of average severity are especially well managed by anterior instrumentation and fusion (63).

An anterior fusion is often indicated in neurogenic scoliosis to gain correctability of the spine and to enhance the likelihood of fusion. Distinct improvements in the rate of successful fusion of neuromuscular deformities have been shown by many authors (9,46,56,59). Achieving an anterior fusion is essential in conditions such as myelomeningocele, where the absence of posterior elements makes posterior fusion difficult or impossible (5,15,41,49,65) (Fig. 4).

The stabilization of kyphosis often requires an anterior fusion because the biomechanics of a supporting graft under compression are much more favorable for fusion than those of a posterior graft under tension (35,64,68). Anterior fusion is usually recommended for any kyphosis greater than 50 degrees, but it may

J. A. Herring: University of Texas Southwestern Medical School, Texas Scottish Rite Hospital for Crippled Children, Dallas, Texas 75219.

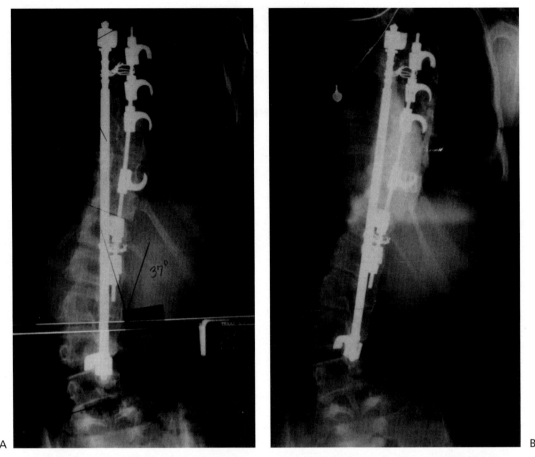

FIGURE 1. A case illustrating the crankshaft phenomenon. **A:** Anteroposterior radiograph of a 14-year-old girl 1 year after Harrington instrumentation and fusion. The Risser sign is still zero, and the patient is premenarchal. **B:** Anteroposterior radiograph of the patient 3 years after surgery showing progressive rotation of the spine, an increase in the Cobb angle, and a marked progression of the rib hump deformity. At the time of reinstrumentation, a solid fusion mass was found and osteotomized. The postoperative progression occurred because of continued anterior spinal growth against the posterior fusion mass, the so-called crankshaft phenomenon.

also be necessary for younger patients with less severe deformities (68). Conditions requiring this approach include congenital kyphosis, Scheuermann kyphosis (13,39,55), kyphosis associated with laminectomy and radiation, and the combined deformities of neurofibromatosis (8). An anterior fusion is also indicated when the spinal cord has been decompressed anteriorly for either a kyphotic or a scoliotic deformity (68). In addition, an anterior fusion is often necessary to stabilize the spinal deformity caused by tuberculous or pyogenic destruction of the vertebral bodies as well as by tumor (6,16,20,27,32,38,44,45).

Contraindications

The primary contraindication to anterior fusion is inadequate pulmonary reserve to tolerate the procedure. Patients with extreme weakness, such as those with spinal muscular atrophy or Duchenne muscular dystrophy, may be unable to recover from an anterior fusion because of respiratory insufficiency (23,33). Patients who have other pulmonary disorders, such as pulmonary hypoplasia, cor pulmonale, and congenital heart disease,

may also be poor candidates for anterior surgery. A comprehensive preoperative pulmonary evaluation is necessary for any patient whose cardiopulmonary capacity is in question. The availability of appropriate postoperative care is a prerequisite for this surgery.

Advantages and Disadvantages

One advantage of an anterior fusion is that better correction of deformity can be obtained by combining anterior fusion with posterior instrumentation and fusion for idiopathic scoliosis. In addition, anterior fusion prevents crankshaft progression by removing the anterior growth centers of the spine. Also, an anterior fusion places the fusion mass under compression with kyphotic deformities, allowing better maintenance of correction.

The two major disadvantages of anterior spinal fusion are the added time of surgery and the potential for postoperative complications. Performing the anterior and posterior fusions under the same anesthetic offsets many of the disadvantages of the anterior procedure. It has been shown that there is a signifi-

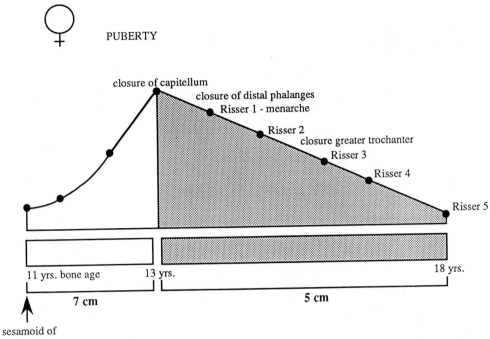

FIGURE 2. A graph of the rate of spinal growth in girls during puberty. Note that closure of the capitellar epiphysis corresponds to the peak rate of spinal growth. There is a mean of 7 cm of spinal growth between the onset of puberty and the closure of the capitellum. Between the closure of the capitellum and the end of growth, there is another 5 cm of spinal growth. (From Dimeglio A, Bonnel F [1990]: *Le rachis en croissance*. Paris: Springer-Verlag, with permission.)

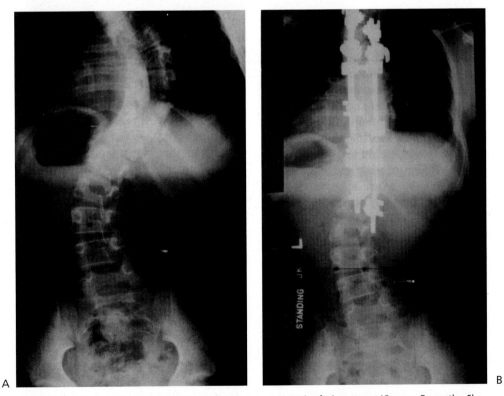

FIGURE 3. An example of a patient treated with anteroposterior fusion at age 12 years, 5 months. She was premenarchal, and the Risser sign was 0 at the time of surgery. Her capitellar epiphysis was still open, suggesting that there was a large amount of spinal growth remaining. **A:** Preoperative anteroposterior radiograph showing an 80-degree scoliosis with a Risser sign of 0. **B:** Radiograph 6 months after anterior and posterior spinal fusion and instrumentation, showing correction of the scoliosis to 23 degrees. The ablation of anterior growth potential should prevent future progression of the deformity.

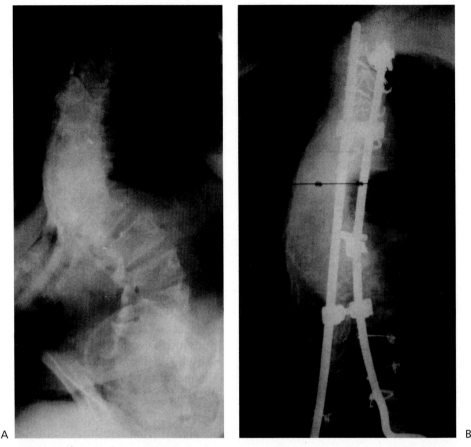

FIGURE 4. A patient with myelodysplasia and scoliosis. **A:** Preoperative radiograph showing a double scoliosis, with curves measuring 70 and 50 degrees. There is a large posterior element defect from T12 to the sacrum. **B:** Radiograph after anterior and posterior fusion with posterior instrumentation showing satisfactory correction and stabilization of the deformity.

cant reduction in morbidity when the same-day approach is used (24,53). When the anterior and posterior procedures are separated by a period of weeks, the patient often has not fully recovered from the first procedure when the second is performed. In this situation, there is a greater likelihood of complications during recovery from the second procedure. At times, it is necessary to stage the anterior and posterior procedures. This is usually true when one stage is complex, such as a repeat anterior exposure with spinal osteotomies or a difficult posterior instrumentation. In these instances, it is important to assess and properly manage the patient's nutritional status before and between surgeries (42).

Techniques

Exposure

The thoracic spine is approached through a thoracotomy, usually on the convex side of the scoliosis. (The spine may also be approached thoracoscopically, which is the subject of another section.) When there is a true kyphotic deformity and a mild scoliosis, the spine should be approached on the concave side of the scoliosis. (The surgeon should be certain that the deformity

is a kyphosis. A severely rotated lordoscoliosis often appears kyphotic on a lateral radiograph, and these must be approached on the convexity.) The disc between T12 and L1 may be reached from above or below the diaphragm by separating the crura of the diaphragm. The thoracolumbar spine is approached with a thoracoabdominal approach, peripherally incising the diaphragm. The lumbar spine may be approached retroperitoneally beneath the diaphragm. When instrumentation is required, wide exposure is necessary so that the insertion instruments may be placed at a right angle to the spine. Thus, instrumentation of the first lumbar vertebra requires a thoracoabdominal approach, but instrumentation from the second lumbar vertebra distally may be performed beneath the diaphragm. In exposing the lower lumbar spine, the surgeon should avoid injuring the inferior mesenteric ganglion of the sympathetic chain. This ganglion, which is ill defined, is found at the level of the third or fourth lumbar vertebra on the left side in 80% of cases (22,30). Damage to the sympathetic chain at this level may cause retrograde ejaculation in male patients, a complication that occurred in 0.45% of cases reviewed by Flynn and Price (22).

The two uppermost thoracic vertebrae are difficult to approach through a traditional thoracotomy. Transsternal and claviculomanubrial approaches have been used to reach this area anteriorly (58,59).

The first step in the exposure of the vertebrae is direct dissection over the intervertebral discs. The bulge of the disc is easily palpated, and there are few vessels at the disc level. Next, the segmental vessels are located between the discs, where they lie on the concave anterior surface of the vertebral bodies. The vessels are elevated with a right-angle clamp, and vessel loops are placed around the vessels. In most cases in which no instrumentation is used, the vessels may be left intact. If greater exposure is required, or if instrumentation is used, most surgeons doubly ligate the vessels. Apel and coworkers reported three cases in which paraplegia followed ligation of segmental vessels (4). They subsequently reported an additional seven cases in which temporary vessel occlusion produced complete loss of somatosensory evoked potentials. They advocate temporary occlusion of segmental vessels with vessel loops and evaluation of spinal cord monitoring to be certain that no vascular compromise to the spinal cords exists. If monitoring reflects no change, the vessels are then doubly ligated (Fig. 5). The exposure of the lumbar vertebrae needs to be fairly wide, requiring careful elevation of the psoas (Fig. 6). Cautery should be used with care in the psoas because of possible injury to the lumbar plexus. The cautery should also be used with care in the lower lumbar area to minimize the risk of injury to the sympathetic chain. If the surgeon plans to elevate the periosteum of the vertebral body,

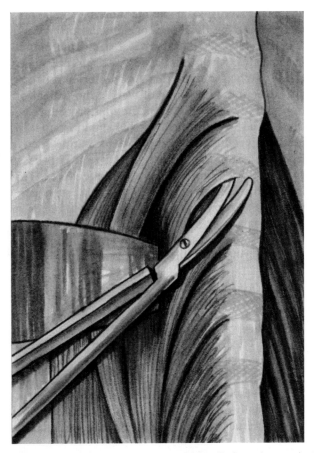

FIGURE 6. The psoas muscle is dissected laterally from the vertebral bodies and disc. Cautery should be used with great care because the lumbar plexus courses within the substance of the psoas.

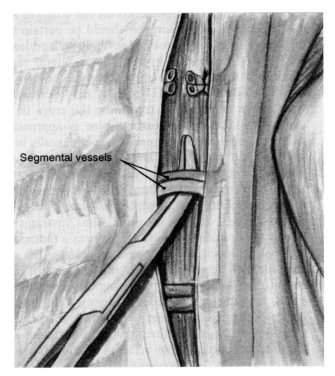

FIGURE 5. The segmental vessels should be elevated from the vertebral bodies over a 1-cm area. They may be controlled with vessel loops and retracted to allow disc excision. If instrumentation is to be used, or if greater control is required, they may be doubly ligated. Temporary occlusion has been recommended to evaluate somatosensory evoked potential changes that might indicate spinal cord ischemia.

it is best to do this toward the end of the procedure to minimize bleeding.

Disc Excision

Excision of the intervertebral disc begins with an elliptical incision in the annulus fibrosus over four fifths of its exposed surface (Fig. 7). Through this incision, the nucleus pulposus is removed with rongeurs. The remainder of the annulus is removed using rongeurs of increasing size until the dense annular tissue has been excised throughout the circumference of the disc. It is helpful to leave intact a thin layer of perichondrium over the periphery of the disc to protect the surrounding structures. The surgeon's finger can readily palpate the rongeur beneath this layer of anterior ligament. In addition, a small posterior portion of the annulus fibrosus protecting the canal should be left intact. Spreaders are used to open the disc space so that the cartilaginous end plate of the vertebra may be removed with ring curets. A Cobb elevator may also be turned 90 degrees in the interspace to improve exposure. If the bony end plate of the vertebra is to be removed, this is done with osteotomes and rongeurs. Excision of the end plate should be done as late in the procedure as possible to minimize blood loss. Some surgeons believe that re-

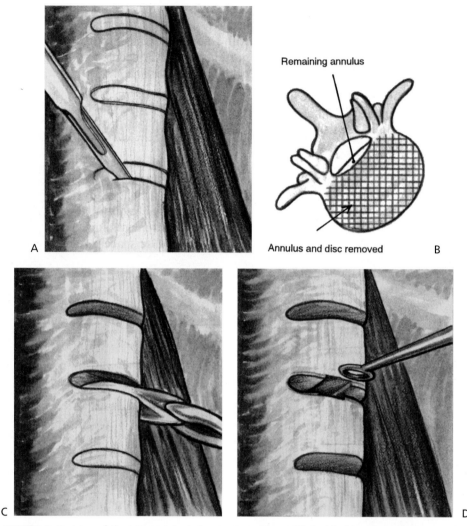

FIGURE 7. Excision of the intervertebral discs begins with an elliptical incision through the annulus fibrosus (**A**). Rongeurs are used to extract the nucleus pulposus and remove the annulus fibrosus (**C**). A thin rim of annulus is left intact just anterior to the spinal canal as a safety precaution (**B**). After removal of the annulus, the cartilaginous end plate is completely removed with ring curets (**D**).

moval of the end plate is essential to achieve fusion; others deem it unnecessary. When the end plate is removed, the vertebral strength for purchase of screws and staples is lessened. Thus, when we plan instrumentation of the spine, we do not remove the bony end plate.

Fusion

The rib that is removed during the thoracotomy usually provides sufficient bone graft for intervertebral fusion. If extensive grafting is necessary, the iliac crest may also be used. The bone graft is cut into small pieces and packed into the disc spaces. The surgeon may obtain additional fusion surface by elevating the periosteum of the vertebral bodies to lay strips of rib across the disc spaces on the surface of the vertebrae (Fig. 8). When a structural graft is needed, such as the replacement of a vertebral body, a tricortical iliac crest graft may be wedged between the remaining vertebral bodies.

Another useful fusion technique is to create a trough in the vertebral bodies with a burr and lay rib graft in the trough. Either whole or half rib segments are wedged into the vertebral slots deep enough so that they are level with the surface of the vertebral bodies.

Pitfalls

Excision of a disc requires a right-angle approach to the disc space. It is difficult to excise a disc when it lies either under the rib margin or below the iliac crest. Whenever possible, the exposure should be wide enough to allow visualization of the depths of the excised disc space. The surgeon should not expect to be able to remove discs that are cephalad to the excised rib. Thus, the tenth rib approach allows exposure of the disc between the tenth and eleventh thoracic vertebrae but not the more cephalad disc spaces.

When many segments of the thoracic spine require anterior

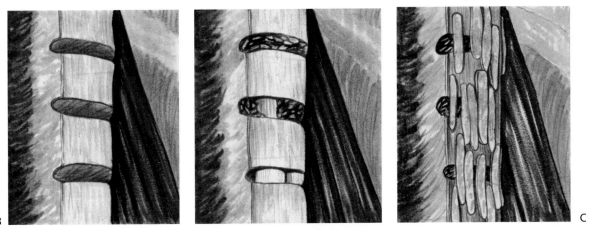

A,B   C

FIGURE 8. A: Disc and annulus have been completely removed. **B:** The rib is cut into 1-cm blocks that are inserted into the disc spaces as bone graft. **C:** Strips of cancellous bone are placed across the vertebral bodies and disc spaces to enhance fusion.

fusion, it may be impossible to excise the discs over the entire curve through a single thoracotomy. When this is the case, a double thoracotomy may be performed (Fig. 9). This may be done through a single skin incision, using a second intercostal incision. The rib is excised at the higher level, and the interspace is incised without rib removal at the lower level to facilitate closure.

The segmental vessels should be doubly ligated with nonab-sorbable suture. Vascular clips should be used with care because they may be pulled during the procedure, resulting in significant hemorrhage. At all times, the surgeon and assistants must guard against injury to any adjacent structures by retractors or other instruments. Cautery should not be used near the vertebral foramen or the lumbar plexus. Even excessive retraction may cause a neurapraxia of the lumbar nerves.

Before closure of the thorax, a chest tube is placed in an

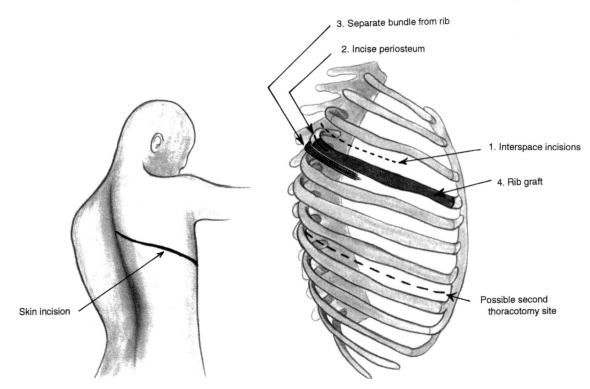

FIGURE 9. A double thoracotomy can usually be performed through a single skin incision placed between the rib levels. After removal of the rib at the first incision, the interspace is opened without rib removal at the second level.

intercostal space several levels above or below the thoracotomy. It should lie in the midaxillary line so that the patient may lie supine without occluding the tube. Tunneling the tube beneath the skin for several centimeters beyond the interspace helps prevent air leakage. The chest tube should be sutured to the skin with a nonabsorbable wrap-around stitch, and all connections should be secured with tape to avoid disconnection or contamination.

Complications

The most dreaded complication of any spinal surgery is paralysis. Fortunately, this complication is rare after anterior fusion. Inadvertent penetration of the dura is a potential hazard that must be avoided. Small, sharp instruments such as fine curets should not be used in the disc spaces. Adequate visualization of the interspace is the best way to minimize the risk of entering the neural canal. Spinal cord monitoring may aid in detection of an injury to the cord. In the event of a direct spinal cord injury, immediate treatment should be considered, including direct cooling of the spinal cord and the use of pharmacologic agents such as dopamine to reduce spinal cord edema (10,25,60). Corticosteroid pretreatment of high-risk patients may raise the threshold for spinal cord injury.

Neurologic dysfunction may also occur as a result of injury to the lumbar plexus. Transient quadriceps weakness after anterior lumbar exposures has been observed, probably representing a neurapraxia caused by retraction of the lumbar plexus. Recovery can occur without treatment.

Lower lumbar exposures may be complicated by injury to the superior hypogastric sympathetic plexus, resulting in retrograde ejaculation in male patients. This may be avoided by carefully protecting this nerve plexus, which usually lies just in front of the third or fourth lumbar vertebra. It has been recommended that vascular clips or ligatures be used instead of cautery to control vessels in the presacral area. Electrocautery may injure the nerve plexus, but bipolar cautery is safer to use if cautery is necessary. Between one fourth and one third of patients with retrograde ejaculation recover normal sexual function over a 6-month to 2-year period (22). Pharmacologic agents may also improve sexual function after such an injury (30,47,61).

A dural leak may occur and is more likely in cases in which there is dural ectasia, as is seen in neurofibromatosis. These leaks usually cease with compression packing and rarely require dural repair.

Other surgical complications, such as hemothorax, pneumothorax, and chylothorax, may occur (17,43). Atelectasis is a common postoperative problem, and aggressive pulmonary physiotherapy in the early postoperative period reduces its incidence (2). Diaphragmatic rupture is also a potential complication, although it is extremely rare with proper suturing techniques. Acute renal obstruction has been reported and was caused by blood clots in the ureter (54). Immediate and delayed ruptures of the spleen have also occurred in anterior spinal procedures (26). These complications are best avoided by taking extreme care with the exposure and retraction of the viscera. If splenic injury is suspected, direct observation of the spleen at the time of surgery is recommended (26).

The development of a pseudarthrosis may complicate any fusion, but the chance of its occurrence is reduced by careful fusion techniques. The diagnosis is confirmed when there is progression of deformity, pain, and radiographic evidence of pseudarthrosis. At times, a disc space may appear unfused in a patient who has no other manifestations of pseudarthrosis, and this finding alone is not an indication for reoperation.

ANTERIOR STRUT GRAFT

Indications

Strut grafting is indicated for kyphotic spinal deformities (35,68). The purpose of the anterior strut is to maintain correction of the kyphotic deformity and to place the bone graft in a compression construct (Fig. 10). The strut graft for a kyphotic deformity should extend from the upper and lower end vertebrae of the kyphosis if possible. Anterior strut grafts are also used to reconstruct the anterior column of the spine after destruction or resection of a vertebral body (40). Vascularized strut grafts have been shown to incorporate into the end vertebrae rapidly and to provide early structural support (11,13,38,40,50,51) (Fig. 11). Nonvascularized strut grafts do not fully incorporate to support the spine for many months. Thus, whenever possible, vascularized graft is preferred.

Contraindications

Strut grafting is contraindicated when a second procedure is planned that would produce enough correction to dislodge the graft. In that case, the strut should be placed after the more corrective posterior procedure. A relative contraindication to the use of a strut graft is a deformity in which the bone is so soft that the graft would likely penetrate the posterior vertebral cortex and enter the neural canal. This can occur in osteogenesis imperfecta because of generalized osteopenia or in neurofibromatosis with dural ectasia.

Advantages and Disadvantages

The strut graft provides the best alternative for stabilizing a kyphotic deformity by placing a compression arthrodesis in the line of axial stress of the spine. Kyphoses are poorly stabilized by posterior fusion alone, and postoperative progression is frequent (39,55,68). The vascularized graft heals rapidly to the vertebrae, and there is no period of creeping substitution in the graft (11,28,38). Nonvascularized grafts must be slowly replaced by new bone before gaining significant strength. The vascularized rib does not require an anastomosis and is thus much simpler to use than a vascularized fibula. The fibula is preferred when great initial strength is required to restore spinal stability (28) (Fig. 12).

The placement of a vascularized rib requires a modest increase in operative time. The interspace is slightly harder to close because the intercostal muscles are taken, but these disadvantages are easily overcome. A vascularized fibula requires a vascular anastomosis, which can be difficult and time-consuming. Also,

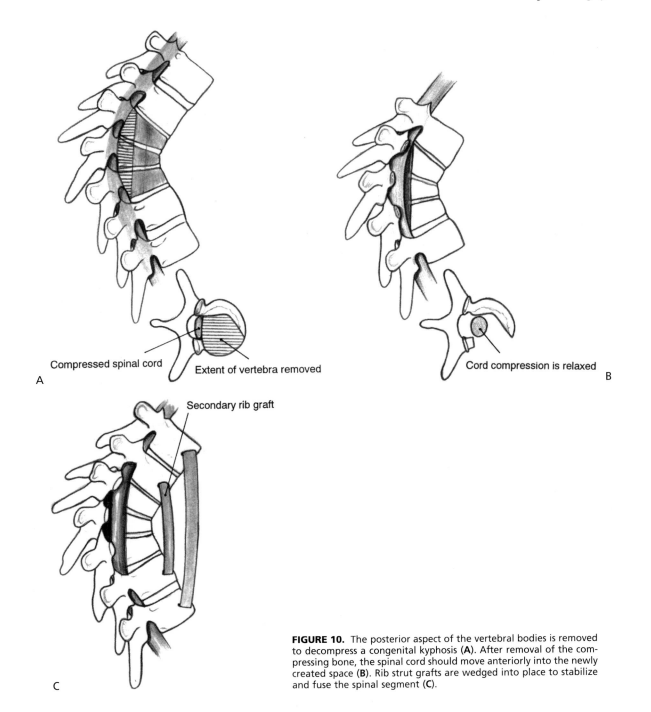

Compressed spinal cord   Extent of vertebra removed

A

Cord compression is relaxed

B

Secondary rib graft

C

FIGURE 10. The posterior aspect of the vertebral bodies is removed to decompress a congenital kyphosis (**A**). After removal of the compressing bone, the spinal cord should move anteriorly into the newly created space (**B**). Rib strut grafts are wedged into place to stabilize and fuse the spinal segment (**C**).

there may be problems with ankle valgus after removal of the fibula; this should be done with caution in growing children.

Techniques

The surgeon should make the thoracotomy over the rib of the upper vertebra to be fused. If the ribs droop excessively, a rib one level higher should be used to improve exposure of the upper vertebra. The rib is excised subperiosteally and removed posteriorly at the level of the costotransverse joint.

To prepare for the strut graft, a canal is made into the body of the end vertebra through the disc space using burrs and curets. The rib or fibula is step-cut at the end to fit into the vertebral cavity under the anterior lip of the body. The strut graft must be keyed into the end vertebra under compression, and the final cut of the strut is the most critical step (Fig. 10). Before the rib graft is shortened to fit the deformity, it is seated at one end while the spine is maximally corrected by external pressure over the apex of the kyphosis. The graft is marked for length and is shortened somewhat less than marked. Maximal correction is applied again, and the graft should just seat into the vertebral bodies. When the external pressure is released, the graft should

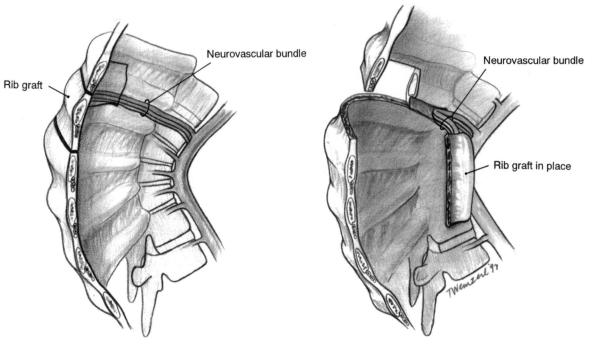

A

B

FIGURE 11. Vascularized rib strut graft. The neurovascular bundle is separated from the rib proximal to the angle of the rib so that the rib may be transected. Usually, the rib chosen corresponds to the upper vertebra to be fused. For fusions above the fourth thoracic vertebra, the rib graft may be reversed (**A**). When the rib is seated, the vascular pedicle should not be kinked or occluded. The ends of the rib should be exposed over a 1-cm segment that is inserted into the vertebral body (**B**).

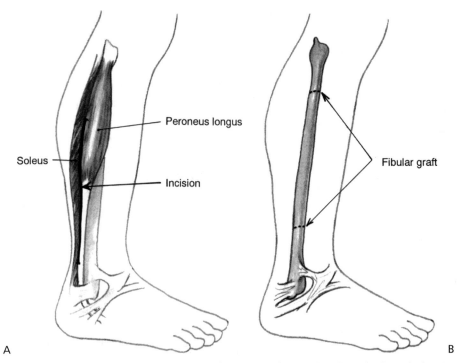

A

B

FIGURE 12. Fibula graft. When the fibula is used for a strut graft, it is taken through a lateral subperiosteal approach (**A**). The distal one fourth of the fibula should be left intact for ankle stability (**B**).

not be removable. Smaller struts may be placed beneath the primary graft and should be placed before seating it.

If a vascularized rib is to be used, the choice of levels is even more specific (Fig. 11). For a kyphosis with its apex between T2 and T5, a rib two or three segments below the apex of the kyphosis is chosen. This rib is then rotated proximally on its vascular pedicle. When the apex is below T6, it is preferable to use the rib of the proximal vertebra into which the graft will be placed. That rib is then rotated distally across the kyphosis.

The thoracotomy for a vascularized rib is performed by incising the intercostal muscles above and below the rib (Fig. 11). The incision caudal to the rib must be as far away from the rib as possible to avoid injury to the intercostal vessels. After the intercostals are incised, a chest retractor is placed so that the vasculature to the rib may be visualized. The neurovascular bundle is dissected away from the rib proximal to the angle of the rib so that the base of the rib may be transected. The distal end of the rib may then be transected. The vessels at the distal end should be ligated. The periosteum may be peeled back about 1 cm at each end of the rib to allow seating.

During the exposure of the spine, the surgeon must not ligate the segmental vessels at the level of the vascularized rib because this would devascularize the rib. Otherwise, the discs are removed and the fusion performed as previously described. As the rib is rotated into position, the surgeon must avoid twisting the vascular pedicle. After insertion of the rib, the vascularity of the graft should be assessed by incising the intercostal muscle. If the muscle fails to bleed, the surgeon must evaluate the course of the segmental vessel to exclude kinking and external occlusion.

Pitfalls

Dislodgment of the strut graft is a major pitfall that is best prevented by ensuring that the graft is keyed in place under maximum compression. If the graft is overshortened, there is little recourse other than to take a longer graft using another rib. Inadvertent ligation, compression, or kinking of the segmental vessels that supply the vascularized rib must be avoided. If the vascularized rib loses its blood supply, the surgeon will have little choice other than to use the rib as an avascular graft. Removal of another rib and intercostal space is usually not an option because the gap in the thorax would be impossible to close. An alternative would be to use a vascularized fibula.

Complications

The complications of strut grafting are much the same as the pitfalls. Cast immobilization is usually necessary to protect a strut graft from dislodgment unless the spine has been instrumented posteriorly. When the vertebral bone is soft or when the posterior vertebral cortex is perforated, it is possible for the graft to intrude into the neural canal. This is best avoided by carefully preserving the posterior vertebral cortex as the graft is inserted. Late progression of the deformity may happen if the strut grafts resorb and collapse. This is less likely to occur with a vascularized graft.

ANTERIOR HEMIEPIPHYSIODESIS AND HEMIARTHRODESIS

Indications

The goal of an anterior hemiarthrodesis is ablation of growth on the convexity of a scoliosis in a young patient while maintaining growth on the concavity of the deformity (3,66,67) (Fig. 13). This allows gradual straightening of the deformity as the spine grows. To be successful, the anterior hemiarthrodesis must usually be combined with a posterior hemiarthrodesis and some form of instrumentation. Young patients with progressive infantile and juvenile scolioses are candidates for this procedure. The etiology of these deformities may be idiopathic, or they may be associated with another diagnosis such as syringomyelia, spinal cord tethering, or neurofibromatosis. In addition, some patients with congenital scoliosis are candidates for this procedure. In several series, the procedure was shown to be likely to succeed if the spinal deformity is not severe, there is no kyphosis, and the patient is young (less than 5 or 6 years old) (3,66,67). Treatment of scoliosis due to a hemivertebra is successful when the patient is 5 years old or younger, the curve is less than 70 degrees, the curve involves five or fewer segments, and there is no significant kyphosis (67). When there is a congenital bar, the involved segment lacks growth potential, and this procedure will fail. Keller and associates have reported performing anterior hemiepiphysiodesis through a transpedicular approach (31). In their se-

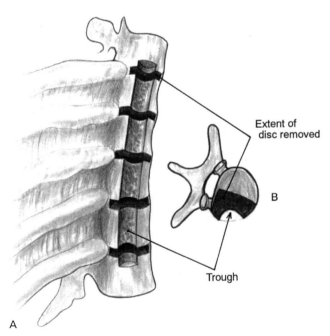

FIGURE 13. Anterior hemiepiphysiodesis. Half of the intervertebral disc and end plate is excised to produce a partial growth arrest and an intervertebral fusion (**A**). A burr is used to make a trough in the vertebral bodies so that rib graft may be placed across the interspaces. The rib should be inserted about 1 cm deep into the vertebral bodies (**B**).

ries, as in others, a fusion was achieved but true hemiepiphysiodesis occurred rarely. I have no experience with this technique.

Contraindications

The major contraindications to this procedure are kyphotic deformities and deformities greater than 70 or 80 degrees. Although the exact upper age limit has not been determined, children older than 5 or 6 years of age usually do not have significant improvement after this procedure (3,66,67). In these situations, progression of the deformity overshadows the possible benefits of growth on the concavity of the curve.

Advantages and Disadvantages

The major advantage of an anterior hemiepiphysiodesis is that the spine may continue to grow, allowing for gradual correction of the deformity. The thorax and spine may be expected to have better growth potential with this procedure than with an early circumferential fusion.

The most common disadvantage is that the procedure may be partially successful, with slowing of the progression of the deformity, or it may fail completely. The procedure is not effective for large deformities, for kyphotic deformities, or for older children. Another disadvantage is that even though the frontal plane correction appears to be well maintained, there may be continued rotatory deformity as the spine grows. This may occur as a variation of the crankshaft phenomenon (19,62).

Another major disadvantage is that the spine must be protected in a brace or cast while it is growing to avoid loss of fixation of the posterior instrumentation. Long-term wear of an orthosis may cause gradual rib deformity, resulting in a disproportionately small thorax. Another disadvantage is that these children usually require revision procedures to lengthen or reinsert posterior instrumentation. Some require spinal fusion as they approach maturity.

Techniques

In performing a hemiepiphysiodesis, the vertebrae are exposed through a transthoracic approach, and the segmental vessels are ligated. Between one third and one half of each disc is excised with rongeurs (3,66) (Fig. 13). In this same area, the cartilaginous end plate is excised. At least one third but not more than one half of the vertebral end plate should be excised (67). To achieve a fusion, the convex halves of the vertebral bodies are exposed subperiosteally. A trough is cut into the adjacent vertebral bodies, and a rib graft is inserted deeply into the trough, crossing the disc space.

To perform the posterior portion of the fusion, only the convex half of the spine is exposed. A standard arthrodesis is performed on that portion of the spine, including facetectomy, decortication, and placement of autologous bone graft. If instrumentation is used, it should be easily revisable for lengthening and later fusion procedures. For this reason, instrumentation with removable hooks is preferable to sublaminar wire techniques. Some concave exposure is necessary to perform instru-

mentation, but this should be limited to only the hook sites. In earlier techniques, hooks were placed only at the ends of the major curve, and gradual loss of fixation was common. We now prefer to use a four-hook pattern with two intermediate hooks and two end hooks. Some rotational correction is performed as well as distraction. The rods should be carefully contoured to the sagittal spinal curvature.

Pitfalls

The most common pitfall is not achieving an arthrodesis, which may be due to an inadequate fusion technique. It is also possible to fuse so much of the disc space that there will be no further growth at that level.

Complications

Loss of instrument fixation is a common complication. Even while the patient is wearing an orthosis, there is movement of the instrumentation at the sites of attachment to the spine. Hooks may gradually erode the soft, immature bone of the lamina and become dislodged. Repetitive cyclic loading of the implant may cause the hooks to disconnect from the rod or the rod to fracture. Each of these complications is corrected by reinstrumentation. Unfortunately, when there has been lamina fracture, it may be necessary to add one or two levels to the initial construct.

COSTOTRANSVERSECTOMY
Indications

Costotransversectomy is a useful approach to the spine when the main objective is decompression of the spinal canal (Fig. 14). Spinal cord compression due to congenital kyphosis or neurofibromatosis kyphosis may be relieved through the costotransverse approach. When there is a severe kyphosis, the costotransverse approach to the spinal cord is more direct than an anterior approach because the apex of a severe kyphosis is so far posterior that it is hard to reach from an anterior transthoracic approach. A costotransversectomy of several apical levels provides a direct approach to the area of maximal cord compression and greatly simplifies decompressive procedures.

Costotransversectomy is a time-honored approach for decompression of spinal column infections (1,21). This approach may also be used to perform anterior fusion when the spine is so severely rotated that the vertebrae lie beneath the angles of the ribs.

Contraindications

There is not sufficient access to the anterior spine through a costotransversectomy to perform a strut graft. Thus, if such a graft is necessary, a secondary thoracotomy is required.

Advantages and Disadvantages

The major advantage is the ease of spinal cord decompression. Our neurosurgical colleagues find that this approach provides

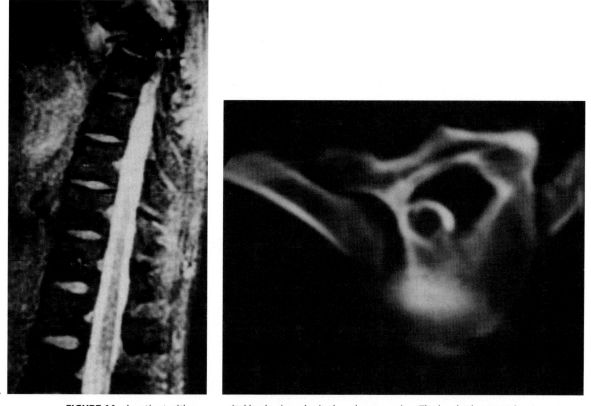

A   B

FIGURE 14. A patient with a congenital kyphosis and spinal cord compression. The boy had progressive leg weakness and pyramidal tract findings. **A:** A preoperative lateral magnetic resonance imaging scan showing marked spinal cord compression by a kyphosis at the third thoracic level. **B:** A computed tomographic myelogram showing that the spinal cord is maximally compressed by the pedicle and posterior vertebral body. Note the proximity of the base of the third rib. A decompression is optimally performed by excising the base of the rib, after which the transverse process and pedicle may be excised. This may be done at several adjacent levels. This patient had complete recovery after decompression and fusion.

excellent access for use of a microscope. The more severe the kyphotic deformity, the better the access through this approach and the worse the access directly anteriorly. Another advantage is that a posterior approach to the spine may be done through the same skin incision.

A disadvantage of the costotransversectomy is that it is impossible to place a strut graft through this approach. Only an interdiscal fusion can be performed. Another disadvantage is that the intercostal neurovascular bundle is ligated at several levels, producing areas of anesthesia over the thorax.

Techniques

The apical vertebra is located, and a longitudinal incision is placed just medial to the angle of the rib (Fig. 15). This area can be reached from a midline skin incision by elevating a flap of skin and subcutaneous tissue over the ribs. This is useful when the spine will also be exposed posteriorly. The overlying muscles are divided longitudinally, and the rib is exposed by subperiosteal dissection (Fig. 15). The costotransverse junction is exposed, and the rib is transected. The intercostal neurovascular bundle is separated from the rib and ligated. The retropleural space is dissected bluntly, taking care not to enter the pleura. The rib

is removed from its connections with the transverse process and also with the vertebral body. The vertebral body can now be exposed by enlarging the retropleural space. The segmental vessels can be ligated as they cross the vertebral body. Several ribs can be taken if wider exposure is required.

The spinal canal is exposed by excision of the transverse process and the pedicle. Several adjacent levels can be exposed in a similar fashion. The portion of the vertebral body producing cord compression is easily visualized and removed with rongeurs and burrs. An osteotomy across vertebral bodies or previous fusion masses can also be performed at this stage of the procedure.

Pitfalls

Occasionally, inadequate exposure is obtained through the initial rib excision. The exposure may be extended by taking adjacent ribs when necessary.

Complications

An inadvertent entry to the pleural space may create a pneumothorax or a hemothorax, which requires the placement of a chest

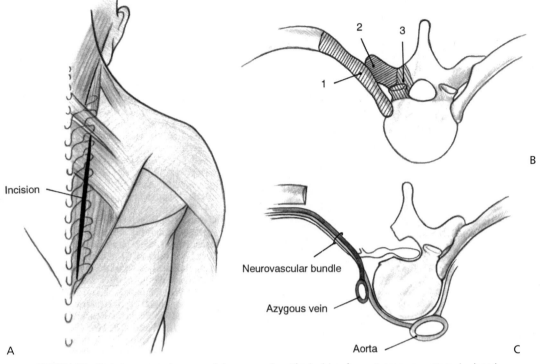

FIGURE 15. Costotransversectomy canal decompression. The incision for costotransversectomy is placed just lateral to the midline, over the costotransverse junction (**A**). This area may also be reached by dissecting laterally from a midline approach. The plane of dissection is between the subcutaneous tissue and the erector spinae muscles. The base of the rib *(1)* and its junction with the transverse process *(2)* are approached subperiosteally and excised (**B**). The neurovascular bundle and the pedicle *(3)* may be excised to expose the dura (**C**).

tube. Numbness over the intercostal distribution is common but usually well tolerated.

REFERENCES

1. Alici E (1989): *The treatment of tuberculosis of the spine.* Presented at the 24th annual meeting of the Scoliosis Research Society, Amsterdam.
2. Anderson PR, Puno MR, Lovell SL (1985): Postoperative respiratory complications in non-idiopathic scoliosis. *Acta Anaesthesiol Scand* 29: 186–192.
3. Andrew T, Piggott H (1985): Growth arrest for progressive scoliosis: combined anterior and posterior fusion. *J Bone Joint Surg Br* 67: 193–197.
4. Apel DM, Marrero G, King J, et al. (1991): Avoiding paraplegia during anterior spinal surgery: the role of somatosensory evoked potential monitoring with temporary occlusion of segmental spinal arteries. *Spine* 16[Suppl 8]:S365–S370.
5. Banta JV (1989): *Combined anterior and posterior fusion for spinal deformity in myelomeningocele.* Presented at the 24th annual meeting of the Scoliosis Research Society, Amsterdam.
6. Bednar DA, Brox WT, Viviani GR (1991): Surgical palliation of spinal oncologic disease: a review and analysis of current approaches. *Can J Surg* 34:129–131.
7. Bergoin M, Bollini G, Gennari JM (1989): *One stage hemivertebral excision and arthrodesis for congenital scoliosis in infants.* Presented at the 24th annual meeting of the Scoliosis Research Society, Amsterdam.
8. Betz RR, Iorio R, Lombardi AV, et al. (1989): Scoliosis surgery in neurofibromatosis. *Clin Orthop* 245:53–56.
9. Boachi-Adjei O, Lonstein JE, Winter RB, et al. (1989): Management of neuromuscular spinal deformities with Luque segmental instrumentation. *J Bone Joint Surg Am* 71:548–562.
10. Bracken MB, Shepard WF, Holford TR, et al. (1990): A randomized controlled trial of methylprednisolone or naloxone in the treatment of acute spinal cord injuries. *N Engl J Med* 322:1405–1461.
11. Bradford DS (1980): Anterior vascular pedicle bone grafting for the treatment of kyphosis. *Spine* 5:318.
12. Bradford DS, Ahmed KB, Moe JH (1980): The surgical management of patients with Scheuermann's disease: a review of twenty-four cases managed by combined anterior and posterior spine fusion. *J Bone Joint Surg Am* 62:705–712.
13. Bradford DS, Daher YH (1986): Vascularized rib grafts for stabilization of kyphosis. *J Bone Joint Surg Br* 68:357.
14. Cambridge W, Drennan JC (1987): Scoliosis associated with Duchenne muscular dystrophy. *J Pediatr Orthop* 7:436–440.
15. Carstens C, Paul K, Niethard FU, et al. (1991): Effect of scoliosis surgery on pulmonary function in patients with myelomeningocele. *J Pediatr Orthop* 11:459–464.
16. Chakirgil GS (1991): Evaluation of anterior spinal fusion for treatment of vertebral tuberculosis. *Orthopedics* 14:601–607.
17. Colletta AJ, Mayer PJ (1982): Chylothorax: an unusual complication of anterior thoracic interbody spinal fusion. *Spine* 7:46–49.
18. Dimeglio A, Bonnel F (1990): *Le rachis en croissance.* Paris: Springer-Verlag.
19. Dubousset J, Herring JA, Shufflebarger H (1989): The crankshaft phenomenon. *J Pediatr Orthop* 9:541–550.
20. Emery SE, Chan DP, Woodward HR (1989): Treatment of hematogenous pyogenic vertebral osteomyelitis with anterior debridement and primary bone grafting. *Spine* 14:284–291.
21. Floman Y, Liebergall M, Chaimsky G, et al. (1989): *Pyogenic spondylitis with neurologic involvement.* Presented at the 24th annual meeting of the Scoliosis Research Society, Amsterdam.
22. Flynn JC, Price CT (1984): Sexual complications of anterior fusion of the lumbar spine. *Spine* 9:489–492.

23. Gibson DA, Winlins KE (1975): The management of spinal deformities in Duchenne muscular dystrophy. *Clin Orthop* 108:41–51.

24. Grimm JO, Bui V, Shufflebarger HL (1989): *Anterior and posterior spinal fusion: staged versus same day surgery.* Presented at the 24th annual meeting of the Scoliosis Research Society, Amsterdam.

25. Hasenbout RR, Tanner JA, Romero-Sietta C (1984): Current status of spinal cord cooling in the treatment of acute spinal cord injury. *Spine* 9:508–511.

26. Hodge WA, DeWald RL (1983): Splenic injury complicating the anterior thoracoabdominal surgical approach for scoliosis. *J Bone Joint Surg Am* 65:396–397.

27. Hsu LC, Cheng CL, Leong JC (1988): Pott's paraplegia of late onset: the cause of compression and results after anterior decompression. *J Bone Joint Surg Br* 70:534–538.

28. Hubbard LF, Herndon JH, Bounanno AR (1985): Free vascularized fibula transfer for stabilization of the thoracolumbar spine: a case report. *Spine* 10:891–893.

29. Jewell L (1978): The pathophysiology of spinal cord trauma. Springfield, IL: Charles C. Thomas.

30. Johnson RM, McGuire EJ (1981): Urogenital complications of anterior approaches to the lumbar spine. *Clin Orthop* 154:114–118.

31. Keller PM, Lindseth RE, DeRosa GP (1994): Progressive congenital scoliosis treatment using a transpedicular anterior and posterior convex hemiepiphysiodesis and hemiarthrodesis. *Spine* 19(17):1933–1939.

32. Korkusuz Z, Binnet MS, Isiklar ZU (1989): Pott's disease and extrapleural anterior decompression: results of 108 consecutive cases. *Arch Orthop Trauma Surg* 108:349–352.

33. Kurz LT, Mubarak SJ, Schulz P, et al. (1983): Correlation of scoliosis and pulmonary function in Duchenne muscular dystrophy. *J Pediatr Orthop* 3:347–353.

34. Lapinski AS, Richards BS (1995): Preventing the crankshaft phenomenon by combining anterior fusion with posterior instrumentation: does it work? *Spine* 20(12):1392–1398.

35. Laurain JM, Onimus M, Fiore N (1989): *Biomechanical aspects of anterior spinal reconstruction.* Presented at the 24th annual meeting of the Scoliosis Research Society, Amsterdam.

36. Little DG, Song KM, Katz D, et al. (1995): *Use of peak growth age in idiopathic scoliosis.* Presented at the 30th annual meeting of the Scoliosis Research Society, Ashville, NC.

37. Lonstein JE, Winter RB, Moe JH, et al. (1980): Neurologic deficits secondary to spinal deformity: a review of the literature and report of 43 cases. *Spine* 5:331–335.

38. Louw JA (1990): Spinal tuberculosis with neurological deficit: treatment with anterior vascularized rib grafts, posterior osteotomies and fusion. *J Bone Joint Surg Br* 72:686–693.

39. Lowe TG (1987): Double L-rod instrumentation in the treatment of severe kyphosis secondary to Scheuermann's disease. *Spine* 12:336–341.

40. McBride GG, Bradford DS (1983): Vertebral body replacement with femoral neck allograft and vascularized rib strut graft: a technique for treatment of post-traumatic kyphosis with neurologic deficit. *Spine* 8:406.

41. McMaster MJ (1987): Anterior and posterior instrumentation and fusion of thoracolumbar scoliosis due to myelomeningocele. *J Bone Joint Surg Br* 69:20–25.

42. Mandelbaum MD, Tolo VT, McAfee PC, et al. (1988): Nutritional deficiencies after staged anterior and posterior spinal reconstructive surgery. *Clin Orthop* 234:5–11.

43. Nakai S, Zielke K (1986): Chylothorax: a rare complication after anterior and posterior spinal correction. Report on six cases. *Spine* 11:830–833.

44. Omari B, Robertson JM, Nelson RJ, et al. (1989): Pott's disease: a resurgent challenge to the thoracic surgeon. *Chest* 95:145–150.

45. Rajasekaran S, Soundarapandian S (1989): Progression of kyphosis in tuberculosis of the spine treated by anterior arthrodesis. *J Bone Joint Surg Am* 71:1314–1323.

46. Rinsky LA (1990): Surgery of spinal deformity in cerebral palsy: twelve years in the evolution of scoliosis management. *Clin Orthop* 253:100–109.

47. Sacks S (1966): Anterior interbody fusion of the lumbar spine. *Clin Orthop* 44:163–170.

48. Sanders JO, Herring JA, Browne RH (1995): Posterior arthrodesis and instrumentation in the immature (Risser-grade-0) spine in idiopathic scoliosis. *J Bone Joint Surg Am* 77:39–45.

49. Savini R, Cervellati S, Bettini N, et al. (1991): Surgical treatment of vertebral deformity due to myelomeningocele. *Ital J Orthop Traumatol* 17:55–63.

50. Schaberg SJ, Petri WH, Gregory EW, et al. (1985): A comparison of freeze-dried allogenic and fresh autologous vascularized rib grafts in dog radial discontinuity defects. *J Oral Maxillofac Surg* 43:932–937.

51. Shaffer JW, Davy DT, Field GA (1988): The superiority of vascularized compared to nonvascularized rib grafts in spine surgery shown by biological and physical methods. *Spine* 13:1150.

52. Shufflebarger HL, Clark CE (1990): *Prevention of the crankshaft phenomenon.* Presented at the 25th annual meeting of the Scoliosis Research Society, Honolulu.

53. Shufflebarger HL, Grimm JO, Bui V, et al. (1991): Anterior and posterior spinal fusion: staged versus same day surgery. *Spine* 16:930.

54. Slawshi DP, Bridwell KH, Manley CB (1990): Acute renal obstruction after combined anterior and posterior arthrodesis on the convex side of the spine. *J Bone Joint Surg Am* 72:1259–1261.

55. Speck GR, Chopin DC (1986): The surgical treatment of Scheuermann's kyphosis. *J Bone Joint Surg Br* 68:189–193.

56. Sponseller PD, Wiffen JR, Drummon DS (1986): Interspinous process segmental spinal instrumentation for scoliosis in cerebral palsy. *J Pediatr Orthop* 6:559–563.

57. Swank SM, Cohen DS, Brown JC (1989): Spine fusion in cerebral palsy with L-rod segmental spinal instrumentation: a comparison of single and two-stage combined approach with Zielke instrumentation. *Spine* 14:750–759.

58. Sundaresan N, Shah J, Feshali JG (1984): A transsternal approach to the upper thoracic vertebrae. *Am J Surg* 148:473–477.

59. Sundaresan N, Shah J, Foley KM, et al. (1984): An anterior surgical approach to the upper thoracic vertebrae. *J Neurosurg* 61:686–690.

60. Tator CH, Fehlings MG (1991): Review of the secondary injury theory of acute spinal cord trauma with emphasis on vascular mechanisms. *J Neurosurg* 75:15–26.

61. Taylor TKF (1970): Anterior interbody fusion in the management of disorders of the lumbar spine. *J Bone Joint Surg Br* 52:784.

62. Terek RM, Wehner J, Lubicky JP (1991): Crankshaft phenomenon in congenital scoliosis: a preliminary report. *J Pediatr Orthop* 11:527–532.

63. Trammell TR, Benedict F, Reed D (1991): Anterior spine fusion using Zielke instrumentation for adult thoracolumbar and lumbar scoliosis. *Spine* 16:307–316.

64. van der Heijden KWAP, van Ooy A, Slot GH, et al. (1989): *Operative treatment of Scheuermann's kyphosis.* Presented at the 24th annual meeting of the Scoliosis Research Society, Amsterdam.

65. Ward WT, Wenger DR, Roach JW (1989): Surgical correction of myelomeningocele scoliosis: a critical appraisal of various spinal instrumentation systems. *J Pediatr Orthop* 9:262–268.

66. Winter RB (1981): Convex anterior and posterior hemiarthrodesis and hemiepiphysiodesis in young children with progressive congenital scoliosis. *J Pediatr Orthop* 1:361–366.

67. Winter RB, Lonstein JE, Denis F, et al. (1988): Convex growth arrest for progressive congenital scoliosis due to hemivertebrae. *J Pediatr Orthop* 8:633–638.

68. Winter RB, Moe JH, Lonstein JE (1985): Congenital kyphosis: a review of 94 patients age 5 years or older with 2 years or more follow-up in 77 patients. *Spine* 10:224–235.

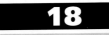

VERTEBRECTOMY AND SPINAL CORD DECOMPRESSION

NORBERT BOOS
KAN MIN

Spinal cord compression in children is an infrequent finding and in most cases is related to spinal trauma or tumor. The principles of treatment are the same as in adult patients. However, surgical treatment of traumatic and tumorous spinal cord compression must take into account that the spine is immature and still growing. Therefore, iatrogenic spinal deformity must be avoided.

Progressive severe spinal deformities may also rarely cause spinal cord compromise by a distortion of the spinal canal (30). In those patients, who often present with severe congenital or idiopathic scoliosis, the compromise occurs at the concavity of the curve. Similarly, severe kyphotic deformity may also lead to a compromise at the apex of the curvature. In these cases, decompression of the spinal cord is achieved by vertebrectomy, often in conjunction with a corrective osteotomy. MacLennan (33) was the first to describe vertebral body resection in 1922. Since that time, several authors have reported on vertebrectomy for spinal cord decompression (4,24), and it has become a standard surgical technique in spinal surgery (4,7,21,29,39). It is obvious that such a procedure, particularly in children, is technically demanding and hazardous and should only be done by an experienced spine surgeon. However, the risks associated with this surgical procedure can be significant with the use of intraoperative spinal cord monitoring. Rigid internal fixation today allows mobilization of patients in the immediate postoperative period.

This chapter reviews the literature on vertebrectomy and spinal cord decompression in children and provides some technical hints in performing these technically demanding procedures.

FRACTURES

Spinal fractures associated with neurologic deficits are infrequent in children and range from 2% to 5% of all cases admitted to specialized paraplegic centers, depending on whether the upper age is set at 10 or 15 years (16). Of 4,470 patients admitted to the National Spinal Injuries Center, 29 patients younger than

14 years of age had traumatic paraplegia between the years 1948 and 1969 (35). Hubbard (23) reported on 42 consecutive children and adolescents treated at the Children's Orthopedic Hospital and Medical Center in Seattle, Washington for a spinal injury between 1955 and 1971. Six of the 42 patients suffered from a concomitant spinal cord injury (four complete and two incomplete paraplegia or quadriplegia).

In neonates and infants, the cervical spine is more frequently affected, whereas in adolescents, the trauma is more often located in the thoracic and lumbar spine (18). Yngve and associates (40) reported that patients with spinal cord injury with osseous spine fracture (mean age, 16 years) are usually older than those without osseous injury (mean age, 6 years). Because patients with bony spinal injuries are usually older, their fracture pattern resembles that of an adult population. Therefore, treatment recommendations are similar to those developed for adults but have to take into account that the spine is still growing.

Spinal cord compression without neurologic deficit does not necessarily require a surgical decompression because remodeling of the spinal canal can be expected (15), and conservative treatment of incomplete burst fractures has been reported with satisfactory results in adults (36). However, compound fractures, dislocations, and fracture-dislocations compromising the growth plate necessitate an anatomic reduction and stable fixation to avoid growth disturbances such as progressive scoliosis and kyphosis originating from unreduced fractures (25). Incomplete quadriparesis or paraparesis due to anterior canal encroachment requires emergency decompression of the spinal cord by the anterior approach, similarly to adult spinal fractures (4,22,26). Laminectomy without fusion to decompress the spinal cord has been reported to result in pain and progressive kyphosis and is therefore not advised (34). After decompression of the cord by partial vertebrectomy, the anterior column should be reconstructed with a tricortical iliac bone graft. Technical details of anterior cord decompression are depicted in Figure 1. Postoperative management requires cast fixation until fusion has occurred. Depending on the age of the patient, posterior instrumentation can be considered to facilitate postoperative treatment. In adolescent patients, plate fixation of the cervical spine (Fig. 2) or a short segmental pedicle screw fixation of the thoracolumbar spine allows early mobilization of the patient without cumbersome external support.

N. Boos and K. Min: Orthopedic University Hospital Balgrist, Zurich, Switzerland.

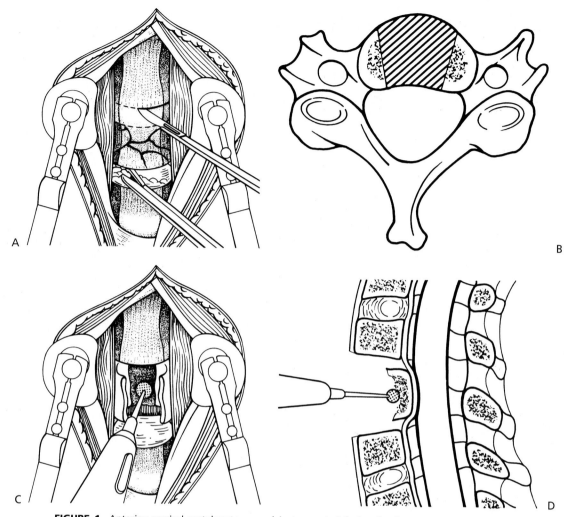

FIGURE 1. Anterior cervical vertebrectomy and instrumented fusion for fractures with spinal cord compression. **A:** The fractured vertebral body and the two adjacent intervertebral discs are exposed by a standard anterolateral approach. The discs are then incised with a knife, and the disc material is resected with a fine rongeur. **B:** Schematic drawing of the part of the vertebral body that is to be removed; the lateral vertebral wall remains intact to protect the vertebral arteries. **C:** After disc excision, the vertebral body is resected with a high-speed air drill up to the posterior wall, which is still left intact. **D:** Lateral view. While drilling to the posterior vertebral wall, great care must be taken not to press loose fragments into the spinal canal. *(Figure continues.)*

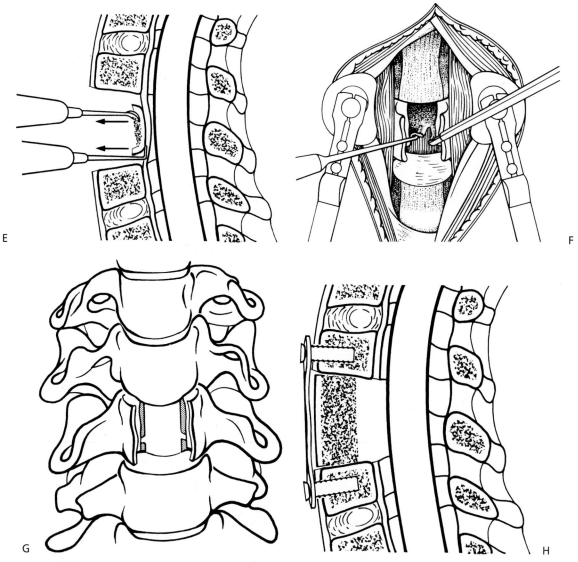

FIGURE 1. *Continued.* **E:** Alternatively, a curette can be used to resect the cancellous part of the verte-bral body. When only a thin cortical layer of the vertebral wall is left, the posterior wall is lifted off the posterior longitudinal ligament with a dissecting hook. **F:** While lifting the posterior vertebral wall, it can be resected in a piecemeal fashion with a Kerrison rongeur. Similarly, the posterior longitudinal ligament is resected. **G:** The posterior longitudinal ligament should be resected to ensure that spinal cord decompression is complete. View after partial vertebrectomy and exposure of the dura. **H:** After removal of the vertebral end plate cartilage of the adjacent vertebral bodies, a tricortical iliac (horseshoe) bone graft is press-fitted, and the affected segments are stabilized with a plate (refer to Fig. 2).

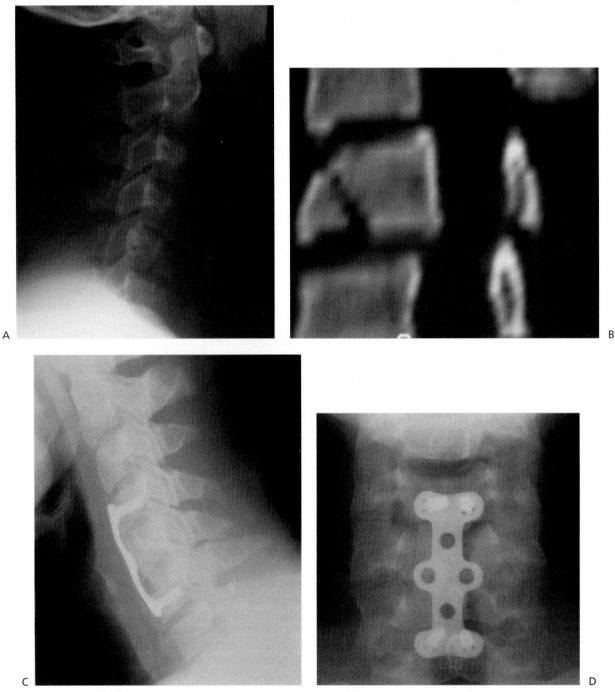

FIGURE 2. This 16-year-old boy sustained an incomplete quadriparesis below C5 subsequent to a diving accident. **A:** Lateral radiograph showing a teardrop fracture of C5. **B:** Computed tomography reconstruction demonstrating the posterior dislocation of the vertebral body. **C:** Lateral postoperative radiograph. Partial vertebrectomy, spinal cord decompression, reconstruction of the anterior vertebral column, and plate fixation were performed according to the technique describe in Fig. 1. **D:** Anteroposterior postoperative radiograph. Three months after surgery, the patient has completely recovered from his neurologic injury.

spinal deformity was mentioned, 68% of patients had kyphoscoliosis, 17% had kyphosis, and 15% had scoliosis, with 81% of the deformities occurring in the thoracic spine. A paraplegia was encountered in 49% and a paralysis in 41%.

A large variety of treatment modalities were employed. Most of the patients (32%) underwent laminectomy. In 26% of cases, treatment consisted of a nonoperative curve correction by bed rest, traction, or application of a cast, corset, or brace, followed by a posterior arthrodesis after neurologic improvement had occurred. Thirteen percent of patients underwent a Hyndman-Schneider radical posterior decompression (24,38), 13% had a Capener posterolateral rhachotomy (12), and only 2% were treated by an anterior transthoracic cord decompression (20). In only 77 cases, a follow-up was mentioned averaging 2.8 years. When each treatment group was analyzed, 89% of patients who underwent curve correction showed improvement, whereas 87% who underwent Hyndman-Schneider decompression and 69% who had a laminectomy had neurologic improvement. However, the authors have emphasized that these figures may be misleading because they refer to only 77 of 282 patients.

The same authors (30) provided the largest series (43 patients) to date on cord compression as result of untreated spinal deformities, reinforcing the findings of their literature review. The main causes were congenital deformity in 17 patients, previously treated inactive tuberculosis in seven, and neurofibromatosis in six. A kyphotic deformity averaging 95 degrees (range, 50 to 180 degrees) was present in all but one patient. The deformities were noted in most patients at a young age but remained untreated. With progression of the kyphosis, presentation of the cord compression occurred an average of 13 years later. The complication was more common in male patients, in the presence of thoracic deformities, and in the second decade of life. Treatment consisted of anterior spinal cord decompression in 25 patients, laminectomy in ten, Capener decompression in six, correction and fusion in five, and Hyndman-Schneider decompression in three. The authors made a strong argument against laminectomy because the compression is anterior and a simple posterior decompression does not remove the cause of the spinal cord compression. Furthermore, a laminectomy desta-

bilizes the spine, and the kyphosis will increase. In their series, six of the ten patients who underwent laminectomy deteriorated. The best statistical results occurred in a small group of patients (*n* = 5) who had mild paraparesis and a flexible kyphosis that corrected with gentle, controlled traction and were subsequently treated by posterior fusion. As the treatment of choice for more significant neurologic deficits, the authors recommend anterior spinal cord decompression by direct removal of the compression followed by anterior and posterior fusion.

Idiopathic Scoliosis

In children with idiopathic scoliosis, the curves are commonly still flexible, and correction can be achieved by posterior instrumentation with or without anterior release. Neurologic deficits in juvenile or adolescent scoliosis prompts the search for an underlying intraspinal pathology. However, the routine use of spinal cord monitoring has indicated that patients with severe curves often show subtle abnormalities of the spinal cord function. In severe curves, the spinal cord is located along the concavity of the deformity because it occupies the shortest route in the spinal canal. Such curves may therefore lead to spinal cord compromise as a result of an impingement with the pedicles and the costotransversal joints and consecutively cause a spinal cord distortion (Fig. 4). We sometimes observe slightly delayed somatosensory evoked potentials (SSEPs) at the side of the concavity of curves measuring more than 70 to 80 degrees. The clinical significance of such minor alterations as a risk factor for future myelopathy still needs to be explored. In our clinical practice, we recommend curve correction in patients presenting with a distorted cord, particularly in light of the risk for further curve progression.

Decompression of the spinal cord is achieved indirectly by a correction of the curvature. This is performed by anterior release and posterior instrumentation using pedicle screw fixation in conjunction with a combined anterior and posterior fusion. Spinal cord monitoring often normalizes during surgery or shortly after surgery.

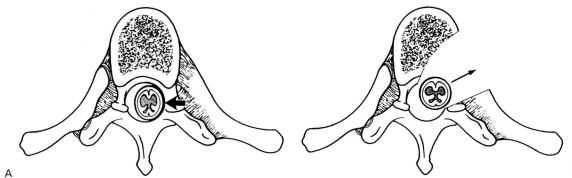

A   B

FIGURE 4. Spinal cord compression in severe scoliosis. **A:** In severe scoliosis, the spinal cord is located along the concavity of the deformity. Spinal cord compromise results from an impingement with the pedicles and the costotransversal joints and consecutively causes a spinal cord distortion. **B:** Decompression of the spinal cord is achieved by partial anterolateral vertebrectomy and resection of the impinging pedicles and costotransversal joints.

Kyphosis

Surgery is only rarely needed in patients with juvenile kyphosis (i.e., Scheuermann kyphosis). Lowe (31) has recommended surgery only for patients with back pain unresponsive to nonoperative treatment and curves measuring more than 75 degrees. Although they are rare, severe progressive curves (more than 90 degrees) may lead to spinal cord compromise because the cord is stretched over the posterior aspect of the vertebral bodies, taking the shortest route across the deformity (Fig. 5). Lonstein and associates (30) reviewed the cases of the Twin Cities Scoliosis Center (1938 to 1974) with neurologic deficits secondary to untreated spinal deformity. They reported only two cases with Scheuermann kyphosis that presented with a neurologic deficit, indicating that significant spinal cord compression is rare in

this disease. SSEPs, however, now routinely used in deformity surgery, have indicated that patients with severe kyphosis demonstrate abnormalities as a result of the kyphosis related to spinal cord distortion. Treatment in those patients is performed by curve correction after anterior release and posterior instrumentation in conjunction with combined anterior and posterior fusion (Fig. 6). Anterior and posterior osteotomy may sometimes be necessary to correct the curve, whereas vertebrectomy is hardly ever needed.

Rigid Decompensated Spinal Deformity

The management of a severe spinal deformity becomes challenging when associated with rigid coronal or sagittal trunk decom-

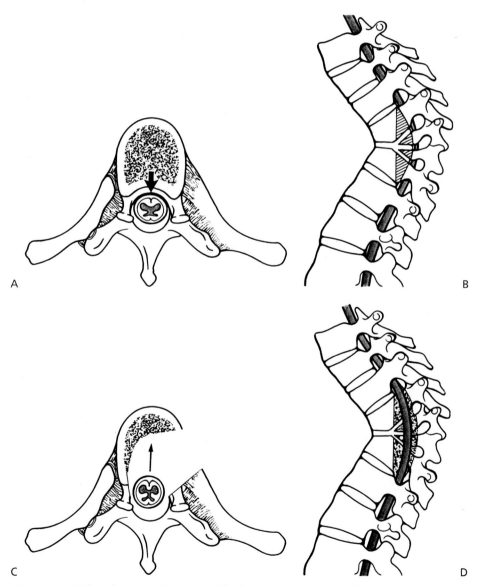

FIGURE 5. Spinal cord compression in severe kyphosis. **A, B:** In severe kyphosis, the spinal cord is stretched over the posterior aspect of the vertebral bodies, taking the shortest route across the deformity. **C, D:** Decompression of the spinal cord is achieved by partial anterior vertebrectomy, allowing the spinal cord to relocate and relax.

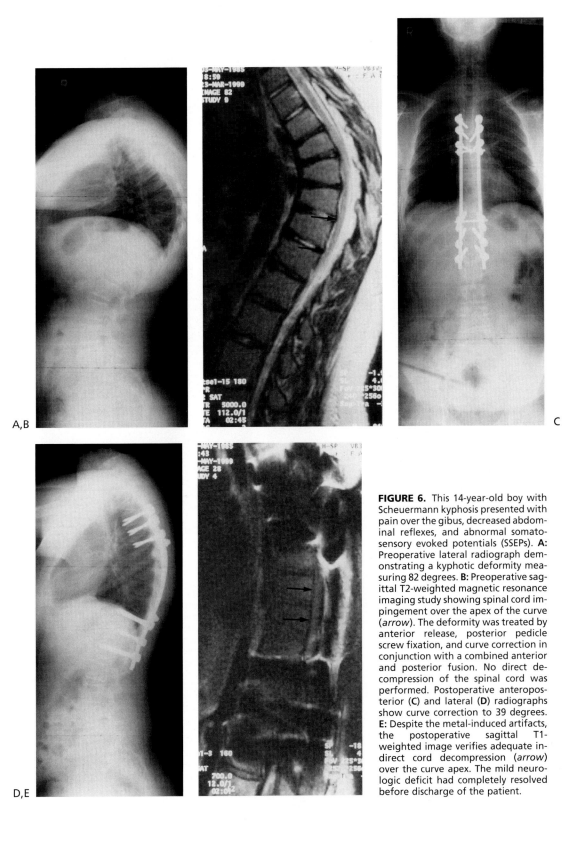

A,B

C

D,E

FIGURE 6. This 14-year-old boy with Scheuermann kyphosis presented with pain over the gibus, decreased abdominal reflexes, and abnormal somatosensory evoked potentials (SSEPs). **A:** Preoperative lateral radiograph demonstrating a kyphotic deformity measuring 82 degrees. **B:** Preoperative sagittal T2-weighted magnetic resonance imaging study showing spinal cord impingement over the apex of the curve (*arrow*). The deformity was treated by anterior release, posterior pedicle screw fixation, and curve correction in conjunction with a combined anterior and posterior fusion. No direct decompression of the spinal cord was performed. Postoperative anteroposterior (**C**) and lateral (**D**) radiographs show curve correction to 39 degrees. **E:** Despite the metal-induced artifacts, the postoperative sagittal T1-weighted image verifies adequate indirect cord decompression (*arrow*) over the curve apex. The mild neurologic deficit had completely resolved before discharge of the patient.

pensation. Rigid unbalanced scoliosis that deforms not only in the sagittal but also in the coronal plane is a challenging treatment problem. This problem is most frequently encountered in patients with neglected fixed congenital deformity (Figs. 7 and 8) and in patients who had a posterior spinal fusion at a very young age and subsequently developed crankshaft phenomenon or pseudarthrosis with curve progression (8).

In particular, severe kyphosis can lead to significant spinal cord compression. Lonstein and associates (30) reported in their review of 43 cases with neurologic deficits secondary to spinal deformity that all but one patient presented with kyphosis. With increasing kyphosis, there is great tension in the posterior dura, which compresses the spinal cord against the anterior wall (Fig. 5). Severe kyphosis in the upper thoracic spine places the cord

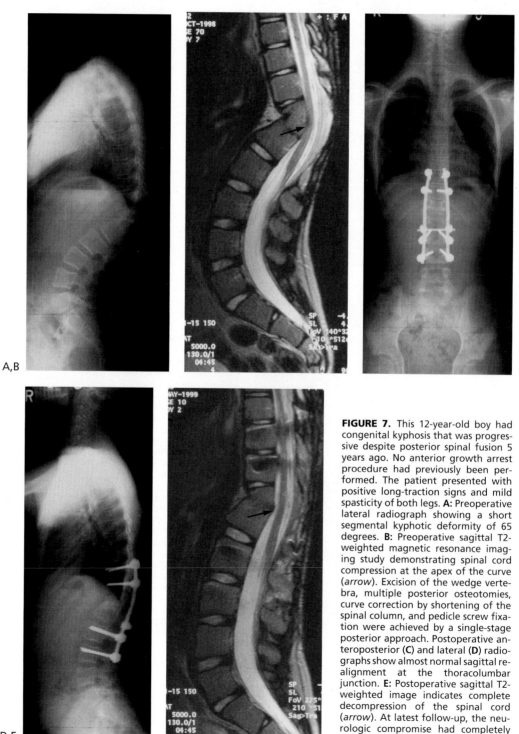

FIGURE 7. This 12-year-old boy had congenital kyphosis that was progressive despite posterior spinal fusion 5 years ago. No anterior growth arrest procedure had previously been performed. The patient presented with positive long-traction signs and mild spasticity of both legs. **A:** Preoperative lateral radiograph showing a short segmental kyphotic deformity of 65 degrees. **B:** Preoperative sagittal T2-weighted magnetic resonance imaging study demonstrating spinal cord compression at the apex of the curve (*arrow*). Excision of the wedge vertebra, multiple posterior osteotomies, curve correction by shortening of the spinal column, and pedicle screw fixation were achieved by a single-stage posterior approach. Postoperative anteroposterior (**C**) and lateral (**D**) radiographs show almost normal sagittal realignment at the thoracolumbar junction. **E:** Postoperative sagittal T2-weighted image indicates complete decompression of the spinal cord (*arrow*). At latest follow-up, the neurologic compromise had completely resolved.

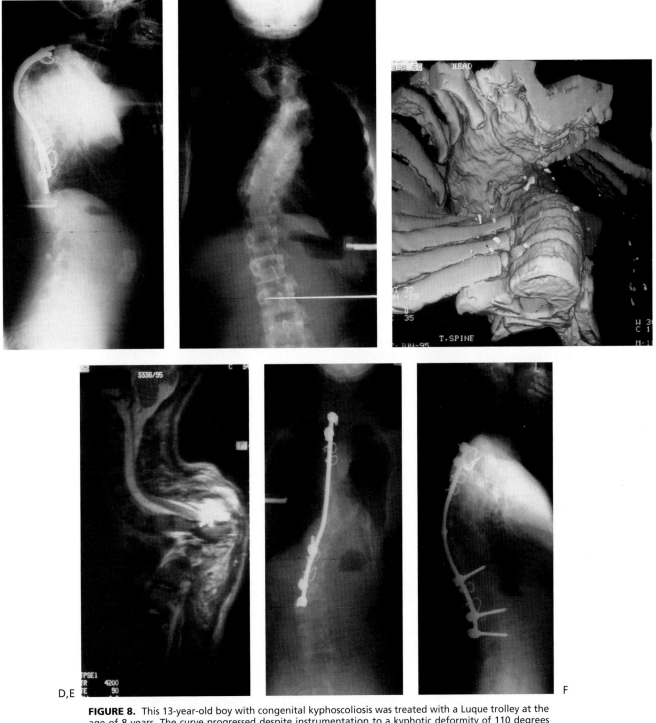

FIGURE 8. This 13-year-old boy with congenital kyphoscoliosis was treated with a Luque trolley at the age of 8 years. The curve progressed despite instrumentation to a kyphotic deformity of 110 degrees (**A**). He presented with decreased abdominal reflexes, mild Babinski sign on the right side. In a first step, the implant was removed and the spinal cord decompressed posteriorly. A preoperative diagnostic workup included computed tomography (CT) and magnetic resonance imaging (MRI) studies. **B:** Preoperative anteroposterior radiographs demonstrating a severe kyphoscoliosis. **C:** CT-guided reconstruction of the thoracic spine illustrating the severity of the deformity. **D:** Sagittal T2-weighted MRI study demonstrating the severe kyphotic deformity and distortion of the spinal canal. In a second step, anterior two-level vertebrectomy was performed, releasing the spinal cord. Anterior autologous bone (rib) chips were applied after adequate cord decompression to generate anterior fusion. Subsequently, the patient was kept in halo-extension for 4 weeks, and the deformity was gradually corrected. In a last step, the spine was instrumented from a posterior approach with pedicle screw fixation caudally and a claw fixation cranially, supplemented with sublaminar wires. Because of the severe deformity, only a single rod could be applied. Anteroposterior (**E**) and lateral (**F**) radiographs at 2-year follow-up show satisfactory curve correction, reestablishing the sagittal and coronal balance. (Courtesy of the Center for Spinal Studies and Surgery, Queen's Medical Center, Nottingham, U.K.)

at risk and can result in a significant neurologic deficit (30). The blood supply to the cord exhibits a critical vascular zone from the fourth to the ninth thoracic segment. Dommisse (14) has shown this area to have the fewest radicular branches and the fewest cord perforators. In addition, the spinal canal is narrowest in this area, and the spinal cord has its least flexibility or elasticity between flexion and extension (10). Rapid curve progression, as in the adolescent growth spurt, rapidly results in an increased anterior compression from the posterior vertebral body wall. It may result in the most severe spinal deformities encountered and often poses significant problems for treatment. Spinal cord compromise in these deformities may result from the severe curvature with vertebral body rotation (Fig. 8). The limitations of conventional procedures are evident (8). Anterior release and posterior curve correction with or without osteotomy may not sufficiently correct the coronal imbalance and necessitate more extensive surgical procedures. In these cases, the treatment of rigid decompensated coronal deformity requires vertebrectomy to reestablish truncal balance in the coronal and sagittal planes (Fig. 7).

Bradford and Tribus (9) summarized indications for anteroposterior vertebral body resection as follows: fixed truncal translation, rigid spinal deformities of greater than 80 degrees in the coronal plane, and asymmetry between the length of the convex and concave column of the deformity precluding achieving balance by osteotomies alone. As a prerequisite, the physical, social, and psychological status of the patient must be satisfactory, the complaints severe, and nonoperative treatment unsuccessful. As a general rule, the risks to benefits ratio must be appropriate for this type of surgery (8).

The literature on vertebrectomy to correct rigid spinal deformity is sparse, and only a few surgeons have sufficient experience with this technique. In 1983, Luque (32) reported on eight cases with a primary deformity of greater than 90 degrees undergoing multiple vertebrectomies and rib resection, with an average correction of 86%. Boachie-Adjei and Bradford (3) modified this technique and presented the first series of 16 cases in 1991. As a follow-up and extension of this first series, Bradford and Tribus (9) reviewed a series of 27 patients between the ages of 7 and 54 years to determine whether patients with rigid coronal decompensation can be safely and successfully treated by anteroposterior vertebral column resection, spinal shortening, posterior instrumentation, and fusion to correct their deformities. The follow-up ranged from 2 to 10 years, with an average of 5 years. The patient population presented with severe fixed deformities requiring extensive surgery as indicated by an average blood loss of 3,000 mL and an average operative time of 7 hours, 30 minutes. Coronal (3 to 25 cm) and sagittal (-4 to 22 cm) decompensation were corrected in an average of 82% and 87% of cases, respectively. T1 tilt and pelvic obliquity were improved in 65% and 53% of cases, respectively. Scoliosis averaged 103 degrees before surgery (range, 44 to 157 degrees) and 49 degrees at follow-up (range, 8 to 92 degrees), representing an improvement of 52%. A total of 31 complications occurred in 14 patients, including three radiculopathies with transient motor weakness and three wound infections. All patients rated their subjective outcome as good or excellent. This study has demonstrated that the benefits of this complex surgery outweigh its inherent risks.

Technical Aspects and Complications

In severe rigid spinal deformity, anterior cord decompression with spinal reconstruction is one of the most challenging procedures in spinal surgery. The importance of adequate preoperative evaluation and a unit experienced in the postsurgical care of these patients cannot be overemphasized (30). Today, spinal cord monitoring is the standard when such a procedures is carried out. The key for successful surgery is adequate exposure by a thoracotomy or a thoracoabdominal approach, which is usually carried out from the convex side of the kyphoscoliosis (Fig. 9). The apex of the deformity is identified and the intervertebral discs at the apex, above, and below are first completely excised to the posterior longitudinal ligament.

Great attention must be paid to the facts that the normal anatomy may be severely distorted and the spinal cord is often dislocated. The vertebral bodies are then resected with a rongeur to the posterior vertebral wall. Curettes and a high-speed air drill are useful to complete vertebral body resection when the posterior vertebral wall is approached. Bleeding from a vertebral vessel can be controlled with the use of bone wax and usually stops when the posterior vertebral wall is reached. The posterior vertebral border must be exposed over an adequate length before the cortical shells of the vertebrae are removed.

When the spinal canal is opened, the cord usually prolapses forward and may obstruct the surgeon's view for further decompression (30). When decompression is perform only over a limited distance, the cord impinges cranially or caudally with the remnants of the vertebral bodies, which must be avoided. Likewise, sharp edges that may impinge with the spinal cord must be avoided (30). Epidural bleeding can be significant but is controlled with thrombin-soaked Gelfoam. After adequate decompression, the spinal cord is covered with Gelfoam and the remaining cavity is filled with autologous bone chips and rib grafts to generate fusion.

After closure, a posterior approach is carried out whenever possible during the same surgery. During the posterior surgery, the spine is instrumented, and partial reduction is attempted when deemed appropriate (Fig. 8). If possible, we use pedicular screw fixation because these implants are a powerful tool to achieve reduction (if desired) and strong stabilization of the unstable spine (Fig. 7). So far, we have observed no screw-related complications in more than 100 cases of adolescent deformity surgery (unpublished data). In small children, in whom pedicle screw fixation is not possible because of the small diameter of the pedicle laminar, claw fixation and sublaminar wires are used in the upper thoracic spine (Fig. 8). Our goal is a rigid fixation, allowing for early mobilization of the patient without cast fixation.

One technical question is related to hypotensive anesthesia during such procedures. Bridwell and colleagues (11) reviewed a series of 1,090 cases undergoing spinal deformity correction for scoliosis, kyphosis, or a combination of the two. They reported on four neurologic deficits that occurred in this series. Three of the four deficits were purely vascular in etiology. The fourth may have had a vascular and mechanical etiology. All four patients had anterior and posterior surgery with harvesting of the unilateral convex segmental vessels, and each had a compo-

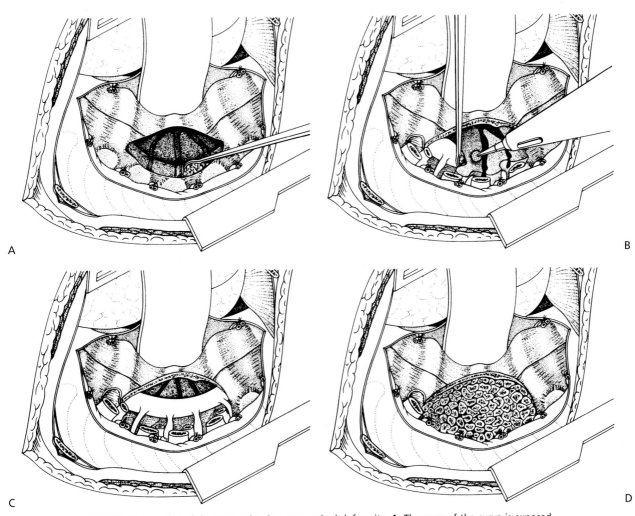

FIGURE 9. Spinal cord decompression in severe spinal deformity. **A:** The apex of the curve is exposed by a thoracotomy or a thoracoabdominal approach. After disc excision, the vertebral bodies are resected with rongeurs and curettes up to the posterior vertebral wall. **B:** After exposure of the posterior vertebral walls, the cortical bone is thinned up to a thin bony shell using a high-speed air drill and then lifted off the posterior longitudinal ligament and thecal sac using curettes. **C:** After adequate decompression of the spinal cord, the remnants of the intervertebral discs on the far side are resected to release the anterior column (not shown). **D:** The spinal cord is covered with Gelfoam, and the remaining cavity is filled with autologous bone chips and rib grafts.

nent of hyperkyphosis as well as intraoperative controlled hypotension. The authors identified combined anterior and posterior surgery and hyperkyphosis as risk factors for neurologic complications.

We concur with Bridwell and colleagues in terms of the practical guidelines emerging from that paper (11). If the patient with spinal deformity is undergoing anterior and posterior surgery on the same day, the anesthesia should not be performed in hypotension, particularly when reduction is attempted. In case of a neurologic complication, the patient's hemoglobin and blood pressure should immediately be normalized in a first approach. Removal of the instrumentation is not absolutely necessary under the prerequisite that a postoperative myelography has ruled out a mechanical spinal cord compression and the spinal canal length was shortened. Bridwell and colleagues (11) have indicated that SSEP monitoring may not be sensitive enough

to pick up anterior spinal artery syndrome. This has to be kept in mind, and the surgeon should make deliberate use of a wake-up test in equivocal cases. We now routinely use motor evoked potentials. This increases the safety margin during surgery, but the surgeon must anticipate that a putative neurologic deficit may not be reversible in all cases at the time when decreased MEPs occur.

REFERENCES

1. Aebi M, Dick W (1990): The application of the internal fixator in spinal tumor surgery. In: Sundaresan N, ed. *Tumors of the spine.* Philadelphia: WB Saunders, pp. 520–530
2. Betz RR, Gelman AJ, DeFilipp GJ, et al. (1987): Magnetic resonance imaging (MRI) in the evaluation of spinal cord injured children and adolescents. *Paraplegia* 25:92–99.

3. Boachie-Adjei O, Bradford DS (1991): Vertebral column resection and arthrodesis for complex spinal deformities. *J Spinal Disord* 4:193–202.

4. Bohlman HH, Eismont FJ (1981): Surgical techniques of anterior decompression and fusion for spinal cord injuries. *Clin Orthop* 154:57–67.

5. Boos N, Goytan M, Fraser R, et al. (1997): Solitary plasma cell myeloma of the spine in an adolescent: case report of an unusual presentation. *J Bone Joint Surg Br* 79:812–814.

6. Bouffet E, Marec-Berard P, Thiesse P, et al. (1997): Spinal cord compression by secondary epi- and intradural metastases in childhood. *Childs Nerv Syst* 13:383–387.

7. Bradford DS, Boachie-Adjei O (1990): One-stage anterior and posterior hemivertebral resection and arthrodesis for congenital scoliosis. *J Bone Joint Surg Am* 72:536–540.

8. Bradford DS, Tribus CB (1994): Current concepts and management of patients with fixed decompensated spinal deformity. *Clin Orthop* 306:64–72.

9. Bradford DS, Tribus CB (1997): Vertebral column resection for the treatment of rigid coronal decompensation. *Spine* 22:1590–1599.

10. Breig A (1964): Biomechanics of the spinal cord in kyphosis and kyphoscoliosis. *Acta Neurol Scand* 40:196.

11. Bridwell KH, Lenke LG, Baldus C, et al. (1998): Major intraoperative neurologic deficits in pediatric and adult spinal deformity patients: incidence and etiology at one institution. *Spine* 23:324–331.

12. Capener N (1954): The evolution of lateral rachotomy. *J Bone Joint Surg Br* 36:173–179.

13. Conrad EUD, Olszewski AD, Berger M, et al. (1992): Pediatric spine tumors with spinal cord compromise. *J Pediatr Orthop* 12:454–460.

14. Dommisse GF (1974): The blood supply of the spinal cord: a critical vascular zone in spinal surgery. *J Bone Joint Surg Br* 56:225–235.

15. Ha KI, Han SH, Chung M, et al. (1996): A clinical study of the natural remodeling of burst fractures of the lumbar spine. *Clin Orthop* 210–214.

16. Hachen HJ (1977): Spinal cord injury in children and adolescents: diagnostic pitfalls and therapeutic considerations in the acute stage. *Paraplegia* 15:55–64.

17. Heary RF, Vaccaro AR, Benevenia J, et al. (1998): "En-bloc" vertebrectomy in the mobile lumbar spine. *Surg Neurol* 50:548–556.

18. Hensinger RN (1991): Fractures of the thoracic and lumbar spine. In: Rockwood CA, Wilkins KE, King RE, eds. *Fractures in children.* Philadelphia: JB Lippincott, pp. 958–989.

19. Hernigou P, Djindjian M, Ricolfi F, et al. (1994): Neuro-aggressive dorsal vertebral hemangioma and vertebrectomy: apropos of 2 cases. Review of the literature. *Rev Chir Orthop* 80:542–550.

20. Hodson AR (1965): Correction of fixed spinal curves. *J Bone Joint Surg Am* 47:1221–1227.

21. Holte DC, Winter RB, Lonstein JE, et al. (1995): Excision of hemivertebrae and wedge resection in the treatment of congenital scoliosis. *J Bone Joint Surg Am* 77:159–171.

22. Hu SS, Capen DA, Rimoldi RL, et al. (1993): The effect of surgical decompression on neurologic outcome after lumbar fractures. *Clin Orthop* 288:166–173.

23. Hubbard DD (1974): Injuries of the spine in children and adolescents. *Clin Orthop* 100:56–65.

24. Hyndman OR (1947): Transplantation of the spinal cord: the problem of kyposcoliosis with cord signs. *Surg Gynecol Obstet* 84:460–464.

25. Jani L (1987): Spinal fractures in children and adolescents. *Z Kinderchir* 42:333–338.

26. Kaneda K, Abumi K, Fujuja M (1984): Burst fractures with neurological deficits of the thoraco-lumbar spine: results of anterior decompression and stabilization with anterior instrumentation. *Spine* 9:209–218.

27. Kramer ED, Lewis D, Raney B, et al. (1989): Neurologic complications in children with soft tissue and osseous sarcoma. *Cancer* 64:2600–2603.

28. Lewis DW, Packer RJ, Raney B, et al. (1986): Incidence, presentation, and outcome of spinal cord disease in children with systemic cancer. *Pediatrics* 78:438–443.

29. Lindseth RE, Stelzer L (1979): Vertebral excision for kyphosis in children with myelomenigocele. *J Bone Joint Surg Am* 61A:699–704.

30. Lonstein JE, Winter RB, Moe JH, et al. (1980): Neurologic deficits secondary to spinal deformity: a review of the literature and report of 43 cases. *Spine* 5:331–355.

31. Lowe TG (1990): Current concepts review: Scheuermann disease. *J Bone Joint Surg Am* 72:940–945.

32. Luque ER (1983): Vertebral column transposition. *Orthop Trans* 7:29.

33. MacLennan A, (1922): Scoliosis. *Br Med J* 2:864–866.

34. Mayfield JK, Erkkila JC, Winter RB (1981): Spine deformity subsequent to acquired childhood spinal cord injury. *J Bone Joint Surg Am* 63:1401–1411.

35. Melzak J (1969): Paraplegia among children. *Lancet* 2:45–48.

36. Mumford J, Weinstein JN, Spratt KF, et al. (1993): Thoracolumbar burst fractures: the clinical efficacy and outcome of nonoperative management. *Spine* 18:955–970.

37. Raffel C, Neave VC, Lavine S, et al. (1991): Treatment of spinal cord compression by epidural malignancy in childhood. *Neurosurgery* 28:349–352.

38. Schneider RC (1960): Transposition of the compressed spinal cord in kyphoscoliotic patients with neurological deficit. *J Bone Joint Surg Am* 42:1027–1039.

39. Slabough PB, Winter RB, Lonstein JE, et al. (1980): Lumbosacral hemivertebrae: a review of twenty-four patients with excision in eight. *Spine* 5:234–244.

40. Yngve DA, Harris WP, Herndon WA, et al. (1988): Spinal cord injury without osseous spine fracture. *J Pediatr Orthop* 8:153–159.

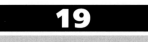

OSTEOTOMY AND THE PEDIATRIC SPINE

SAMUEL J. CHEWNING, JR.
CHARLES F. HEINIG

Surgical management of deformity is designed to bring the spine as close as possible to the normal anatomic alignment in all three planes. One of the techniques for realigning the spine is spinal osteotomy. Spinal osteotomies can accomplish angular displacement of the spine. They can result in a lengthening or shortening of the spinal column. An osteotomy can also accomplish a rotational change in the spine.

OSTEOTOMY DESIGN CONSIDERATIONS

Osteotomies involving the spine should include all three columns of the spine. The pediatric spine differs from the adult spine in size and growth potential; thus, the remaining growth potential of the spine must be taken into consideration when planning and performing an osteotomy. In its simplest form, an osteotomy may be considered to be an opening or closing wedge; either way, there will be a net change in the length of one or more columns of the spine (Fig. 1).

Consider the geometry of three tubes eccentrically oriented one inside the other (Fig. 2). The largest tube will be considered the body as a whole, consisting of the rib cage and chest wall anteriorly and the muscles of the back posteriorly. The second tube will be the spinal column itself. The third tube is the spinal canal. All three tubes are closely approximated to each other posteriorly. As can be seen from Figure 3, moving the axis of the rotation of an osteotomy has a substantial effect on the lengthening or shortening of the walls of these three tubes.

Consider a posterior closing wedge osteotomy (Fig. 4). If the wedge is only taken out of the lamina and the osteotomy is allowed to pivot around the posterior wall of the body, the net effect will be a closing of the interlaminar distance posteriorly. The interdiscal distance at the anterior body will be widened equal to about that of a closing wedge posteriorly. Assume that the sternum is 10 cm anterior to the body and the anterior body is 3 cm anterior to the spinal canal. The canal is another 2 cm anterior to the posterior elements. A 20-degree angular correc-

tion may be obtained by removing 5 cm of the posterior elements and 3 cm of the anterior body to allow the osteotomy to pivot around the sternum and obtain the desired angular correction (Fig. 3A). The geometry of this osteotomy would also indicate that if we are to carry out our osteotomy (as in Fig. 3C) and if the above measurements are for a 1 cm shortening at the laminar level, a 5 cm lengthening must take place at the anterior chest wall. Later, we discuss the secondary stabilizers, particularly in the thoracic spine, that must be considered to carry out this type of osteotomy.

The primary consideration for an osteotomy is protection of the neural elements and their vascular supply within the spinal canal. Overdistraction of the spinal canal has a well-known record of producing catastrophic complications in the form of paralysis (2–4,7,15–18). In contrast, neural elements tolerate shortening relatively well (8–11). Therefore, regardless of the deformity to be corrected, the net effect must be to maintain the length of the neural column or allow for its overall shortening.

Before performing an osteotomy, the surgeon must consider the forces and implants that are available to move and maintain the position of the spine after the osteotomy has been completed. Four basic forces can be applied across an osteotomy site (Fig. 5): distraction, compression, translation, and rotation. Any one of these or all of these may be used depending on the defect to be corrected. Consider again the example of three eccentric tubes when dealing with a kyphotic deformity. If distraction is to be a viable force, it must be anterior to the pivot point for the correction of the deformity. If not anterior to the pivot point, the distraction will only make the deformity worse (Fig. 6). Therefore, to obtain correction of a kyphotic deformity through a distractive force in the thoracic spine, it will be necessary to use anterior instrumentation, such as the Harrington-Kostuik construct. To obtain correction of kyphosis with a closing wedge osteotomy, the compressive force must be posterior to the axis of rotation of the osteotomy. Several systems (Harrington compression rods, Texas Scottish Rite, Isola, Cotrel-Dubousset) can provide this compressive force.

Translatory correction can be used to translate directly at the two sides of the osteotomy. An example would be the case with the translatory effect of pedicle screws on moving or reducing a spondylolisthesis. The other translatory effect can be a distal

S. J. Chewning Jr. and C. F. Heinig: Orthopaedic Surgeons, Miller Orthopaedic Clinic, Charlotte, North Carolina 28203.

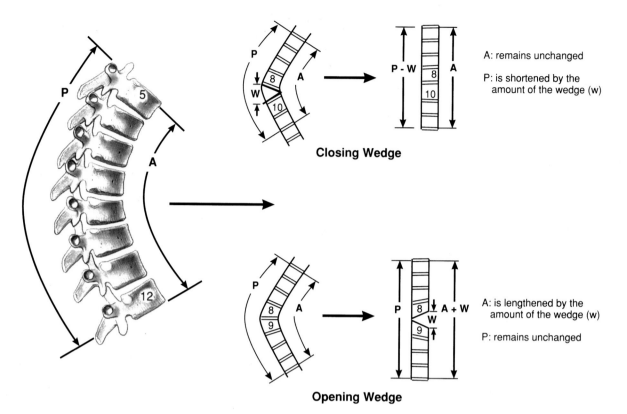

Closing Wedge

A: remains unchanged

P: is shortened by the amount of the wedge (w)

Opening Wedge

A: is lengthened by the amount of the wedge (w)

P: remains unchanged

FIGURE 1. In a closing wedge, the anterior length *(A)* remains unchanged, and the posterior length *(P)* is shortened by the amount of the wedge *(W)*. In an opening wedge, *A* is lengthened by the amount of the wedge and *P* remains unchanged.

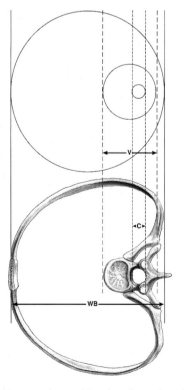

FIGURE 2. The chest may be considered as three tubes: the whole body (WB; the rib cage); the spinal canal (C); and the vertebra (V).

one. The extension moment applied through the Luque sublaminar wire technique is an example of translation at a distance from the osteotomy (14) (Fig. 7). Again returning to the three eccentric tube model, translation could be applied over a short segment, as in the case of spondylolisthesis requiring a translation for reduction (Fig. 5B). A translation force can provide a hyperextension moment across a kyphosis. The Harrington distraction instrumentation and the Edwards distraction instrumentation with rod sleeves provide a three-point bending moment on the spine that can give an extension moment that translates the ends of the spine. This can also be accomplished with sublaminar wiring such as Luque instrumentation (5,13).

In the axial plane, rotation around a given pivot point may be accomplished through an osteotomy site. It must again be emphasized that no forces can be applied to the spinal cord itself and that any translation, rotation, or bending moment must allow either a shortening of the spinal canal or no net change.

Anatomic constraints must also be considered when performing an osteotomy. For example, the surgeon must consider the secondary stabilization effect that the rib cage has on the spinal column. The rib heads at the costovertebral junction span two vertebral segments and further stabilize a given motion segment. The ribs are also a space-occupying structure. Despite doing a complete vertebrectomy anteriorly and posteriorly, complete compression across this site is not possible unless the space-occupying ribs are partially or completely removed. The rib cage

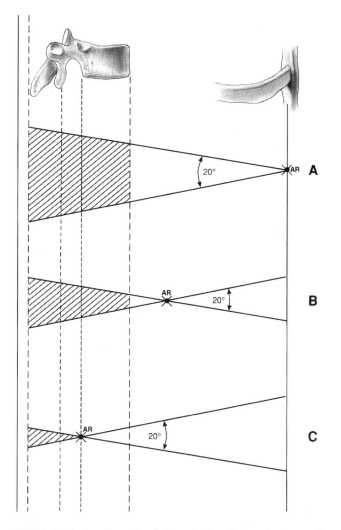

FIGURE 3. Moving the axis of the rotation of an osteotomy will lengthen or shorten the "three tubes" (see Fig. 2) of the chest. **A:** The axis of rotation *(AR)* is in the sternum or anterior chest wall. **B:** The *AR* is in the posterior third of the chest cavity. **C:** The *AR* is along the posterior wall of the vertebral body.

itself and the sternum are strong secondary stabilizers of the spine.

A theoretical pivot point may be designed into an extension osteotomy system that puts the pivot point someplace in the middle of the chest cavity. This would then cause an elongation moment across the sternum or rib cage (Fig. 3B). Although this theoretical condition can work in the lumbar spine where the only anterior constraints are from muscle tension, it may be difficult to get the kind of correction desired as a result of the tethering effect of the sternum and the chest wall anteriorly.

In the lumbar spine, the duodenum and the superior mesenteric artery must be considered. The cast syndrome or superior mesenteric artery syndrome is well described (6). An osteotomy that would put an extension moment around a pivot point posterior to the anterior longitudinal ligament would result in direct compression of the duodenum by the superior mesenteric artery (Fig. 8); this would result in a small bowel obstruction. The

aorta and inferior vena cava are directly anterior to the vertebral bodies in the lumbar spine. An osteotomy with its axis of rotation at the posterior margin of the vertebral body will have a lengthening effect on the anterior body and the aorta (Fig. 4). Adams (1) and Lichtblau and Wilson (12) reported either rupture or obstruction of the aorta as a complication of anterior opening wedge osteotomies.

When planning a correction in the coronal plane, the surgeons must consider the tethers that could potentially block correction. Multiple fused ribs are an example of this kind of problem. A long-standing scoliosis with contracture of the lateral flank musculature can effectively tether the ribs to the iliac crest. This may be a good reason to separate anterior and posterior stages. Ten to 14 days in traction after the anterior release can mobilize these soft tissues.

We have discussed the four basic corrective forces that can be applied to the spinal column. These may be applied in concert to achieve the desired effect. Rotation has taken on a new meaning in light of the posterior derotation instrumentation systems. However, the derotation maneuver used to correct scoliosis is more often a translatory motion than a true derotation (6). True rotational change of one segment relative to another can be accomplished with an osteotomy and soft tissue releases.

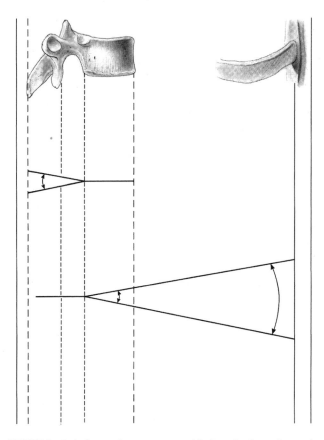

FIGURE 4. A closing wedge osteotomy with the axis of rotation at the posterior longitudinal ligament causes equal amount of opening in the anterior longitudinal ligament. This places considerable force on the anterior chest wall.

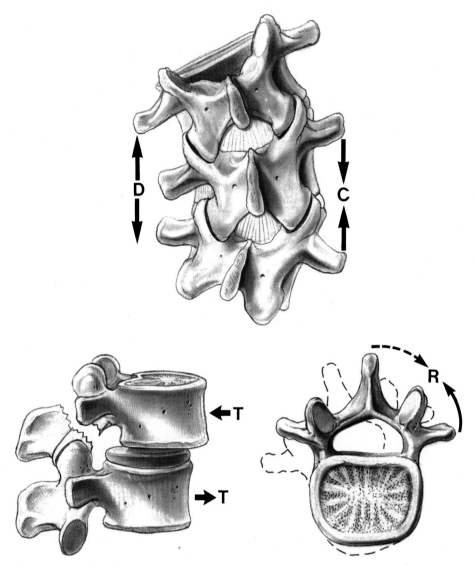

FIGURE 5. Four basic forces that can be applied to an osteotomy: distraction (D); compression (C); translation (T); rotation (R).

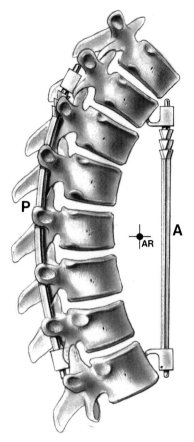

FIGURE 6. Distraction posterior *(P)* to the axis of rotation *(AR)* makes the kyphosis worse. Distraction anterior *(A)* to the *AR* reduces the kyphosis.

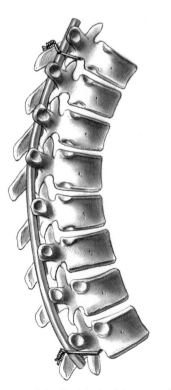

FIGURE 7. Translation of the distal ends of the curve yields correction with the Luque system.

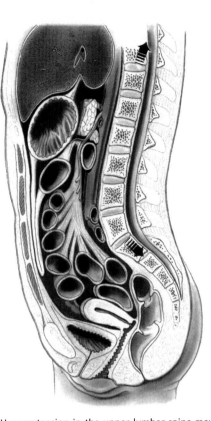

FIGURE 8. Hyperextension in the upper lumbar spine may allow the superior mesenteric artery to compress the duodenum.

SURGICAL TECHNIQUE

There are several important basic considerations with respect to surgical technique when performing spinal osteotomies on children. For example, spinal osteotomies are lengthy procedures, and small children do not tolerate as much blood loss as adults. Therefore, extra consideration should be given to blood loss control, padding of bony prominences, access to airways, access to central venous monitoring, and central venous fluid and blood replacement. Conservation of body temperature is also important in children.

Position

Surgical considerations, such as padding and abdominal decompression, are related to proper positioning of the patient. Special emphasis must center around the osteotomy itself. It is assumed that a significant to severe deformity exists. The goal of the procedure is to decrease or eliminate that deformity. At the beginning of the case, positioning and body support must take the deformity into account. As the osteotomy is completed, the body must be well supported on both sides of the osteotomy to prevent unwanted shifts in the osteotomy segments (and potential catastrophic injury to the neural elements). The support system for the body must also allow for change in position as the deformity is corrected.

TABLE 1. HYPOTHETICAL PEDIATRIC CANDIDATE FOR OSTEOTOMY OF THE SPINE

Sex: Female
Age: 13 y
Maturity: Risser 1, menarche 4 mo
Pathology: Progressive congenital kyphoscoliosis
Neurology: Normal; magnetic resonance imaging revealed no intracanal pathology
Spinal morphology:
   T7 normal
   T7–T8 facets normal
   T8 (L) facet hypoplastic
   T8–T9 (R) facet deformed and enlarged
   T9 (L) inferior and superior facets missing
   T9–T10 (R) facet deformed and enlarged
   T10–T11 facets normal
   T8–T10 (L) bar bridging the bodies
   T9 (L) pedicle missing
   T9 (R) pedicle long and narrow
   T9 body hemivertebra causing scoliosis and kyphosis
   58 degree (Cobb) T7 to T11 (R) scolisis
   53 degree (Cobb) T7 to T11 kyphosis
   T8 and T9 (L) rib heads fused

Consider, for example, a 90-degree pelvic obliquity that is undergoing lumbar osteotomy. The pelvis will lie in a plane of 90 degrees relative to the long axis of the spine when the patient is placed on the table, and the legs will not line up with the trunk. After removal of bone and release of soft tissue, the pelvis (and to some degree the lower extremities) must be moved through 90 degrees to obtain proper alignment. Consider also a 105-degree short-segment congenital kyphotic deformity at the thoracolumbar junction. If adequate support (external as well as internal) is not provided as the osteotomy is completed, a sudden uncontrolled translation of the two segments relative to each other could have tragic consequences on the spinal cord. It becomes clear that flexibility of position as well as support are prime considerations in patient positioning.

Hypothetical Case

A hypothetical patient is described in Table 1 and Figure 9. If surgical correction of the deformity is desired, all three columns of the spine must be involved. The approach may either be combined anterior and posterior or posterior alone. Both approaches are presented.

Combined Anterior and Posterior Approach

The patient undergoes the anterior procedure first. The position is for a right thoracotomy through the T7 rib. In this case, the seventh rib thoracotomy was selected because the apex of the deformity is T9. The seventh rib slopes anteriorly and inferiorly. A T9 thoracotomy would not have allowed exposure above the

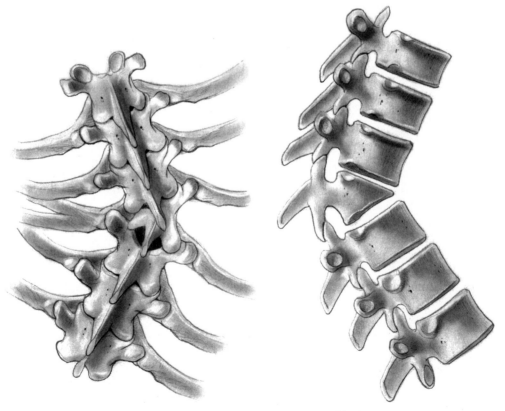

FIGURE 9. T9 hemivertebra causing scoliosis and kyphosis.

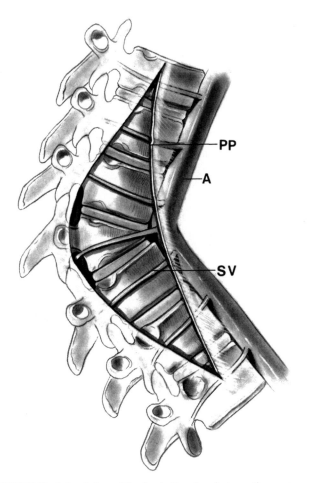

inspected and all bleeding controlled. The rib that was harvested during exposure is prepared as a bone graft to be placed in the T7–8 and T10–11 interspaces. The end plates are decorticated and the bone graft placed in these two interspaces. The end plates of T8 and T10 are also decorticated. A bone graft should not be placed here because any bone in this position may prevent correction from the posterior approach. The graft material could also displace posteriorly into the canal as the deformity is corrected. Gelfoam may be backed in this space to control bleeding from the end plates. This Gelfoam can be removed posteriorly. Anterior instrumentation can also block correction posteriorly. Bone may be placed anteriorly and laterally in a subperiosteal position lateral to T8 and T10 (Fig. 11).

The parietal pleura is then closed. A chest tube is inserted, and the wound is closed in standard fashion. At this point, a conference is held with all persons involved with the operative care of the child (e.g., surgeons, anesthesiologists, neuromonitoring), and a decision is reached either to continue with the poste-

FIGURE 10. Lateral view of the kyphotic spine during a thoracotomy. The parietal pleura *(PP)* is incised over the midportion of the vertebral body. The segmental vessels *(SV)* arising from the aorta *(A)* should be preserved.

hemivertebra. A transpleural approach is performed. The parietal pleura is transected in a longitudinal direction over the middle of the vertebral bodies from T7 to T11 (Fig. 10). The segmental arteries and veins should be left intact. Retropleural dissection is continued to expose the right side and anterior surface of the discs and bodies of T7, T8, T9, T10, and T11. The annulus is incised, and discectomy is performed at the T7–8 level. This interspace is then packed with Gelfoam and a cottonoid. The T10–11 interspace is addressed in a similar fashion. With the same technique, the abnormal T8 to T9 and T9 to T10 discs are resected. Subperiosteal dissection is completed circumferentially to expose the T9 hemivertebra. The T9 segmental vessels should not be sacrificed. The rib head and 8 to 12 cm of the proximal end of the T9 rib should be removed. Osteotomes, curets, and rongeurs are used to remove the deformed T9 hemivertebra completely. The anterior third of the right T9 pedicle should also be removed.

Epidural bleeding is controlled with bipolar electrocautery. Bone wax may be used on the base of the pedicle removed from the posterior approach. At this point, the operative site should be

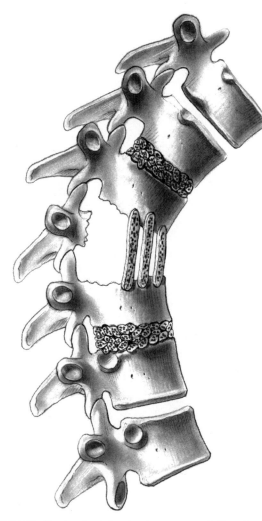

FIGURE 11. The hemivertebra has been removed. Bone is placed in the disc spaces above and below the osteotomy site. No bone is placed in the osteotomy site. Bone may be placed anteriorly and in a subperiosteal position laterally.

rior procedure or to stop and perform the second stage at a later date.

Posterior Approach (Second Stage of Combined Anterior and Posterior Osteotomy)

The child is positioned on the operating table in the prone position. Chest rolls may be used for chest and abdominal support. A table that allows for flexion and extension can be helpful in controlling the deformity on the table. The thoracolumbar junction should be positioned over the angle of the bed. The bed is placed in a flexed position. The prep and drape are standard for a midline approach and exposure of the posterior iliac crest. The spine is exposed from T6 to T12 in a subperiosteal fashion. Anchor sites for the instrumentation are then prepared. Depending on the patient's anatomy, it may be necessary to include an additional level above or below to secure the spine.

In the case being described, the anchor sites are hooks in a claw pattern: the superior sites are T6 to T7 claws; control of inferior sites is achieved with T11 to T12 claws (Fig. 12). The facets of all involved levels are denuded of soft tissue. A provisional or working rod is placed on the concave side of the spine

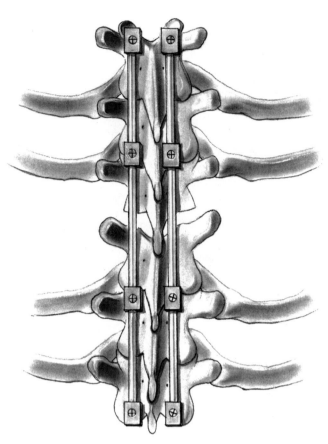

FIGURE 13. Normal alignment after removal of the T9 posterior elements.

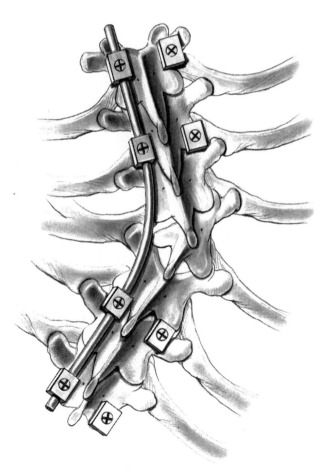

FIGURE 12. All anchor sites have been prepared. A provisional or working rod is inserted on the concave side.

to control the spine as the osteotomy is completed (Fig. 12). A complete laminectomy of the abnormal T9 segment is carried out. The inferior edge of T8 is also removed. The inferior and superior facets of the right side of T9 are removed next. The spinal column is now becoming progressively more unstable. Care should be taken to ensure that the provisional rod and the operating table are providing adequate support to prevent unwanted motion of the spine. Decompression and soft tissue removal should continue on the concave (left) side of the spine until the dura and nerve roots of T8, T9, and T10 have been exposed. The upper 2 to 3 mm of the lamina and the facets of T10 should also be resected. Careful subperiosteal dissection is now necessary to expose and remove the remaining posterior two thirds of the right T9 pedicle and its transverse process.

The convex (right) rod is now placed. Either the superior or inferior claw is firmly attached to the rod. Slow progressive contraction (compression) is now placed on the convex rod. The Gelfoam that was placed between the bodies of T8 and T10 during the anterior procedure is removed through the opening created by removal of the T9 pedicle. If desired, a small amount of cancellous bone (from the iliac crest) may be placed anteriorly in place of the Gelfoam. Compression is continued along the convex rod. The operating room table can be taken out of flexion and placed in neutral or slight extension to help reduce the kyphosis in the spine. The dura is constantly observed to ensure no kinking or pressure is being applied to the neural elements. Compression on the right-hand rod is continued until the desired correction has occurred. The inferior facet of T8 is in close approximation to the superior facet of T10 (Fig. 13). Both claws are now firmly affixed to the convex rod. The concave (provisional) rod may be changed as necessary to the final rod. Some final compression on both rods may be necessary.

Neuromonitoring (evoked potentials or a wake-up test) should be normal at this time. We prefer the wake-up test. If the preoperative planning was correct and the necessary amount of bone has been removed, the patient's scoliosis should be gone and the kyphosis returned to normal. Bone grafting is carried out in a standard posterior-posterolateral fashion. Depending on the instrumentation used, the rods may be transfixed. The wound is closed in the standard fashion. A molded thoracolumbosacral orthosis (TLSO) may be used for 3 to 6 months posteriorly.

Technique for Entire Osteotomy from a Single Posterior Approach

The child is positioned on the operating table in the prone position. Chest rolls may be used for chest and abdominal sup-port. A table that allows for flexion and extension can be helpful in controlling the deformity on the table. The thoracolumbar junction should be positioned over the angle of the bed. The bed is placed in a flexed position. The prep and drape are standard for a midline approach and exposure of the posterior iliac crest. The spine is exposed from T6 to T12 in a subperiosteal fashion. Anchor sites for the instrumentation are then prepared. Depending on the patient's anatomy, it may be necessary to include an additional level above or below to secure the spine.

In the case being described, the anchor sites are hooks in a claw pattern: the superior sites are controlled with T6 to T7 claws; control of inferior sites is achieved with T11 to T12 claws (Fig. 12). The facets of all involved levels are denuded of soft tissue. Subperiosteal dissection is undertaken to expose 6 to 10 cm of the right side of the ninth rib. The transverse process, rib head, and the proximal portion of the ninth rib are removed. The removal of the transverse process of T9 exposes the posterior portion of the T9 pedicle (Fig. 14). A probe is placed into the body of T9 through the pedicle. The body of T9 is enucleated using progressively larger curets passed through the pedicle. At this point, it is important to maintain the medial pedicle wall (Fig. 15). This wall acts as a natural retractor to keep the dura out of the operative field and the surgeon out of the dura. To gain adequate exposure

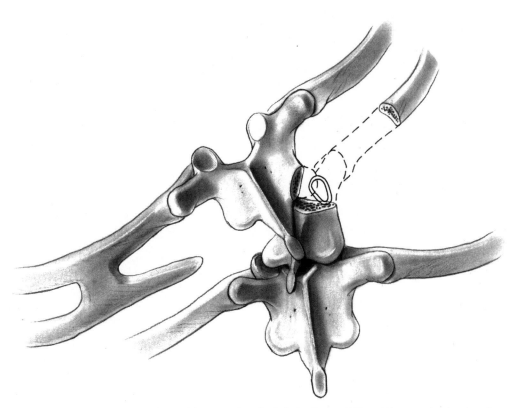

FIGURE 14. The pedicle is located by removing the inferior facet of T8 and the superior facet and transverse process of T9. The proximal end of the ninth rib has also been removed.

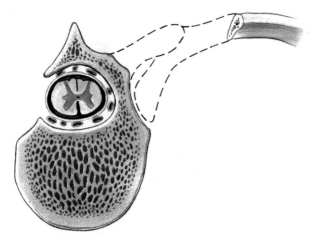

FIGURE 15. The medial wall of the pedicle provides retraction of the neural elements.

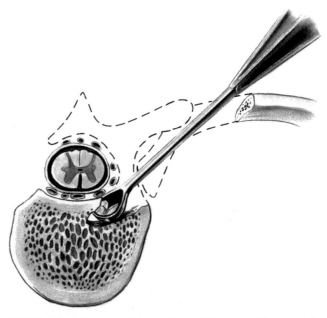

FIGURE 16. A large bowled curet is used to remove the remaining posterior wall of the vertebral body.

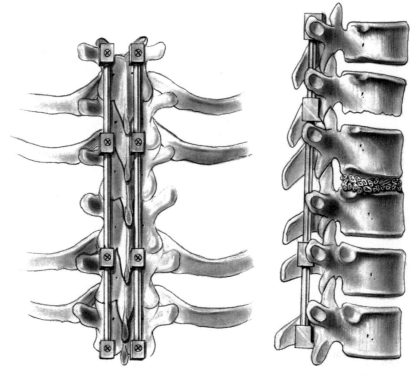

FIGURE 17. Posteroanterior and lateral view after osteotomy showing correction of the deformity and instrumentation.

of the vertebral body, it may be necessary to remove the lateral wall of the pedicle (Fig. 15).

After the cancellous bone is removed, curets are used to remove the superior and inferior end plates of T9. The T8 to T9 and T9 to T10 discs are also removed through the pedicle. This space is packed with Gelfoam. A provisional or working rod is now placed on the concave side of the spine to control the spine as the osteotomy is completed. A complete laminectomy of the abnormal T9 segment is carried out. The inferior edge of T8 is removed. The inferior and superior facets of the right side of T9 are removed. The spinal column is now becoming progressively more unstable. Care should be taken to ensure that the provisional rod and the operating table are providing adequate support to prevent unwanted motion of the spine. Decompression and soft tissue removal should continue on the concave (left) side of the spine until the dura and nerve roots of T8, T9, and T10 have been exposed. The upper 2 to 3 mm of the lamina and facets of T10 are resected. The remaining medial wall of the right T9 pedicle is removed. The edge of a large curet (directed from the right side through the void created by removing the rib, transverse process, and pedicle) is used to remove the remaining posterior wall of the T9 vertebra (Fig. 16). The convex (right) rod is now placed. Either the superior or inferior claw is firmly attached to the rod. Slow progressive contraction (compression) is now placed on the convex rod. The Gelfoam that was placed between the bodies of T8 and T10 is removed. If desired, a small amount of cancellous bone (from the iliac crest or the removed vertebral body) may be placed anteriorly in place of the Gelfoam. Compression is continued along the convex rod. The operating room table can be taken out of flexion and placed in neutral or slight extension to help reduce the kyphosis in the spine. The dura is constantly observed to ensure that no kinking or pressure is being applied to the neural elements. Compression on the right rod is continued until the desired correction has occurred. The inferior facet of T8 should be in close approximation to the superior facet of T10. Both claws are firmly affixed to the convex rod. The concave (provisional) rod may be changed as necessary to the final rod. Some final compression on both rods may also be necessary.

Neuromonitoring (evoked potentials or a wake-up test) should be normal at this time. We prefer the wake-up test. If the preoperative planning was correct and the necessary amount of bone has been removed, the patient's scoliosis should be gone and the kyphosis returned to normal (Fig. 17). Bone grafting is carried out in a standard posterior-posterolateral fashion. Depending on the instrumentation used, the rods may be transfixed. The wound is closed in standard fashion. A molded TLSO may be used for 3 to 6 months postoperatively.

DISCUSSION

The procedures described previously use a biplane osteotomy of the spine. Rotation or translation could also have been accom-

plished; however, these two corrective maneuvers are more dependent on bending the rod and the anchor attachment to the rod. Correction of the kyphoscoliosis was accomplished by shortening the bony column. In this way, tension was not placed on the spinal cord or its vascular supply.

Surgical treatment of our hypothetical patient was addressed from two approaches. One was a combined anterior and posterior approach; the other was strictly a posterior approach. Both have advantages and disadvantages. The advantage of the combined anterior and posterior procedure is the direct visualization of the deformed anterior vertebral body and the discs above and below. Because a thoracotomy and rib resection are performed, an additional bone graft is obtained from the rib. Also, the ribs themselves act as a secondary stabilizer of the spine. A more complete resection of the ribs may be carried out from an anterior procedure. A disadvantage of the combined procedure is that two operative procedures must be performed. This involves increased operating time (for two sets of prep and drape) as well as the time required to reposition the patient between anterior and posterior procedures. The thoracotomy itself is another insult to the patient's body, and thus the overall physical condition of the patient may affect the recovery period. An additional scar is also a result. Conservation of body temperature, particularly in smaller children, is mandatory. A thoracotomy exposes the highly vascularized lung and the pleura to the atmosphere of the operating room. This can lead to significant heat loss from the patient. Heat loss from irrigating this incision with saline at less than body temperature can also be a source of heat loss in these children.

Carrying out the entire operation from the posterior procedure has the advantage of not requiring repositioning of the patient. In addition, surgical trauma to the patient from the thoracotomy is avoided, and we believe that there is better control of bleeding using the posterior approach. The transpedicular approach into the body—keeping all of the soft tissue coverings of the vertebral body intact, including the pleura, periosteum, and anterior and posterior longitudinal ligament—allows the surgeon to tamponade bleeding by simply placing a finger into the opening of the pedicle or packing it with bone wax or Gelfoam. Disadvantages of this procedure center on the technical requirements of doing the transpedicular or posterolateral approach; this is somewhat of a blind procedure compared with the anterior thoracotomy.

Osteotomy Through a Previous Posterior Fusion

In certain circumstances, an osteotomy may be required through a previous posterior fusion. This may be needed to address problems related to curve progression secondary to bending of a fusion mass or a pseudarthrosis or to correct an iatrogenically induced deformity such as lumbar flat-back syndrome.

After exposure of the fusion mass, the tips of the transverse process are identified in the region of the intended osteotomy

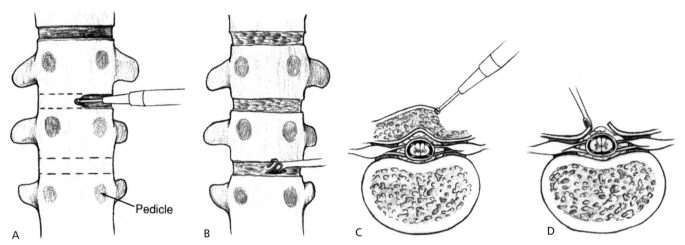

FIGURE 18. Osteotomy through a previous fusion mass. See text for details.

(osteotomies). The transverse processes serve as markers orienting the surgeon for the osteotomy. Because the pedicles lie at the base of the transverse processes, the osteotomy courses between the transverse processes and across the previously fused facet joints. Mobility of the osteotomy occurs through the unfused disc spaces anteriorly.

A high-speed burr is used to define the bony outline of the osteotomy (Fig. 18A). The burr may be used to remove the entire outer cortex and medullary bone down to the deep cortex (Fig. 18C). Alternatively, curets, gouges, and rongeurs may be used to remove the medullary bone and expose the cortical bone overlying the spinal canal (Figs. 18B and C).

A small penetration is made through the deep cortex in the midline into the spinal canal using a burr. Great care must be exercised not to injure the neural structures. In many instances, remnants of the ligamentum flavum remain in the midline, aiding entry into the spinal canal.

The remainder of the deep cortex must then be carefully removed using rongeurs or curets (Fig. 18D). The surgeon should work in a midline to lateral direction staying midway between the transverse processes and pedicles. After the osteotomy is completed, a cervical lamina spreader or Harrington distracter aids in the exposure of the osteotomy site to allow for further decompression. Enough bone mass must be removed to accomplish the intended correction of deformity and to ensure that the neural elements are not impinged. Hemostasis during the procedure is accomplished by generous use of bone wax and thrombin-soaked Gelfoam.

If instrumentation is planned, purchase sites for hooks may be developed in the fusion mass. If the mass is thick, the outer cortex provides sufficient bone stock for purchase of hooks or sublaminar wires. If the fusion mass is thin, the deep cortex must be used as the fixation site, and any sublaminar wires used must pass under the deep cortex in the epidural space.

Osteotomy of spine is the most demanding procedure re-

quired of the spinal surgeon. This procedure requires a complete understanding of the patient's normal and pathologic anatomy. The surgeon must be proficient with bone removal and decompressive techniques. Skill in inserting and manipulating the instrumentation is also required. These procedures are often time-consuming and very tiring to the surgeon. A team approach to these cases is strongly recommended.

REFERENCES

1. Adams JD (1952): Technique, dangers and safeguards in osteotomy of spine. *J Bone Joint Surg Br* 34:226–232.
2. Chaklin VD (1960): Surgery of the spine. *Ortop Travmatol Protez* 21: 3–13.
3. Compere EL (1932): Excision of hemivertebrae for correction of congenital scoliosis. *J Bone Joint Surg* 14:555–562.
4. Dommisse GF, Enslin TB (1970): Hodgson's circumferential osteotomy in the correction of spinal deformity. *J Bone Joint Surg Br* 52: 778.
5. Gaines RW Jr, Carson WL, Satterlee CC, et al. (1991): Experimental evaluation of seven different spinal fracture internal fixation devices using nonfailure stability testing: The load-sharing and unstable-mechanism concepts. *Spine* 16:902–909.
6. Gray JM, Smith BW, Ashley RK, et al. (1991): Derotational analysis of Cotrel-Dubousset instrumentation in idiopathic scoliosis. *Spine* 16[Suppl]:S391–S393.
7. Hodgson AR, Stack FE (1956): Anterior spinal fusion. *Br J Surg* 44: 266–275.
8. Leatherman KD (1969): Resection of vertebral bodies. *J Bone Joint Surg Am* 51:206.
9. Leatherman KD (1972): Resection of vertebral bodies: a new perspective. American Orthopaedic Assoc. Fellowship Thesis.
10. Leatherman KD (1973): The management of rigid spinal curves. *Clin Orthop* 93:215–224.
11. Leatherman KD, Dickson RA (1977): Two stage corrective surgery for congenital spine deformities. *J Bone Joint Surg Br* 59:497.
12. Lichtblau PO, Wilson PD (1956): Possible mechanism of aortic rupture in orthopaedic correction of rheumatoid spondylitis. *J Bone Joint Surg Am* 38:123–127.

13. Luque ER (1984): In: Luque ER, ed. *Segmental spinal instrumentation.* Thorofare, NJ: Charles Slack, pp. 1–11.

14. Luque ER (1984): In: Luque ER, ed. *Segmental spinal instrumentation.* Thorofare, NJ: Charles Slack, pp. 147–163.

15. Roaf R (1955): Wedge resection for scoliosis. *J Bone Joint Surg Br* 37: 97–101.

16. Von Lackum HL, Smith A de F (1933): Removal of vertebral bodies in the treatment of scoliosis. *Surg Gynecol Obstet* 57:250–256.

17. Wiles P (1951): Resection of dorsal vertebrae in congenital scoliosis. *J Bone Joint Surg Am* 33:151–153.

18. Winter RB (1983): *Congenital deformities of the spine.* New York: Thieme-Stratton.

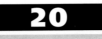

THORACOPLASTY

JOHN MCCLELLAN
MICHAEL GREVITT
JOHN WEBB

The development of a scoliotic deformity is associated with a complex series of vertebral displacements most marked at the apex. Rotation and translation occur around all three orthogonal axes. The rib cage adapts to these abnormal stresses imposed by the spinal curvature and develops altered shape. This is clinically apparent as a rib hump on the curve convexity and best seen in the forward-bending test (Fig. 1).

The ribs on the convexity are rotated backward and acquire an increased angulation at the level of the posterior angle. The coronal plane diameter is reduced, reducing the overall chest volume on this side. Reciprocal changes occur on the concavity, with flattening of the posterior rib angles and forward displacement of the ribs. This accentuates the rib prominence on the other side and reduces the anteroposterior dimensions of the chest. These volumetric changes in the rib cage are responsible for the cardiopulmonary complications arising from "malignant" spinal deformity in infancy (Fig. 2).

The exact etiology of the rib hump remains unclear; there is no clear linear relationship between the degree of lateral curvature (as measured by the Cobb angle) nor the amount of vertebral rotation and the size of the rib hump (23). Cosmetically apparent rib prominence may exist without significant coronal plane deformity. Even with a solid posterior arthrodesis after scoliosis correction, there may be some reassertion of the rib hump (Pratt R, Burwell R, Webb J, unpublished data).

The rib hump is an important sign in screening for scoliosis and is the most significant cosmetic feature of scoliosis. It is this that often alerts the parents to the spinal deformity. Scoring of back shape by lay assessors showed significant correlation between these scores and the severity of the rib hump. There was poor correlation between these cosmetic scores and Cobb angle or lateral asymmetry (22).

Methods of measuring the rib hump have included a spinal pantograph (25), contour devices (7,18,23), scoliometer (6), and sophisticated computerized stereo photogrammetric techniques (8). These latter methods have been used in predicting and identifying curve progression (9,24).

The number of reports on the effect of treatment on rib deformity is small, given its cosmetic importance. In a group of 22 patients with adolescent idiopathic scoliosis (AIS) treated with Boston brace, the rib hump improved significantly (22). Harrington instrumentation does not significantly reduce the rib hump except when a distraction rod is used (1). Luque segmental instrumentation does not confer an additional advantage in rib hump correction. In a series of 40 adolescent thoracic curves, Hullin and colleagues (12) found that the rib hump was reduced in only six patients, unchanged in 27, and worsened slightly in seven. Using a H-frame construct, Hosman and associates (11) demonstrated average Cobb angle correction for King type II and III curves of 68% and 64%, respectively. Corresponding rib hump corrections, however, were only 49% and 27%, respectively. These results indicate that correction of the coronal plane deformity in AIS, even with fourth-generation instrumentation, will not always satisfactorily address the main cosmetic issue. It is important that surgeons treating spinal deformity consider including thoracoplasty as part of the overall surgical strategy.

INDICATIONS, CONTRAINDICATIONS, AND TIMING OF SURGERY

Indications

The most common indication for thoracoplasty is patient dissatisfaction with appearance. There is no objective measure of the size of costal deformity necessary to produce a cosmetic problem. A rib hump as small as 3 cm on forward-bending test has been reported as an indication for thoracoplasty in patients undergoing scoliosis correction (10).

Functional limitation of scapular movement and pain are uncommon indications for thoracoplasty. In adults with progressive spinal deformities, the costal margin may impinge on the iliac crest to produce pain. The rigidity of these curves may make correction difficult. In this situation, thoracoplasty and fusion in situ of the underlying spinal deformity may help relieve pain.

Contraindications

Thoracoplasty should be avoided in the very young, skeletally immature patient. Recurrent rib deformity and crankshaft phenomenon may be expected in certain patients undergoing poste-

M. Grevitt and J. Webb: Centre for Spinal Studies and Surgery, University Hospital, Queen's Medical Centre, Nottingham, U.K.

J. McClellan: Nebraska Spine Center, Omaha, Nebraska 68154.

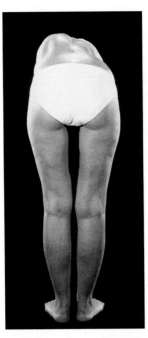

FIGURE 1. Forward-bending test illustrating rib hump.

rior fusion alone. Residual curve of more than 30 degrees, initial apical vertebral rotation of greater than 30 degrees, premenarchal, Tanner grade 2 or less, and Risser 0 patients are all at risk for crankshaft phenomenon without a concomitant anterior arthrodesis (26). In these situations, thoracoplasty can be delayed until skeletal maturity.

Thoracoplasty should also be avoided in patients with poor preoperative pulmonary function. Those with pulmonary function of less than 30% of the predicted values can be expected to have a more difficult postoperative course if thoracoplasty is added to the procedure.

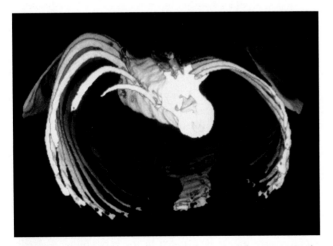

FIGURE 2. Three-dimensional computed tomography reconstruction showing typical rib hump deformity on curve convexity and reciprocal changes in concavity of spine.

Timing

There are no definitive data demonstrating the most appropriate time to perform thoracoplasty. It may add time and blood loss to an already lengthy procedure when combined with instrumented correction and fusion of the scoliosis. However, the resected ribs are an excellent source of bone graft and have provided fusion rates of 96% to 98% when combined with modern scoliosis instrumentation (10,21).

The availability of rib autograft may obviate the need for bone harvest elsewhere and thus save time. Geissele and coworkers (10) found no significant difference in the estimated blood loss, operative time, or duration of inpatient stay when comparing posterior correction alone with posterior correction combined with thoracoplasty. If an anterior release is required, an internal thoracoplasty may be considered. It adds little to the blood loss and operating time and improves the exposure for the anterior release; the rib sections can be used as autologous bone graft for the posterior procedure.

TECHNIQUES

The spine surgeon should be familiar with the variety of techniques of performing thoracoplasty. This allows the most appropriate method to be tailored to the specific needs of the patient and the planned surgical approach for the scoliosis.

The extent of the deformity can be assessed preoperatively. The cephalad and caudal limits, as well as the medial to lateral extent of the rib hump, can be estimated using the forward-bending test. The preoperative assessment is important because the mediolateral extent of the rib hump dictates the amount of rib resection required. It may also influence the decision to move the ribs caudad after resection or to create a rib hump in the spinal concavity (see later). The size of the rib deformity may also be minimized when the patient is placed prone on the operating table, making subsequent intraoperative planning unreliable.

The more complex "razor-back" deformities should be assessed by computed tomography (CT). Apical sections demonstrate the amount of costal angulation and the proximity of the vertebral convexity to the rib. Three-dimensional CT is particularly valuable in visualizing these cases and may demonstrate the need to perform additional excision of the transverse processes to obtain the best cosmetic result.

The most common technique uses a midline dorsal incision with exposure of the medial portion of the ribs. Thoracoplasty can also be performed from within the chest either through a thoracotomy or using video-assisted endoscopic methods.

Dorsal Thoracoplasty

Dorsal thoracoplasty can be performed as an adjuvant procedure during the primary scoliosis correction or at a later stage. It may also be indicated in skeletally mature patients with minor curves. In these patients with minimal risk for curve progression, the rib hump may be the only complaint.

The standard technique involves midline exposure of the rib deformity from the transverse process to the lateral edge of the rib deformity. Steel (21) described an additional separate incision starting at the inferior border of the scapula extending distally to the extent of the costal deformity. We have not used this incision because an additional scar seems to us cosmetically undesirable.

Retraction of paraspinous muscles using Langenbeck retractors may provide adequate exposure if only short medial segments of ribs require resection. More extensive rib resection requires a plane to be developed between the paraspinous muscles and the thoracolumbar fascia. To avoid extensive muscle dissection, after the medial portion of the rib is located, this plane can be developed by blunt finger dissection over the respective rib. This plane can be extended to the posterior axillary line. Electrocautery is used to incise the periosteum over the rib along the length of the planned resection. Periosteal elevators are used to strip the periosteum off the rib, taking care to avoid damaging the neurovascular bundle along its inferior border. In addition, strict adherence to the subperiosteal plane reduces the risk of breaching the parietal pleura.

The amount of rib resection recommended has varied among several authors. Steel (21) resected an average of 12 cm at each level from 1,840 ribs in 392 patients. Others have described resecting the deformity from the articulation with the transverse process to the lateral extent of the deformity, usually 2 to 3 cm at each rib (3,14). The amount of rib resection may also be influenced by the amount of bone graft required (13). If they are contributing to the deformity, prominent transverse processes and costotransverse joints should be excised.

Some authors have described leaving the ends of the ribs apart after resection. There are several disadvantages to this approach. A flail chest may develop, some postoperative bracing may be required, and it is our impression that these patients have more postsurgical pain. We prefer to reapproximate the ribs when possible (15). If the preoperative assessment indicates a rib hump with a broad-based convexity, a resection of more than 3 cm over the most prominent ribs may be required. In these instances, reapproximation at the same level may be difficult or produce an unacceptable dimple in the chest wall through traction on the lateral rib segment. By moving the lateral portion of rib one or two segments caudally to its original location, wire suturing to a medial rib stump may be easier and has the added advantage of further flattening the previous costal deformity. Small drill holes are made in each of the ends, and 20-gauge wire is used to tie the ends together (Fig. 3).

Translocation of the resected ribs for severe rib hump has been described (3,4). In cases of razor-back deformity, flattening of the convex rib hump may still leave an unsatisfactory asymmetry in the back contour. In this situation, the resected rib portions may be used to manufacture a rib hump in the spinal concavity. The ribs opposite the residual rib hump are selected and divided 1 cm lateral to the transverse process. For each rib, an AO/ASIF $\frac{1}{3}$ semitubular plate is bent into a Z shape. A four- or five-hole plate usually suffices. A resected rib portion is fixed in the midportion of the plate with a 3.5-mm cortical screw. The plate is then fixed to the divided rib ends such that the lateral end is elevated (Figs. 4 to 6).

Testing for a pleural tear involves installation of saline into the wound and inspection for bubbles when the lung is maximally inflated. If these are present, a chest tube should be inserted before wound closure. It is our own practice to insert a

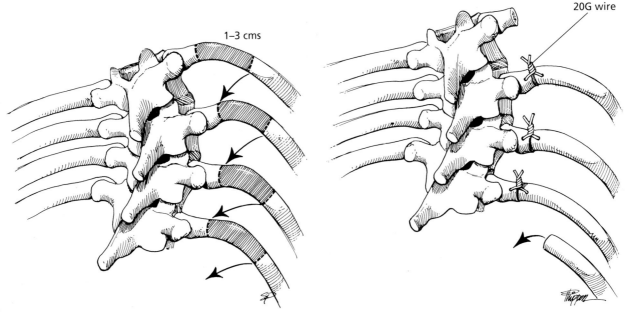

1–3 cms

20G wire

A

B

FIGURE 3. Diagram illustrating rib resection, caudal displacement, and suture of approximated ends with 20-gauge wire.

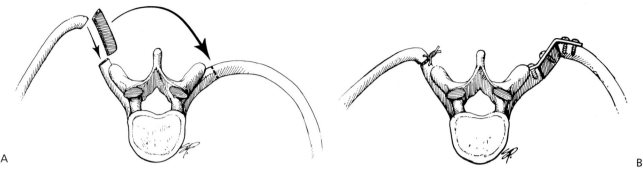

FIGURE 4. Diagram illustrating principle of rib segment translocation to create rib hump in spinal concavity. AO/ASIF ⅓ semitubular plates (bent into Z shape) and screws are used for fixation.

chest drain routinely because even without a pleural tear, there is risk for a pleural effusion that may require drainage.

The inferomedial portion of the scapula may be deformed because of the previous underlying rib deformity. This may be prominent after rib hump resection and rarely cause impingement and pain. Steel (21) performed reduction scapuloplasty in 50% of adults and 4% of adolescents undergoing thoracoplasty. He thought that the children's scapulae had the potential for remodeling to the flattened ribs. Up to half of the scapula may be excised without apparent functional deficit (5). We have not performed this procedure as part of a thoracoplasty. We question, however, if it is a benign operation because we have seen long-term shoulder morbidity from high thoracotomy. This is due in part to the large amount of periscapular muscle division inherent in this approach.

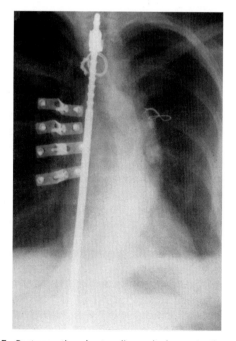

FIGURE 5. Postoperative chest radiograph demonstrating wiring of resecting rib ends and use of rib segments and metal plates to elevate chest wall in spinal concavity.

Internal Thoracoplasty

Internal thoracoplasty can be performed before anterior releases and anterior correction for scoliosis. Internal thoracoplasty during open growth arrest was described by Shufflebarger and colleagues (20). The rib of the superior vertebra to be included in the fusion was resected for the anterior exposure. This rib often corresponds with the superior rib involved in the rib hump. Internal thoracoplasty is done on the next three to four ribs. Subperiosteal exposure of the ribs is performed and osteotomized at the posterior axillary line. The lateral divided portion is pulled medially; 2 to 3 cm of rib is then removed to leave a gap between the remaining rib ends. These ends may be left apart or alternatively sutured together with two Dexon or wire sutures. Intercostal nerve blocks may be performed (0.25% bupivacaine) at each osteotomized rib level. The latter reduces the postoperative analgesic requirement.

Video-assisted endoscopic techniques are gaining popularity in scoliosis surgery. Thoracoscopic costoplasty was first mentioned in the literature by Regan and coworkers (19) and later described by Mehlman and associates (16). In this technique, the ribs are exposed by electrocautery and a small rib elevator (Fig. 7). A high-speed burr is used for the rib osteotomies (Fig. 8). The resected rib segments can be delivered through the endoscopic portals (Fig. 9). Our preference is to stabilize the rib ends. The burr is used to make holes in the respective ends of ribs (Fig. 10). An outside-in suturing technique similar to that used in meniscal repairs with burying of the knot subcutaneously is used to tie the rib ends together (aided by external chest compression before tying the knot) (Fig. 6).

The thoracoscopic technique also lends itself to thoracoplasty after posterior scoliosis correction when thoracotomy has been avoided. It avoids the extensive dorsal dissection and has a shorter rehabilitation period.

Bracing

Casting or bracing has been advocated to help remold the rib cage and reduce the incidence of hemothorax. Betz and Steel (5) described use of a clam shell held in place with Ace wraps or Velcro straps for the first 48 hours. They believed this reduced the incidence of hemothorax in the immediate postoperative period. Absence of a flail chest and with a resected area less

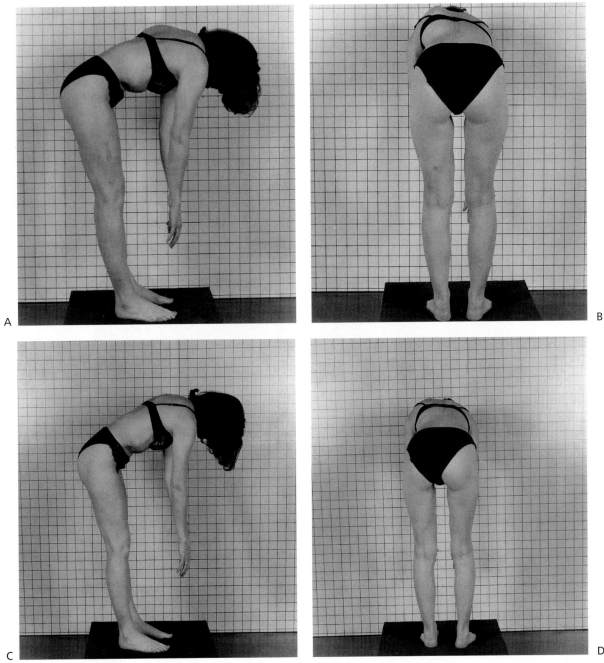

FIGURE 6. Preoperative (**A, B**) and postoperative (**C, D**) views of patient shown in Figure 5 after rib resection and translocation.

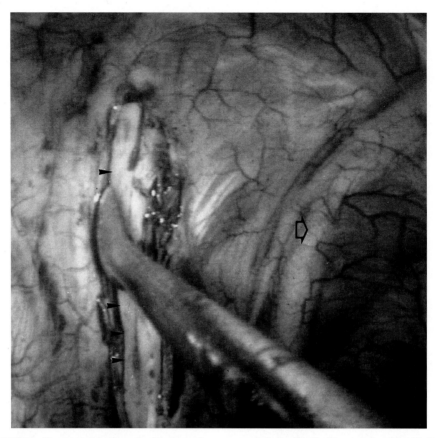

FIGURE 7. Thoracoscopic view of subperiosteal exposure of rib (outlined with *arrowheads*) with Cobb elevator. Second rib is visible (*broad arrow*).

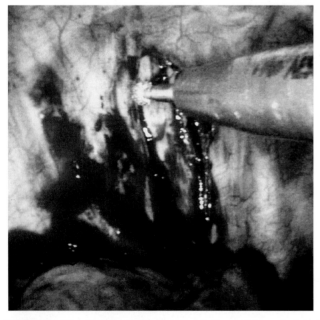

FIGURE 8. Rib osteotomy with high-speed diamond burr. Deflated lung at bottom of visual field (*broad arrows*).

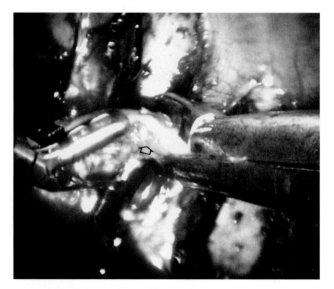

FIGURE 9. Removal of resected rib segment (*arrow*).

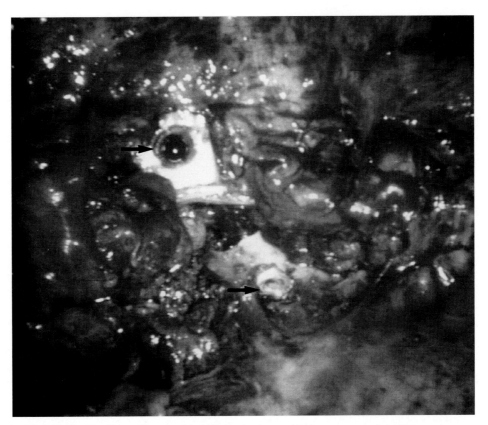

FIGURE 10. Remaining rib ends with drilled holes (*arrows*) before passage of stabilizing sutures.

than the width of a palm led to discontinuance of the brace. If necessary, the brace was worn for 3 months in adolescents and for 6 months in adults. Risser casts have also been used after thoracoplasty (14,21).

RESULTS

There have been few objective assessments of the results of thoracoplasty using validated outcome measures.

Geissele and coauthors (10) found that 93% of patients noted cosmetic improvement in the rib hump and that 86% were willing to go through with the procedure again if given the opportunity. The largest personal series of thoracoplasty had only 3% of cases with unsatisfactory results, half of which were due to inadequate rib resection (21).

Using back-surface measurements, Barrett and colleagues (2) evaluated the results of thoracoplasty in 55 patients (age range, 12 to 35 years). The best correction was achieved in patients undergoing short-segment (average 1.6 cm) thoracoplasty at the same time as scoliosis correction. In adults, a larger (3 cm) segment of rib extended beyond the apex for adequate correction of deformity. Reformation of the resected rib segment was found in all patients at an average 3.4 months after surgery. A *Z*-shaped pattern of regrowth suggested some caudal migration of the cut rib ends.

There was no difference in the 2-year results in the immature

patients (Risser 1 or 2) compared with the more skeletally mature patients. At final follow-up, there was no difference in loss of correction whether the thoracoplasty was done during scoliosis or as a separate procedure.

PITFALLS AND COMPLICATIONS

Incomplete Resection of the Rib Hump

Incomplete resection of the rib hump is a complication that has been reported in 4% of patients (10) and has accounted for 69% of unsatisfactory results (21). The extent of the deformity may be less apparent when the patient is prone on the operating table. This fact emphasizes the importance of marking the extent of the deformity preoperatively.

A deformed medial scapular border may produce symptoms when it articulates with the flattened chest wall or an unsightly prominence. Consideration should be given to a partial resection if there is significant chest wall and scapular incongruence in an adult.

Flail Chest

Although flail chest is the most-often quoted reason for the use of postoperative bracing, it has not been extensively reported in the literature. We have not seen it in our practice.

Hemothorax, Pneumothorax, and Pleural Effusion

Hemothorax, pneumothorax, and pleural effusion are common complications, and their incidence may be reduced if there is no pleural breach at the time of rib dissection and osteotomy. Even when the saline test demonstrates no apparent leakage, we have encountered pleural effusions and hemothoraces in the first few postoperative days. Insertion of a chest drain or thoracocentesis at this stage is uncomfortable for the patient; we routinely insert a chest drain at the time of wound closure.

Chest Wall Hypoesthesia and Neuralgia

Chest wall hypoesthesia or neuralgia may be present in 15% to 24% of patients after thoracoplasty (2,10). When thoracoplasty was performed as separate procedure, the incidence rates of neuralgic pain were 62% of patients at 3 months and 29% at 6 months (4). The incidence may be reduced by attention to strict subperiosteal exposure of the ribs and avoidance of incorporation of the neurovascular bundle in the suture line if closing the periosteum.

Impairment of Pulmonary Function

Steel (21) found a 12% decline in maximum voluntary ventilation, vital capacity (VC), and total lung capacity (TLC) 2 weeks after surgery. By 3 months, most were approaching preoperative levels, and by 1 year, 90% had reached or exceeded their preoperative function. The age range of the patients in this study was 7 to 51 years, but Steel did not distinguish the results of children from those of adults, and the 3-year follow-up rate was poor.

Patients undergoing Harrington instrumentation alone have significant reductions in VC and forced expiratory volume in one second (FEV_1). Those having a thoracoplasty before instrumentation had reductions in the latter parameters as well as TLC and peak expiratory flow rate (17). This was thought to represent loss of functional lung tissue beneath the rib hump and alteration in the total volume of the thoracic cage.

Broome and colleagues (4) noted a 17% reduction in forced vital capacity (FVC) and 14% reduction in FEV_1 at 3 months. A more comprehensive review by Lenke and associates (13) of posterior instrumentation and thoracoplasty in adolescents noted a 16% decline in pulmonary function (FVC, FEV_1, TLC) at 3 months. There was near-normal return of the same parameters at 2 years. In contrast, adults showed a 27% reduction in lung function at 3 months, with 23% persistent deterioration at 2 years. This deficit was clinically insignificant during normal daily activities and demanding aerobic exercise.

In summary, thoracoplasty does appear to compromise pulmonary function in the first few months after surgery. In adolescents, this deficit recovers by 2 years, but in adults, some restriction persists. Although not clinically relevant in healthy subjects, caution should be exercised in thoracoplasty when lung function is less than 30% predicted. We have operated on spinal deformities in children with lung capacities lower than this figure (e.g., Duchenne neuromuscular dystrophy). However, in cases of major thoracic cage deformity, rib resection and resultant post-operative splinting of the intercostal muscles have produced significant pulmonary problems in the postoperative period when this guideline was ignored.

SUMMARY

The exact relationship between rib deformity and scoliosis remains unclear. The rib hump is an important element in the cosmetic problem associated with scoliosis. Modern instrumentation systems for deformity correction do not completely address the rib hump. There is also evidence for some late reassertion of the rib despite a solid posterior arthrodesis.

Thoracoplasty is an essential procedure in the spinal surgeon's armamentarium. The better cosmetic results and psychological advantages over rib resection should prompt the spine surgeon to consider thoracoplasty either as an adjuvant procedure at the time of scoliosis correction or at a later stage.

The various techniques need to be mastered so that the appropriate option can be applied to any given patient and approach. Dorsal and internal thoracoplasties are well established, with the latter being modified using endoscopic techniques.

Careful preoperative assessment and imaging determine the levels of required resection. Severe pulmonary dysfunction should be a contraindication for the thoracoplasty. Careful attention to detail minimizes complications. A decrease in pulmonary function is to be expected in the first months after surgery. In adults, there is a permanent deficit that is not clinically significant.

REFERENCES

1. Aaro S, Dahlborn M (1982): The effect of Arrington instrumentation on the longitudinal axis rotation of the apical vertebra and on the spinal and rib cage deformity in idiopathic scoliosis studied by computer tomography. *Spine* 7(5):456–462.
2. Barrett DS, MacLean JGB, Bettany J, et al. (1993): Costoplasty in adolescent idiopathic scoliosis: objective results in 55 patients. *J Bone Joint Surg Br* 75:881–885.
3. Briard JL, Chopin D, Cauchoix J (1980): Surgical correction of rib deformity in scoliosis. *Orthop Trans* 4:25.
4. Broome G, Simpson AHRW, Catalan J, et al. (1990): The modified Schollner costoplasty. *J Bone Joint Surg Br* 72:894–900.
5. Betz RR, Steel HH (1997): Thoracoplasty for rib deformity. In: Bradford DS, ed. *Master techniques in orthopaedic surgery: the spine.* Philadelphia: Lippincott-Raven, pp. 209–227.
6. Bunnell WP (1984): An objective criterion for scoliosis screening. *J Bone Joint Surg Am* 66:1381–1387.
7. Burwell RG, James NJ, Johnson F, et al. (1983): Standardized trunk asymmetry scores: a study of back contour in healthy schoolchildren. *J Bone Joint Surg Br* 65:452–463.
8. Carr AJ, Jefferson RJ, Turner-Smith AR (1991): Familial back shape in adolescent scoliosis. *Acta Orthop Scand* 62(2):131–135.
9. Duvall-Beaupere G (1996): Threshold values for supine and standing Cobb angles and rib hump measurements: prognostic factors for scoliosis. *Eur Spine J* 5:79–84.
10. Geissele AE, Ogilvie JW, Cohen JW, et al. (1994): Thoracoplasty for the treatment of rib prominence in thoracic scoliosis. *Spine* 19:1636–1642.
11. Hosman AJF, Slot GH, van Limbeek J, et al. (1996): Rib hump correction and rotation of the lumbar spine after selective thoracic fusion. *Eur Spine J* 5:394–399.

12. Hullin MG, McMaster MJ, Draper ERC (1991): The effect of Luque segmental sublaminar instrumentation on the rib hump in idiopathic scoliosis. *Spine* 16(4):402–408.
13. Lenke LG, Bridwell KH, Blanke K (1995): Analysis of pulmonary function and chest cage dimension changes after thoracoplasty in idiopathic scoliosis. *Spine* 20:1343–1350.
14. Laughlin TT (1980): Rib hump resection in scoliosis surgery *Orthop Trans* 4:24–25.
15. Manning CW, Prime FJ, Zorab PA (1973): Partial costectomy as a cosmetic operation in scoliosis. *J Bone Joint Surg Br* 55:521–527.
16. Mehlman CT, Crawford AH, Wolf RK (1997): Video-assisted thoracoscopic surgery (VATS): endoscopic thoracoplasty technique. *Spine* 22:2178–2182.
17. Owen R, Turner A, Bamforth JSG, et al. (1986): Costectomy as the first stage of surgery for scoliosis. *J Bone Joint Surg Br* 68:91–95.
18. Pun WK, Luk KDK, Lee W, et al. (1987): A simple method to estimate the rib hump in scoliosis. *Spine* 12(4):342–345.
19. Regan JJ, Mack MJ, Picetti G, et al. (1994): A comparison of video-assisted thoracoscopic surgery (VATS) with open thoracotomy in thoracic spinal surgery. *Today's Therapeutic Trends* 11:203–218.
20. Shufflebarger HL, Smiley K, Roth HJ (1994): Internal thoracoplasty: a new procedure. *Spine* 19:840–842.
21. Steel HH (1993): Rib resection and spine fusion in correction of convex deformity in scoliosis. *J Bone Joint Surg Am* 65:920–925.
22. Theologis TN, Jefferson RJ, Simpson AHRW, et al. (1993): Quantifying the cosmetic defect of adolescent idiopathic scoliosis. *Spine* 18(7):909–912.
23. Thulborne T, Gillespie R (1976): The rib hump in idiopathic scoliosis: measurement, analysis and response to treatment. *J Bone Joint Surg Br* 58:64–71.
24. Weisz I, Jefferson RJ, Turner-Smith RJ, et al. (1988): ISIS scanning: a useful technique in the management of scoliosis. *Spine* 13(4):405–408.
25. Wilner S (1983): Spinal pantograph: a non-invasive anthropanetric device for describing postures and asymmetries of the trunk. *J Paediatr Orthop* 3:245–249.
26. Winter RB (1992): Surgical correction of rigid thoracic lordoscoliosis. *J Spinal Disord* 5:108–110.

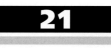

KYPHECTOMY

J. IVAN KRAJBICH

Surgical treatment of spinal deformities in children with spina bifida with myelomeningocele is a relatively new field. Consequently, one does not find the usual volume of North American and European literature from the turn of the century describing operative procedures performed on these children. Before World War II, the vast majority of these children died early in infancy of sepsis. This was particularly true of children with kyphotic deformity and spina bifida as this particular deformity is usually associated with relatively high-level lesions, and these children almost never survived early infancy. It was not until after the war, with the development and wide use of antibiotics and early surgical closure of the neural tube defect, that these children survived. And it was not until they reached childhood and adolescence in the 1950s and 1960s that the problems associated with the concomitant spinal deformities became apparent and required the attention of physicians and surgeons (41).

The first step in dealing with these abnormalities was to learn about their incidence, natural history, and structural and anatomical characteristics (40). In 1967, Hoppenfeld (16) reviewed a large number of patients with spina bifida. He examined their radiographs and in several instances necropsy material to provide the first scientific description of kyphosis in meningomyelocele. His findings, later confirmed by the work of Sharrard (36), showed that the kyphosis was associated with spina bifida with meningocele in approximately 12% of these children at birth. Hoppenfeld's description of the spinal abnormality is probably still the best in the literature. He found that the kyphosis is fixed and not reducible. The posterior element defect starts in the lower thoracic area and extends distally over the lumbar area and sacrum. Widely separated, splayed pedicles are oriented essentially in the coronal plane; the lamina or portion of lamina is completely inverted, with the normally anterior surface of the lamina actually facing posteriorly and laterally (Fig. 1).

The pedicles are widest apart at the apex of the deformity. The dural sac lies on the surface of the vertebral bodies with no bony coverings. The roots exit almost directly anteriorly through the vertebral foramina. The paraspinal muscles are displaced anteriorly next to the vertebral body, functioning essentially as flexors of the spine over the kyphotic segment rather than as extensors, which is their normal anatomical function. Further

deforming force can be generated by the action of psoas muscles, which have retained their innervations (6).

The lower ribs assume a relatively horizontal position, frequently flaring out, particularly in older children. The ribs start to rest on the pelvis and the thoracic cavity has to accommodate the abdominal viscera as they are pushed against the diaphragm in the lower part of the chest (Fig. 2).

Hoppenfeld (16) also described the compensatory thoracic lordosis that these patients develop above the level of the kyphosis. This can become quite a rigid structural deformity; it is difficult to treat and occasionally limits what can be accomplished by corrective surgery. Sharrard (36) shed further light on the natural history of the kyphotic deformity by analyzing data on nearly 500 patients. Only those patients with a thoracic neurologic level had a significant incidence of kyphosis at birth. They also demonstrated a steady increase in kyphosis during childhood. It is relatively uncommon for a patient with a lower neurologic level to develop kyphosis. The difference between thoracic and lumbar lesions was even more striking when the radiographs were examined. Essentially 100% of patients with a radiographic thoracic level developed kyphosis, but fewer than 20% of patients with a lumbar defect did so. Hoppenfeld also found that kyphosis greater than 65 degrees progressed relentlessly in all patients. It is therefore obvious that the kyphosis in children with spina bifida with meningomyelocele is usually associated with the thoracic lesion, and such children are severely affected both neurologically and skeletally. In these higher level lesions, the incidence of associated central nervous system abnormalities, such as Chiari malformation, hydrocephalus, and other spinal dysraphism, above the level of the spina bifida rises as well. Associated increase in bony spinal abnormalities (congenital scoliosis) is also seen.

These factors, together with a significant structural deformity of the spine, make treatment of these children a formidable undertaking. Nevertheless, since the 1960s, relatively aggressive surgical correction has been tried and recommended (4,9, 10,13,14,23, 36–39) mostly because of the problems and complications associated with this deformity.

To address the problems of progressive kyphosis, and in the hope of preventing further neurologic deterioration and perhaps provide some improvement, surgical correction of the congenital kyphosis was originally performed and described by Sharrard (36). He advised surgery in the newborn infant in the hopes of

J. I. Krajbich: Department of Orthopedic Surgery, Shriners Hospital for Children, Portland, Oregon 97201-3095.

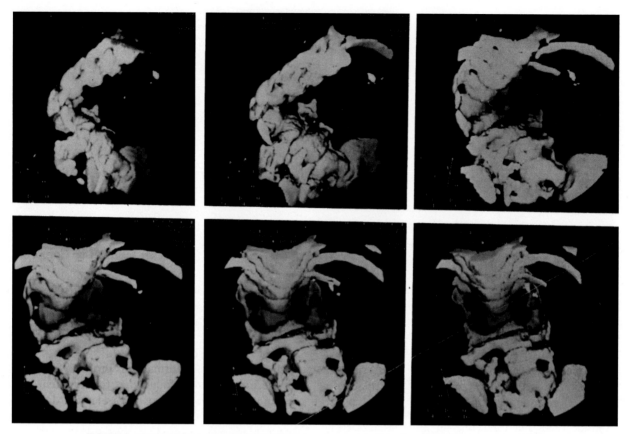

FIGURE 1. Computed tomography three-dimensional reconstruction of moderately severe spina bifida kyphosis, demonstrating the sharp gibbus, widely splayed lateral elements, and loss of normal truncal height.

improving both the soft-tissue coverage of the meningomyelocele defect and the neurologic status. He suggested excision of 1½ vertebral bodies from the apex of the deformity, preserving all of the neuroelements by careful dissection. Fixation was carried out with sutures only. He was encouraged by the early results, but the deformity had a tendency to recur. For older children, he suggested a transverse osteotomy with bayonet apposition of the spine and fixation with screws. In spite of the technical difficulty of this procedure, the high rate of complications, and high recurrence rate reported in the initial series, it became a popular procedure. A number of authors reported their results in the 1970s (2,9,10,13,14,20,21,24,37–39).

The procedure initially suffered from less than ideal internal fixation. Kirschner wires, wire sutures, Blount staples and screws were all being used with predictably less than optimal results. Because of the poor results with this type of internal fixation, some authors recommended using external immobilization in a cast as the only means of fixation. Even with the internal fixation, most children needed braces or casts postoperatively to improve the chance of maintaining the spinal alignment. This brought on the additional challenge of looking after insensitive skin under a cast and the increased risk of lower extremity fractures due to immobilization osteoporosis (27).

It was Hall et al. who pointed out the advantage of performing the surgery at an older age or using more adequate instru-

mentation (14). This and the development and wider use of reliable spinal instrumentation led to renew interest in surgical treatment in these children. From then on, the story of kyphectomy closely parallels the developments in spinal instrumentation (4,8). Initially, Harrington instrumentation, involving a combination of compression and distraction rods and frequently augmented by anterior strut bone grafting, yielded better results. However, it became obvious that unless the spinal deformity was almost completely corrected and a reasonable biomechanical axis restored, the procedure had little chance of accomplishing most of the goals of treatment. The deformity would frequently reoccur over the ensuing months or years.

The real significant improvement came with the use of segmental instrumentation as described by Luque (25). Luque rods fixed to the pelvis and to the lumbar spine by segmental wires allowed the application of correction forces to obtain a straight or nearly straight alignment of the spine and hold it by reasonably rigid fixation. This avoided a prolonged immobilization in a cast or brace, allowing the young patient to be mobilized relatively early in the postoperative course, avoiding secondary complications. The technique of Luque rod instrumentation with segmental wiring and fixation to the pelvis is to date the most widely used procedure in association with kyphectomy and is the one preferred by the author. In the majority of cases it allows for excellent correction of the spinal deformity and rigid fixation

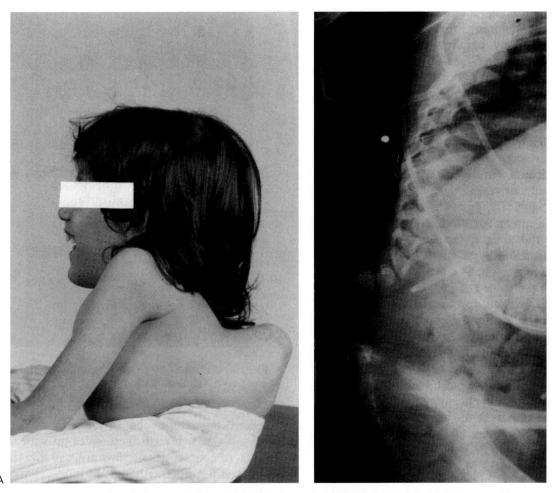

A   B

FIGURE 2. Clinical photograph **(A)** and lateral sitting radiograph **(B)** of a young girl with a thoracic level spina bifida and kyphosis. Ribs become horizontal in orientation as the rib cage rests on the pelvis and anterior thighs. Marked decrease in trunk height and elevation of the diaphragm well into the thoracic cavity are apparent. Note shunt tubing of two ventriculoperitoneal shunts on the radiograph **(B)**. The kyphosis is close to 170 degrees. The compensatory lordosis in the lower thoracic area is the part of the deformity that is frequently the most difficult to correct.

without the need for postoperative external immobilization (15,17,29,30,31,43).

INDICATIONS FOR SURGERY

Kyphectomy with segmental spinal instrumentation is a formidable procedure even in the most experienced hands, with potentially significant complications. One must have a clear picture regarding the pros and cons of this surgery for each individual patient. The only absolute or nearly absolute indications for this procedure are either a persistent pressure sore over the spinal gibbus, with underlying infection of the bone that fails to respond to conservative treatment (Fig. 3), or inability to secure safe urinary diversion access, which threatens the integrity of the patient's upper urinary tract. All other indications are relative.

One such indication is the gradual compromise of pulmonary function from pressure of the abdominal viscera against the dia-

phragm as the trunk height gradually diminishes and the child's rib cage is left resting on his or her pelvis or thighs (Fig. 2). The trunk height itself could be a problem for a child attending school. Inability to provide a child with an adequate seating device and reasonable sitting balance is another relative indication. Many of these children need elaborate inserts to accommodate the spinal gibbus, and they cannot sit upright without resting their abdomen and lower chest against the anterior thighs. The only way for them to sit upright is to push themselves up with their arms. This, of course, ties up their arms so that they cannot be used for other activities. The effort to keep the upper torso upright forces the lower thoracic spine into a compensatory lordosis, which can gradually become fixed.

Recurrent pressure sores and skin breakdowns over the gibbus constitute further relative indications, as does pain either at the lower end of the rib cage as it impinges on the pelvis or in the upper region of the kyphotic deformity. Another relative indication is a gradual progression of a secondary spinal deformity, namely, a compensatory lordosis above the gibbus. This

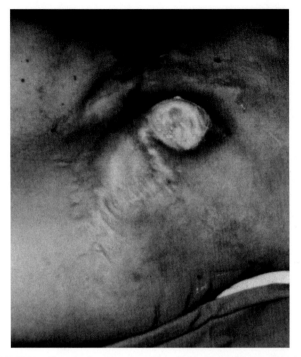

FIGURE 3. Chronic ulcer over the gibbus deformity of a child with spina bifida kyphosis.

Fixed extension deformity of the child's hips is a rare contraindication, as straightening of the spine would result in inability of the child to sit upright in a chair. On the positive side, a successful operation leaves the child able to sit up straight in a chair, resulting in easier seating, a decrease in pressure sores and skin breakdown over the posterior aspect of the spine, better cosmesis, and easier access to the genitourinary tract. The majority of patients also improve their physical fitness as their pulmonary function improves once the abdominal viscera are no longer pressing on the diaphragm (Fig. 4). The child is taller, can sit better, and has a significantly improved self-image. But the child needs to adjust to the fact that because of the increased trunk height, his or her center of gravity is higher than it used to be. Reestablishment of the new sitting balance requires practice and time, with the majority of children adjusting within a few weeks. Increased space for the abdominal viscera and thus ability to eat larger meals can occasionally lead to more than average weight gains, and some children may require nutritional and recreational guidance because of it. Quite frequently, we see children progress from being marginal manual chair ambulators to active participants in wheelchair sports and athletics.

The age of the patient when the operation is performed depends to some extent on the treating surgeon, but it is usually dictated by the severity of the complications associated with the

deformity is initially somewhat flexible but later becomes rigid—further compromising the normal shape of the thorax. In older children or teenagers, cosmesis becomes an important factor that comes into play as they become aware of their abnormal appearance and are embarrassed by the spinal deformity.

These relative indications have to be balanced against the potential complications of kyphectomy, some of which are significant and serious. The most important and most serious is an acute neurologic decompensation with increased intracranial pressure, leading to death (44). This has been reported in a number of series and in some institutions; a fatal outcome was common enough to result in abandonment of the procedure. However, this complication can be prevented by careful preoperative evaluation (35), careful postoperative monitoring of the child's neurologic function, and adherence to a meticulous surgical technique. It is essential that the child's shunt be evaluated for patency and function. This is particularly important in cases in which the remnant of the spinal cord in the area of the kyphosis is to be transected. Even a neurologically nonfunctioning cord is part of the cerebrospinal fluid circulatory pathway. Its disruption, by tying or mishandling, can precipitate an acute increase in the intracranial pressure, which if not promptly relieved by a shunt will lead to brain herniation and death (44).

Other significant complications include infection, difficulty with a soft-tissue coverage in patients with ulcerated skin over the posterior spinal area, and a recurrent breakdown of the skin over sometimes prominent hardware. Loss of fixation and recurrence of the deformity with nonunion have also been reported, but these are relatively uncommon with the newer surgical techniques (27,43).

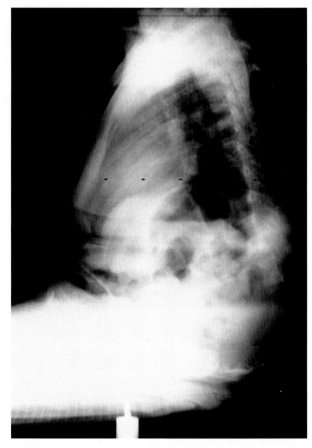

A

FIGURE 4. A 9-year-old girl with thoracic level meningocele and progressive kyphosis. **A:** Preoperative lateral radiograph. *(Figure continues.)*

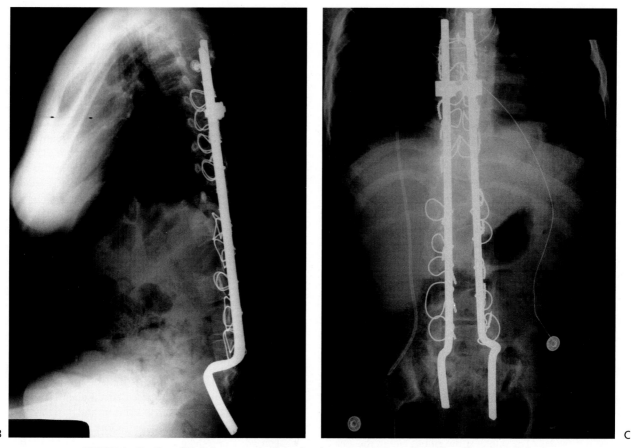

FIGURE 4. *Continued.* **B, C:** Postoperative lateral and anteroposterior radiographs with patient sitting. Spinal instrumentation into the sacrum is by a technique described by Fackler, with the distal ends of the rods in the first sacral foramina. Note the increase in the height of the trunk.

gibbous deformity. Persistent skin breakdown and infection of the underlying bone and/or difficulty in genitourinary tract care can make the operation mandatory at an early age. However, the more common picture is progression of the deformity during childhood, with loss of trunk height, decrease in pulmonary function, and problems of seating and cosmesis. These children are probably best operated on when they are between 8 and 12 years of age—occasionally older—as the operation on more mature spines allows for better fixation and future spinal growth becomes less of a factor. Some authors recommend operation at a younger age using nonrigid fixation with only partial correction and expectation of some degree of deformity recurrence (27,32). It has been this author's experience that better lasting correction with less extensive spinal resection can be achieved in slightly older children using rigid spinal fixation (15,19,29,43).

PREOPERATIVE ASSESSMENT

Once the decision has been made to proceed with surgical correction of the kyphotic deformity, careful preoperative evaluation of the patient and planning of the procedure are undertaken. It is preferable to have the child assessed by both a neurosurgeon

and a urologist (33). It is important that the child not have an ongoing urinary tract infection at the time of the planned surgery. Also, any necessary urologic diversion surgery can be planned in coordination with the orthopaedic intervention. Postoperative neurosurgical consultation regarding evaluation of shunt function must also be secured to guard against the catastrophic complication of sudden central nervous system pressure decompensation.

The child is evaluated by magnetic resonance imaging (MRI) for any previously unrecognized intraspinal anomalies above the level of the lesion, such as syringomyelia, hydromyelia, or diastematomyelia (35). The extent of the Chiari malformation, which is almost invariably present in these children, is also assessed. Sitting anteroposterior and lateral radiographs of the spine are secured for adequate planning of the surgery. Decisions have to be made regarding the extent of the resected segment. The surgeon has to determine whether resection of one vertebrae at the apex is sufficient or if the resection should be more extensive or perhaps more proximal to secure a longer distal fragment to improve fixation. The extent and rigidity of the compensatory thoracic lordosis must be assessed. In rare instances, the procedure can be combined with anterior release and discectomies over the prominent lordotic thoracic segment to allow for better correction. Recently developed techniques of endoscopic disce- ctomies can be employed to accomplish this.

Resection of the apical vertebrae is recommended by most authors, including us. If the apex is a disc space, the vertebra proximal to the apex is resected. A small amount of the vertebral body on each side of this apical resection is also removed to allow good cancellous bone apposition of the two adjacent portions of the spine. Avoiding resection of a larger segment preserves spinal column length and improves the stability of the spinal fixation; the two flat osteotomized ends have a tendency to compress against each other when the deformity is reduced. This is impor- tant, as trunk height improvement is one of the goals of surgery (Fig. 18). Extensive resection of a lordotic portion of the spine as described by some (21,27,37) is in the author's opinion coun- terproductive because it further compromises the height of the trunk. On the other hand, resection of a larger segment makes the correction easier and is preferable to undercorrection.

Some authors argue against spinal length preservation on the basis of possible stretching of great vessels, which were shown to bowstring across the kyphotic curve (12,22). To the author's knowledge, this has never been reported in the literature and has never occurred in more than 30 patients operated on by the author using this technique, suggesting that vessels are elastic enough to accommodate the spinal deformity corrections. Close monitoring of the lower limb circulation during and the follow- ing the procedure is, of course, mandatory.

The patient is carefully evaluated for any active pressure sores and, if present, these are allowed to heal. If necessary, inpatient treatment is provided. The skin over the gibbus and in the adja- cent area is evaluated for quality, as well as for the presence of chronic ulcerations, defects, and infections. A decision is made whether the child needs a supplementary skin coverage tech- nique following the surgery. In cases of difficult skin problems, we have employed a soft-tissue expander prior to the kyphec- tomy with good success (19). When the surgeon is satisfied that the procedure is well planned, the child has been cleared by both the urologist and the neurosurgeon, and the skin is in optimal shape, the surgical procedure is implemented.

SURGICAL TECHNIQUE

Our basic surgical technique of kyphectomy followed by spinal segmental instrumentation varies little from the techniques de- scribed in the literature by various authors (10,15,17,29,30, 31,43). The patient is positioned prone on the operating table on Hall-Relton spinal frame, with care taken to avoid pressure against the abdomen. A straight midline incision is made over the spine, and skin flaps are elevated. Not infrequently, some modifications to the skin incision are necessary to accommodate the previous incisions and scars. Care is taken not to enter the dural sac. The skin, which in many instances is adherent to the dural sac, is carefully dissected; the skin flaps must not be buttonholed.

The spine is exposed well into the thoracic area over the lordotic segment of the spine proximally. Distally it is exposed down to the sacrum. Subperiosteal technique is used to strip the spine of the overlying muscles in the lordotic segment in the area of the intact lamina. In the area of the posterior element defect, careful subperiosteal stripping and dissection are carried out over the lateral elements, proceeding laterally and anteriorly, staying out of the spinal canal area and not disturbing the neural tube. At the apex of the gibbus, the dissection is carried out past the inverted pedicles to the vertebral bodies. The anterior aspects of the three apical vertebral bodies are carefully exposed subperi- osteally. The spine is thus exposed circumferentially (Fig. 5).

Next the periosteum is stripped from the posterior aspect of the vertebral bodies over the three or four apical vertebrae. Care is taken not to produce a tear in the dural sac. The nerve roots with accompanying blood vessels in this area are secured and tied off with sutures and divided, allowing mobilization of the dural sac. Some authors choose to mobilize the neural plaque and neural tube in a different fashion (Fig. 6) and prefer to divide the dural sac at this point, allowing for better exposure. The author believes that dividing the dural sac can compromise the precarious cerebrospinal fluid circulation or, occasionally, bladder function, as observed by Pontari et al. (33). Because of this the author prefers to work around the dural sac and has

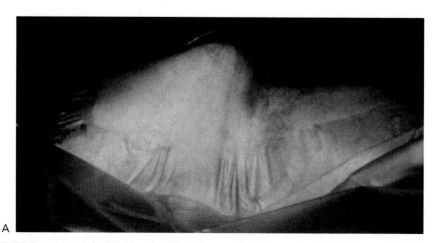

A

FIGURE 5. A 33-month-old girl with T10 meningomyelocele, a progressive 100-degree kyphosis, and skin breakdown. **A:** The patient is prone in a spinal frame, with her head to the right. *(Figure continues.)*

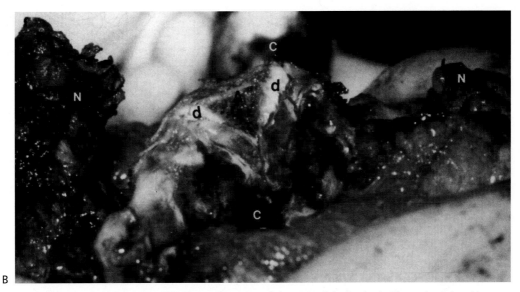

FIGURE 5. *Continued.* **B:** Subperiosteal dissection of the apex of the kyphosis. The patient's head is to the left. In this case, the neural sac was divided over the apex and reflected (Hall JE, Poitras B (1977): The management of kyphosis in patients with myelomeningocele. *Clin Orthop* 128:33). *a,* apical vertebra; *d,* discs; *c,* Cobb elevator; *N,* reflected neural sac. (Courtesy of S. L. Weinstein, University of Iowa.)

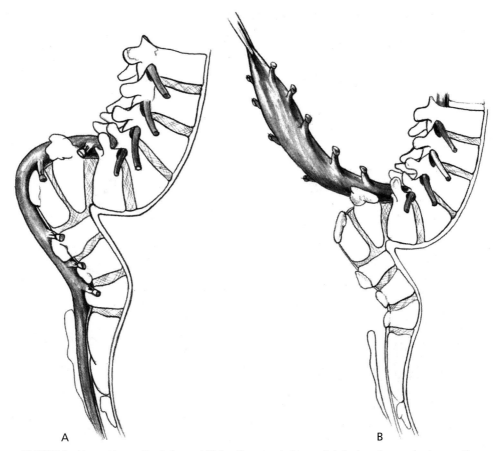

FIGURE 6. Alternative methods for mobilizing the neural plaque. **A:** Intact anatomy prior to resection. **B:** Neural plaque can be divided distally and reflected proximally, with ligation of roots and vessels at each segment. It may be resutured distally upon completion of the bony kyphectomy. *(Figure continues.)*

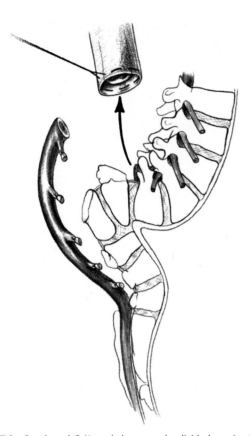

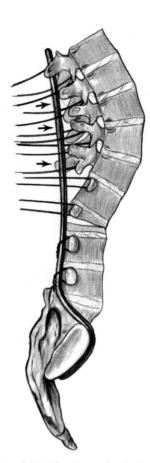

FIGURE 6. *Continued.* **C:** Neural plaque can be divided proximally, with the cord remnant resected proximal to the distal end of the intact dura. The dura must then be oversown with purse-string sutures. It is important in this technique to avoid suturing the distal end of the intact cord remnant, as this may precipitate hydrocephalus.

FIGURE 7. Drawing of distal fixation and reduction of the kyphosis by levering the rod against the thoracic spine and tightening the segmental wires.

had no acute neurologic decompensation in patients treated by this technique. If the decision is made to divide the spinal cord, then care should be taken to suture the dural sac water tightly independent of the neural tube, leaving the end of the neural tube open inside the dural sac to allow for SCF to circulate. Next the dissection is carried out distally over the sacrum exposing the sacroiliac Sone (S1) foramina. Using a blunt elevator, Sone (S1) roots remnants are pushed out of the foramina and from the anterior aspect of the sacrum where the foramina exit. This allows for insertion of a rod through the foramina to rest against the anterior aspect of the sacrum, as described by Fackler (Fig. 4); alternatively, rods can be inserted anterior to sacral ala as described by Dunn (Figs. 7 and 8). Both of these "sacral anchors" provide excellent fixation to resist flexion forces on the instrumentation and can be used quite interchangeably. Once the sacral sites are prepared, sites for wire fixation are selected and prepared. Usually we try to pass wires around the pedicles in the lumbar and thoracolumbar spine in the area of the posterior element defect. Sublaminar wires are used in the more proximal part of the spine where the posterior elements are intact. In the transitional zone between the intact lamina and a wide-open defect, the fixation is more difficult; we sometimes use Drummond buttons to pass through a hole made in the lamina or the pars interarticularis. Occasionally, spinal hooks or even pedicular

screws can be used to supplement the fixation to the rod in this area. Three of four pairs of wires are used in the lumbar segment, and at least five or six pairs are used proximally (Fig. 9).

Next, the actual kyphectomy is carried out, usually involving resection of a single apical vertebra (Fig. 10). This is easily accomplished by cutting through the adjacent intervertebral discs. A small portion of each adjacent vertebra is also removed, using a ronguer or an osteotome (Fig. 11). The resected vertebral body is used as an autogenous bone graft. Fixation is carried out using modification of a Luque rod, with the distal part of the rod being bent to fit anteriorly to the sacral ala or through the sacral S1 foramina. To produce an appropriately fitting rod, we use a standard *U*-shaped (hairpin) Luque rod, or two single Luque rods connected proximally by a cross-link device, and make the required bends with bending irons and tubular rod benders. Two bends are usually required. Working from proximal (U end) to distal, the first bend is usually anterior and slightly lateral. The second bend realigns the distal aspect into a straight sagittal plane, perhaps with the distal portion being a few degrees posterior and gently curved to conform to the anterior shape of the sacrum (Figs. 7 and 12). In younger, smaller patients, a $\frac{3}{16}$-in.-diameter rod can be used. In older patients, a $\frac{1}{4}$-in. rod is preferable. If it is too difficult to bend the heavier rod under sterile conditions in the operating room, a template of the rod

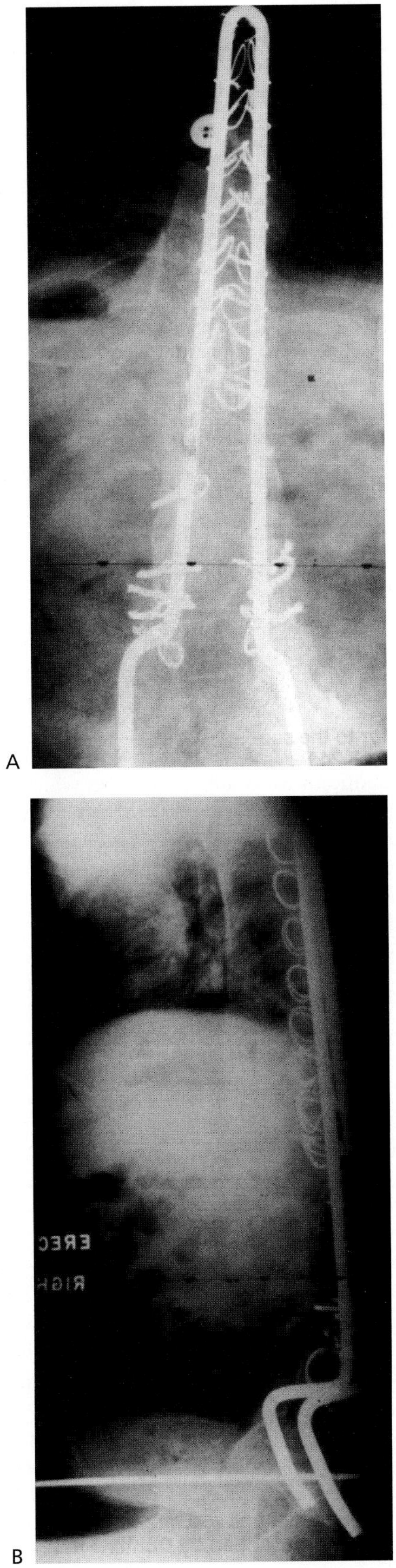

A

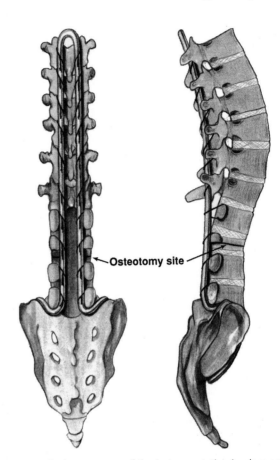

FIGURE 9. Final appearance of the instrumentation in place and the kyphosis reduced.

B

FIGURE 8. Anteroposterior **(A)** and lateral **(B)** radiographs demonstrate postoperative appearance of the instrumented spine after a kyphectomy.

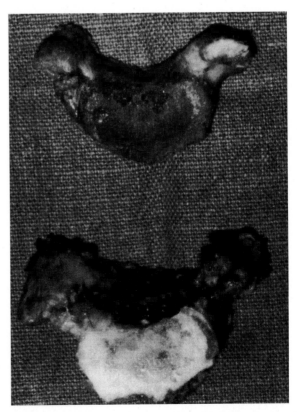

FIGURE 10. Apical vertebra from a patient with meningomyelocele.

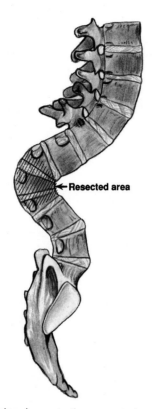

FIGURE 11. Drawing demonstrating suggested area of spinal resection. The apical vertebra is excised together with a small portion of the vertebra above and below.

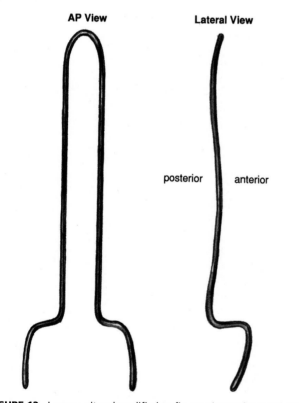

FIGURE 12. Luque unit rod modified to fit anterior to the sacral ala, as described by Dunn. (From refs. 7, 15, 30.)

shape can be made from pliable wire, and the rod can be bent outside the sterile field or even outside the operating room and autoclaved. Once the rod is prepared, it is gently inserted anterior to the sacral ala or SI foramina along the previously prepared passages, with care taken to stay close to the anterior aspect of the sacrum away from the major intrapelvic structures. The proximal portion lies in the gutter between the posterior aspect of the vertebral bodies and the dysplastic lateral elements. In his description of the technique, Dunn suggests bending the rods in the machine shop prior to surgery and even prestocking rods of different sizes (7,30). This can be very helpful, particularly if two Luque rods are used—one on each side—rather than one U-shaped unit rod, which is somewhat easier to control during bending.

The rod is wired to the distal lumbar segment of the spine. The kyphosis is then reduced by approximating the proximal portion of the rod to the thoracic spine. This sometimes has to be done gradually, allowing for relaxation of the soft tissues and correction of any secondary spinal deformity (i.e., thoracic lordosis) (Fig. 7). Care is taken not to overtighten any individual wires so as not to cause wire pullout. Gradually, the completed reduction is achieved with the rod lying flush against the whole length of the instrumented spine and being firmly held in place by wires. Spinal fusion over the instrumented segment is then carried out. The bone graft is placed both anterior and lateral to the osteotomy site as well as along the spine proximally and distally to achieve solid fusion. Wires are carefully bent so that there is no significant hardware prominence, which could lead to skin breakdown (Fig. 9).

Fascia and paraspinal muscles are partially mobilized, and an attempt is made to cover the hardware with muscle or fascia; however, this is not always possible, as there is a large muscle and fascial defect over the wide-open spinal canal defect. The subcutaneous tissue and skin are closed without tension, usually over a drain. In children who had a soft-tissue expander placed prior to surgery, the skin closure is somewhat simplified because relatively healthy skin can be brought over to cover the surgical site and the hardware. A dressing is applied, and the child is awakened and carefully monitored during the postoperative phase (Figs. 8 and 13).

This basic surgical technique can be modified for certain specific situations and sometimes according to the surgeon's preference. For example, in a very young child, one tries to fuse only a relatively short segment of the spine so as not to interfere with the further growth of the vertebral column. A technique called Luque trolley can be utilized to achieve this. The proximal and distal part of the spine exposed extraperiosteally and Luque wires are passed using minimal exposure. The spine is not fused, so that growth can continue with the wires sliding along the rod.

Alternative fixation to the distal segment has been found to be effective. It is an intermedullary technique of drilling holes down the middle of the vertebral bodies of the distal segments once the osteotomies are completed. First Hyndman (18) and later Torode (42) reported their experience with this variation and found it a satisfactory form of distal fixation. Our experience with this technique has been somewhat mixed, with recurrence of the kyphosis at lumbosacral junction, distal to the rods in at least one patient. If used, care should probably be taken to insert

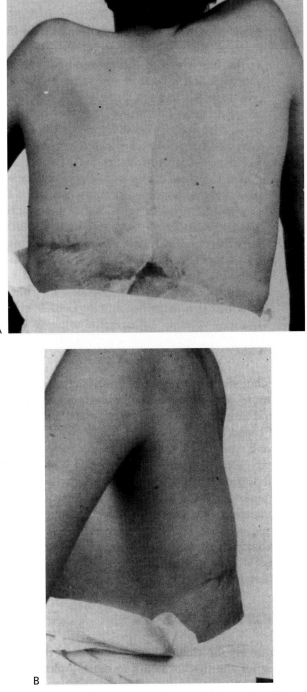

A

B

FIGURE 13. A and **B:** Clinical postoperative photographs of the same child as in Figure 8.

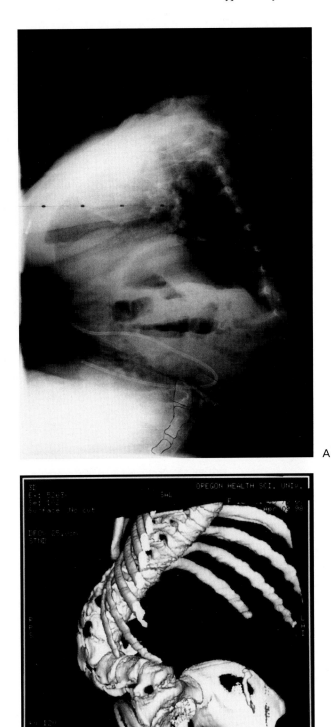

A

B

FIGURE 14. A 12-year-old girl with thoracic level spina bifida and marked kyphosis in the upper lumbar area and a marked lordosis at the lumbosacral junction. **A:** Sitting lateral radiograph. **B:** Three-dimensional computed tomography scan of the spine with much clearer demonstration of the deformity, particularly at the lumbar-sacral junction. *(Figure continues.)*

the rods past the L5–S1 junction. In most cases, we prefer the more conventional fixation with segmental wires and rod insertions into the S1 foramina or anterior to the sacral ala. However, this technique can be very useful in the very occasional case of marked compensatory lordosis at the L-S junctions. In this instance, the flexion movement at the L-S junctions produced by the rods will aid in the correction of this secondary deformity (Fig. 14).

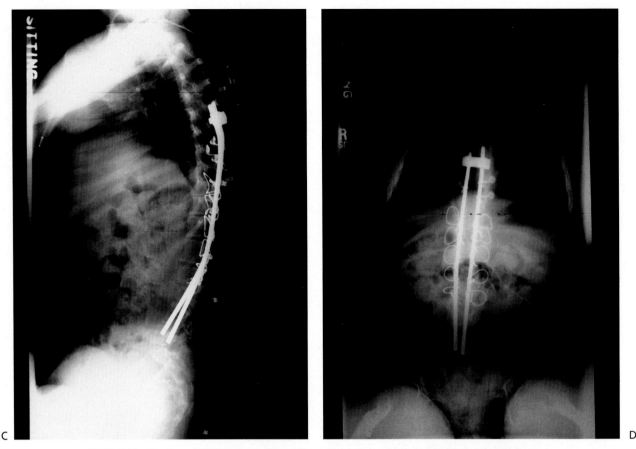

C   D

FIGURE 14. *Continued.* **C, D:** Postoperative radiographs demonstrating intramedullary spinal fixation in the distal spinal segment. Note secondary corrections of the lumbar-sacral lordosis.

POSTOPERATIVE COURSE

Postoperatively the child is kept in an area of intensive nursing for the first 24 hours to closely monitor his or her neurologic and hemodynamic status. The child receives prophylactic antibiotics during surgery and for 48 hours postoperatively. With the slightest evidence of increased intracranial pressure, the child is evaluated by a neurosurgeon on an emergency basis and a decompressive procedure is carried out if needed.

Once the child's condition is stable, he or she is transferred to the orthopaedic ward. Most of these patients are young children, and healing of the osteotomy site and the fusion occurs rapidly. Because the fixation is segmental and relatively stable, external immobilization is not used. The child is allowed to sit in a chair within a few days of the surgical procedure. However, there are restrictions in terms of activity; self-transfers and all other activities that require bending, lifting, or significant physical effort are prohibited. After 6 to 8 weeks the child is usually allowed to gradually increase activities. Six to eight months after surgery—provided that healing is proceeding satisfactorily as demonstrated on radiographic examination—the child is allowed to resume full activity, including wheelchair sports.

TECHNIQUE MODIFICATIONS FOR DIFFICULT OR COMPROMISED CASES

The technique described above is adequate for most patients, but further modification is occasionally required. This is the case when the deformity is especially severe or when the condition of the skin and the soft tissues above the kyphosis is poor.

In children who have an extreme degree of kyphotic deformity with a corresponding rigid compensatory lordosis above the kyphosis, the technique is frequently modified. If the lordosis is so extreme that it is deemed uncorrectable, discectomies over the lordotic segment allow a better correction. This can be done as the first stage of the procedure, with an anterior approach and release of the spine followed by a second-stage posterior approach and a formal kyphectomy, as described above. Another option is a technique described by Dunn (7) of posterior release of the lordotic segment by a costotransversectomy approach working under an intact cord.

However, reduction of the lordosis with simultaneous concomitant reduction of the kyphosis with only apical segment resection can be a formidable undertaking (Fig. 15). In extreme cases, part of the lordotic segment can be resected, as reported by Lindseth and Stelzer (21). However, in this author's opinion,

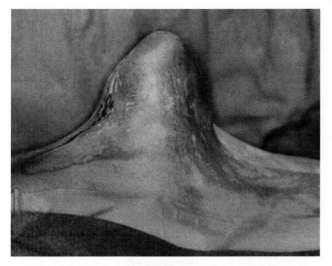

FIGURE 15. This patient's photograph demonstrates an extreme form of spinal kyphosis with adjacent marked lordosis, requiring modifications of the basic technique if trunk height is to be optimized.

reestablishment of truncal height is an important aspect of this procedure; therefore, reduction of the lordotic segment rather than its resection is recommended. In the most rigid cases we have found two *U*-shaped Luque rods useful in facilitating the reduction and improving the fixation. This technique employs one *U*-shaped Luque rod wired to the lumbar spine segment and anchored distally, anterior to the ala of the sacrum, as described for the basic technique. However, the proximal portion of the rod is temporarily left unwired. Another *U*-shaped Luque rod is wired to the proximal portion of the spine above the osteotomy site, spanning the length of the intended instrumentation of the thoracic spine, with the lower portion of the rod extending beyond the osteotomy site by approximately the length of the lumbar spine segment. This rod is wired to the thoracic spine, with the emphasis being reduction of the lordosis. Again, the distal portion of the rod is not wired. Once the two rods have been securely fastened to the thoracic and lumbar spine, respectively, they overlap and criss-cross at the kyphectomy site, forming an angle of around 45 to 50 degrees.

Next, the wires are passed under the already wired rods in the thoracic and lumbar areas and passed around the overlapping segments of the opposite rods, which are presently unwired and sticking out of the wound above the rod underneath (Fig. 16).

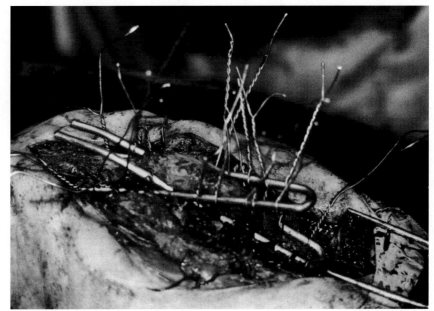

B

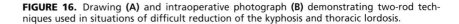

A

FIGURE 16. Drawing **(A)** and intraoperative photograph **(B)** demonstrating two-rod techniques used in situations of difficult reduction of the kyphosis and thoracic lordosis.

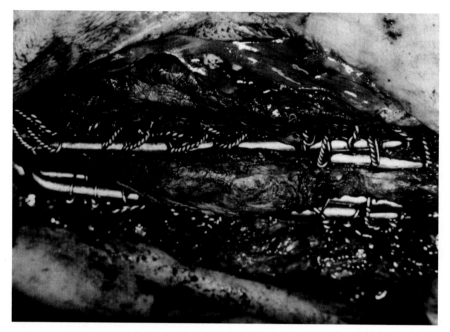

FIGURE 17. Final intraoperative appearance of the two-rod construct.

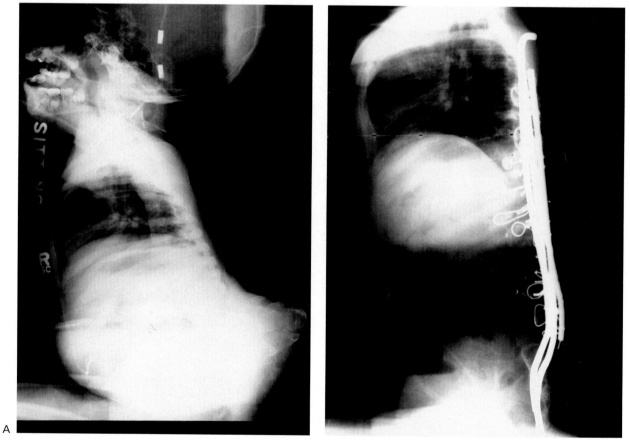

A

B

FIGURE 18. A 7-year-old girl with midthoracic level spina bifida and upper lumbar spine kyphosis of almost 180 degrees. **A:** Preoperative lateral radiographs demonstrating the kyphosis compensatory thoracic lordosis and very short trunk with abdominal viscera displacing the diaphragm cranially. **B, C:** Postoperative lateral and anteroposterior radiographs demonstrating double-rod counter-level construct with desired improvement in the sagittal plane deformities and increase in the trunk height. (Figure continues.)

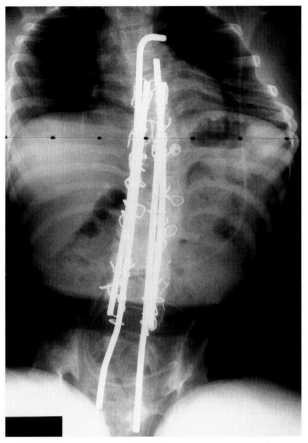

FIGURE 18. *Continued.*

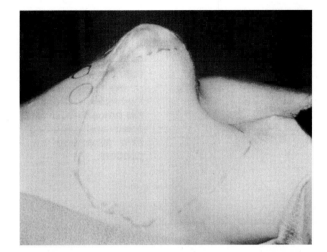

FIGURE 19. Intraoperative planning of the soft-tissue expander procedure. Outline of the pockets for the expanders and the sites for the injection valves are marked on the skin. Note the distal position of the injection sites in the area of anesthetized skin.

Reduction is achieved by gradually pushing on the prominent ends of the rod and tightening the wires in both the thoracic and lumbar areas until the reduction is complete and the two rods are lying on top of each other in a parallel fashion. They are securely fastened together, holding the spine in the reduced position (Fig. 17). Significant forces can be generated by this technique and reduction achieved. The critical part of the procedure is to wire the rods securely to the primary area (i.e., the lumbar rod to the lumbar spine and the thoracic rod to the proximal portion of the spine, with good correction of the lordosis in the proximal segment). We have used this technique successfully in several cases with no complications (Fig. 18). However, this technique requires slightly more soft-tissue coverage due to the additional hardware involved, but this is not prohibitive.

The other problem one encounters when dealing with children with marked kyphosis secondary to meningomyelocele is chronic ulcerations over the gibbus and extremely poor skin coverage over the area of the kyphosis. In the case of extensive skin ulceration or damage compromising the eventual closure of the surgical wound, soft-tissue expanders can be employed to improve the skin closure (19). The technique requires careful planning, as the soft-tissue expanders must be inserted into the paraspinal flank areas 8 to 12 weeks prior to the kyphectomy

procedure (Fig. 19). Silastic tissue expanders are inserted in the subcutaneous tissues and then gradually inflated with injections of saline over a period of 6 to 8 weeks (Fig. 20), thus gradually stretching the overlying skin (Fig. 21). Injections are performed through an injection valve; in children with spina bifida, this can be located in the anesthetized area of the skin so that the injections are painless. They can be done on an outpatient basis or at a physician's office (Fig. 21).

During the planned kyphectomy procedure, the midline incision is used and the silastic pouches, now fully inflated, are removed. The standard kyphectomy procedure is then carried out.

Postoperatively, the compromised skin is excised and the expanded skin used to provide closure of the operative wound (Fig. 22) . In most cases, excellent closure can be achieved, with uncompromised, unscarred, healthy skin providing coverage over the instrumented spine. Suction drains are left in the wound postoperatively because the pocket where the expander was in place is a potential dead space, where serous fluid or hematoma

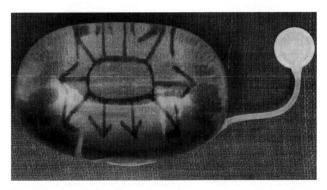

FIGURE 20. Partially inflated silastic tissue expander with its injection valve.

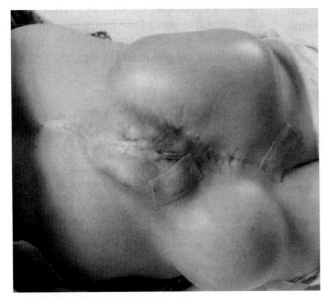

FIGURE 21. Clinical photograph of fully inflated skin expanders just prior to kyphectomy procedure.

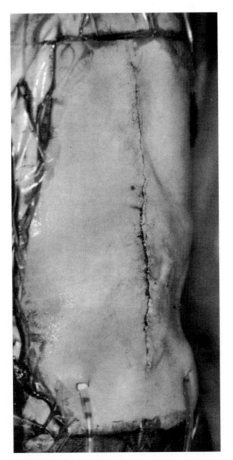

FIGURE 22. Intraoperative photograph of the final skin closure following kyphectomy and soft-tissue expander procedure. Ulcerated skin is excised and replaced with healthy skin generated by the skin expanders.

can easily accumulate. Although this technique is very useful in many cases of extreme skin compromise, it should not give one a sense of security. The child still has insensitive skin over his or her spine, as well as little or no fascial layer between the hardware and the skin. Therefore, these children are still prone to pressure sores and breakdowns if they do not receive the appropriate care.

PITFALLS AND COMPLICATIONS

The procedure of kyphectomy is extensive and frequently formidable. It is helpful to keep in mind potential problems that may arise during the surgery or in the immediate postoperative period and guard against them. Bleeding can be fairly substantial from the epidural vessels, the segmental vessels accompanying the nerve roots, and the exposed cancellous bone.

Some children have large vascular venous channels in this area. We find that working around the dural sac, dividing only the minimal number of roots to perform the resection, can keep bleeding from the epidural veins and segmental vessels to a minimum. Gelfoam padding under the dural sac in the half-open spinal canal helps to control bleeding once it starts. Bone wax is used to control bleeding from bone. Careful subperiosteal dissection anterior to the spine and placement of the rod anterior to the sacrum or sacral ala, staying close to the bony surface, can avoid any significant bleeding from the larger vessels of the abdomen or pelvis.

The second aspect of kyphectomy requiring close attention is the overall neurologic picture. As a rule, we do not divide the dural sac, thereby minimizing any disturbance to cerebrospinal fluid circulation, which can lead to a catastrophic postoperative complication. Great care should be taken not to create cerebrospinal fluid leaks or to compromise the neural elements above the kyphectomy level. If a spinal fluid leak occurs during the surgical procedure, it is best to close it immediately by appropriate dural sutures. This will minimize the chance of a postoperative leak and possible infection. During the postoperative period, the neurologic function of the patient needs to be closely monitored for any sign of shunt malfunction and increased intracranial pressure. Any evidence of altered neurologic function or level should be investigated aggressively and treated without delay to avoid the catastrophic complication of a brain herniation.

Pontari et al. recently pointed out that some of these children have preservation of useful bladder and/or bowel function (33). This may be lost if the cord is divided. On the other hand, some children have spastic bladder and would benefit from division of the distal nerve roots to render the bladder flaccid. It is therefore advisable to assess the urologic function prior to the planned surgery so as to select the most appropriate way of dealing with the neural elements (32).

The complication encountered most frequently in our group of patients is skin breakdown over the prominent hardware. Careful attention to the placement of wires and rods and their soft-tissue coverage during wound closure is essential. Failure to do so invariably leads to erosion of the skin and reoperation for removal of the offending hardware. Mobilization of the paraspinal muscles and available lumbar fascia and, occasionally, latissimus dorsi muscles is sometimes helpful in improving the overall soft-tissue coverage.

REFERENCES

1. Antonyshyn O, Gruss JS, Mackinnon SE, et al. (1988): Complications of soft tissue expansion. *Br J Plast Surg* 41:239–250.
2. Banta JV, Park SM (1983): Improvement in pulmonary function in patients having combined anterior and posterior spine fusion for myelomeningocoele scoliosis. *Spine* 8:765–770.
3. Brown PH (1978): Management of spinal deformity in myelomeningocele. *Orthop Clin N Am* 9:391–402.
4. Channon GM, Jenkins DHR: (1981) Aggressive surgical treatment of secondary spinal deformity in spina bifida children—Is it worthwhile? *Z Kinderchir* 34(4):395–398.
5. Christofersen MR, Brooks AL (1985): Excision and wire fixation of rigid myelomeningocele kyphosis. *J Pediatr Orthop* 691–696.
6. Drennan JC (1970): The role of muscles in the development of human lumbar kyphosis. *Dev Med Child Neurol* 12(Suppl 22): 33.
7. Dunn HK (1992): Personal communication.
8. Dunn HK (1982): Kyphosis of myelodysplasia: Operative treatment based on pathophysiology. Presented at the Annual Meeting of the Scoliosis Research Society, Denver.
9. Eckstein HB, Vora RM (1972): Spinal osteotomy for severe kyphosis in children with myelomeningocele. *J Bone Joint Surg Br* 54:328.
10. Eyring RJ, Wanken JJ, Sayers MP (1972): Spine osteotomy for kyphosis in myelomeningocele. *Clin Orthop* 88:24.
11. Fackler CD, Warner W Jr, VanderWoude L (1992): Instrumentation technique for kyphectomy in myelodysplasia. Exhibit at the Annual Meeting of the American Academy of Orthopaedic Surgery, Washington, DC.
12. Fromm B, Carstens C, Graf J. (1994): Aorographic findings in children with myelomeningocele and lumbar kyphosis. *Z Orthop* 132:56–61.
13. Hall JE, Bobecko WP (1973): Advances in the management of spinal deformities in myelodysplasia. *Clin Neurosurg* 20:1964.
14. Hall JE, Poitras B (1977): The management of kyphosis in patients with myelomeningocele. *Clin Orthop* 128:33.
15. Heydemann JS, Gillespie R (1987): Management of myelomeningocele kyphosis in the older child by kyphectomy and segmental spinal instrumentation. *Spine* 12:37–41.
16. Hoppenfeld S (1967): Congenital kyphosis in myelomeningocele. *J Bone Joint Surg Br* 49:276.
17. Huang TJ, Lubicky JP (1994): Kyphectomy and segmental spinal instrumentation in young children with myelomeningocele kyphosis. *J Formos Med Assoc* 93:503–508.
18. Hyndman JC (1990): Kyphosis myelomeningocele: an anterior-posterior approach. Presented at the Annual Meeting of the Pediatric Orthopaedic Society, San Francisco.
19. Krajbich JI, Zuker R (1990): Use of the soft tissue expanders in surgical treatment of spina bifida children with spinal kyphosis. Presented at the Annual Meeting of the Scoliosis Research Society. Honolulu.
20. Leatherman KD, Dickson RA (1978): Congenital kyphosis in myelomeningocele, vertebral body resection and posterior spinal fusion. *Spine* 3:22.
21. Lindseth RE, Stelzer L (1979): Vertebral excision in children with myelomeningocele. *J Bone Joint Surg Am* 61:699.
22. Loder RT, Shapiro P, Towbin R, et al. (1991): Aortic anatomy in children with myelomeningocele and congenital lumbar kyphosis. *J Pediatr Orthop* 11(1):31–35.
23. Lorder J (1971): Results of treatment of myelomeningocele. *Dev Med Child Neurol* 13:279.
24. Lowe GP, Menelaus MB (1978): The surgical management of kyphosis in older children with myelomeningocele. *J Bone Joint Surg Br* 60:40.
25. Luque ER (1982): The correction of postural curves of the spine. *Spine* 7:270.
26. Manders EK, Schenden MJ, et al. (1984): Soft tissue expansion: Concepts and complications. Plast Reconstr Surg 74:493.
27. Martin J Jr, Kumars J, Guille JT, et al. (1994): Congenital kyphosis in myelomeningocele: results following operative and nonoperative treatment. *J Pediatr Orthop* 18(6):820–823.
28. Mayfield JK (1981): Severe spinal deformity in myelodysplasia and sacral agenesis, an aggressive surgical approach. *Spine* 6:498.
29. McCall RE (1998): Modified luque instrumentation after myelomeningocele kyphectomy. *Spine* 23(12):1406–1441.
30. McCarthy RE, Dunn HK, McCullough FL (1989): Luque fixation to the sacral ala using the Dunn-McCarthy modification. *Spine* 14: 281–283.
31. McMaster MJ (1988): The long-term results of kyphectomy and spinal stabilization in children with myelomeningocele. *Spine* 13:417–424.
32. Pang D (1995): Surgical complications of open spinal dysraphism. *Neurosurg Clin N Am* 6(2):243–257.
33. Pontari MA, Bauer SB, Hall JE, et al. (1998): Adverse urologic consequences of spinal cord resection at the time of kyphectomy: value of preoperative urodynamic evaluation. *J Pediatr Orthop* 18(6):820–823.
34. Raycroft JF, Curtis BH (1972): Spinal curvature in meningocele: natural history and etiology. In: *Proceedings of the American Academy of Orthopaedic Surgery Symposium on Myelomeningocele.* St. Louis: CV Mosby, p. 186.
35. Sammelson L, Bergstroem K, Thuomas KA, et al. (1987): MR imaging of syringomydromyelia and Chiari malformations in myelomeningocele patients with scoliosis. *Am J Neuroradiol* 8:539–546.
36. Sharrard WJW (1968): Spinal osteotomy for congenital kyphosis in myelomeningocele. *J Bone Joint Surg Br* 50:466.
37. Sharrard WJW, Drennan JC (1972): Osteotomy-excision of the spine for lumbar kyphosis in older children with myelomeningocele. *J Bone Joint Surg Br* 54:50–60.
38. Sherk HH, Ames MD, Charney EB, et al. (1997): Kyphectomy in myelodysplasia. *Z Kinderchir* 28(4):396–401.
39. Sriram K, Bobechko WP, Hall JE (1972): Surgical management of spinal deformities in spina bifida. *J Bone Joint Surg Br* 54:666–676.
40. Shurtleff DB, Goiney R, Gorson LH, et al. (1976): Myelodysplasia: The natural history of kyphosis and scoliosis: a preliminary report. *Dev Med Child Neurol* 18(Suppl 37):126–133.
41. Shurtleff DB, Hayden PW, Loeser JD, et al. (1974): Myelodysplasia: decision for death or disability. *N Engl J Med* 291:1005.
42. Torode I, Godette G (1995): Surgical correction of congenital kyphosis in myelomeningocele. *J Pediatr Orthop* 15:202–205.
43. Warner WC, Fackler CD (1993): Surgical correction of congenital kyphosis in myelomeningocele. *J Pediatr Orthop* 13:704–708.
44. Winston J, Hall JE, Johnson D, et al. (1977): Acute elevation of intracranial pressure following transection of nonfunctional spinal cord. *Clin Orthop* 128:41.

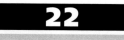

THE DECOMPENSATED SPINE

DAVID S. BRADFORD
JASON A. SMITH

Visual and proprioceptive cues functioning through the cerebellum ensure upright posture, with the head centered over the pelvis. With lesser degrees of spinal deformity, the body is able to maintain head-centered posture. In patients with more severe spinal deformity, normal compensating mechanisms are not sufficient in restoring coronal and sagittal plane balance. Correcting these deformities and rebalancing the spine may prove the most technically demanding reconstructive procedures performed by the spine surgeon.

The causes for decompensation of the spine are varied and include both de novo and iatrogenic causes. Although most often the result of congenital scoliosis and kyphosis, other causes include crankshaft phenomenon, adding on of previous spine fusions, postlaminectomy kyphosis, neuromuscular scoliosis, idiopathic scoliosis, or scoliosis associated with fixed L5 obliquity secondary to spondylolisthesis. The surgical correction of the coronal decompensation following previous fusion may be managed in select cases by merely extending the instrumentation. Two-plane deformity with decompensation in virgin or redo cases may be managed with two-stage surgery consisting of anterior discectomies and fusion followed by posterior instrumentation and fusion. However, in more severe cases, management requires osteotomies, partial vertebrectomy, or vertebral column resection, depending on the severity of the deformity (1,4,5,9, 11,12,14,17,18,19,21,22,26,27,29,31–33). In this chapter, we discuss the evaluation and management of the fixed, decompensated spine.

HISTORY

MacLennan reported the first posterior spine osteotomy for the correction of scoliosis in 1922 (25). A decade later, Compere reported excision of hemivertebrae in two patients requiring correction of congenital scoliosis (8). In 1933, Von Lacham and Smith reported the results of vertebrectomy for the treatment of lumbar scoliosis in 10 patients, in which an anterior procedure preceded posterior arch excision and fusion (36). In 1951, Wiles reported severe post-operative kyphosis as a complication of two-

stage resection in two patients with congenital scoliosis (38). In 1965, Hodgson, utilizing both anterior and posterior fusions after anterior wedge osteotomies, reported successful correction of fixed deformities secondary to tuberculosis in two patients (16).

Leatherman and Dickson supplemented their two-stage procedure with posterior compression and distraction instrumentation to gain correction, followed by fusion (23). Their report of 24 patients appeared in 1979. Luque, in 1983, described his novel two-stage procedure in which a decancellation procedure through fenestrations in the apical vertebrae was performed without removal of the segmental vessels or discs (24). This was followed by correction through spinal shortening with posterior segmental instrumentation and fusion.

In 1984, Heinig and Boyd, utilizing an approach to the vertebral body first described by Michele and Krueger (28), described a spine shortening "eggshell" osteotomy through a single posterior approach (13). Their decancellation vertebrectomy allowed shortening and angular correction without formally entering the chest or retroperitoneum. A variation of this procedure was reported in 1985 by Thomasen, in which partial vertebrectomy was performed involving removal of all of the posterior arch, the pedicles bilaterally, and a posterior-based wedge of the vertebral body, all through the posterior approach for treatment of primarily kyphotic deformities (35).

Because of the difficulties encountered in efforts to correct severely decompensated spines, Bradford developed the vertebral column resection procedure (1), first reporting his results in 1987 (2). A modification of the technique reported by Luque, it involved resection of the entirety of one or more vertebral bodies while maintaining a convex osteoperiosteal flap, with replacement by morselized cancellous bone and reattachment of the flap. This is followed several days later by posterior resection, translational and angular correction through spine shortening, and segmental fixation and fusion. Rib resections and/or releases on both the convex and concave sides of the deformities are a component of this procedure, along with anterior discectomies and anterior and posterior osteotomies maximal and distal to the resected area.

The results of vertebral column resection were reported for 52 patients in 1998 (3,6) (Fig. 1). The surgical time for the anterior procedure averaged 4 to 5 hours, whereas the posterior procedure averaged 7 to 8 hours. The coronal plane decompensation improved from 8.5 cm preoperatively to 1.5 cm postoperatively. The sagittal plane decompensation improved from 8 cm

D. S. Bradford: Department of Orthopedic Surgery, University of California, San Francisco, California 94143-0728.

J. A. Smith: Department of Orthopedics, University of California, San Francisco, California 94143-0728.

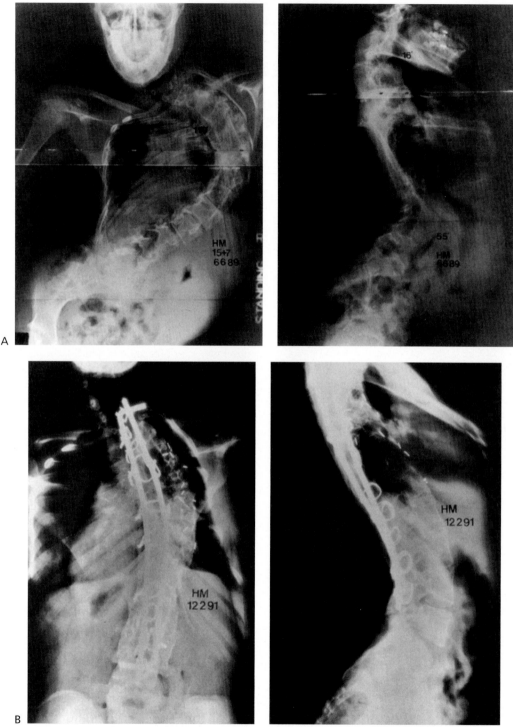

FIGURE 1. A 15-year-old girl with congenital scoliosis who had undergone previous posterior fusion in situ. **A:** Preoperative anteroposterior *(left)* and lateral *(right)* radiographs reveal significant coronal curvature with fixed decompensation, as well as decreased thoracic kyphosis and lumbar hyperlordosis. **B:** Postoperative anteroposterior *(left)* and lateral *(right)* radiographs demonstrate improvement of coronal and sagittal balance following combined anterior and posterior resection procedure. *(Figure continues.)*

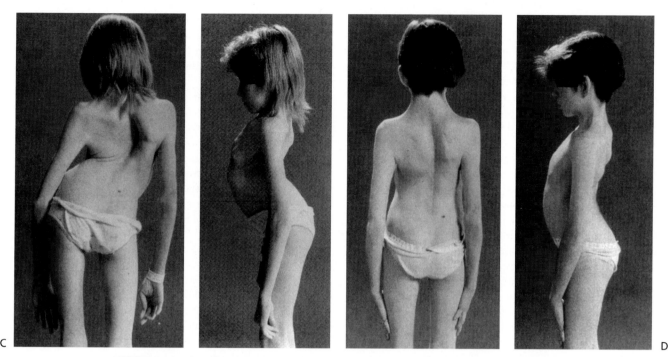

FIGURE 1. *Continued.* **C:** Preoperative clinical photographs. **D:** Postoperative clinical photographs 2 years after surgery. (From Bradford DS, Tribus CB [1997]. Vertebral column resection for the treatment of rigid coronal decompensation. *Spine* 22(14):1590–1599, with permission.)

preoperatively to 1 cm postoperatively. Scoliosis improved from 103 degrees preoperatively to 49 degrees postoperatively. Complications occurred in five patients. These included three deep-wound infections, two transient neurologic deficits, and one permanent quadraceps paresis (grade IV/V) with subsequent arachnoiditis. Two patients required prolonged ventilation, and three patients developed pseudarthrosis. Two of these three suffered deep infections. All three patients with pseudarthrosis had L-rod fixation, which is no longer used.

EVALUATION

A thorough history and physical examination is undertaken. Frequently, these children present with complaints of sitting or upright imbalance, and they may have localized pain in their back or neck secondary to failed attempts to stand in an upright posture. There may be complaints of progression of deformity, or of a short limb as pelvic obliquity worsens.

Identification and management of concomitant medical problems is necessary prior to consideration of surgical intervention. The nutritional status of the patient likewise is evaluated. If malnutrition is suspected, consultation with a nutritionist and pre-operative nutritional supplementation may be required. Similarly, the respiratory status of the patient is thoroughly evaluated (and optimized preoperatively, if possible).

The physical examination focuses on flexibility of the deformity, as well as evaluation of coronal and sagittal plane decompensation. The neurologic status of the patient is determined and further evaluated by imaging if deficits are noted. All patients with congenital deformities are evaluated by magnetic resonance imaging (MRI).

Radiologic evaluation includes standing full-spine posteroanterior and lateral views on 14-in. × 36-in. cassettes or, if the patient is nonambulatory, seated full-spine views. The magnitude of curves in both the coronal and sagittal planes using the standard Cobb technique is determined. Truncal balance is determined by measuring the deviation from the midline at the sacrum of a plumb line dropped from the spinous process of C7 on the posteroanterior view and from the body of C7 on the lateral projection. Supine bending films are required as well. MRI and/or computed tomography (CT)–myelography are used selectively to evaluate intraspinal anatomy. Syringomyelia, diastematomyelia, or tethering, if discovered, must be dealt with prior to correction of the deformity.

It is of paramount importance to have highly skilled anesthesia and critical care teams assist with the management of these patients. Blood loss often is substantial, and pulmonary function requires careful monitoring and support during the immediate postoperative period. Preoperative evaluation by the anesthesia team several weeks prior to surgery is useful and is encouraged when feasible. If such skilled ancillary services are unavailable or if the surgeon has limited experience in these procedures, we recommend referral to a center where procedures such as these are performed frequently.

MANAGEMENT

The indications for surgical intervention are similar to those of other spinal deformities (i.e., progression, pain poorly controlled by nonoperative measures, neurologic deficit, and deterioration of pulmonary function) (37). Decompensation, when severe, especially in the growing child, may in itself prove to be an indication for surgery.

The goals of surgery are as follows: three-plane balance; solid arthrodesis; rigid internal fixation; minimal postoperative external support; and improvement of quality of life in terms of increased activities of daily life, decreased pain, and improvement of pulmonary function.

Traction preoperatively, intraoperatively, or between staged procedures should be avoided. Since resection of any structural component necessarily destabilizes the spine, stable fixation is necessary. Preoperative autologous blood donation is recommended, and hypotensive anesthesia helps to lessen intraoperative blood loss. Use of the cell saver is likewise recommended. These procedures may be time consuming and associated with significant blood loss, so that separation of procedures by 4 to 7 days may prove necessary. When a two-stage operation is separated by several days, some form of nutritional supplementation is desirable. Enteral feeding is preferred, if tolerated, as it has been proven in general surgical and trauma patients to decrease bacterial translocation in the gut, thereby decreasing the risk of sepsis. If, however, enteral feeding is not tolerated or feasible, intravenous hyperalimentation should be provided between stages and should be continued following the second stage until the patient has resumed a normal diet. Some form of neuromonitoring is necessary intraoperatively, either in the form of multiple wake-up tests or with combined monitoring of somatosensory and motor evoked potentials.

The initial evaluation and primary treatment of congenital deformity has been discussed elsewhere and will not be discussed in detail here. In this and all other deformities, every effort is made to avoid fusion to the sacrum. However, in cases of neuromuscular scoliosis, deformity associated with significant pelvic obliquity, and deformity centered at the lumbosacral junction, fusion to the sacrum may be required. Limited degrees of decompensation (less than 2 to 3 cm in either the sagittal or coronal planes) may be managed by standard techniques, such as posterior instrumentation and fusion, with or without osteotomies (11,15). Minor degrees of fixed imbalance secondary to a lumbosacral curve or an oblique lumbar take-off without structural deformity above may be managed by a combined anterior/posterior procedure with fusion of L4 to the sacrum. Such a situation may occur in spondylolisthesis with a significant rotational component. On the other hand, a fixed oblique take-off, secondary to a lumbosacral congenital wedged hemivertebra, is best managed, in our experience, with a hemivertebra excision anteriorly, followed by posterior resection of the remnants of the hemivertebra, instrumentation, and fusion (4).

Moderate decompensation (3 to 4 cm) secondary to fixed thoracic or lumbar deformity may be successfully managed by combined approaches, in which total discectomies with fusion anteriorly is followed by posterior osteotomies, facetectomies, and fusion, with rigid segmental fixation (15,34).

In cases in which the deformity is primarily uniplanar, and in cases with previous arthrodesis in which there has been prior anterior surgery resulting in scarring that may make an anterior approach unnecessarily difficult, a pedicle resection osteotomy as described by Thomasen (35) may be utilized to gain correction. Thirty to forty degrees of correction can be gained in the sagittal plane with removal of the pedicles of a single vertebra and with wedge resection of the vertebral body. We have also found that with this approach coronal correction of 15 to 30 degrees may be gained by removal of both pedicles, and by asymmetric resection of the vertebral body with a posterolateral wedge being removed from the convexity. This technique, though allowing less correction in the coronal plane, allows shortening of the spine with correction of the deformity through a single approach. Obviously, translational correction is not possible with this technique, and proximal and distal anterior fusion cannot be accomplished through the posterior approach. The advantages of a single-stage procedure should therefore be weighed with this in mind.

Severe coronal, or mixed coronal and sagittal, decompensation, especially with fixed translational deformity, is best managed by spine resection procedures. The indication for this procedure occurs under the following conditions: (a) a patient with greater than 6 cm of fixed coronal imbalance; (b) a fixed upper thoracic curve and pelvic obliquity and/or a lumbosacral oblique take-off; (c) asymmetric length between the concave and convex sides of the vetebral column. In these cases, surgery consisting only of combined osteotomies with instrumentation may bring the head over the sacrum in the coronal and sagittal plane, but in the coronal plane the upper shoulder asymmetry may actually be increased along with the cervical deformity. Resection with spinal shortening coupled with osteotomies above the resected area may achieve the necessary balance. The apparent need in these cases is spinal shortening with angulation correction to furnish balance.

PROCEDURE

The more traditional techniques for correction of decompensation, including posterior instrumentation and fusion, anterior discectomies and fusion followed by posterior instrumentation, and pedicle subtraction osteotomies, have been described elsewhere and will not be described here. This section will focus on the surgical technique of vertebral column resection.

Careful preoperative planning is required to determine the number of vertebrae to be removed during the first stage of the anterior procedure. If the deformity is sharply angulated, removal of one vertebra may be sufficient. If the deformity is long and sweeping, it may be necessary to resect two or three apical vertebrae to achieve sufficient correction.

First-stage surgery consists of an anterior approach on the convex side of the area to be resected on either the thoracic or thoracoabdominal approach. The rib conforming to the uppermost level of the spine to be approached is removed. Following segmental vessel ligation and division, anterior discectomies and/or osteotomies are carried out throughout the length of the curvature as much as feasible through the particular approach. The disc spaces are then packed with Gelfoam soaked in thrombin solution to promote hemostasis.

An osteoperiosteal flap is elevated over the vertebral body or bodies to be resected using a sharp slightly curved osteotome.

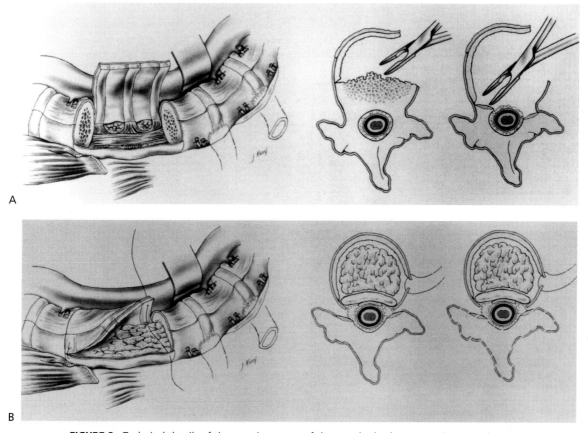

FIGURE 2. Technical details of the anterior aspect of the vertebral column resection procedure. **A:** A standard thoracotomy has been performed, and segmental vessels over the convexity have been taken. The apical vertebrae have been removed back to the posterior longitudinal ligament, removing as much of the pedicles as feasible. **B:** Morselized cancellous bone from the resected vertebrae is laid loosely over Gelfoam protecting the dura. (Reproduced with permission from Bradford DS, Tribus CB [1997]: Vertebral column resection for the treatment of rigid coronal decompensation. *Spine* 22(14):1590–1599, with permission.)

Then the vertebra is transferred to the posterior cortical shell with a variety of rongeurs and curettes (Fig. 2). The convex pedicle is easily removed during the anterior procedure, whereas removal of the concave pedicle may be more difficult. A small portion of the pedicle may remain, subsequently to be removed during the posterior procedure. The posterior cortical shell of the vertebral body is then removed. The underlying epidural veins may bleed profusely, and hemostasis is secured again with Gelfoam soaked in thrombin solution or a generous use of Surgicel or Oxycel. If an additional vertebra must be removed, it is done at this time, again maintaining hemostasis before proceeding with an additional resection.

The resected bone is combined with the rib that was removed during the thoracotomy and morselized. The dura is protected with Gelfoam soaked in thrombin solution and the morselized bone is placed loosely in the resected area. Then the osteoperiosteal flap is sewn down loosely over the vertebral column to retain the morselized bone and reconstitute the "vertebral body."

If the blood loss has been minimal (less than 25% of the total blood volume) and the anterior procedure has taken less than 3 hours, the posterior procedure then may follow under the same anesthetic. This situation is uncommon. Most patients will require a two-stage procedure 5 to 7 days apart. The patient is then placed on supple mental nutrition, either enteral or parenteral, to maintain caloric intake. The residual posterior stability determines the patient's activity status. If the spine is rigid due to a previous posterior fusion, the patient is allowed out of bed in a chair and may even ambulate. It has been our experience that temporary stabilization, even in a patient whose spine was not previously fused posteriorly, is unnecessary. Rather, such a patient is restricted to bed rest with spine precautions; log rolling is performed every 2 to 3 hours until the second stage is undertaken.

The posterior procedure is carried out through a routine subperiosteal exposure to the spine. Rib resection (thoracoplasty) is performed on the convex side of the deformity. Osteotomies are done throughout the spine to ensure flexibility and mobility at each spinal segment.

The posterior elements of the previous excised anterior vertebrae are then removed, including the residual pedicle on both the concave side of the deformity and the convex side of the deformity. Segmental instrumentation, using a combination of hooks, wires, and, in the lumbar spine pedicle, screws, is carried out first on the convex side, using cantilever bending forces to correct coronal as well as sagittal deformity. Redundancy of the dura is noted, and dural pulsations are expected and carefully evaluated. Multiple wake-up tests are performed during the corrective stage of the procedure. If the concave ribs are fused either congenitally or iatrogenically over the apical portion of the spine, these should be osteotomized or resected at their bases subperiosteally. If this is not done, correction of the deformity will be hindered.

It is important to remember that during the corrective stage with instrumentation, correction is done slowly and carefully, accompanied by monitoring of neurologic function. The function of the instrumentation is to obtain balance both in the sagittal and coronal planes while shortening the spinal column. Total correction of the deformity, though possible, is neither necessary nor advisable. The goal is to achieve occiput/C7 centering over the sacrum, both in the coronal and sagittal planes. Although some surgeons prefer to template such cases preoperatively to help predict the amount of bone resection necessary to carry out this function, we determine the appropriate correction intraoperatively and then check, post correction, intraoperative long films in both the anteroposterior and lateral projections for balance. If the intraoperative films demonstrate residual imbalance in the sagittal or coronal plane, further correction is undertaken.

Postoperatively patients are allowed to ambulate in 2 to 3 days. A thoracolumbar sacral orthosis is sufficient, unless the resection is performed in the upper thoracic spine. In such cases, use of a Milwaukee brace is recommended. Patients are followed with serial radiographs until healing is obtained. Reformation of the vertebral column within 6 months is to be expected.

DISCUSSION AND CONCLUSION

The surgical treatment of the decompensated spine runs the gamut from the routine to the highly complex. Limited degrees of decompensation, less than 2 to 3 cm in either plane, may be managed by posterior instrumentation and fusion, with or without osteotomies. More severe decompensation of up to 6 cm may be managed by combined anterior discectomies/osteotomies followed by posterior osteotomies, instrumentation, and fusion. Uniplanar or biplanar deformity can often be managed with a pedicle subtraction osteotomy (Fig. 3), as described by Thomasen (35). However, severe combined coronal and sagittal deformity associated with marked spinal translation may require the spinal shortening technique as described. This is a demanding procedure with limited indications. The indications include truncal translation, rigid deformity in the coronal plane, asymmetry in the length of the convex and concave columns of the spinal deformity, precluding achieving balance by routine combined osteotomies and instrumentation. One should consider this a shortening procedure, more involved than vertebrectomy.

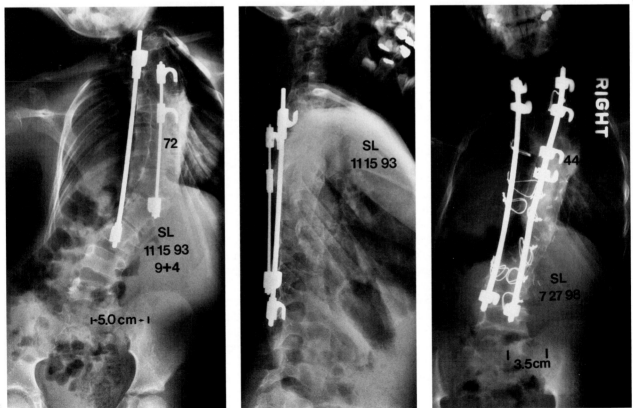

FIGURE 3. A–C. *(Figure continues.)*

A,B

C

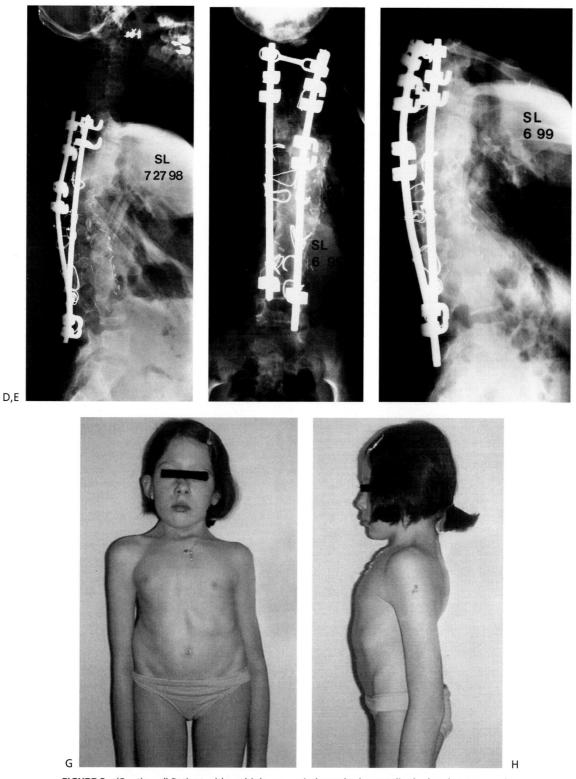

FIGURE 3. *(Continued)* Patient with multiple congenital vertebral anomolies had undergone previous posterior instrumented fusion of the thoracic curve. **A, B:** Continued growth (i.e., crankshaft phenomenon) resulted in marked decompensation in the coronal plane. **C, D:** Patient underwent vertebral column resection of the thoracic curve, resulting in improvement of the curve and decompensation, as seen in this 48-month follow-up series. However, because of residual decompensation, she had developed upper thoracic and neck pain, as well as headaches. **E, F:** Postoperative radiographs following asymmetric pedicle subtraction osteotomy, with multiple concave and convex rib osteotomies of the upper thoracic curve, reveal balancing of the spine in both the coronal and sagittal planes. **G, H:** Clinical radiographs reveal a well-balanced spine, although the patient has obvious trunk shortening secondary to the congenital anomolies and surgical procedures. Her back pain and headaches had resolved at 6-month follow-up.

The components include anterior vertebral resection, followed by total removal of the posterior arch and the pedicles at the site of the resection, as well as the lamina above and below the resection. Anterior osteotomies and discectomies above and below the resection along with posterior osteotomies and facetectomies above and below the resection are necessary as is thoracoplasty on the convex and, often, the concave sides of the deformity. Although this is a demanding procedure, we believe that for the select patient who meets our criteria it is the procedure of choice for severely decompensated deformity.

REFERENCES

1. Boachie-Adjei O, Bradford DS (1991): Vertebral column resection and arthrodesis for complex spinal deformities. *J Spinal Disord* 4:193–202.
2. Bradford DS (1987): Vertebral column resection. *Orthop Trans* 11: 502.
3. Bradford DS (1998): Vertebral column resection for the management of rigid, decompensated spinal deformity. *Semin Spine Surg* 10(4): 381–386.
4. Bradford DS, Boachie-Adjei O (1990): One-stage anterior and posterior hemivertebral resection and arthrodesis for congenital scoliosis. *J Bone Joint Surg Am* 72:536–540.
5. Bradford DS, Hu SS (1997): Excision of hemivertebrae. In: Bradford DS, ed. *The spine.* Philadelphia: Lippincott-Raven Publishers.
6. Bradford DS, Tribus CB (1994): Current concepts and management of patients with fixed decompensated spinal deformity. *Clin Orthop* 306:64–72.
7. Bradford DS, Tribus CB (1997): Vertebral column resection for the treatment of rigid coronal decompensation. *Spine* 22:1590–1599.
8. Compere EL (1932): Excision of hemivertebrae for correction of congenital scoliosis: Report of two cases. *J Bone Joint Surg* 14:555–562.
9. Dewald RL (1997): Osteotomy of the thoracic lumbar spine. In: Bradford DS, ed. *The spine.* Philadelphia: Lippincott-Raven Publishers.
10. Doherty JH (1972): Complications of fusion in lumbar scoliosis. *J Bone Joint Surg Am* 55:438.
11. Floman Y, Micheli LJ, Penny N, et al. (1982): Combined anterior and posterior fusion in seventy-three spinally deformed patients: Indications, results and complications. *Clin Orthop* 164:110–122.
12. Grobler J, Moe JH, Winter RB, et al. (1978): Loss of lumbar lordosis following surgical correction of thoracolumbar deformities. *Orthop Trans* 2:239.
13. Heinig CF, Boyd BM (1985): One stage vertebrectomy or egg-shell procedure. *Orthop Trans* 9:130.
14. Herbert JJ (1948): Vertebral osteotomy: technique, indications, and results. *J Bone Joint Surg Am* 30:680–689.
15. Herndon WA, Sullivan JA, Yngve DA, et al. (1987): Segmental spinal instrumentation with sublaminar wires. *J Bone Joint Surg Am* 69: 851–859.
16. Hodgson AR (1965): Correction of spinal curves. *J Bone Joint Surg Am* 47:1221–1227.
17. Holte DC, Winter RB, Lonstein JE, et al. Excision of hemivertebrae and wedge resection in the treatment of congenital scoliosis. *J Bone Joint Surg Am.*
18. Kostuik JP, Maurais GR, Richardson WJ, et al. (1988): Combined single-stage anterior and posterior osteotomey for correction of iatrogenic lumbar kyphosis. *Spine* 13:257–266.
19. Lagrone MO, Bradford DS, Moe JH, et al. (1988): Treatment of symptomatic flatback after spinal fusion. *J Bone Joint Surg Am* 70:569–580.
20. Lauerman WC, Bradford DS, Transfeldt EE, et al. (1991): Management of pseudoarthrosis after arthodesis of the spine for idiopathic scoliosis. *J Bone Joint Surg Am* 73:222–236.
21. Law WA (1969): Osteotomy of the spine. *Clin Orthop* 66:70–76.
22. Leatherman KD (1969): Resection of vertebral bodies. *J Bone Joint Surg Am* 51:206.
23. Leatherman KD, Dickson RA (1979): Two-stage corrective surgery for congenital deformities of the spine. *J Bone Joint Surg Br* 61:324–328.
24. Luque ER (1983): Vertebral column transposition. *Orthop Trans* 7: 29.
25. MacLennan A (1922): Scoliosis. *Br Med J* 2:865–866.
26. McMaster MJ (1985): A technique for lumbar spinal osteotomy in ankylosing spondylitis. *J Bone Joint Surg Br* 67:204–210.
27. Meiss WL (1955): Spinal osteotomy following fusion for paralytic scoliosis. *J Bone Joint Surg Am* 37:73–77.
28. Michele AA, Krueger FJ (1949): Surgical approach to the vertebral body. *J Bone Joint Surg Am* 31:873–876.
29. Moe JH, Denis F (1977): The iatrogenic loss of lumbar lordosis. *Orthop Trans* 1:131.
30. Perra JH (1994): Techniques of instrumentation in long fusions to the sacrum. *Orthop Clin N Am* 25:287–99.
31. Royle ND (1928): The operative removal of an accessory vertebra. *Med J Aust* 1:467–468.
32. Schmidt AC (1969): Osteotomy of the fused spine and the use of halo traction apparatus. In: *American Academy of Orthopaedic Surgeons Symposium on the Spine.* St. Louis, pp. 265–282.
33. Smith-Petersen MN, Larson CB, Aufranc OE (1945): Osteotomy of the spine for correction of flexion deformity in rheumatoid arthritis. *J Bone Joint Surg* 27:1–11.
34. Sponseller PD, Cohen MS, Nachemson AL, et al. (1987): Results of surgical treatment of adults with idiopathic scoliosis. *J Bone Joint Surg Am* 69:667–675.
35. Thomasen E (1985): Vertebral osteotomy for correcting kyphosis in ankylosing spondoylitis. *Clin Orthop* 194:142–152.
36. Von Lackumn HL, Smith ADF (1933): Removal of vertebral bodies in the treatment of scoliosis. *Surg Gynecol* 57:250–256.
37. Weinstein SL, Ponseti IV (1983): Curve progression in idiopathic scoliosis. *J Bone Joint Surg Am* 65:447–455.
38. Wiles P (1951): Resection of dorsal vertebrae in congenital scoliosis. *J Bone Joint Surg Am* 33:151–154.

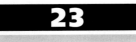

23

THORACOSCOPIC SPINAL SURGERY

PETER O. NEWTON

The anterior approach to the spine via open thoracotomy is straightforward and provides excellent exposure to the vertebral bodies, the discs, and, when required, the spinal canal. This approach has become standard in the treatment of many spinal conditions and allows reconstructive options not possible from either a posterior or a costotransversectomy approach. When the pathology is anterior, the approach generally should be anterior as well. However, the traditional open transthoracic approach requires extensive dissection of the chest wall. Thoracoscopic surgery now makes this same direct anterior approach possible with minimally invasive methods.

HISTORY OF THORACOSCOPY

The thoracic cavity is an ideal location for utilization of endoscopic surgical methods, particularly with regard to the thoracic spine. With a lung deflated, the chest cavity is spacious and access to the anterior spine is wide. Thoracoscopic surgery is also known as video-assisted thoracic surgery (VATS). In the early 1900s, thoracoscopic surgery was performed in the treatment of pulmonary tuberculosis, although widespread use did not occur until the 1980s. As with endoscopic surgery in other parts of the body, optic and video technological advancements allowed great strides to be made in minimally invasive endoscopic approaches.

PRINCIPLES OF MINIMALLY INVASIVE SURGERY

The purpose of all minimally invasive procedures is to limit the extent of the surgical exposure while reaching and treating the pathology within the body with the same accuracy and completeness as is possible by open approach. This principle must never be forgotten as we put effort into developing techniques involving smaller skin and muscle incisions. The same surgery on the inside, in this case the surgical treatment of the spine, should be accomplished whether performed by open or thoracoscopic

means. The quality of the procedure should not be compromised in order to complete a procedure endoscopically.

The first large series of spinal thoracoscopic cases was reported in 1993 by Mack et al. (12). Since that time the number of published articles reporting on spinal thoracoscopy has been growing rapidly. Many of these reports are related to adult spinal pathology (2,7,13,21,22,24–26), yet the best indication for the thoracoscopic approach to the spine may be in the pediatric age group in cases of spinal deformity (1,5,6,9,14,18,19,23,27,29).

INDICATIONS

The indications for a thoracoscopic anterior spinal surgery are essentially the same as those for any open anterior thoracic spinal procedure, with a few specific contraindications that will be highlighted below. In the pediatric age group, the treatment of spinal deformity makes up the most common indication, though the technique is also useful in the workup and management of vertebral tumors (14,28) and infections (3,14,21). This method has also been used in performing internal thoracoplasty for chest deformities associated with scoliosis (15).

Spinal Deformity

In the treatment of spinal deformities, an anterior approach with discectomy and fusion is beneficial in several circumstances. For the purpose of spinal release, removing the discs anteriorly increases curve flexibility in both severe scoliosis and kyphosis. The quality of the anterior release performed thoracoscopically is often criticized, yet several experimental (8,16,30) and clinical (18) studies have suggested that it is possible to match the results of open surgery. Arthrodesis is performed as with any open anterior spinal surgery, with bone grafting of the evacuated disc spaces to increase the rate of solid fusion. Increasing the likelihood of fusion may be the primary indication for an anterior procedure if pseudarthrosis is likely with isolated posterior surgery (e.g., neurofibromatosis, Marfan syndrome). Prevention of anterior crankshaft growth (4) is another common indication for an anterior fusion, limiting the vertebral growth by anterior arthrodesis (11). Congenital scoliosis treatment is also amenable to thoracoscopic methods when anterior fusion or hemiepiphysiodesis is to be performed. Anterior hemivertebra excision, though technically feasible thoracoscopically, may be best done

P. O. Newton: Department of Orthopedic Surgery, Children's Hospital and Health Center, and University of California, San Diego, California 92123.

319

with open surgery unless one has extensive thoracoscopic spinal surgical experience.

Tumor and Infection

Thoracoscopy is a useful method for performing minimally invasive vertebral body biopsies when either a tumor or an infection is suspected. In many cases, however, a computed tomographic percutaneous approach may be simpler and more precise. If a corpectomy is required for infection debridement or tumor resection, the thoracoscopic approach becomes more difficult as spinal reconstruction becomes a larger factor. Short-segment instrumentation systems are available for endoscopic implantation and vertebral body reconstruction.

CONTRAINDICATIONS

The contraindications to performing an anterior thoracoscopic procedure include all of the contraindications for performing an open thoracotomy approach in addition to those specific to the thoracoscopic method. A patient with poor pulmonary function who is not a candidate for an open thoracotomy should not be recommended for thoracoscopy because it is a "less invasive" approach. The thoracoscopic approach may be less invasive and less taxing to the pulmonary system, but any patient must be able to be converted to an open thoracotomy approach at any time if the need arises (e.g., bleeding). Those patients who will not tolerate single-lung ventilation (sufficient oxygen saturation cannot be maintained), as may occur in patients with congenital diaphragmatic hernia and an underdeveloped contralateral lung, should not be treated thoracoscopically.

The specific contraindications for thoracoscopic spinal surgery relate to the technical aspects of the surgery. Thoracoscopic procedures require an adequate space or cavity in which to work. Therefore, the lung on the operative side must be completely collapsed. If this is not possible because of substantial pleural adhesions or an inability to selectively block ventilation, the endoscopic procedure should be abandoned.

Pleural Adhesions

Pleural adhesions should be expected in patients with prior intrathoracic surgery (open or endoscopic). In addition, prior pulmonary infection, especially if an empyema develops, may have a large amount of pleural scarring. Children with severe neuromuscular disorders who have a history of frequent bouts of pneumonia commonly have some degree of pleural adhesion, the severity of which will determine the difficulty of the exposure. Minor adhesions can easily be divided allowing retraction of the lung, whereas a severe pleural symphysis may make this and subsequent visualization of the spine impossible.

Small Children

Thoracoscopic spinal surgery is generally contraindicated in small children (less than 20 kg) because of the difficulty in ob-

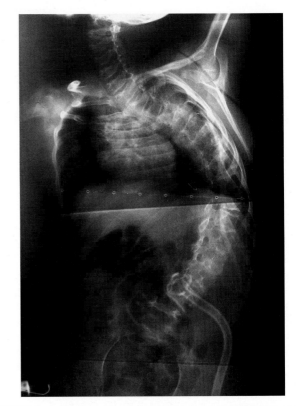

FIGURE 1. In this case of severe scoliosis, the apical vertebrae are rotated 90 degrees and nearly in contact with the ribs laterally. The working distance for the instruments is markedly restricted.

taining selective lung deflation, as well as problems associated with the small working space and the reduced distance from the chest wall to the spine. The relative benefit of thoracoscopy over thoracotomy in these patients is often reduced because generally in young patients very few anterior levels require fusion (hemivertebra, hemiepiphysiodesis), which can be performed open through a limited thoracotomy.

Severe Scoliosis

Severe scoliosis poses difficulties with substantially limited distances between the portal and the spine. Working the instruments is difficult because the field of view is reduced as the distance from the tip of the endoscope to the spine decreases. In the extreme situation, the vertebral bodies at the apex of a severe scoliosis may touch the chest wall laterally (Fig. 1). When introduced through the chest wall, the endoscope contacts the vertebra, thus preventing visualization of any other area of the spine.

THORACOSCOPIC SURGICAL TECHNIQUE

In properly selected patients, the thoracoscopic technique provides excellent visualization from the upper thoracic spine to the thoracolumbar junction. The technique for performing a thoracoscopic multilevel anterior spinal release (discectomy) and arthrodesis is summarized in the text that follows. There are several subtly different ways to perform this operation in an open fashion, and similar variations exist for the endoscopic technique.

Anesthesia Requirements

Thoracoscopic spinal surgery begins with obtaining selective ventilation of the lung. If the lung in the operative side of the chest is not deflated, thoracoscopic surgery on the spine cannot be safely performed. Deflation of the lung is required to allow visualization within the chest, as well as provide a clear path for instruments placed in the chest to reach the spine. An incompletely deflated lung is at risk for perforation with an instrument.

Single-lung ventilation can be obtained with one of several methods. The anesthesiologist (and the surgeon) needs to be familiar with each and facile in operating a flexible bronchoscope to verify placement of either a bronchial blocker or double-lumen endotracheal (ET) tube.

Bronchial Blocker

Placement of a balloon within the mainstem bronchus just distal to the carina is a relatively straightforward method of blocking ventilation to a lung. In this method of lung isolation a standard tracheal intubation is performed. A bronchoscope placed within the ET tube is utilized to accurately place the blocking balloon in the appropriate bronchus at the correct level. If the balloon is placed too distally, the right upper lobe may remain ventilated (this may or may not be problematic, depending on the levels of the spine to be operated); if placed too proximally, the entire trachea will be blocked, preventing all ventilation.

The Univent (Fuji Systems Corp., Tokyo, Japan) ET tube includes a blocking balloon that can be advanced within a side channel of the ET tube (Fig. 2A). In smaller patients (younger than 8 to 10 years), the Univent tube diameter may be too

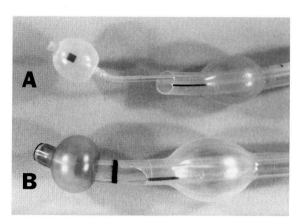

FIGURE 2. A: The Univent endotracheal tube. The distal balloon is positioned within the mainstem bronchus to prevent ventilation to that lung. **B:** The double-lumen endotracheal tube is positioned with the distal opening within the bronchus and the proximal opening in the trachea.

large to pass through the vocal cords. In this case, a standard, appropriately sized ET tube is placed and a small balloon-tipped catheter (Foley or Fogarty) can be inserted in the trachea alongside the ET tube and positioned in the mainstem bronchus as described for the Univent tube.

Double-Lumen Endotracheal Tube

Some anesthesiologists are more familiar with the double-lumen ET tube and prefer this to a bronchial blocker. The double-lumen ET tube is made of two tubes attached side to side, with one longer (bronchial tube) than the other (tracheal tube). When properly placed, the longer tube extends into the mainstem bronchus (usually on the left) and the other remains proximal to the carina. By clamping the individual tubes, ventilation to either or both lungs is possible (Fig. 2B). The smallest double-lumen tube will fit most teenagers; however, smaller patients require either use of a bronchial blocker or mainstem bronchial intubation.

Mainstem Bronchial Intubation

Direct placement of an ET tube into the mainstem bronchus is a technique that can be used to isolate ventilation to one lung. The limitation of the method comes from the fact that it is difficult to determine under bronchoscopic visualization the depth beyond the carina at which the tube has been placed. A chest radiograph can be used to confirm ET tube placement.

With each of these methods, accurate placement within the trachea/bronchus is required to ensure complete collapse of the lung and exposure of the spine. In most cases, the oxygen saturation can be maintained at 100% with only the dependent lung ventilated.

Endoscopic Equipment

Video

Specialized tools have been developed to perform endoscopic surgery. The most important of which provides the visualization of the operative field. Rigid solid crystal endoscopes (similar to those used for standard knee arthroscopy) provide clear sharp images. The endoscope in thoracoscopic procedures is identical to those used in laparoscopy. They are typically 5 or 10 mm in diameter and 40 to 50 cm in length. Directional viewing is possible at angles of 0, 30, 45, and 70 degrees. Camera technology is ever advancing, with the image displayed on a video monitor opposite the surgeon (Fig. 3).

Endoscopic Instruments

The working instruments have been sized to fit inside 5.5- to 11.5-mm portals. Nearly all of the tools to which a surgeon is accustomed are available in an endoscopy version. Expanding retractors are available in a variety of designs. Similarly, scissors and grasping instruments (usually with a connection directly to electrocautery) have been designed. Tissue dissection and vessel coagulation can be performed with unipolar or bipolar cautery,

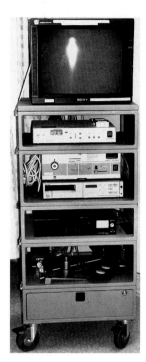

FIGURE 3. Video equipment includes a monitor, camera, light source, and endoscope.

as well as ultrasonic devices (Fig. 4A). The ultrasonic dissection devices create less smoke and tissue charring than electrocautery. In addition, these devices coagulate relatively large-caliber segmental vessels, allowing division without the need for endoscopic vessel clips.

Orthopaedic Instruments

Orthopaedic tools typical of spinal surgery are available in long narrow forms for endoscopic use. Cobb elevators, curettes, rongeurs (pituitary, Kerrison), as well as osteotomes provide the

surgeon with instruments commonly employed with the open technique (Fig. 4B).

Surgical Technique: Thoracoscopic Anterior Spinal Release and Fusion

Thoracoscopic spinal surgery requires the presence of two surgeons whose skills cover endoscopic surgery and spinal surgery. In addition, there must always be available a surgeon capable of converting to an open thoracotomy. The instruments for open conversion should be available in the operating room.

Patient Positioning

Following intubation and isolation of the lung ventilation, the patient is placed in the lateral decubitus position. The operative side is placed up, and draping is done as for a thoracotomy. Rolling the patient slightly forward of the true lateral position allows the atelectatic lung to fall forward and away from the spine.

The surgeons generally stand on the anterior side of the patient, looking across the body at a video monitor (Fig. 5). This is the most natural orientation for most surgeons, with the camera orientation "looking" in the same direction as the surgeon is facing. An assistant (third surgeon) may be positioned on the opposite side of the patient with a second monitor; however, this individual must adjust to the "mirror" motions, which occur when the endoscopic camera direction and video monitor viewing direction are opposite.

Portal Placement

Access to the inside of a chest cavity begins with the insertion of plastic cannulas through the chest wall between the ribs. The diameter of the portal depends on the size of the patient and the planned procedure, though generally portals are sized to allow passage of 10-mm-diameter instruments. The number and orientation of the portals is dictated by the nature of the procedure, deformity of the spine, and number of levels to be ad-

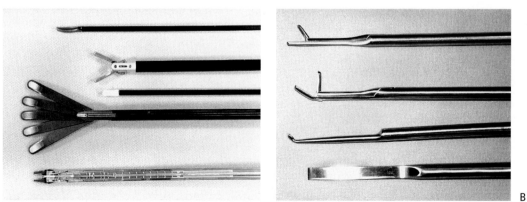

FIGURE 4. A: Typical endoscopic instruments used in thoracoscopic spinal surgery (vessel clip applier, expandable fan retractor, peanut dissector, suturing device, grasper). **B:** Modified orthopaedic instruments for endoscopic spinal surgery.

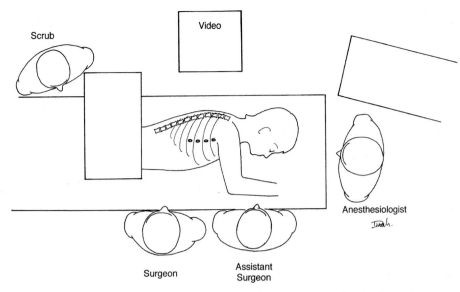

FIGURE 5. Patient and surgeon positioning during thoracoscopic spinal surgery.

dressed. In most spinal deformity cases, three to five portals are placed along the anterior axillary line (Fig. 6). This allows exchange of the endoscope, retractors, and working instruments (ultrasonic device, rongeurs, curette, etc.) between the portals, with each giving access or visualization to a different segment of the thoracic spine. The ports for thoracoscopic surgery are not sealed as they are for pressurized laparoscopic surgery. This greatly simplifies the ports used in thoracoscopy, and in smaller patients they may not be required for instrument passage if the chest wall soft tissues are relatively thin.

The technique for portal insertion is similar to placing a chest tube. After incising the skin, blunt dissection between the chest muscles over the superior margin of the rib allows safe entrance into the chest. The first portal is placed in the mid-chest at approximately the sixth or seventh rib interspace. An endoscope is introduced and the lack of lung ventilation confirmed. Even without active ventilation, the lung may remain relatively inflated. This can be expected to decrease as resorptive atelectasis

occurs with time. Initial inspection should identify any pleural adhesions and the level of the diaphragm (Fig. 7). Subsequent portal placement can be done with visualization from within the chest. This is especially important inferiorly to ensure that the portals are not placed below the level of the diaphragm.

Exposure of the Spine

The extent of spinal exposure necessary varies with the goals of the procedure. In deformity surgery, typically five to eight or more levels are exposed for disc removal and fusion. A retractor is used to protect the lung and allow visualization of the spine (Fig. 8A). The initial exposure of the spine requires reflection of the parietal pleura. A longitudinal division along the spine makes pleural closure at the end of the procedure possible. Blunt dissection of the pleura exposes the segmental vessels. These segmental vessels may be divided (Fig. 8B) or left intact (Fig. 8C), depending on the extent of the anterior and far side exposure of the spine required. When desired, ligation of the vessels can be accomplished with clips, bipolar or ultrasonic coagulation. When the segmental vessels are divided, the great vessels can be safely retracted well anterior to the spine.

Disc Excision

Removal of the intervertebral discs is begun by circumferentially incising the annulus fibrosis with either the electrocautery or ultrasonic blade (Fig. 9A). The soft nuclear material can then be removed with a pituitary rongeur (Fig. 9B). The cartilaginous end plate of each vertebral body should be excised exposing cancellous bone. This is accomplished with a rongeur, curette, Cobb elevator, or a combination of these instruments. The depth of disc space evacuation should be comparable to that performed with an open technique. The working portal should be in line (or nearly so) with the axis of the disc space utilizing an angled

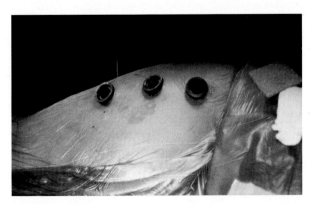

FIGURE 6. Thoracoscopic ports are placed along the anterior axillary line.

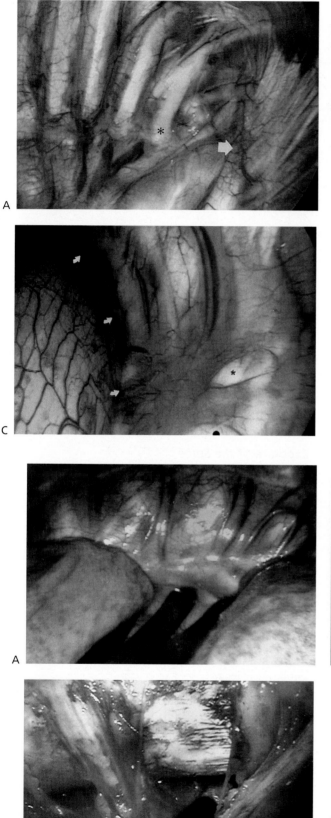

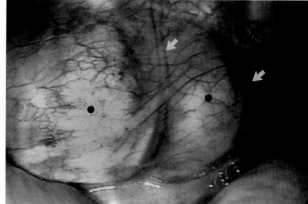

FIGURE 7. A: Initial thoracoscopic view of the proximal aspect of the thoracic spine. The white arrow points to the apex of the chest cavity and the asterisk marks the second rib head. **B:** A close-up view of the midthoracic spine is shown with the discs marked with black dots and the segmental blood vessels identified with white arrows. **C:** The distal extent of the thoracic spine is seen with the diaphragm outlined with white arrows. The disc *(black dot)* and corresponding rib head *(asterisk)* are marked.

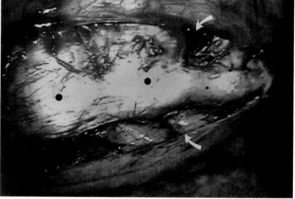

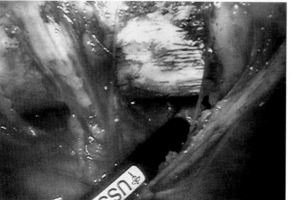

FIGURE 8. A: Fan retractor being used to protect the lung and expose the spine. **B:** With division of the segmental vessels, wide exposure of the anterior spine is possible. The cut edges of the pleura are identified with white arrows and the discs with black dots. **C:** Exposure of the disc is also possible when the vessels are maintained.

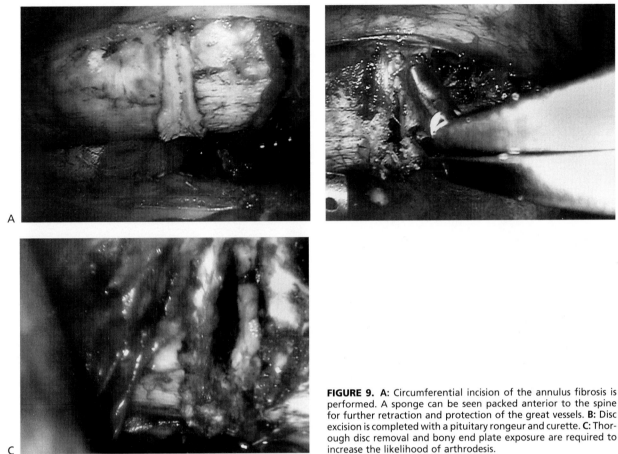

A

B

C

FIGURE 9. A: Circumferential incision of the annulus fibrosis is performed. A sponge can be seen packed anterior to the spine for further retraction and protection of the great vessels. **B:** Disc excision is completed with a pituitary rongeur and curette. **C:** Thorough disc removal and bony end plate exposure are required to increase the likelihood of arthrodesis.

(45-degree preferably) endoscope to provide visualization into the full depth of the disc space during removal of the disc tissue (Fig. 9C).

Bone Grafting

To facilitate a solid arthrodesis, bone graft is placed within the disc space. The source for this bone may be either autogenous (iliac crest, rib) or allogenous (freeze-dried cancellous chips, fresh-frozen cancellous). In most cases, structural grafting is not required and cancellous bone can be delivered to the disc space either one piece at a time or in large aliquots via a cannula-plunger device (Fig. 10). In either case, complete filling of the space with bone graft gives the greatest chance for subsequent arthrodesis.

Pleural Closure

Once each of the discs has been thoroughly debrided and grafted, closure of the pleura is recommended. This is not mandatory; however, when possible it restores the intrathoracic anatomy and prevents the bone graft from migrating throughout the chest cavity. Pleural closure may help to decrease blood loss.

The EndoStitch device (U.S. Surgical Corp., Norwalk, CT) allows a relatively simple running closure to be performed endo-

scopically. This closure is also utilized to repair any opening of the diaphragm (Fig. 11A) that may have been performed to gain access to the T12–L1 or L1–2 levels. A sliding fisherman's cinch knot is utilized to secure the suture to the pleura or diaphragm. This knot is tied by hand outside the chest and slides down the suture when tension is applied (Fig. 11B). The EndoStitch is

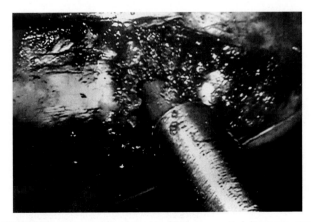

FIGURE 10. Bone graft is packed to fill the evacuated disc space completely. In this case, it has been delivered through a long tube with a central plunger/tamp.

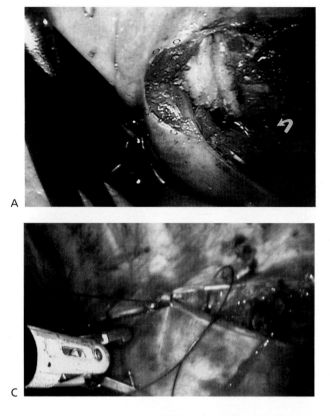

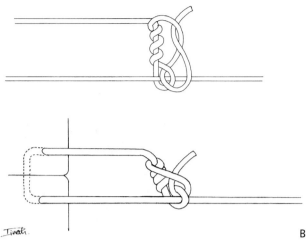

FIGURE 11. **A:** Division of the diaphragm insertion allows exposure of the T12–L1 disc. Open black arrows outline the split fibers of the diaphragm. The white arrow points to a sponge used for additional retraction. The fan retractor is reflecting the diaphragm inferiorly. **B:** A three-turn fisherman's cinch knot is used to create a sliding knot to initiate the diaphragm and pleural closure. **C:** A running pleural closure is possible with the EndoStitch device.

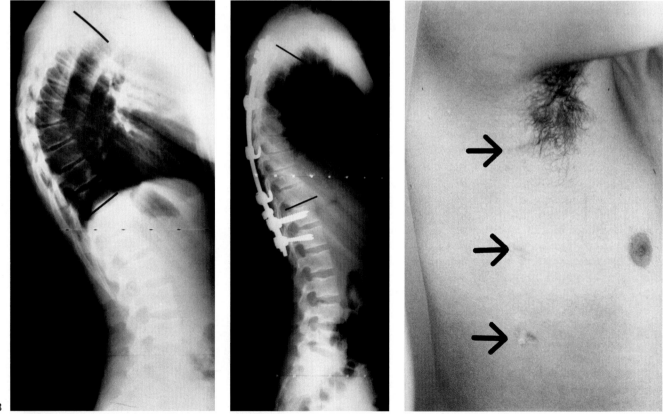

FIGURE 12. **A:** Preoperative lateral radiograph of a 15-year-old boy with Scheuermann kyphosis measuring 85 degrees. **B:** Postoperative lateral radiograph after thoracoscopic anterior spinal release and fusion, as well as posterior instrumentation and fusion performed on the same day. The kyphosis was reduced to 43 degrees. **C:** Clinical appearance of the three thoracoscopic incisions 9 months postoperatively.

used to pass a double-ended needle back and forth between the jaws of the device, creating a running closure (Fig. 11C). A series of half hitches can be tied internally to finish the closure.

Postoperative Management

Following the thoracoscopic procedure, a chest tube is placed through an inferior portal. This may be removed when the drainage becomes serous and the output slows to 50 to 75 ml per 8-hour period. In most deformity cases the anterior release and fusion is followed by a posterior procedure (instrumentation and/or fusion) either on the same day or as a staged surgery (Fig. 12).

COMPLICATIONS OF THORACOSCOPIC SPINAL SURGERY

In general, the potential complications of thoracoscopic anterior spinal surgery are the same as those of open anterior spinal surgery. However, some may be more challenging to deal with endoscopically, particularly excessive bleeding.

Intraoperative Complications

Complications that may occur during a thoracoscopic procedure include injury to the heart, great vessels, spinal cord, lung parenchyma, diaphragm, or thoracic duct. Excessive bleeding may come from segmental vessels, epidural veins, or directly from exposed bone. Each source of bleeding should be minimized as much as possible with appropriate use of electrocautery, ultrasonic coagulation, bone waxing, early disc space bone grafting, and, at times, use of substances such as Endo-Avitene (Med-Chem Products Inc., Woburn, MA).

Prevention of Complications

The greatest likelihood for injury to a critical structure comes when visualization is suboptimal. As such, the most important aspect of any endoscopic procedure is maintaining ideal visualization. The most common hindrance to visualization is bleeding, and it is critical to maintain as dry a field as possible. In most cases, the exposure of the spine can be accomplished without any substantial bleeding. Disc excision is always associated with some blood loss once the vertebral end plates are exposed. Packing the discs with bone graft immediately after excision limits this bleeding.

Injury to the lung is possible if there is inadequate deflation or retraction of the lung. As discussed, pleural adhesions may prevent retraction of the lung, as seen in Figure 13. In this case, the adhesions were divided endoscopically and excellent exposure of the spine was possible. In more significant cases of adhesion this may become quite challenging. Direct sighting down the portal from outside to inside the chest is one way to ensure there is no lung tissue in the path of the instrument

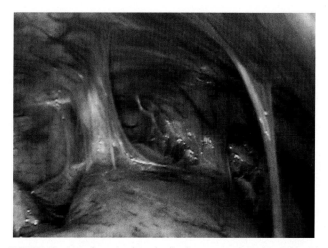

FIGURE 13. Intrathoracic pleural adhesions are seen in this child with cerebral palsy. She had a history of many prior pneumonias, but no prior chest surgery or chest tube placement had been done.

being placed to the spine. Alternatively, each instrument can be visualized endoscopically to ensure that a clear path exists from the portal to the spine.

Thoracic duct injury with chyle leakage has been reported after both open and thoracoscopic spinal procedures (17). If recognized at the time of surgery, by noting cloudy fluid, the area may be oversewn or ligature clips applied. If a chylous effusion develops post-operatively, a nonfat diet and/or thoracic duct ligation may be required.

Spinal cord injury during anterior disc excision may result either from direct trauma during entrance into the spinal canal or from vascular insufficiency attributable to segmental vessel ligation. Prevention of direct injury is largely dependent on visualization, especially into the depths of the disc space. Particularly in the scoliotic spine, this is often not possible with a 30-degree angled scope, and for this reason a 45-degree angle is recommended. The safety of routine segmental vessel ligation remains controversial. Visualization of the anterior and contralateral aspect of the spine is certainly enhanced when these vessels are divided. In high-risk patients (e.g., congenital kyphosis), an attempt to maintain the segmental vessels should be made or monitoring of spinal cord function after placing an endoscopic vessel clip at each level may be performed. If monitoring changes occur, the clips may be removed, though a thoracotomy may be required to remove them.

Conversion to Open Thoracotomy

In some instances, conversion to open thoracotomy may be required (14,17). The surgeon should not be reluctant to switch if the procedure is not going as desired thoracoscopically. One must ask: Is the exposure/visualization adequate to support safe performance of the procedure? Is the procedure being carried out effectively? If at any point the answer to either question is no, a change in approach (i.e., conversion to an open thoracotomy) should be considered.

Additionally, if rapid bleeding develops that cannot be controlled endoscopically, the surgeon should be capable of expeditiously performing a thoracotomy. The thoracotomy instruments should be in the operating room, ready if needed. In our initial series of 65 patients, 2 patients required conversion to open thoracotomy. In both cases, a combination of bleeding and inadequately released pleural adhesions began to obstruct endoscopic visualization (17).

OUTCOMES OF THORACOSCOPIC SPINAL DEFORMITY PROCEDURES

The efficacy of thoracoscopic spinal procedures has not been proven in long-term outcome studies. Because the technique is relatively new, long-term data are lacking. Several reports of the early results, however, are encouraging. The adequacy of anterior spinal release, as well as the complication rate and learning curve, seem acceptable and comparable to the open method.

Deformity Correction Outcome

In our early clinical series comparing the degree of deformity correction following anterior release and posterior instrumentation, similar degrees of correction occurred with thoracoscopic and open anterior techniques. The average preoperative angle of scoliosis was 84 ± 23 degrees in the thoracoscopic group, compared with 73 ± 18 degrees in the open thoracotomy group, and the postoperative percent correction was 56% and 60%, respectively. Similar trends were noted in patients with kyphosis undergoing anterior release with both techniques (18).

Experimental studies have also suggested that the degree of increased spinal motion is comparable when disc excision is performed by thoracoscopic and open approaches (16,30). In addition, the extent of experimental end plate exposure is similar with each of the methods (8,30).

In our initial experience with the thoracoscopic approach for patients treated for spinal deformity, 65 consecutive cases were analyzed. The indications for the anterior procedure were as follows: idiopathic scoliosis, 13; kyphosis, nine; neuromuscular deformity, 35; congenital, four; tumor/syrinx, four. Complications occurred in six patients, two of whom required conversion to a thoracotomy. The percentage deformity correction was similar to that reported in the earlier series, 59 ± 17% for scoliosis and 92 ± 12% for kyphosis (17).

The rate of arthrodesis with thoracoscopic procedures has not been well studied. The success of crankshaft prevention has also not been confirmed. There have been few reported failures due to pseudarthrosis when a posterior procedure was included. However, this is not the case for those scoliosis patients treated with instrumentation entirely from the anterior side. Careful long-term assessment of the success of the anterior fusion and its prevention of crankshaft growth remains to be performed.

The Learning Curve

Thoracoscopy requires acquisition of new surgical skills and is associated with a learning process. With increasing experience, the time to perform the operation decreases and the quality

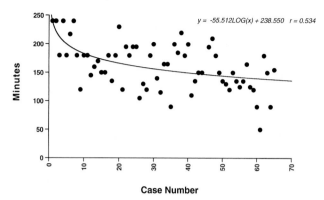

FIGURE 14. One measure of the learning curve for thoracoscopy is the time required to perform the operation as it relates to the greater operative experience. This graph demonstrates total anterior operative time compared to the case number in a consecutive series of patients. A decrease occurred as experience was gained.

with which it is performed increases. In the series of patients mentioned above, there was a decrease in the operative time throughout the experience (Fig. 14). When total operative time was normalized based on the number of discs excised, the time decreased from 29 minutes per disc in the first 30 patients to 22 minutes per disc for the second 35 patients (17). The additional clinical measures for these two groups are presented in Table 1.

Quantifying the changes in the quality of the disc excision, anterior release, and spinal fusion as surgical experience is gained is difficult. There is, however, no question that the learning curve in this regard is also real and likely parallels that of the operative time. The number of cases needed by any one surgeon to master the technique will vary based on numerous factors. There is, however, a substantial learning process associated with this procedure that must be recognized.

TABLE 1. OPERATIVE AND POSTOPERATIVE DATA

Parameter	All 65 Cases	Cases 1–30	Cases 31–65
Age (years)	14 ± 3.4	14.4 ± 4.2	13.7 ± 2.5
Number of Portals	3.8 ± .6	3.6 ± .7	3.9 ± .4
Discs excised	6.5 ± 1.5	6.2 ± .9	6.9 ± 1.8
Anterior Operative Time (min)	161 ± 41	177 ± 39	147 ± 38
Operative Time per Disc (min)	25.7 ± 7.2	29.3 ± 7.7	22.3 ± 4.7
Anterior Blood Loss (ml)	301 ± 322	262 ± 216	336 ± 393
Anterior Blood Loss per Disc (ml)	46 ± 50	43 ± 35	48 ± 60
Hospital Days	9.5 ± 4.1	9.2 ± 3.1	9.7 ± 4.8
ICU Days	2.3 ± 3.1	1.9 ± 3.3	2.6 ± 3.0
Chest Tube Days	3.9 ± 1.6	4.2 ± 1.8	3.6 ± 1.4
Chest Tube Output (ml)	796 ± 452	888 ± 508	718 ± 388
Chest Tube Output per Disc (ml)	123 ± 67	143 ± 82	106 ± 46

Operative and postoperative data on 65 consecutive thoracoscopic anterior spinal release and fusion cases. (From Newton PO, Shea KG, Granlund KF (2000): Defining the pediatric spinal thoracoscopy learning curve: sixty–five consecutive cases. *Spine* 25:1028–1035.

ADVANTAGES OF THORACOSCOPIC SPINAL SURGERY

The primary advantages of the thoracoscopic approach relate largely to the limited dissection of the chest wall. The muscles of the chest (latissimus dorsi, serratus anterior, and intercostals) are split by blunt dissection rather than cut transversely. The return of shoulder girdle and thoracic respiratory muscle function is affected to a much lesser degree than by open thoracotomy.

Postoperative pain is milder in thoracoscopic approaches than in open exposures. This has been demonstrated in cases of pulmonary biopsy using both methods (10). This fact has been more difficult to confirm in spinal surgery when much of the postoperative pain results from the accompanying posterior instrumentation procedure.

Cosmesis related to the wounds is felt by most patients to be improved with the thoracoscopic approach even if four to five portals are required. The incisions lie beneath the arm and are less visible than a standard thoracotomy incision.

Another important advantage of the thoracoscopic approach is the ease in which the exposure can be extended either proximally or distally. As many as 12 levels (T2 to L1) can be fused, compared with the 5 or 6 levels possible with a single thoracotomy. In many cases, the visualization and access of the end levels is better with the endoscopic than the open procedure.

DISADVANTAGES OF THORACOSCOPIC SPINAL SURGERY

The advantages of the thoracoscopic approach when properly applied are substantial, but the disadvantages must also be recognized. This technique, like all new methods, has not yet stood the test of time. Because it involves surgical skills not in the repertoire of most pediatric spinal surgeons, a concerted effort in learning the method is required by those interested in safely using this approach. This is not a "see one, do one" procedure. The tactile sense that surgeons are so accustomed to having is missing with the thoracoscopic method. This, in addition to the altered means of "seeing" the spine (with an endoscope projected on a monitor), requires adjustment and practice. The attendance at specialized courses, tutorials, and workshops is the first step in gaining this skill (20).

The specialized equipment and imaging technology that make this approach possible also preclude its use when they malfunction. This technology is also expensive. The cost of thoracoscopic procedures was compared to open procedures with similar indications at the Children's Hospital in San Diego. In the initial thoracoscopic experience the cost was estimated to be 15% greater in thoracoscopy cases. The additional cost was related to longer operative times, increased use of disposable endoscopic instruments, and the rental of several high-cost items (endoscopic orthopaedic instruments, video equipment, ultrasonic device). Since that time, fewer disposable tools are being used (a retractor, EndoStitch, and endoscopic peanuts are the only disposables currently used routinely), and the equipment costs have decreased since purchase was made of the video equipment, orthopaedic tools, and ultrasonic device. In addition, the cost of operative time has decreased approximately 25%. These changes over time have made the cost of thoracoscopy nearly equivalent to open thoracotomy procedures.

INSIGHT INTO THE FUTURE OF PEDIATRIC SPINAL THORACOSCOPY

The number of surgeons who are utilizing the thoracoscopic spinal approach in their practice continues to grow, despite the fact that this group remains in the minority. For a surgeon to gain expertise in this approach it is necessary that there be a sufficient number of patients to support his or her progress along the learning curve in a timely fashion. For this reason, it seems likely that experience will be amassed in centers that have the critical volume of cases to warrant the investment of time and effort needed to foster mastery of the procedure (20).

Just as technological advances have made this procedure possible, similar advances will make it simpler to apply as well as broaden the applications. Minimally invasive surgery is now part of all surgical specialties, and cross-fertilization of new ideas continues to lead to innovations in each field.

As with arthroscopy, thoracoscopy will not entirely replace the open approach. In the knee, meniscectomy and anterior cruciate ligament reconstruction, once open operations, are now routinely performed endoscopically, though arthroplasty continues to require an arthrotomy. Over time, the indications for thoracoscopy and open thoracotomy will become more clearly defined. It is relatively early in the developmental stages of thoracoscopy, and substantial progress should be expected.

One example of this is the thoracoscopic introduction of anterior spinal instrumentation for the correction of thoracic scoliosis. Thoracoscopic anterior discectomy, fusion, and insertion of multilevel anterior screw/rod systems are being investigated at several centers. Although clearly requiring additional refinement and study, early reports suggest this will likely become an option for some patients with thoracic scoliosis requiring fusion. This will allow for the first completely minimally invasive endoscopic approach to the surgical treatment of scoliosis.

REFERENCES

1. Burgos J, Rapariz JM, Gonzalez-Herranz P (1998): Anterior endoscopic approach to the thoracolumbar spine. *Spine* 23:2427–2431.
2. Dickman CA, Mican CA (1996): Multilevel anterior thoracic discectomies and anterior interbody fusion using a microsurgical thoracoscopic approach. Case report. *J Neurosurg* 84:104–109.
3. Dickman CA, Rosenthal D, Karahalios DG, et al. (1996): Thoracic vertebrectomy and reconstruction using a microsurgical thoracoscopic approach. *Neurosurgery* 38:279–293.
4. Dubousset J, Herring JA, Shufflebarger H (1989): The crankshaft phenomenon. *J Pediatr Orthop* 9:541–550.
5. Gonzalez Barrios I, Fuentes Caparros S, Avila Jurado MM (1995): Anterior thoracoscopic epiphysiodesis in the treatment of a crankshaft phenomenon. *Eur Spine J* 4:343–346.
6. Holcomb GW III, Mencio GA, Green NE (1997): Video-assisted thoracoscopic diskectomy and fusion. *J Pediatr Surg* 32:1120–1122.
7. Huang TJ, Hsu RW, Liu HP, et al. (1999): Video-assisted thoracoscopic surgery to the upper thoracic spine. *Surg Endosc* 13:123–126.

8. Huntington CF, Murrell WD, Betz RR, et al. (1998): Comparison of thoracoscopic and open thoracic discectomy in a live ovine model for anterior spinal fusion. *Spine* 23:1699–1702.

9. Kokoska ER, Gabriel KR, Silen ML (1998): Minimally invasive anterior spinal exposure and release in children with scoliosis. *J Soc Laparoendosc Surg* 2:255–258.

10. Landreneau RJ, Hazelrigg SR, Mack MJ, et al. (1993): Postoperative pain related morbidity: Video assisted thoracoscopy versus thoracotomy. *Ann Thorac Surg* 56:1285–1289.

11. Lapinksy AS, Richards BS (1995): Preventing the crankshaft phenomenon by combining anterior fusion with posterior instrumentation. Does it work? *Spine* 20:1392–1398.

12. Mack MJ, Regan JJ, Bobechko WP, et al. (1993): Application of thoracoscopy for diseases of the spine. *Ann Thorac Surg* 56:736–738.

13. McAfee PC, Regan JR, Fedder IL, et al. (1995): Anterior thoracic corpectomy for spinal cord decompression performed endoscopically. *Surg Laparosc Endosc* 5:339–348.

14. McAfee PC, Regan JR, Zdeblick T, et al. (1995): The incidence of complications in endoscopic anterior thoracolumbar spinal reconstructive surgery. A prospective multicenter study comprising the first 100 consecutive cases. *Spine* 20:1624–1632.

15. Mehlman CT, Crawford AH, Wolf RK (1997): Video-assisted thoracoscopic surgery (VATS). Endoscopic thoracoplasty technique. *Spine* 22:2178–2182.

16. Newton PO, Cardelia JM, Farnsworth CL, et al. (1998): A biomechanical comparison of open and thoracoscopic anterior spinal release in a goat model. *Spine* 23: 530–535.

17. Newton PO, Shea KG, Granlund KF (2000): Defining the pediatric spinal thoracoscopy learning curve: sixty-five consecutive cases. *Spine* 25:1028–1035.

18. Newton PO, Wenger DR, Mubarak SJ, et al. (1997): Anterior release and fusion in pediatric spinal deformity. A comparison of early outcome and cost of thoracoscopic and open thoracotomy approaches. *Spine* 22: 1398–1406.

19. Nymberg SM, Crawford AH (1996): Video-assisted thoracoscopic releases of scoliotic anterior spines. *AORN J* 63:561–2, 5–9, 71–5.

20. Olinger A, Pistorius G, Lindemann W, et al. (1999): Effectiveness of a hands-on training course for laparoscopic spine surgery in a porcine model. *Surg Endosc* 13:118–122.

21. Parker LM, McAfee PC, Fedder IL, et al. (1996): Minimally invasive surgical techniques to treat spine infections. *Orthop Clin N Am* 27: 183–199.

22. Regan JJ, Ben-Yishay A, Mack MJ (1998): Video-assisted thoracoscopic excision of herniated thoracic disc: description of technique and preliminary experience in the first 29 cases. *J Spinal Disord* 11:183–191.

23. Regan JJ, Mack MJ, Picetti GD III (1995): A technical report on video-assisted thoracoscopy in thoracic spinal surgery. Preliminary description. *Spine* 20:831–837.

24. Regan JJ, Yuan H, McCullen G (1997): Minimally invasive approaches to the spine. *Instr Course Lect* 46:127–141.

25. Rosenthal D, Dickman CA (1998): Thoracoscopic microsurgical excision of herniated thoracic discs. *J Neurosurg* 89:224–235.

26. Rosenthal D, Marquardt G, Lorenz R, et al. (1996): Anterior decompression and stabilization using a microsurgical endoscopic technique for metastatic tumors of the thoracic spine. *J Neurosurg* 84: 565–572.

27. Rothenberg S, Erickson M, Eilert R, et al. (1998): Thoracoscopic anterior spinal procedures in children. *J Pediatr Surg* 33:1168–1170.

28. Tan HL, McMurrick PJ, Merriman TE, et al. (1994): Thoracoscopic biopsy of a pathological vertebral body. *Aust N Z J Surg* 64:726–728.

29. Waisman M, Saute M (1997): Thoracoscopic spine release before posterior instrumentation in scoliosis. *Clin Orthop* 336:130–136.

30. Wall EJ, Bylski-Austrow DI, Shelton FS, et al. (1998): Endoscopic discectomy increases thoracic spine flexibility as effectively as open discectomy. A mechanical study in a porcine model. *Spine* 23:9–15.

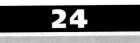

POSTERIOR DISTRACTION SYSTEMS AND COMBINATIONS: HARRINGTON RODS

NEIL E. GREEN

HARRINGTON INSTRUMENTATION SYSTEMS

History

The Harrington system, named for Paul Harrington, was the original system for instrumentation of the deformed spine. It provided surgeons the ability to increase correction of the spinal deformity and achieve an increased rate of fusion of the spine. Harrington developed his system for correction and stabilization of scoliosis in the late 1950s and reported a series of patients in 1962 (30). His earliest experience was with patients who had poliomyelitis, but later he began to use the system for idiopathic scoliosis. At first, spinal fusion was not used; however, it became evident to Harrington that fusion of the instrumented spine was essential. The original fusion was performed using only local bone for grafting. Although Harrington was careful to perform excellent decortication of the posterior elements of the spine, he realized that addition of autogenous bone increased the fusion mass and decreased the risk of pseudarthrosis (30–34).

Advantages

The Harrington system is relatively inexpensive, especially in comparison with the newer segmental instrumentation systems. It is easy to use, and the principles of its application are well defined. The fusion levels can usually be determined with ease and accuracy.

Because of ease of use, the surgical procedure can be performed quickly with little blood loss. The rate of neurologic injury is very low with the Harrington distraction system. Because there are only two points of hook fixation with this system, much bone is free for decortication, which allows greater surface area to be fused. With the newer segmental systems, much less of the spine is decorticated because of the increased points of fixation.

N. E. Green: Department of Orthopaedics and Rehabilitation, Vanderbilt University Medical Center, Nashville, Tennessee 37232-2550.

Disadvantages

The disadvantage of the Harrington system is that it constitutes nonsegmental fixation to the spine. Because the Harrington distraction rod is secured to the spine at only the cephalad and caudad vertebrae included in the fusion area, it is less rigid than segmental fixation. Because of the decreased stability of the Harrington distraction rod, the patient requires postoperative immobilization, whereas because of increased stability, the tendency is not to immobilize the patient who has undergone spine fusion with a segmental fixation system of instrumentation.

The pure distraction force of the Harrington distraction rod tends to flatten the spine between the hook sites, thereby not reducing the hypokyphosis of the instrumented thoracic spine and producing kyphosis of the instrumented lumbar spine (1,2,10) (Fig. 1). The Harrington system of fixation to the sacrum has not proven satisfactory. Instrumentation to the sacrum with Harrington hooks that attach to the alae of the sacrum produces kyphosis at the lumbosacral level because the distraction force not only flattens the lumbar spine but extends the pelvis, producing a lumbosacral kyphosis. Neither is the rate of fusion across the lumbosacral articulation as reliable as expected with the use of Galveston fixation to the pelvis.

Instrumentation

The distraction rod (stainless steel) consists of a ratchet end and a collar end. The ratchet end is intended to lock the hook and rod together. Once the hook and rod are engaged, further distraction is accomplished with ease; however, there is significant resistance to loss of the distraction gained. At the end of the surgical procedure, a C ring is placed between the cephalad hook and the exposed ratchet below the hook to prevent loss of the distraction gained (Fig. 2).

The collar end of the rod is designed in both round and square ends. The square-ended rod fits into a specially designed hook that accepts square-ended rods. This square design prevents rotation of the rod, making possible better maintenance of the normal sagittal plane contour of the spine, and was an early attempt to prevent creation of kyphosis of the instrumented lumbar spine.

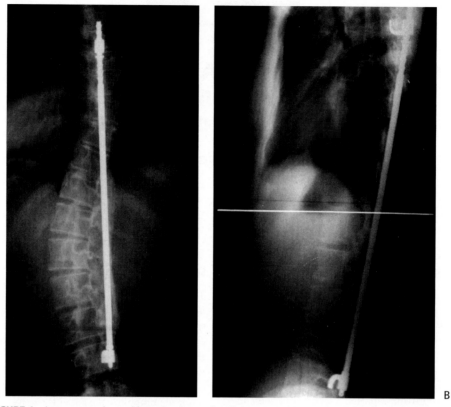

FIGURE 1. Anteroposterior and lateral radiographs of a 17-year-old girl who had undergone posterior spinal fusion for adolescent idiopathic scoliosis 2 years previously. **A:** Anteroposterior radiograph of both the thoracic and lumbar scoliosis with a "dollar sign" Harrington rod. Both the thoracic and lumbar curves were structural double primary curves. The Harrington rod crosses the spine between the thoracic and lumbar curves. Both curves measured 50 degrees preoperatively. A solid arthrodesis is evident clinically and radiographically. **B:** The lateral radiograph taken at the same time shows lack of contouring of the round-ended Harrington rod and flattening of the lumbar spine.

Technique

Harrington described the so-called stable zone, which indicated the area where hooks should be inserted in the spine. Use of this area for hook insertion should allow a balanced spine postoperatively. According to Harrington, the lower hook site should be within the stable zone, which is determined by drawing two parallel vertical lines perpendicular to a line drawn between the two iliac crests. The vertical lines begin at the two lumbosacral

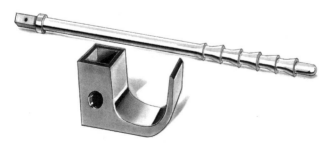

FIGURE 2. Square-ended distraction rod and hook. The square-ended hook and rod fit together, preventing rotation of the rod. This allows contouring of the rod for better control of the sagittal plane of the body.

facets (Fig. 3A). The lower hook site should lie between these two vertical lines (36).

King et al. (40,41) also determined the ideal fusion levels in patients with adolescent idiopathic scoliosis. They defined the level of the lower hook insertion more narrowly than did Harrington, believing that the lower hook should be inserted into the stable vertebra, which they defined as the first vertebra at the caudal end of the curve to be instrumented that is bisected by a vertical line drawn cephalad through the middle of the sacrum. This vertical line must be perpendicular to a line drawn between the top of the iliac crests (40,41) (Fig. 3B).

Because of the importance of preserving the mobility of the lumbar spine, one should instrument only the absolutely necessary portion of the lumbar spine. Fusing only the thoracic spine even in face of curves in both the thoracic and the lumbar areas of the spine is advocated if the criteria of King et al. are followed. These investigators described five types of curves. For all curves, the stable vertebra should be used to determine the lower extent of the fusion. In the type 2 curve, in which both a thoracic and a lumbar curve exist, they advocate fusion of only the thoracic curve if the lumbar curve is equal to or smaller than the thoracic curve and if the lumbar curve is more flexible. The flexibility of the curves is determined by measuring the individual curves

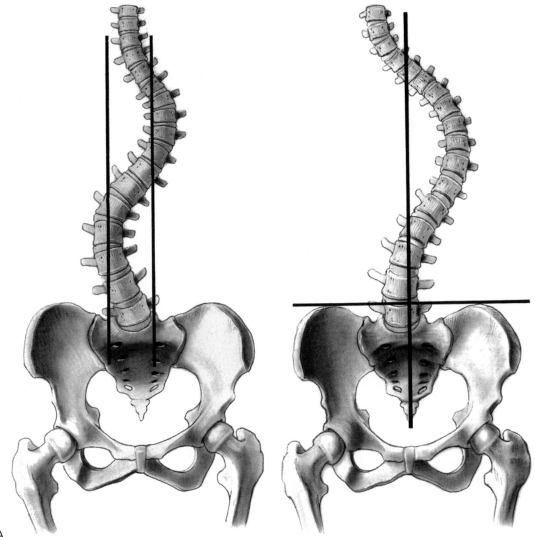

A

B

FIGURE 3. **A:** The stable zone of Harrington is outlined by two vertical lines beginning at the lumbosacral facets and drawn vertically perpendicular to a line across the iliac crest. The vertebra should be included, and the lower end of the spinal fusion should lie within the zone. **B:** The stable vertebra is defined by drawing a line perpendicular to a horizontal line through the iliac crest. This vertical line bisects the midpoint of the sacrum and then is drawn vertically. The vertebra bisected by the line is termed the stable vertebra. In this example, the stable vertebra is L3.

on side bending radiographs. Therefore, if the lumbar curvature corrects more than the thoracic curve, it is deemed more flexible and will meet the criteria for performance of a selective thoracic fusion, leaving the lumbar spine mobile. Because of the flexibility of the lumbar spine, one should expect sufficient correction of the lumbar curve so that the spine will be balanced postoperatively. In addition, the lumbar curve should not progress even though it has not been instrumented and fused (40,41).

The cephalad bifid hook site is prepared by notching the inferior articular process of the most cephalad vertebra to be included in the fusion. A small (¼-in.) osteotome is placed 2 to 3 mm from the inferior edge of the joint perpendicular to the longitudinal axis of the spinous process. This 2 to 3 mm of the inferior portion of the superior articular process is removed, exposing a small portion of the facet joint. The bone resection also renders the surface against which the hook sits square, thereby resisting the tendency for the hook to dislodge in a lateral direction (Fig. 4).

The caudad hook is inserted under the lamina of the most

distal vertebra to be instrumented and fused. First, a laminotomy is performed by removing the interspinous ligament and the ligamentum flavum from the side that is to be instrumented. A Lexsell rongeur may be used to remove the interspinous ligament and enough of the ligamentum flavum to allow entry under the ligament with a Kerrison rongeur. The remainder of the ligamentum flavum on the concave side of the spine is removed. The hook to be used is placed on a hook holder and, with a motion that rotates the hook under the lamina, inserted into the spinal canal (Fig. 5).

While these two hooks are stabilized with hook holders, the outrigger is applied to the spine. The outrigger consists of a bar and screw mechanism with prongs at the cephalad and caudad ends. These prongs are inserted into the two hooks, and the screw mechanism is twisted, distracting the spine. This is done slowly, with care taken not to overdistract the spine (Fig. 6). Once a moderate amount of tension has been accomplished, the spine will be more stable, thus facilitating facet excision and decortication of the posterior elements. Throughout the process

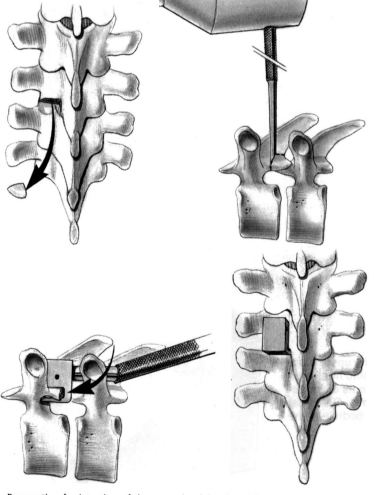

FIGURE 4. Preparation for insertion of the upper hook begins with notching of the inferior articular process of the cephalad vertebra. The notch is made by excising a small piece of the inferior articular process with a ¼-in. osteotome. Enough bone is removed to allow the bifid hook to engage the pedicle.

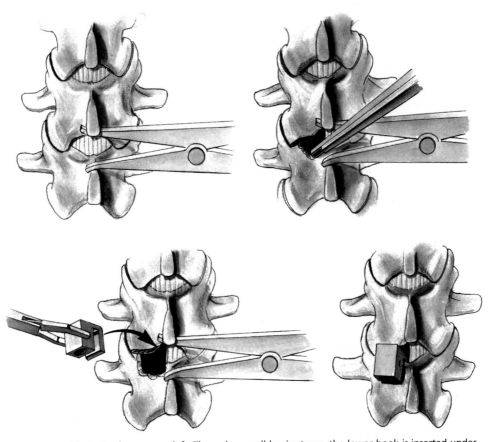

FIGURE 5. *Clockwise from upper left:* Through a small laminotomy, the lower hook is inserted under the lamina of the most caudad vertebra to be included in the fusion. A Lexsell rongeur is used to remove the overhanging spinous process from the cephalad vertebra if it is obstructing the view of the interspinous ligament. The interspinous ligament is then removed with the Lexsell rongeur. The ligamentum flavum may also be partially removed with the Lexsell rongeur until the spinal canal is visible. Epidural fat will be apparent, protruding through the opening in the ligamentum flavum. Next, with a Kerrison rongeur, the ligamentum flavum is removed from the concave side of the spine. A small amount of bone is also removed from the lamina to allow square seating of the lower hook.

of decortication and facet excision, the distraction on the outrigger is increased gradually. One should not attempt to obtain maximum distraction because of the risk of spinal cord injury or lamina fracture; if too much distraction force is used, the cephalad hook may cut through the superior articular process.

Once the desired distraction has been obtained and the facet excision and decortication is complete, the outrigger is removed and replaced with a distraction rod of appropriate length. Accurate measurement is best accomplished with the outrigger in place and the spine distracted to the desired length. A square-ended rod is generally used to allow control of the sagittal contour of the spine. The rod is contoured with French rod benders to produce a normal thoracic kyphosis and lumbar lordosis. The cephalad end of the rod is first inserted into the cephalad hook and pushed far enough into this hook that the caudal end of the rod can be inserted into the caudal hook. Once the rod is inserted into both hooks, the spine is distracted with the Harrington distractor. This device is placed between the ratchets that are exposed below the cephalad hook and the inferior end of this hook. The cephalad hook is pushed cephalad on the rod as the distractor handles are squeezed together. If no ratchets

are exposed below the hook, a specially designed Gaines distractor that attaches to the ratchets above the hook and grasps the hook from below is used (Fig. 7). When the handles of this distractor are squeezed, the hook is pulled forward on the rod, exposing ratchets below the hook. The regular distractor may then be used. As the hook passes each ratchet, the hook self-stabilizes, resisting loss of the distraction gained. Once the desired distraction has been obtained, a C ring is placed between the bottom of the hook and the next ratchet below the hook. Squeezing the rings of the C ring locks it to the rod, preventing loss of the distraction obtained.

Use of a compression rod on the convexity of the curve is optional (25). This rod helps correct the spine by compressing the convexity of the curve and provides segmental fixation of the spine. It is also useful for helping to maintain lordosis of the instrumented lumbar spine. By far its greatest use is for correction of thoracic kyphosis such as exists in Scheuermann kyphosis, in which it is used on both sides of the spine without a distraction rod.

The compression rod consists of a 3.2-mm rod and corresponding no. 1259 hooks. A larger (4.8-mm) rod with no. 1256

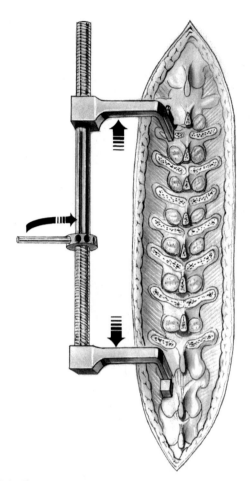

FIGURE 6. The Harrington outrigger is applied to both the upper and lower hooks and, with distraction of the outrigger, the spine is straightened.

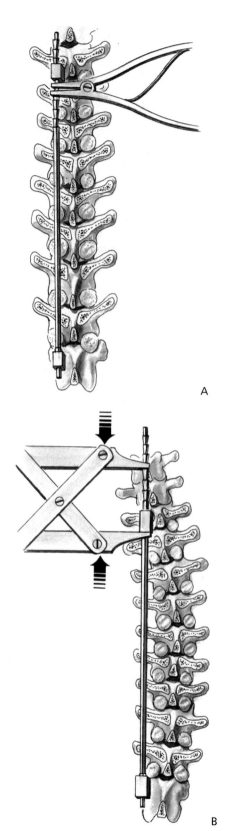

FIGURE 7. Two distractors, the Harrington spreader and the Gaines distractor, may be used to distract and lock the upper Harrington hooks on the ratchet end of the Harrington rod. **A:** The routine Harrington spreader is applied beneath the upper hook. **B:** The Gaines distractor should be used if no ratchets are exposed below the upper hook; it distracts the spine until ratchets are exposed below the upper hook, at which time the regular Harrington distractor may be used.

hooks is also available. The larger rod is used for larger patients and especially for correction of thoracic kyphosis when only compression rods are used. Six hooks are attached to the compression rod for its use. Three hooks, facing caudad, will be inserted around transverse processes cephalad to the apex of the curvature or kyphosis. The three hooks inserted on the caudad side of the apex of the curve face cephalad. They may also be placed around a transverse process in the thoracic area, but in the lumbar spine and even in the lowest thoracic vertebra, where the transverse processes are too small to resist the stress of the hooks, the hooks enter the spinal canal through a small laminotomy.

Insertion of the instrumentation begins with preparation of the rod and hooks. The hooks are placed on the rod with nuts behind each hook. Because the rod is flexible, the hooks can be manipulated into place while positioned on the rod. Sites for the hook insertions are then prepared. A hook attached to a hook holder is placed around the transverse process, cutting the costotransverse ligament (Fig. 8). This facilitates insertion of a hook attached to a rod. This maneuver is repeated at all three levels for thoracic hook insertion. A laminotomy is performed for the lower hook insertion below T10, and transverse process insertion sites are created with a Lexsell rongeur for cephalad-

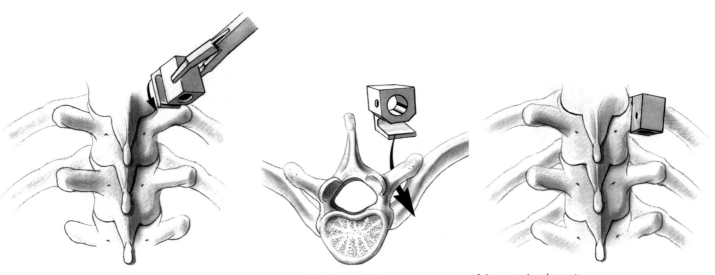

FIGURE 8. The caudad upper hooks are placed around the transverse process of the posterior elements. A sharp no. 1259 hook is used to cut the costotransverse ligament. One must take care that this sharp hook does not cut into the bone of the transverse process.

facing hooks that are to be inserted in the thoracic area above T10. The interspinous ligament and a portion of the ligamentum flavum are removed. Sufficient ligamentum flavum is removed to allow hook insertion.

The three cephalad hooks are inserted first, one at a time. Once they are all in place, the nuts are twisted with a Penfield elevator so as to be against the hooks, which helps resist the tendency of the hooks to slide out of their insertion site. The caudal hooks are then inserted; again, the nuts behind these hooks are twisted to a position just behind the hooks (Fig. 9). Then, beginning with the most cephalad hook, the nuts are tightened further. The rod behind the hook is grasped firmly with a rod holder, and a hook spreader is placed between the rod holder and the hook. As the handles of the distractor are squeezed, the hook slides forward. The nut behind the hook is then turned so that it lies immediately behind the hook, maintaining the compression obtained. This maneuver is repeated for each cephalad- and caudad-facing hook and then is repeated for all the hooks until an appropriate amount of compression has been obtained. A final amount of compression may be obtained by twisting the nuts with a small wrench (Fig. 10). The threads behind each nut are then damaged with pliers to resist untwisting of the nuts (13,14).

Decortication of the spine is then performed, with the hook-bearing laminae and transverse processes left intact. When both a compression rod and a distraction rod are used, they may be linked with a device for transverse traction, which increases the strength of the construct.

When two compression rods are required for correction of thoracic kyphosis, the larger (4.8-mm) rods should be used. The rods and hooks are set up and inserted as described above, but the surgeon may choose to use four hooks above and four below the apex of the kyphosis to increase the strength of the system. Regardless of the number of hooks used, the top vertebra instrumented should probably be T2 or T3. The spine is compressed as described above, decreasing the kyphosis.

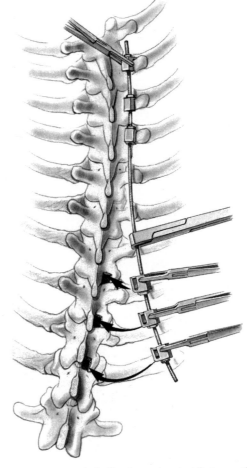

FIGURE 9. The three cephalad hooks are inserted first, over the transverse processes. With these held in place, the lower three hooks are inserted in the spinal canal. The Harrington compression rod is flexible, allowing for insertion of the hooks while they are on the rod.

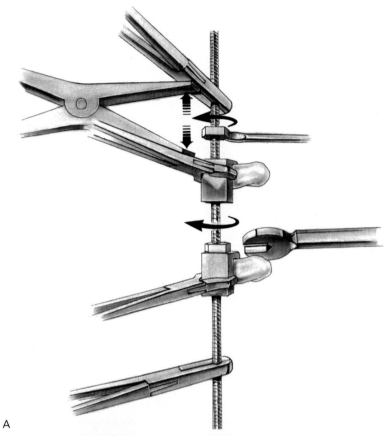

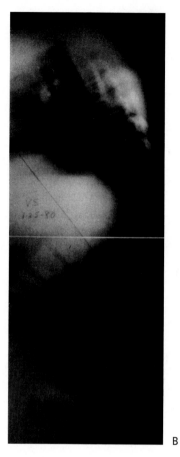

A

B

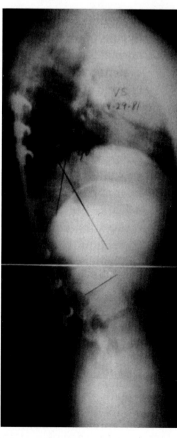

C

FIGURE 10. A: Compression is applied by tightening the hooks on the rods sequentially. A rod holder is placed behind one of the hooks. A hook holder grabs the hook, and a Harrington spreader is used to distract between the rod holder and the hook holder. This pushes the hook toward the apex of the curve and, with a Penfield elevator used first, the nut is spun toward the hook. To ensure secure application of the nut to the hook, a wrench is used to obtain the final amount of tightening. **B:** Lateral radiograph of a 16-year-old boy with a 77-degree thoracic kyphosis secondary to Scheuermann disease. **C:** Lateral radiograph of the same patient more than a year after surgery. The patient had undergone an anterior release and then posterior fusion and stabilization with Harrington compression instrumentation.

If the spine is not flexible enough to reduce the kyphosis to less than 50 degrees on forced hyperextension lateral radiograph, an anterior release and fusion is performed before the posterior approach is used. The anterior release increases the flexibility of the spine, allowing greater correction. The incidence of pseudarthrosis is unacceptably high if only a posterior fusion is performed when kyphosis is greater than 50 degrees (7,8). Thus, anterior release and fusion serves to increase the rate of fusion both by creating an anterior fusion and allowing greater correctability of the spine when it is instrumented posteriorly.

Posterior fusion of the spine is performed in the routine manner with complete facet excision and decortication of the non-hook-bearing portions of the spine. The wounds are closed over a suction drain.

Postoperatively, patients are nursed in a regular bed. Once the patient is sufficiently comfortable (usually after 5 to 7 days), a cast is applied. Early in the evolution of this procedure, a Risser cast was used. This cast extended from the chin to below the iliac crests. To apply this cast, the patient is placed on the Risser table and straps are applied to the patient to pull on the chest across the convexity of the curvature. The cast has now been modified so that it extends from the axilla to below the iliac crest. To lighten the cast, a longitudinally oblique window may be made on the concave side of the spine posteriorly. In addition, a small abdominal window may be made. The cast is worn for 6 months, after which no further bracing is used. One may choose to replace the cast after 3 months with a brace that is worn by the patient when out of bed. Return to activities is allowed slowly during the 6 months after cast removal, so that essentially full activity is allowed at the end of the first year (3,6,12,20,21,23–27,30–34,39,42,43,50,54,58).

Pitfalls and Complications

The most feared complication of spinal instrumentation is neurologic injury (55). To reduce the risk of spinal cord injury, the wake-up test was devised. The patient is prepared for this test preoperatively. After instrumentation is complete, anesthesia is reversed so that the patient can follow commands. Movement of both feet is assessed to ensure intact motor function. The same information may be gained by testing ankle clonus as the level of anesthesia is decreased. If the spinal cord is intact, ankle clonus should be present, but if one or both pyramidal tracts of the spinal cord have been injured, clonus will be absent on the injured side. If either test is positive, the patient should be sufficiently awakened to allow testing of motor function. If neurologic function is abnormal, the instrumentation should be removed and neurologic function should be reassessed. If neurologic function does not return to normal, the instrumentation is not replaced. If neurologic function has returned to normal, the spine may be reinstrumented, but with slightly less distraction force (32). Neurologic function is again tested with the wake-up test. If the result is still abnormal, the instrumentation should be removed and not replaced. Currently, monitoring of spinal cord function through use of evoked cortical responses or motor action potentials is widely used (5,9,19,41,44,48).

HARRINGTON INSTRUMENTATION WITH SUBLAMINAR WIRING

Indications

The indications for Harrington spinal instrumentation with sublaminar wiring are essentially the same as those for routine Harrington instrumentation. Addition of sublaminar wires increases the stability of the system because of the segmental fixation. In addition, sublaminar wires help to decrease thoracic hypokyphosis.

Contraindications

Harrington instrumentation with sublaminar wiring cannot be used if the posterior elements are not intact. Otherwise, the contraindications for its use are similar to those of the routine Harrington instrumentation system.

Advantages

Because the spine is instrumented at multiple levels, greater correction of the scoliotic deformity is possible. The distraction force is supplemented with a lateral force that pulls the spine to the straight Harrington rod. Because of the lateral pull to the rod, the amount of pure distraction force required is reduced, which in turn decreases the unwanted flattening of the sagittal contour of the spine (59). A second advantage of Harrington instrumentation with sublaminar wires is its ability to reduce the thoracic hypokyphosis commonly associated with idiopathic scoliosis. Most adolescent idiopathic thoracic scoliosis is associated with a decrease in normal kyphosis of the thoracic spine. The standard Harrington distraction system does not increase the kyphosis of the spine; however, addition of sublaminar wiring to the Harrington rod reduces hypokyphosis of the thoracic spine, creating a more normal sagittal contour. The third advantage of this system over the standard Harrington system is the increased stability provided by the segmental fixation of the system, which reduces the need for postoperative immobilization (46,49,56,57).

Finally, this system has two advantages over the traditional Luque instrumentation system, which also uses sublaminar wiring for segmental fixation. The Luque instrumentation system does not distract the spine, whereas the Harrington rod does. Axial distraction increases the correction and reduces the risk of loss of correction. In addition, use of double Luque rods with sublaminar wiring leaves little spinal area for decortication and fusion. Because the Harrington system with sublaminar wiring leaves the convex side of the spine uninstrumented, there is greater area for decortication and fusion.

Disadvantages

The major disadvantage of any system that uses sublaminar wiring is the risk of neurologic injury (35,53). Passage of sublaminar wires into the spinal canal increases the risk of injury to the spinal cord. The theoretical risk is probably less than one might expect with the Luque system because there are fewer wires with

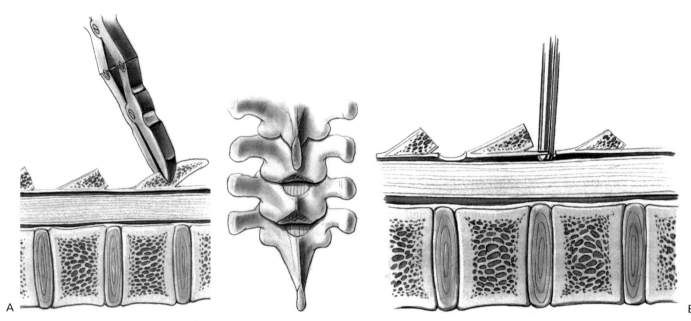

FIGURE 11. A: The posterior one quarter to one half of the overlapping spinous process may have to be removed, especially in the thoracic spine, to enable entry into the spinal canal. **B:** After the interspinous ligament and portion of the ligamentum flavum have been removed with a Lexsell rongeur, the remainder of the ligamentum flavum is removed with a Kerrison rongeur.

which to contend (only the Harrington rod is wired) (40,45,53). As with the Harrington system, the Harrington system with sublaminar wiring decreases normal lumbar lordosis even with use of a square-ended rod because the distraction itself produces flattening of the sagittal contour of the spine (38).

Technique

Preparation of the hook sites for the Harrington system with sublaminar wiring is identical to that used for the standard Harrington system. Once the upper and lower hooks have been inserted, the facet joints on both the concave and convex sides of the spine are excised and filled with bone graft.

The interspinous ligament and ligamentum flavum are excised at each level to be instrumented. Normally no wire is passed under the lamina under which the hooks are inserted, but because wires will be passed under every other lamina, all of the interspinous spaces must be opened from the level of the cranial hook to the caudal hook. In the thoracic spine, the spinous processes face caudad, and the upper third to the upper half of the spinous process must be removed to allow access to the spinal canal. The necessary portion of the spinous process is removed with a Lexsell rongeur. A substantial bite is then taken with the rongeur, removing all of the interspinous ligament and some of the ligamentum flavum. Using this rongeur carefully, the surgeon excises ligamentum flavum until the split in the midline of the ligament is well visualized. A Kerrison rongeur is then inserted into the canal to remove the ligamentum flavum (Fig. 11). Enough of the ligament is removed on both sides of the midline to allow wire passage.

Either 16- or 18-gauge wire may be used. Although 16-gauge wire is stronger, it is not as malleable, and passing it through the spinal canal may be more risky than passing the more flexible 18-gauge wire. A strand of wire approximately 38 to 45 cm long is cut and bent in half. The bent end is compressed tightly together. A small bend of approximately 20 to 30 degrees is made in the distal 0.5 cm of the bent end of the wire. A 180-

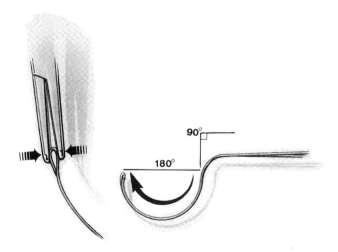

FIGURE 12. A 40-cm strand of 18-gauge wire is bent in half. The two ends are compressed at the bend so that there is no prominent tip. The wire is then bent into a semicircle. The diameter of the semicircle should be slightly larger than the width of the lamina. At the end of the semicircle, the wire is bent back at a 90-degree angle.

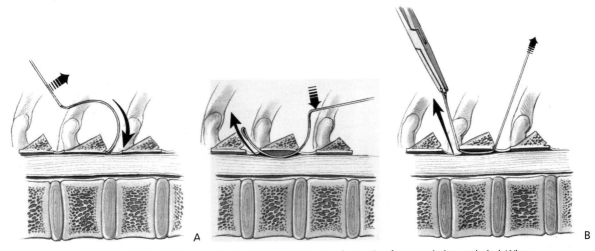

FIGURE 13. **A:** The wire is passed under the lamina in a circular motion from caudad to cephalad. When the wire is passed under the lamina, the arm and wrist of the person passing the wire are rotated, with care taken not to depress that wire. **B:** As the tip of the wire becomes evident just cephalad to the lamina in the next most cephalad intraspinous space, the wire is grabbed with a needle holder. The wire is pulled gently in the caudad direction and then a bit more forcefully from the cephalad position to allow it to continue to move in a cephalad direction until there is an equal amount of wire both caudad and cephalad to the posterior elements under which the wire has passed. One must be careful not to depress the wire during this passage.

degree bend is then made just behind the tip. The bend in the wire is about 3 cm long. At the end of the bend, the wire is bent back acutely in the opposite direction approximately 90 degrees (Fig. 12).

The wires are then passed under each lamina carefully. The surgeon passes the wire from caudad to cephalad under the lamina, trying to keep the wire tightly approximated to the underside of the lamina, thereby minimizing the risk of spinal cord injury. As the tip of the wire begins to exit from the next cephalad

interspinous space, the tip of the wire is grasped by an assistant using a needle holder. The wire is then pulled from that space with the force directed vertically. The surgeon holding the caudal end of the wire keeps sufficient tension on the wire during passage to prevent its depression into the spinal canal (Fig. 13). The wire is pulled out so that there is an equal amount of wire on both sides of the lamina. Both ends of the wire are bent tightly against the lamina to prevent depression of the wire into the spinal canal. The caudal end of the wire is bent cephalad,

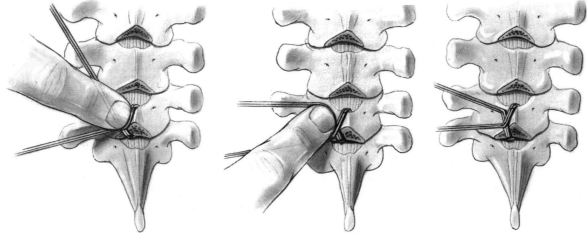

FIGURE 14. The wire is then bent over the lamina. The wire that exits from the inferior side has a sharp end; this is bent over the top of the lamina, and the free end is twisted into the subcutaneous tissue of the back to prevent glove puncture. The bend over the lamina prevents the wire from being depressed into the spinal canal. The doubled cephalad end of the wire is also bent over the lamina; again it is applied very close to the lamina, but this double-ended strand of wire is left midline.

and the cephalic end is bent caudad (Fig. 14). The wire is left doubled; the wire that exits the caudal end of the lamina has the sharp ends. These wire ends are bent laterally into the subcutaneous tissue to prevent injury to the surgical team. The other end that is doubled is left pointing upward and slightly toward the convexity of the curve. Separating the wire ends also facilitates their identification at the time of rod insertion.

The square-ended Harrington distraction rod is then inserted into the cephalad and caudad hooks. Before the rod is inserted, it is contoured to conform to the desired sagittal contour of the spine. The spine is distracted in the usual fashion, but only enough distraction to set the hooks is used. This submaximal distraction allows further correction of the scoliosis and contouring of the sagittal contour of the spine with wire tightening. An assistant on the convex side of the spine pushes on the apical ribs, reducing the severity of the curve. The apical wire is tightened first; cephalad and caudad wires are then successively tightened. Once all the wires have been tightened sufficiently, the distraction force on the distraction rod can

be adjusted if necessary by distracting the rod slightly. To prevent fracture of the inferior articular process of the cephalad vertebra and to avoid risk of injury to the spinal cord, one must be careful not to overdistract the rod. A C ring is locked in place between the caudal end of the cephalad hook and the ratchet caudad to it to prevent loss of distraction (Fig. 15).

Despite the contouring of the square-ended Harrington rod, loss of normal lordosis is still a problem with use of a distraction system. Bradford advocated locking the caudal two spinous processes with a wire to decrease loss of normal lordosis. This also helps reduce the risk of dislodgement of the lower hook (7) (Fig. 16). The wires are cut approximately 2 cm from the rod and bent anterior to the rod to reduce the risk of irritation of the skin or subcutaneous tissues. Autogenous iliac graft is taken from one iliac crest and inserted after complete facet excision and decortication. Postoperative immobilization is generally not required because of the stability of the segmental fixation.

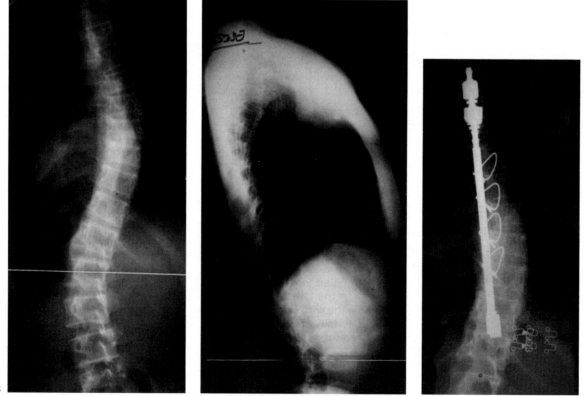

A,B   C

FIGURE 15. A: Anteroposterior (AP) radiograph of a 15-year-old girl with primary right thoracic and compensatory left lumbar scoliosis. **B:** Lateral radiograph shows flattening of the thoracic spine on the sagittal plane, which represents complete loss of normal thoracic kyphosis. **C:** AP postoperative radiograph shows improvement of the scoliosis. The Harrington rod has been inserted into two Bobechko upper hooks, and sublaminar wires have been placed around the laminae of the apical vertebrae. Bobechko self-adjusting hooks were used at one time to provide a second level of fixation for the upper end of the Harrington rod. *(Figure continues.)*

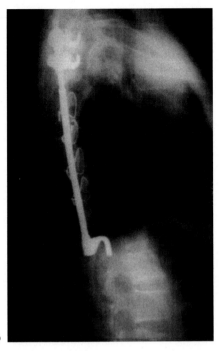

D

FIGURE 15. *Continued.* **D:** Lateral radiograph shows improvement in thoracic kyphosis postoperatively.

Pitfalls and Complications

The risk of neurologic injury is increased with passage of sublaminar wires in conjunction with the Harrington distraction rod more than with the distraction rod alone. Careful passage of the wires is imperative (40,45,53). The wires must be bent over the laminae to prevent accidental depression into the spinal canal until they are twisted over the Harrington rod.

The second problem with use of the distraction rod is flattening of the sagittal plane of the spine. This can be lessened by contouring the square-ended Harrington rod and by wiring the two caudal spinous processes. Wiring of the two caudal spinous processes also reduces risk of dislodgement of the caudal hook.

Implant removal poses another problem. Although the Har-

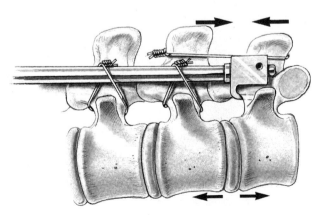

FIGURE 16. The caudal two spinous processes are wired together to prevent dislodgement of the inferior hook.

rington rod may be removed easily, removal of the sublaminar wires poses risk of dural tearing by the sharp end of the wire. The wires should be twisted out with a circular motion, using a needle holder. The needle holder grasps the free cut end of the wire tightly and twists the wire onto the jaws of the needle holder. Further twisting of the instrument pushes it against the lamina. As the instrument is twisted further, the wire should rotate out of its sublaminar location, but the surgeon should keep the instrument against the undersurface of the lamina to decrease the risk of dural tearing.

INTERSPINOUS SEGMENTAL SPINAL INSTRUMENTATION

Indications

The indications for interspinous segmental spinal instrumentation are the same as those for simple Harrington instrumentation. Addition of interspinous wiring increases the stability of the construct by creating segmental fixation. Placement of the segmental wires through the base of the spinous process rather than under the laminae decreases the risk of spinal cord injury (15–18,27,28,47,51,52).

Contraindications

Because interspinous segmental spinal instrumentation corrects the spinal deformity by distraction, it should not be used for congenital scoliosis unless the spinal cord and spinal canal have been studied to establish that the spinal cord is not tethered. Although this system may be used for neuromuscular scoliosis, it does not have universal application. Sacral fixation with the Harrington rod is not secure. However, interspinous wiring may be used with other forms of fixation, such as Luque rods fixed to the pelvis in the Galveston technique, which provides the most secure form of sacral fixation (4). Interspinous wiring is not indicated for correction of kyphosis because of the tendency of the wires to cut out of the spinous process.

Advantages

Interspinous segmental spinal instrumentation provides segmental fixation of the spine without the risk of sublaminar wire passage. Therefore, one may expect correction that is slightly better than that achieved with Harrington distraction alone. In addition, because segmental fixation of the spine is achieved, the amount of stability provided should also be sufficient, obviating the need for postoperative immobilization in most instances.

Disadvantages

Because the main correction force is in distraction, the sagittal plane of the spine tends to be flattened. As with Harrington instrumentation, use of a square-ended distraction rod helps. In addition, if only slight distraction force is used at first, followed by tightening of the interspinous wires, less total distraction is used, which lessens the tendency to flattening of the spine.

The rotational deformity of the spine produces posterior rib prominence in the thoracic spine and lumbar deformity in the lumbar spine. Interspinous segmental spinal instrumentation can increase correction of the rotational deformity more than the pure Harrington distraction system can, but the amount of correction is not as much as can be achieved with other segmental systems that actually produce some derotation of the spine.

Dislodgement of both the upper and lower hooks is also possible. Use of a bifid pedicular upper hook will help prevent this hook from sliding laterally out of the facet joint, with subsequent loss of distraction force. In addition, the button-wire implants pull the rod toward the spinous processes, which also resists the tendency to lateral displacement of the upper hook. The lower hook has a tendency to slide out from under the lamina with forward flexion of the spine, especially if it is placed at the thoracolumbar junction. Use of a hook with a longer shoe (such as the Leatherman hook) aids in stabilization. Wiring together of the last two spinous processes also helps prevent dislodgement of the lower hook.

Technique

Interspinous segmental spinal instrumentation consists of the standard Harrington distraction rod with a square distal end. In addition, a Luque rod is used for the convex side of the curve. These two rods are segmentally fixed to the spine by button-wire implants (Fig. 17). The button is welded to the 18-gauge wire, which is doubled; the two ends of the wire are fused together at the end opposite the button. The button has an extra hole for passage of a wire from the opposite side of the spine.

The preparation and approach to the spine is identical to that used for the routine Harrington instrumentation procedure. Once the spine has been thoroughly exposed from the tip of transverse process to the tip of the opposite transverse process

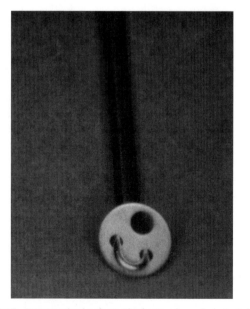

FIGURE 17. Button-wire implant. The button has a hole in it for passage of the wire from the opposite side.

and the facet joints have been excised, the upper and lower hooks are inserted in the routine manner as described above for the routine Harrington procedure. Holes are then placed through the base of each spinous process for passage of the button-wire implants. The spinous process of the two vertebrae that bear the upper and lower hooks does not have wires.

The hole in the base of the spinous process is made with awls. The starting awl is straight and has a sharp point. Several millimeters behind the point is a collar that helps prevent too deep penetration of this awl. The hole is started at the base of the spinous process at the junction of the spinous process and the lamina. If the hole is made more dorsally, the bone in the spinous process will be too thin and will not be able to withstand sufficient stress. On the other hand, one does not want to penetrate too deeply for fear of entering the spinal canal. Although this usually does not occur, caution is urged.

Two different curved awls may be used to complete the passage through the bone. The awl whose curve best approximates the curve of the intended hole in the bone should be used. The hole in the opposite cortex may be made with this curved awl or with the awl used to start the passage (Fig. 18). Once the hole has been made, the awl is passed through it from both sides to ensure that the hole is wide enough to accommodate both wires.

Wires from both the right and left sides are then passed through the holes simultaneously, by the surgeon on one side and by the assistant on the other. The tips of the wires are then grasped with the fingers. The end of the wire is passed through the button of the wire on the opposite side. Enough of the wire is pushed through the button so that the end of the wire can be grasped easily with a needle holder. Both wires are grasped simultaneously with needle holders and are pulled laterally in opposite directions by the surgeon and the assistant. The wires are pulled tightly enough that the buttons fit flush against the spinous process.

Once all of the wires have been inserted through the spinous processes, the rods are inserted. The Harrington distraction rod is inserted first. The wires are separated to make loops so that the rod can pass easily through the wires; the rod is then inserted into the upper and lower hooks in the routine manner previously described for the standard Harrington procedure. With the distraction device, a small amount of distraction force is placed on the rod, but the force is much less than the maximal amount used for the routine Harrington procedure. The surgeon then tightens the wires by twisting them sequentially with a jet wire twister, with care taken not to overtighten any wire for fear of breakage. More tightening of each individual wire can be obtained. One retightens each wire after all of the wires have been twisted (Fig. 19).

As the wires are tightened, the spinous processes are pulled toward the distraction rod, which decreases the curvature of the spine. Next, the Luque rod is cut and bent to conform to the contour of the spine. The two ends of the Luque rod are bent to the same side. The bent portion of the rod is approximately 2 to 3 cm long. The upper bend is placed under the upper end of the Harrington distraction rod cephalad to the upper hook. The lower bend of the Luque rod is placed caudad to the distal

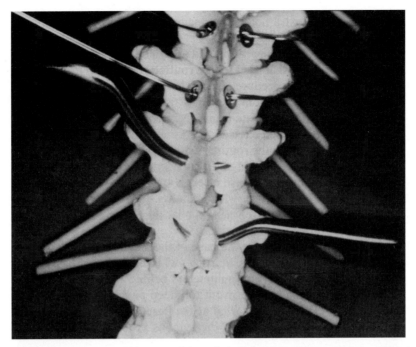

FIGURE 18. Button-wire implants are passed through the base of the spinous processes. A hole is made through the base of the spinous process with an awl. The awls are apparent passing through the base of the spinous process, and the wires have been passed from both sides and pulled tightly against the base of the spinous processes.

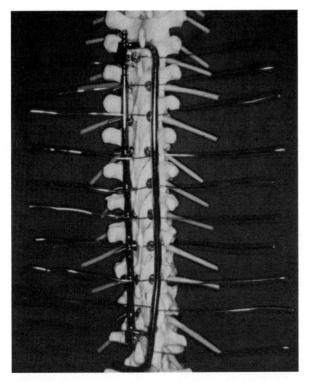

FIGURE 19. All wires have been inserted, and the Harrington and Luque rods have been inserted. Wires are then twisted around both. The upper end of the Luque rod is anterior to the upper end of the Harrington rod.

Harrington hook and between the spinous process of the lower instrumented vertebra and the one below it.

The rod is inserted through the loops of the button-wire implants that are on the convex side of the spine. The upper and lower ends of the Luque rod are positioned as described above. Then the wires are progressively tightened until all have been tightened maximally. The wires on the concave side of the spine are again tightened over the Harrington rod because they may develop some laxity after the wires on the convexity have been tightened. Finally, the upper hook should be checked to determine whether further distraction is possible. This hook should simply be locked in place to prevent hook dislodgement. The posterior elements are decorticated lateral to the buttons all the way to the tip of each transverse process on both sides of the spine. The facet joints are also excised, and autogenous iliac bone graft is placed in each excised facet and along the entire spine.

The ends of the wires are then cut approximately 2 cm above the twisted end of the wire. The wire should be bent over the top of the corresponding rod so that the cut end of the wire is anterior to the rod to prevent it from irritating the skin and subcutaneous tissue. Finally, a C ring should be inserted between the inferior end of the cephalad hook and the ratchet immediately below this hook. The wound is closed in a routine fashion, and the patient is nursed in a regular bed (Fig. 20). Ambulation is allowed when the patient is comfortable (usually 3 to 5 days). Because of the segmental fixation, external immobilization is usually not required, but activities should be restricted until the fusion is judged to be solid.

Crawford described a modification of this instrumentation

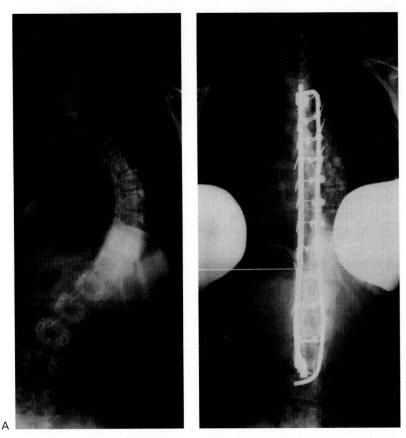

FIGURE 20. A: Anteroposterior radiograph of a patient with a large right thoracic scoliosis. **B:** Postoperative radiograph of the same patient showing significant improvement in degree of curvature after instrumentation and fusion with interspinous segmental spinal instrumentation.

(11). He uses a Harrington compression on the convex side of the spine instead of a Luque rod.

Holes are made with the awls in the base of the spinous processes to allow passage of the button-wires. The compression rod is then inserted by first placing the compression hooks over the transverse processes in the thoracic area. These hooks face caudad. The cephalad-facing hooks are inserted under the laminae of the inferior three or four vertebrae. At this time, only enough compression is used to set the hooks.

The Harrington square-ended distraction rod is then contoured to conform to the normal thoracic kyphosis and lumbar lordosis. The rod is passed through the wires and then into the Harrington hooks that are in place on the concave side of the spine. No distraction is used, but the rod is set into the hooks only to the least distraction used to fix the Harrington distractor. The assistant on the convex side of the spine pushes on the apical ribs toward the spine, thereby reducing the curvature. The button-wire implants are then sequentially tightened. First the cephalad wires are tightened, followed by the caudad wires. The apical wire is then tightened, followed by the other wires. Each wire is then retightened until all of the wires are maximally tight. The wires are then cut and bent over the rod.

The compression rod is tightened sufficiently to set the hooks and lock the rod in place. An 18-gauge wire is then placed superior to the ratchet of the distraction rod located just underneath the upper distraction hook. This prevents dislodgement of the hook from the ratchet. The wire is twisted and placed transversely in a groove made in the superior aspect of the spinous process of the top vertebra in the fusion. This transverse placement of the twisted wire can be used as an indicator of possible dislodgement of the upper hook. Changes in position of the wire are considered hook dislodgement. Finally, a double-looped 18-gauge wire is looped transversely around both rods at the upper and lower ends of the instrumentation to provide transverse fixation for the compression and distraction rods (Fig. 21).

Pitfalls and Complications

Passage of the button-wire implants through the base of the spinous process is safer than passage of a wire under the lamina, but if the hole in the lamina is made too steeply with the awl, the spinal canal might be entered. This complication is

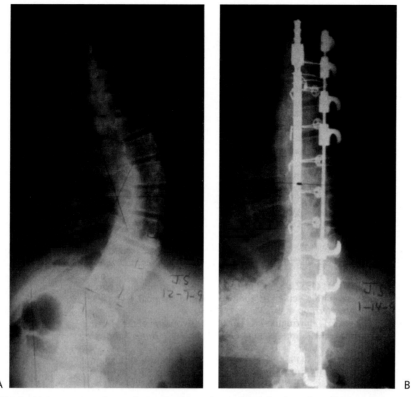

FIGURE 21. **A:** Anteroposterior radiograph of a patient with right thoracic scoliosis. **B:** Postoperative radiograph shows application of the distraction and compression system with interspinous wiring. Extra wires are passed around the two rods at the cephalad and caudad end of the fusion. (Courtesy of Alvin Crawford, M.D.)

rare, however, and is easily avoided by directing the awl correctly.

The button position against the base of the spinous process increases the surface area of the metal applied to the bone, which helps resist the tendency of the wire to cut through the bone when the pull of the wire is lateral, as it is when one is correcting scoliosis. However, when one instruments the spine for correction of kyphosis, the force is in an anteroposterior direction. The button does not provide the same degree of resistance to wire cutout as it does when the pull is directly lateral, as in correction of scoliosis. In addition, correction of the sagittal plane is not accomplished as well as it is with either sublaminar wiring without a distraction force or with CD instrumentation, which provides excellent sagittal plane countouring.

Implant removal, if required, is more difficult than removal of a simple Harrington distraction rod. The button-wire implants become encased in fusion mass, making their removal extremely difficult. If removal of the rod becomes necessary for any reason, the wires may be left in place because their removal might necessitate removal of a significant amount of the fusion mass.

Hook cutout is possible, although the upper hook is inheritantly more stable than is the same hook in a simple Harrington distraction rod because the button wires help anchor the rod and hooks to the spine. Nevertheless, to increase stability of the

upper hook the use of a bifid pedicle hook is advised. The distal hook is at greatest risk for dislodgement because it is placed in the more mobile area of the spine. If the patient is not immobilized postoperatively, the lower hook might slip from its position under the lamina with forward bending. To resist this tendency, one may use a Leatherman-type hook, which has a longer shoe. The extra length of the shoe helps to prevent hook dislodgement. In addition, wiring the two most caudal spinous processes together not only helps lock the caudal hook under the lamina but helps to decrease the tendency of the distraction hook to reduce lumbar lordosis.

REFERENCES

1. Aaro S, Dahlborn M (1982): The effect of Harrington instrumentation on the longitudinal axis rotation of the apical vertebra and on the spinal and rib-cage deformity in idiopathic scoliosis studied by computer tomography. *Spine* 7:456–462.
2. Aaro S, Ohlen G (1983): The effect of Harrington instrumentation on the sagittal configuration and mobility of the spine in scoliosis. *Spine* 8(6):570–575.
3. Akbarnia BA (1988): Selection of methodology in surgical treatment of adolescent idiopathic scoliosis. *Orthop Clin N Am* 19:319.
4. Allen BA Jr (1983): Segmental spinal instrumentation. *Instr Course Lectures* 32:202.

5. Ben-David B (1988): Spinal cord monitoring. *Orthop Clin N Am* 19: 427.

6. Benson DR (1987): Idiopathic scoliosis. The last ten years and state of the art. *Orthopedics* 10:1691–1698.

7. Bradford DS (1987): Techniques of surgery. In: Bradford DS, Lonstein JE, Moe JH, et al., eds. *Moe's Textbook of scoliosis and other spinal deformities.* Philadelphia: WB Saunders, pp. 135–190.

8. Bradford DS, Ahmed KB, Moe JH, et al. (1980): The surgical management of patients with Scheuermann's disease. A review of twenty-four cases managed by combined anterior and posterior spine fusion. *J Bone Joint Surg Am* 62:705–712.

9. Brown RH, Nash CL Jr (1979): Current status of spinal cord monitoring. *Spine* 4:466.

10. Casey MP, Asher MA, Jacobs RR, et al. (1987): The effect of Harrington rod contouring on lumbar lordosis. *Spine* 12:750–753.

11. Crawford A (1991): An analysis of the use of contoured Harrington rods and ISSI to obtain transverse and sagittal plane correction of idiopathic scoliosis. *Orthop Trans* 15:597.

12. DeWald RI (1973): New trends in the operative treatment of scoliosis. In: Ahstrom JP Jr, ed. *Current practices in orthopaedic surgery,* vol. 5. St Louis: CV Mosby.

13. Dickson JH (1982): Spinal instrumentation and fusion in adolescent idiopathic scoliosis: indications and surgical techniques. *Contemp Orthop* 34:397.

14. Dickson JH, Harrington PR (1973): The evolution of the Harrington instrumentation technique in scoliosis. *J Bone Joint Surg Am* 55: 993.

15. Drummond DS (1988): Harrington instrumentation with spinous process wiring for idiopathic scoliosis. *Orthop Clin N Am* 19:281.

16. Drummond DS, Keene JS, Breed A (1984): The Wisconsin system: a technique of interspinous segmental spinal instrumentation. *Contemp Orthop* 8:29–37.

17. Drummond D, Narechania R, Wenger D, et al. (1982): Wisconsin segmental spinal instrumentation. *Orthop Trans* 36:22–23.

18. Drummond D, Guaclagni J, Keene JS, et al. (1984): Interspinous process segmental spinal instrumentation. *J Pediatr Orthop* 4:397.

19. Engler G, Spielhotz NJ, Bernhard WN, et al. (1978): Somatosensory evoked potentials during Harrington instrumentation for scoliosis. *J Bone Joint Surg Am* 60:528.

20. Erwin WD, Dickson JH, Gaines JH III (1986): Utilization of Harrington spinal instrumentation and fusion for scoliosis, surgical technique. Zimmer.

21. Erwin WD, Dickson JH, Harrington PR (1976): The postoperative management of scoliosis patients treated with Harrington instrumentation and fusion. *J Bone Joint Surg Am* 58:479.

22. Gaines RW, McKinley LM, Leatherman DK (1981): Effect of the Harrington compression system on the correction of the rib hump in spinal instrumentation for idiopathic scoliosis. *Spine* 6:489–493.

23. Goldstein LA (1966): Surgical management of scoliosis. *J Bone Joint Surg Am* 48:167–196.

24. Goldstein LA (1969): Treatment of idiopathic scoliosis by Harrington instrumentation and fusion with fresh autogenous iliac bone grafts: results in eighty patients. *J Bone Joint Surg Am* 51:209.

25. Goldstein LA (1971): The surgical management of idiopathic scoliosis. *Clin Orthop* 77:32.

26. Goldstein LA (1973): The surgical treatment of idiopathic scoliosis. *Clin Orthop* 93:131.

27. Green NE (1990): Adolescent idiopathic scoliosis. In: Hsu J, ed. *Spine: state of the art reviews,* vol. 4, no. 1. Philadelphia: Hanley & Belfus, pp. 211–237.

28. Guadagni J, Drummond D, Breed A (1984): Improved post-operative course following modified segmental instrumentation and posterior spinal fusion for idiopathic scoliosis. *J Pediatr Orthop* 4:405.

29. Hall JE, Levine CR, Sudhir KG (1978): Intraoperative awakening to monitor spinal cord function during Harrington instrumentation and spine fusion: descriptions of procedure and report of three cases. *J Bone Joint Surg Am* 60:533.

30. Harrington PR (1962): Correction and internal fixation by spine instrumentation. *J Bone Joint Surg Am* 44:591.

31. Harrington PR (1960): Surgical instrumentation for management of scoliosis. *J Bone Joint Surg Am* 42:1448.

32. Harrington PR (1963): The management of scoliosis by spine instrumentation: an evaluation of more than two hundred cases. *S Med J* 56:1367.

33. Harrington PR (1973): The history and development of Harrington instrumentation. *Clin Orthop* 93:110.

34. Harrington PR, Dickson JH (1973): An eleven-year clinical investigation of Harrington instrumentation: a preliminary report of 578 cases. *Clin Orthop* 93:113.

35. Herring JA, Wenger DR (1982): Early complications of segmental spinal instrumentation. *Orthop Trans* 6:22.

36. King HA (1988): Selection of fusion levels for posterior instrumentation and fusion in idiopathic scoliosis. *Orthop Clin N Am* 19: 247.

37. King HA, Moe JH, Bradford DS, Winter RB (1983): The selection of the fusion levels in thoracic idiopathic scoliosis. *J Bone Joint Surg Am* 65:1302–1314.

38. Leatherman KD, Johnson JR, Holt RT, et al. (1984): A clinical assessment of 357 cases of segmental spinal instrumentation. In: Luque ER, ed. *Segmental spinal instrumentation.* Thorofare, NJ: Slack, pp. 165–184.

39. Lovallo JL, Banta JV, Renshaw TS (1986): Adolescent idiopathic scoliosis treated by Harrington-rod distraction and fusion. *J Bone Joint Surg Am* 68:1326–1330.

40. MacEwen GD, Bunnell WP, Sriram K (1975): Acute neurological complications in the treatment of scoliosis: a report of the Scoliosis Research Society. *J Bone Joint Surg Am* 57:404.

41. Machida M, Weinstein SL, Yamada T, et al. (1985): Spinal cord monitoring: Electrophysiological measures of sensory and motor function during spinal surgery. *Spine* 10:407.

42. Moe JH (1958): A critical analysis of methods of fusion for scoliosis: an evaluation in 266 patients. *J Bone Joint Surg Am* 40:529.

43. Moe JH (1972): Methods of correction and surgical technique in scoliosis. *Orthop Clin N Am* 2:17.

44. Nash CL Jr, Horing RA, Schatzinger HA, et al. (1977): Spinal cord monitoring during operative treatment of the spine. *Clin Orthop* 126: 100.

45. Nicastro JF, Traina J, Lancaster M, et al. (1984): Sublaminar segmental wire fixation: anatomic pathways during their removal. *Orthop Trans* 38:172.

46. Ogilve JW, Millar EA (1983): Comparison of segmental spinal instrumentation devices in the correction of scoliosis. *Spine* 8:416.

47. Phillips WA, Hensinger RN (1988): Wisconsin and other instrumentation for posterior spinal fusion. *Clin Orthop* 229:44.

48. Rappaport M, Hall KM, Hopkins K, et al. (1982): Effects of corrective scoliosis surgery on somatosensory evoked potentials. *Spine* 7: 404.

49. Renshaw TS (1982): Spinal fusion with segmental instrumentation. *Contemp Orthop* 4:413.

50. Renshaw TS (1988): The role of Harrington instrumentation and posterior spine fusion in the management of adolescent idiopathic scoliosis. *Orthop Clin N Am* 19:257.

51. Sponseller PD, Whiffen JR, Drummond DS (1986): Interspinous process segmental spinal instrumentation for scoliosis in cerebral palsy. *J Pediatr Orthop* 6:559–563.

52. Thometz JG, Emans JB (1988): A comparison between spinous process and sublaminar wiring combined with Harrington distraction instrumentation in the management of adolescent idiopathic scoliosis. *J Pediatr Orthop* 8:129–132.

53. Thompson GH, Wilber RG, Shaffer JW, et al. (1985): Segmental spinal instrumentation in idiopathic scoliosis. A preliminary report. *Spine* 10:623–630.

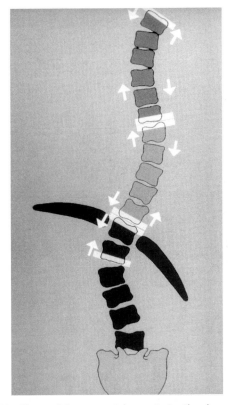

FIGURE 19. The modular concept demonstrates the change of direction in three curves. The middle thoracic is the usual thoracic concave distraction pattern. The left high thoracic pattern is highlighted by the supralaminar hook on the left at thoracic 1, enabling changing to a compression direction on the upper curve. Also note the change of direction at the thoracolumbar junction.

tromyographic stimulus response is employed and is recommended (5).

In general, as many screws as anatomically possible should be used. It is important to place screws bilaterally in at least the two proximal levels and the two distal levels of the construct. It may not be possible to place screws bilaterally at every level between the two proximal and two distal levels.

Figure 20 graphically demonstrates the screw scheme for a thoracolumbar or lumbar idiopathic scoliosis. Figure 21 depicts the radiologic findings of a similar curve.

Figure 22 represents the scheme with screws for a double curve, and the radiologic findings of a similar curve are represented in Figure 23.

Figure 24 represents the scheme with screws for a pure thoracic posterior instrumentation. The author has no experience with this construct.

Several comments are appropriate regarding the use of pure screw constructs in idiopathic scoliosis. The constructs are appealing due to the lack of metal in the spinal canal. This is more theoretical than real. In the past year, three of the author's patients have had thoracic canal stenosis and scoliosis, with significant monitoring change due to intracanal hooks. No permanent deficits resulted, but the potential for significant injury was present. Screws would not confer this risk. However, screws have other associated risks, particularly to the visceral structures in the thorax.

As spinal navigation devices become more sophisticated and

of idiopathic scoliosis. Excellent results were obtained, similar to the hook results noted above by the author. They also report no complications attributable to the thoracic or lumbar pedicle screws.

The author has several years of experience in the use of pedicle screws in adolescent and adult idiopathic scoliosis. Observations follow, as do schemes for the use of screws in idiopathic or other types of scoliosis.

1. It is my unsupported (by scientific evidence) assumption that screws have a significant advantage in the thoracolumbar spine. Correction appears better than with hooks, and it is possible that less distal levels are required.

2. A wide area is present for arthrodesis, both in the midline and in the lateral gutters. Hooks are not present in the interspace, which, I feel may create a barrier to arthrodesis, particularly at the thoracolumbar junction. This is particularly true when two hooks are placed in the same interspace, usually in different directions.

3. Screw placement is facilitated by image intensification. This does require expert and cooperative radiologic technicians. The ability to position the image intensifier in the correct plane on both the anterior and lateral projections is essential.

4. Electrical monitoring of screw placement has proven invaluable in preventing incorrect screw placement. The evoked elec-

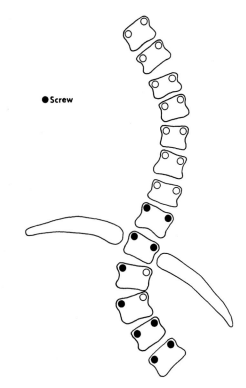

●**Screw**

FIGURE 20. The pattern for placement of screws in a thoracolumbar curve is depicted. Convex-first instrumentation is indicated to produce lumbar lordosis. Note that the two end vertebrae are bilaterally instrumented if possible.

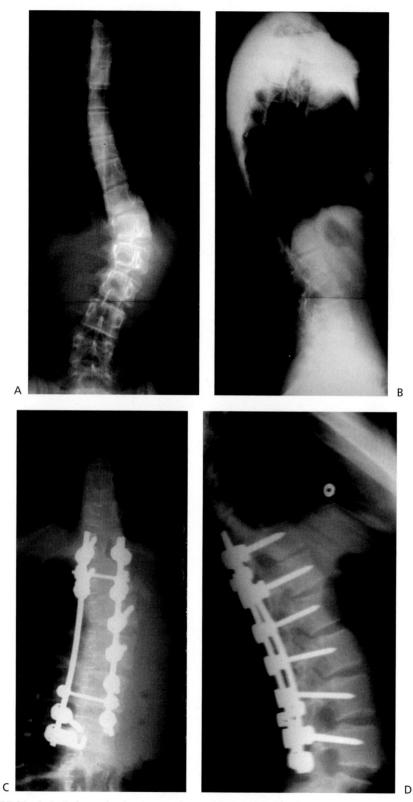

FIGURE 21. A, B: A thoracolumbar curve prior to surgery. **C, D:** An all-screw construct is employed, similar to the strategic drawing. Note the excellent reconstruction of the sagittal plane. The coronal curve is nearly completely corrected, all from the posterior approach.

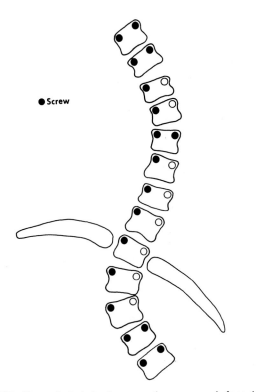

● Screw

FIGURE 22. The projected plan incorporating screws only for a double structural curve. The more screws that could be placed, the better the fixation.

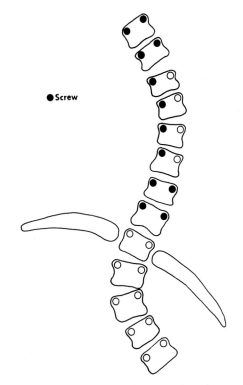

● Screw

FIGURE 24. Screw pattern for a pure thoracic curve.

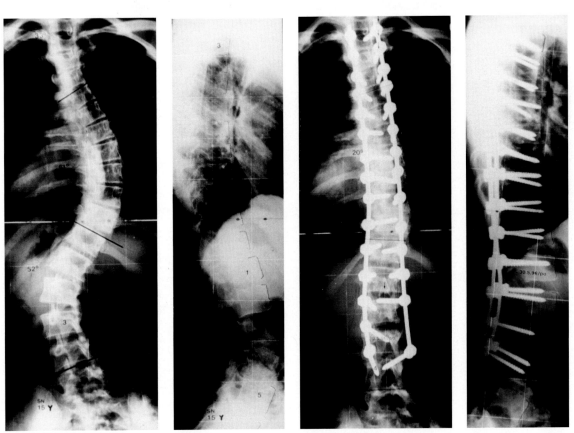

A,B   C,D

FIGURE 23. A, B: This double structural curve is to be instrumented with only pedicle screws. **C, D:** The results of the previous curve using screws at every level are demonstrated. Excellent coronal correction and sagittal reconstruction has been achieved.

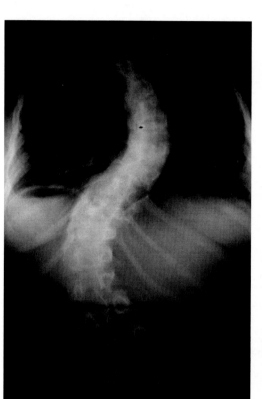

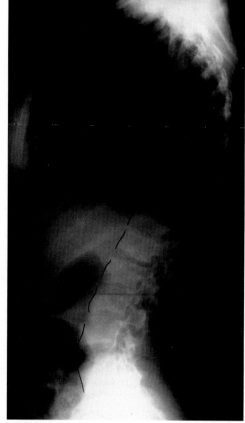

A,B

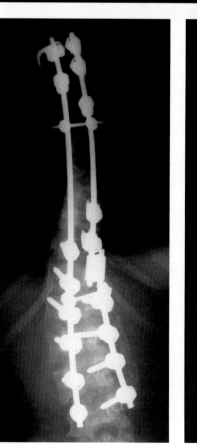

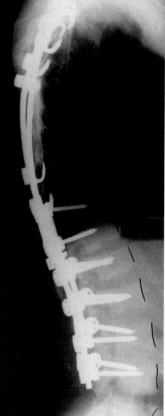

C,D

FIGURE 25. **A, B:** A double structural curve with a thoracic kyphosis. The surgery will be only posterior, with lumbar screws and no hooks in the canal. This will be a combination of hooks and screws. **C, D:** The proposed procedure has been accomplished, with no hooks in the canal. The combination of distal screws and proximal pedicle and transverse process hooks avoids the spinal canal completely. It was felt the thoracic pedicle were too small for 5-mm screws.

affordable, it appears that pedicle screws are the best spinal anchors for the posterior surgical treatment of idiopathic scoliosis. An additional concern is the cost of pedicle screws relative to hooks. A screw construct is approximately 1.75 times the cost of a pure hook construct.

Hook and Screw Combinations

Thoracic hooks and lumbar screws are commonly employed in the surgical treatment of idiopathic scoliosis. All of the principles of implant placement are true for this hybrid of implants. Figure 25 demonstrates the use of a combination of hooks and screws in idiopathic scoliosis. The rod placement sequence and implant tightening sequence is the same as for the pure hook construct.

Scheuermann Kyphosis

Scheuermann kyphosis is usually a pure sagittal plane deformity. The two anatomical variants are well described as being thoracic and thoracolumbar, depending on the apex. If surgery is indicated, anterior and posterior procedures are the standard in most instances. This entails anterior release followed by posterior instrumentation. The posterior procedure usually requires some element of a posterior shortening procedure. This includes excision of interspinous ligament, ligamentum flavum, overhanging edge of superior lamina, and wide-facet excision through the neural foramen. Posterior instrumentation in a compression direction is the norm for this diagnosis. Currently, screws are favored distally. Figure 26 is a radiographic example of Scheuermann kyphosis treated with anterior and posterior surgery.

PITFALLS

As this section is a theoretical or philosophical approach to the theory and mechanics of the surgical treatment of scoliosis from the posterior approach, the pitfalls are mainly in theory or construct design. For spine surgeons practicing currently, concave and convex first or second, distraction and compression, translation and cantilever, and other similar concepts should be second nature.

There may be some pitfalls regarding selection of fusion levels and exact placement of spinal anchors, but these should not have a significant impact on surgical procedure.

The loading sequences of the spinal anchors (hooks or screws) should be well in place. Sequential loading by either distraction or compression forces is easily accomplished. The loading sequences are dictated by either the direction of the implant (hooks) or the nature of the deformity. Screws have the obvious

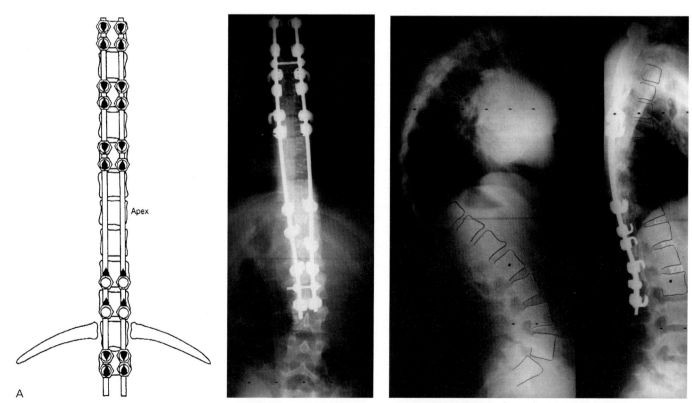

A

B,C

FIGURE 26. A: A plan for instrumentation for Scheuermann kyphosis is depicted. Note that all forces are directed to the apex in compression. **B, C:** The postoperative anteroposterior view approximates the diagram. The before-and-after laterals reflect the significant correction possible with this strategy.

possibility of being loaded in either the distraction or compression direction. Appreciation of the deformity and the sagittal plane requirements of the deformity will dictate the loading sequences for screw constructs.

SUMMARY

1. Analysis of the mechanism of correction of the scoliotic deformity with the rod rotation technique popularized by users of the CD system reveals that rod rotation does not equal spinal derotation. Rather, the change in spinal alignment is by coronal plane translation and sagittal plane angulation. No intersegmental derotation occurs. Axial rotation changes in the periapical zone are produced by the differential rod bend.

2. Systems developed subsequent to the CD, particularly Isola and Moss Miami, permit placement of anatomical rod bends. The mechanics of correction are translation with distraction or cantilever with compression and translation. Periapical rotational changes are produced by the differential rod bend.

3. Analysis of the deformity in the coronal and sagittal plane determines the force directions and which side should be instrumented first. Concave distraction forces produce absolute or relative kyphosis. Convex compression forces decrease kyphosis or produce lordosis. If the need is to correct a thoracic lordoscoliosis, the concave rod should be placed first with distraction direction implants. If the need is to correct a thoracolumbar or lumbar scoliosis, the convex rod should be placed first with compression direction implants.

4. Spinal anchors may be hooks or screws. Using a modular concept of scoliosis, hook placement decisions are simplified. Screws should be placed bilaterally at the terminal two levels. Intermediate screws should be placed in as many levels as possible on the side of the spine that will receive the first rod.

5. Combined constructs—hooks in the thoracic area and screws in the lumbar area—produce the optimum correction in the lumbar area. In addition, the potential hazards of thoracic pedicle screws are avoided.

REFERENCES

1. Akbarnia B, Asher M, Hess W, et al. (1996): Safety of the pedicle screw in pediatric patients with scoliosis and kyphosis. Presented at the Annual Meeting of the Scoliosis Research Society, Ottawa, 1996.
2. Asher M (1998): Isola spinal instrumentation for scoliosis. In: Bridwell K, DeWald R, eds. *Textbook of spinal surgery,* 2nd ed. Philadelphia: Lippincott-Raven Publishers, p. 569.
3. Bernhardt M, Bridwell K (1989): Segmental analysis of the sagittal plane alignment of the normal thoracic and lumbar spine and the thoracolumbar junction. *Spine* 14:117
4. Bridwell K, McAllister J, Betz R, et al. (1991): Coronal plane decompensation produced by Cotrel-Dubousset "derotation" maneuver for idiopathic right thoracic scoliosis. *Spine* 16:769.
5. Calcani B, Madsen P, Lebwohl N (1994): Stimulus evoked EMG monitoring during transpedicular lumbar spine instrumentation. *Spine* 19: 2780.
6. Cotrel Y, Dubousset J, Guillaumat M (1988): New universal instrumentation in spinal surgery. *Clin Orthop Rel Res* 227:10.
7. Ecker M, Betz R, Trent P, et al. (1988): Computer tomography evaluation of Cotrel-Dubousset instrumentation in adolescent idiopathic scoliosis. *Spine* 13:1141.
8. Graf H, Hecquet J, Dubousset J (1983): Three-dimensional approaches to spinal deformities. Application to the study of the prognosis of pediatric scoliosis. *Rev Chir Orthop* 69:407.
9. Ibrahim K, Goldberg B (1990): Cotrel-Dubousset instrumentation for right thoracic type 2 curves-compensation vs decompensation. *Orthop Trans* 14:780.
10. Jackson R, McManus A (1994): Radiographic analysis of sagittal plane alignment and balance in standing volunteers and patients with low back pain matched for age, sex, and size. *Spine* 19:1611.
11. Johnston C, Ashman R, Richards S, et al. (1998): TSRH universal spine instrumentation. In: Bridwell K, DeWald R, eds. *Textbook of spinal surgery,* 2nd ed. Philadelphia: Lippincott-Raven Publishers, p. 535.
12. King H, Moe J, Bradford D, et al. (1983): The selection of fusion levels in thoracic idiopathic scoliosis. *J Bone Joint Surg Am* 65:1302.
13. Lenke L, Bridwell K, Baldus C, et al. (1992): Cotrel-Dubousset instrumentation for adolescent idiopathic scoliosis. *J Bone Joint Surg Am* 74: 1056.
14. Perdriolle R, Vidal J, Bechetti S, et al. (1990): Torsion: the essential factor factor for progression in idiopathic scoliosis. *Orthop Trans* 14: 765.
15. Shufflebarger H (1994): Theory and mechanisms of posterior derotation spinal systems. In: Weinstein S, ed. *The pediatric spine: principles and practice.* New York: Raven Press, pp. 1515–1543.
16. Shufflebarger H (1994): Cotrel-Dubousset instrumentation. In: Weinstein S, ed. *The pediatric spine: principles and practice.* New York: Raven Press, p. 1515.
17. Shufflebarger H (1996): Cantilever and translation mechanics with a 5 mm rod: results in adolescent idiopathic scoliosis. Paper presented at Annual Meeting of the Scoliosis Research Society, Ottawa, 1996.
18. Shufflebarger H, Clark C (1990): Fusion levels and hook patterns in thoracic scoliosis with Cotrel-Dubousset instrumentation. *Spine* 15: 916.
19. Shufflebarger H, Ellis R, Clark C (1989): Cotrel instrumentation in adolescent idiopathic scoliosis. *Orthop Trans* 13:79.
20. Shufflebarger H, Clark C (1998): Effect of wide posterior release on Correction in adolescent idiopathic scoliosis. *J Pediatr Orthop* 7:117.
21. Suk S, Kim J, Kim J, et al. Preservation of distal lumbar motion segments with segmental pedicle screw fixation in King type 1 adolescent idiopathic scolisosi. Presented at the Annual Meeting of the Scoliosis Research Society, St. Louis, 1997.
22. Transfeldt E, Bradford D, Coscia M, et al. (1989): Changes in segmental coupling and vertebral rotation following Cotrel-Dubousset instrumentation for idiopathic scoliosis. *Orthop Trans* 13:80.

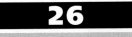

26

COTREL-DUBOUSSET SPINAL INSTRUMENTATION

LAWRENCE G. LENKE

The era of segmental spinal instrumentation was born with the introduction of Cotrel-Dubousset spinal instrumentation, which was first used in 1982 (17,22). The instrumentation was the brainchild of Yves Cotrel, a Frenchman who worked at the Institute Calot in Berck-Plage, France. Dr. Cotrel was always quite interested in scoliosis. As early as 1953, he had introduced the terms *buckled cast* and *distraction cast* of Stagnara design to correct spinal deformity. Once maximal curve improvement was obtained, spinal fusion was performed through a window in the cast. However, Dr. Cotrel realized that this was not the ideal way to care for patients with severe spinal deformity. He undertook a lifelong pursuit to improve the techniques used for this type of reconstructive surgery. He was aided along the way by several visits to the United States, including a fellowship with John Cobb at the Hospital for Special Surgery in New York and another with Joseph Risser in California.

In the 1970s, Cotrel designed a device for transverse traction (DTT) that produced a transverse force on the apex of a thoracic curve. This device was designed to connect a special apical-compression device to a Harrington concave distraction rod. Through this transverse threaded rod, the apex was drawn toward the distraction rod, and curve correction was obtained. In the mid 1970s, Cotrel experienced cardiac difficulties and needed implantation of a pacemaker. He continued on the design of the DTT but was unable to clinically test his theories of spinal instrumentation. In the early 1980s, he persuaded Jean Dubousset of Paris, France, to consider using his designed instrumentation, and the era of Cotrel-Dubousset instrumentation was thus born.

The first Cotrel-Dubousset instrumentation was performed in January of 1983 by Dubousset. In mid 1983, Dubousset began rotating the bent rod and found that doing so had a beneficial effect on both the sagittal plane and coronal correction. In 1984, Cotrel-Dubousset instrumentation was introduced in the United States in both Louisville and Boston, and soon thereafter in Miami. The North American era of Cotrel-Dubousset instrumentation was thus born. The procedure began to proliferate through the mid to late 1980s and by the 1990s

was the accepted standard of care for the surgical treatment of patients with pediatric spinal deformity (5,8,27,46,72,84,86). This is further evidenced by the proliferation of numerous clone segmental instrumentation systems, such as the Isola, Texas Scottish Rite Hospital, and Moss-Miami systems that have followed. In addition, the original Cotrel-Dubousset device has been updated in numerous ways. It now includes a more user-friendly Cotrel-Dubousset Horizon system so that it can be used to treat both pediatric and adult patients. However, the original theories of design of the instrumentation must be credited to Yves Cotrel, and the original segmental and three-dimensional approach to spinal deformity with this implant system must be credited to Jean Dubousset (17,21).

The initial Cotrel-Dubousset system is discussed in regard to implants, techniques, and results. The Cotrel-Dubousset Horizon version is discussed in detail, because it has completely replaced the original Cotrel-Dubousset system at my center and many others for the operative treatment of pediatric spinal problems.

IMPLANTS

Rods

The original Cotrel-Dubousset rod was unique in several respects. The surface of the original Cotrel-Dubousset rod was rough or knurled by multiple, cross-hatched diamond points (Fig. 1). The metal was 316L stainless steel, which was quite malleable compared with the previous Harrington rod. This relatively soft surface allowed easy short-segment contouring of the rod. It also was possible to set screws to mash down the diamond points on the surface of the rod to make a relatively rigid connection to the spinal anchors (hooks and screws).

The initial rod was 7 mm in diameter, and a pediatric set was developed that had a 5-mm rod. In the early 1990s, a 6-mm rod called the *compact Cotrel-Dubousset* became available, made primarily for lumbar procedures. The characteristics of the original 7-mm Cotrel-Dubousset rod offered a considerable advantage in manipulation of the rod. The amount of bending displacement of the rod needed to produce permanent deformation was quite small and allowed easy in situ bending of the rod. At times this Cotrel-Dubousset rod was criticized as being

L. G. Lenke: Department of Orthopaedic Surgery, Washington University School of Medicine, St. Louis, Missouri 63110.

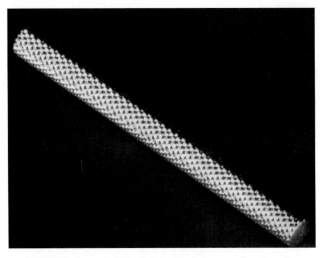

FIGURE 1. Image of 7-mm Cotrel rod shows surface knurling.

too soft and thus not maintaining its orientation during rod manipulation. However, this pliability was a safety mechanism that prevented pullout of the implant or bone failure during manipulation procedures. Eventually, a cold-rolled version of the rod became available that was stiffer and thus made up for many of the shortcomings of the softer rod. However, my colleagues and I rarely used the stiffer rod, tending instead to promote the advantages of the original malleable Cotrel-Dubousset rod. The original rod has been supplanted by the newer 5.5-mm CD Horizon rod.

Hooks

Hooks are available in two distinct types—closed and open. Closed hooks are designed to be used at the proximal and distal ends of instrumentation. Open hooks are placed in the intermediate segments. The open hooks are converted to closed hooks by means of introduction of a blocker device (Fig. 2). This device is a conical implant placed in the open implant only from one side, in the direction the hook is facing either up or down. An

ingenious design mechanism was that once the rod was engaged into the closed hooks above and below and the blockers set in the intermediate hooks, the rod could be freely rotated within the hooks while still maintaining attachment of the hooks to the posterior column of the spine. This allowed the surgeon to control the end of the curves while manipulating the apex in both the coronal and sagittal planes and to a lesser extent, the axial plane simultaneously. This allowed a rod rotation maneuver that could not be performed with previous types of spinal instrumentation. Another distinct advantage of this segmental system was the ability to place different forces (compression, distraction, and translation) on the same rod at different locations. The multitude of hook designs made for the Cotrel-Dubousset system stemmed from two original designs: the pedicle hook and the laminar hook. Once again, each of these was available in a closed and open version.

Pedicle Hooks

Pedicle hooks are designed to be upgoing-only hooks in the thoracic spine between T1 and T10, where the facet orientation is horizontal. Two varieties are available—standard height and decreased height. These differ in the distance between the body and the blade overall, decreasing posterior prominence by 4 mm.

Before placement of the hook, an inferior facet partial osteotomy is performed by means of removal of a small amount of the inferior facet (approximately 4 mm by 4 mm). The cartilage of the superior facet is then exposed and removed (Fig. 3). A pedicle-finding device is carefully laid on top of the superior facet surface. The device is tracked proximally until its prongs reach the inferior border of the pedicle. The location is confirmed by means of moving the pedicle finder and gripping the pedicle in a lateral position away from the spinal canal. The hook is inserted with a hook inserter to seat the hook by means of tapping on the inserter with a mallet to engage the inferior pedicle border. The surgeon must be careful not to crack the superior articular facet, because the underlying spinal canal and spinal cord sit directly beneath this structure, especially on the concavity of scoliosis. Strict attention to detail must be observed while pedicle hooks are prepared and placed.

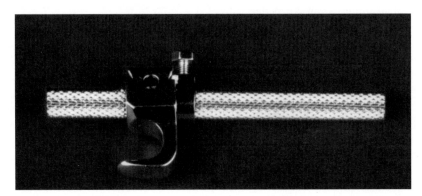

FIGURE 2. The conical blocker is partially seated in an open hook.

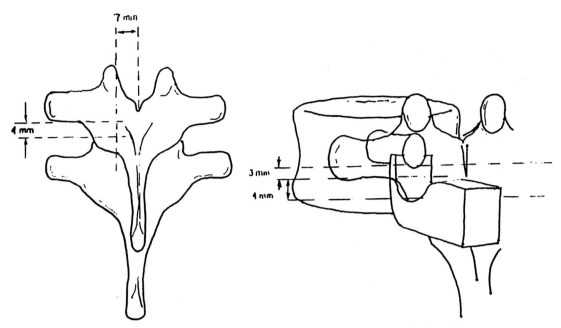

FIGURE 3. The landmark for placement of a thoracic pedicle hook is the facet joint.

Laminar Hooks

Two sizes of laminar hooks initially were available—lumbar (large) and thoracic (small). Originally these differed in throat height, blade diameter, and overall height of the hook. Multiple versions of these two initial laminar hooks since have been developed that have varying throat heights, blade diameters, and overall heights. This was necessary because of the multitude of different anatomic variations in the posterior elements of the spines of both children and adults. These hooks are placed in the lamina and transverse processes.

There are four possible placements for the laminar hooks: supralaminar, infralaminar, supra–transverse process, or infra–transverse process. The supralaminar position requires a canal hook inserted by means of partial ligamentum flavectomy that entails detachment of the distal aspect of the ligament from the proximal edge of the cephalic portion of lamina. Resection of a small portion of the inferior edge of the lamina directly above sometimes is required for appropriate hook placement. The hook body should sit snugly against the posterior cortex with minimal intrusion of the blade to avoid iatrogenic neural injury (4).

The infralaminar position requires a proximally directed hook. This hook is placed between the undersurface of the lamina and the ligamentum flavum, a space produced by the more cephalic attachment of the proximal ligamentum onto the undersurface of the inferior laminar. A laminar developer can be helpful in developing the space onto which the hook blade is seated. It is extremely important to follow the plane of the lamina so that the hook blade is appropriately seated to parallel the laminar surface that is juxtaposed.

Laminar hooks can be placed on the superior or less frequently the inferior surface of the transverse process. A transverse process developer is used to separate the costotransverse ligament between the inferior surface of the transverse process and the superior surface of the adjacent rib. The laminar hook is placed that best fits the anterior-posterior diameter of the transverse process. It can also be placed in the inferior position. In operations on the thoracic spine, however, an upgoing pedicle hook provides much better fixation then an upgoing transverse process hook. In the lower thoracic region, the transverse processes become much softer and less amenable to fixation; the supralaminar position is preferred.

Use of claw constructs at the proximal and distal ends of instrumentation constructs is popular (11,72,74). A claw is two hooks the face in opposite directions. Claws are placed either one or two levels apart. At the proximal end, a pedicle–transverse process or pedicle-supralaminar claw can be spread over one or two vertebral levels. At the distal end, the most common claw is a supralaminar-infralaminar claw usually placed over two levels. Claws are seated with hooks in compression to grip snugly one or two vertebral segments in the posterior aspect to produce a solid proximal or distal foundation.

Transverse Connectors

The DTT is an integral part of the original Cotrel-Dubousset system. It is available in several forms, including three forms for the original 7-mm knurled rod—DTT1, DTT2, and DTT3 (Fig. 4). By connecting the concave and convex rods, these transverse connectors produce a rectangular construct between adjacent rods that increases rigidity (35). This is especially important in longer constructs in which the instrumentation extends into the lumbar spine. With fairly long constructs, longer than 30

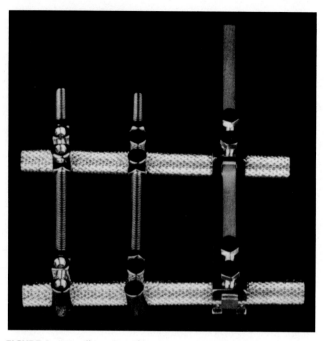

FIGURE 4. A small portion of lamina usually is excised. Three varieties of devices for transverse traction: DTT1 (*left*), DTT2 (*center*), DTT3 (*right*).

cm, often three or even four DTTs may be used to increase the torsional rigidity of the construct (35).

Specialized Hooks

Several custom hooks have been designed to meet specific purposes in user-friendly instrumentation. Several are important enough to merit further discussion. A *lumbar laminar hook* has an extended body and smaller blade than a conventional hook. The modification can be useful for transverse process hooks and for supralaminar hooks in the thoracolumbar and lumbar spine. In the supralaminar position, an extended body is needed to engage the rod into the hook because of the anterior position of this hook and because the blade sits in the spinal canal. An *oblique blade hook* adheres anatomically to the oblique infralaminar region of the lumbar lamina. When a normal rounded blade hook is used, the hook must sit in a very angled direction, thus extensive bending of the distal rod into lordosis is needed to seat the hook appropriately. A *laminar hook with a displaced lateral body* relative to the blade can be used for alignment with more laterally placed pedicle screws. Right and left versions of this hook are needed for access on both sides of the spine. These displaced body hooks are not necessary with screw systems that allow medial displacement of the rod by the screw rod connector.

Screws

Screws are available with the Cotrel-Dubousset system (33). Open sacral screws have been used for transpedicular placement and for placement in the sacrum. These screws, although quite useful, have somewhat limited value in the management of com-

plex spinal deformity because they are minimally versatile. The rod must be perfectly bent to engage directly into the closed or open screw. New versions allow versatility in the rod-screw connection and provide more three-dimensional linkage of the rod to the screws. Other screws, including an iliosacral screw designed for instrumentation constructs that extend into the pelvis and a double-threaded screw for placement into an anteriorly displaced L5 vertebral pedicle or body being treated for spondylolisthesis, can be helpful (10). However, newer instrumentation systems have made the double-threaded screw nearly obsolete.

Axial Extension Devices

Two devices for axial extension are available for use with the Cotrel-Dubousset system—the domino and the axial extension tube. The axial extension tube has not been as popular as the domino has. The domino is available with both open and closed canals and either a single- or double-set bolt-locking device to each rod. A domino with 5-mm and 7-mm canals allows the surgeon to join a portion of the spine instrumented with a 7-mm rod to the portion instrumented with a 5-mm rod. Dominoes are helpful implants. They can be used for salvage of previously failed instrumentation. They also allow proximal or distal extension of previous instrumentation without removal. During primary operations, dominoes can be used in difficult instrumentation sequences to lessen the rod bend necessary to instrument long segments of spinal deformity. A domino is called a *functional domino* when two curves in opposite directions are instrumented separately (as in a double thoracic curve). In kyphosis surgery, the proximal and distal segments can be instrumented independently and then joined at the apex with an apical domino.

Summary

The original Cotrel-Dubousset system comprised a wide variety of implants that were constantly being modified. A wide variety of combinations of hooks, screws, rods, dominoes, and transverse connectors were available. A complete knowledge of the type of implants available and their intended use facilitated instrumentation sequences with the original Cotrel-Dubousset system.

COTREL-DUBOUSSET HORIZON INSTRUMENTATION

Although the original Cotrel-Dubousset system completely revolutionized the principles and techniques of spinal deformity instrumentation, problems with the design made the system less than ideal. The main design flaws were lack of adjustability and removability once the set screws were totally sheared off, locking the rod to the hooks or screws. To remove the device necessitated cutting the rod at multiple locations or destroying the connection of the blocker inside the open hooks. It was especially difficult to remove claw constructs that had closed hooks over a single- or two-level segment.

The second design flaw was the prominence produced by the instrumentation in thin adolescents. Although a 5-mm pediatric system was available, this often was too small for an adolescent of typical size. The posterior prominence of the 7-mm system in thin adolescents occasionally necessitated elective removal of the implants, which carried the risks, although admittedly low, of a second surgical procedure (46).

The third issue revolved around removal of the blockers within the open hooks and possible displacement of the blocker. A C-ring was developed to back up the open-hook blocker to prevent it from backing out. However, use of the C-ring required additional instrumentation and did not always completely prevent the problem. The fourth problem involved threading corrosion caused by micromotion of the rod with its attached diamond burrs against the other screw and hook implants (70).

Because of the design flaws, the Cotrel-Dubousset instrumentation was modified, and the Cotrel-Dubousset Horizon system was developed. The key features of the Cotrel-Dubousset Horizon system, which my colleagues and I began using exclusively in 1995, are revisability, much lower profile, downgrade attachment of the implants to the rod, and entire top loading, making it more user-friendly. The basic rod size is decreased to 5.5 mm (approximately the inner core diameter of the original Cotrel-Dubousset rod without the knurled chips on it). The rod also is stiffened a bit to make it stronger in fatigue, although it does lose some of its in situ bending ability. However, with specialized benders, in-situ contouring is possible for kyphosis (Fig. 5), lor-

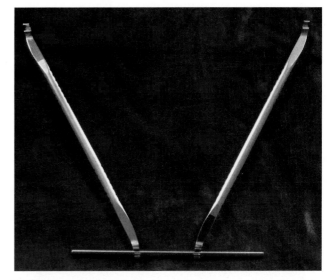

FIGURE 6. In situ lordosis benders positioned on a 5.5-mm Cotrel-Dubousset Horizon rod.

dosis (Fig. 6), and scoliosis benders that straighten the coronal plane (Fig. 7). The original Cotrel-Dubousset hooks are modified to a 5.5-mm rod, and all hooks are open. A variety of hooks, including pedicle (Fig. 8), laminar (Fig. 9), thoracic (Fig. 10), and specialized hooks (Figs. 11, 12) It is possible to make a closed hook by placing the set screw before fastening the hook on the posterior elements. However, not depending entirely on closed hooks at the top and bottom of a construct also becomes

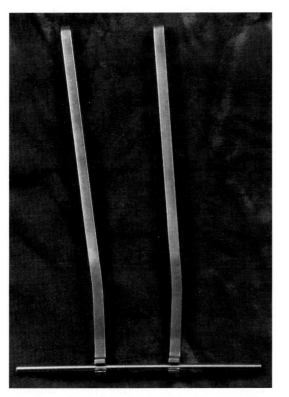

FIGURE 5. In situ kyphosis benders positioned on a 5.5-mm Cotrel-Dubousset Horizon rod.

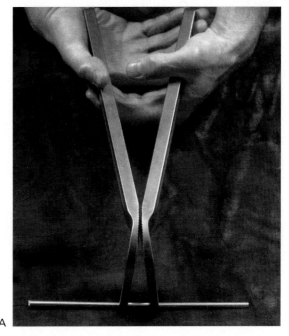

A

FIGURE 7. A: In situ coronal scoliosis benders as positioned on a 5.5-mm Cotrel-Dubousset Horizon rod before placement of a coronal bend. *(Figure continues.)*

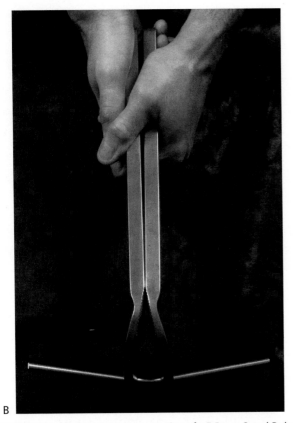

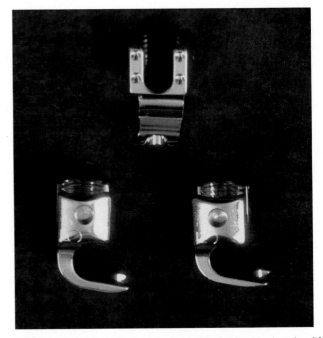

FIGURE 8. Cotrel-Dubousset Horizon pedicle hooks showing the difference between an elongated throat (*bottom left*) and normal throat (*top* and *bottom right*).

B

FIGURE 7. *Continued.* **B:** In situ correction of a 5.5-mm Cotrel-Dubousset Horizon rod with coronal scoliosis benders after creation of a scoliotic bend in the rod.

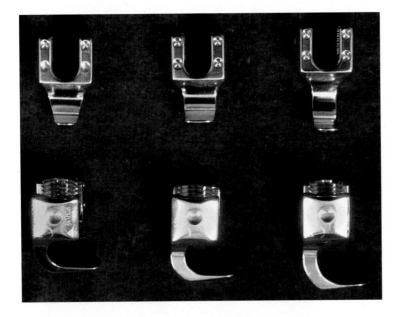

FIGURE 9. Three different varieties of laminar hooks viewed from end on and from the side. *Left to right,* throat height, normal throat and blade, and increased throat height and blade variety.

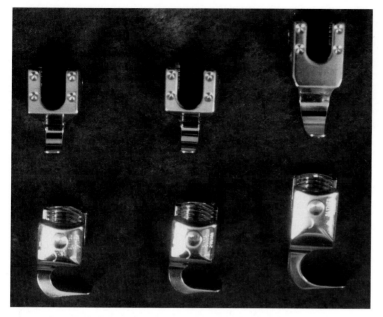

FIGURE 10. Three varieties of slanted-body thoracic hooks viewed from head on and the side. These include a reduced-height throat blade (*left*), normal height thin blade (*center*), and elevated throat and body height and large blade (*right*).

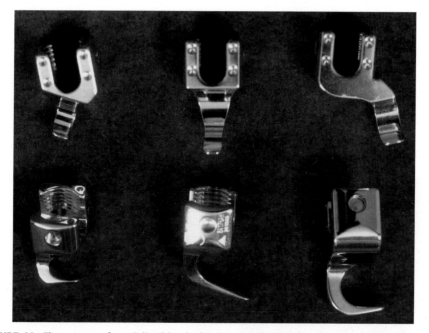

FIGURE 11. Three types of specialized hooks for Cotrel-Dubousset Horizon instrumentation viewed from both head on and side. *Left,* short, oblique blade hook used in the supralaminar position. *Center,* thin-blade, angled laminar hook used in the intralaminar area to accommodate angulation of the cauda portion of the lamina. *Right,* lateral offset hook that allows capture of a laterally placed rod to the head of the hook with the blade going under the more medially positioned lamina.

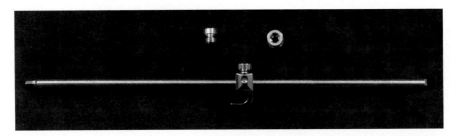

FIGURE 12. Example of a 5.5-mm Cotrel-Dubousset Horizon rod with a standard laminar hook set plug attached. *Top,* lateral and head-on views of an M10 plug device show the hollow core.

helpful in situations in which the rod has to be tunneled from proximal to distal to engage it into completely closed hooks. At times this maneuver is difficult and is obviated by having all hooks open, or only the proximal or distal hooks closed with the rest of the hooks open. Appropriate instruments for the hooks, screws, and rod have been developed to make the system user-friendly. An extremely low profile and contourable cross-link that is entirely top loading and top tightening complements the system and is an extremely valuable feature, as are dominoes that link rods together vertically (Fig. 13).

With the increasing popularity of pedicle screws in operations for pediatric spinal deformities (3,14,30,33,76), uniaxial and multiaxial Horizon pedicle screws of varying diameters and lengths have been developed as well. The Cotrel-Dubousset Horizon system is quite modular in that the rod can connect to Texas Scottish Rite Hospital variable-angle screws with special lateral connectors that accommodate the 5.5-mm rod. A special Liberty connector to iliac screws is helpful in iliac wing fixation with iliac wing screws placed in a Galveston-like position. Thus, the current Cotrel-Dubousset Horizon system is universal for use in the posterior portion of the pediatric spine in the cervical region all the way to the sacrum.

The 5.5-mm Cotrel-Dubousset Horizon rod screw system can be used for anterior instrumentation of the pediatric spine (77). Vertebral body staples are available through which 6.5-mm uniaxial screws are placed at a sufficient length to obtain bicortical purchase of the vertebral body. The 5.5-mm Horizon rod then can be prebent, contoured, and seated in the screws in the appropriate coronal and sagittal alignment by means of cantilever, rod rotation, and intersegmental compression techniques. This system is quite useful in anterior procedures for thoracic, thoracolumbar and lumbar scoliosis.

INDICATIONS

The initial indication for Cotrel-Dubousset instrumentation was adolescent spinal deformity, specifically scoliosis (5,21,22,47, 61,64,68,71). However, over the last 15 years, the use has expanded to include any situation that necessitates anterior or posterior spinal instrumentation in the older juvenile and adolescent age range (23,36,68). The initial theory of use of Cotrel-Dubousset instrumentation, as well as specific implant placement, is discussed elsewhere, and is not repeated here in total. In my practice, the original Cotrel-Dubousset device is of historical interest only. I switched to exclusive use of the updated Cotrel-Dubousset Horizon system in 1996. Thus this discussion includes patients treated with the original Cotrel-Dubousset device but concentrates on the newer Cotrel-Dubousset Horizon system, which is quite versatile and user-friendly. The indications for Cotrel-Dubousset instrumentation in the pediatric age group include spinal deformity of any cause, spinal trauma, and complex reconstruction of the spine.

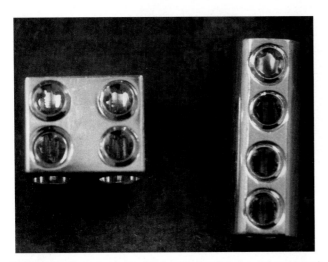

FIGURE 13. Example of a double domino that links two 5.5-mm Cotrel-Dubousset Horizon rods on the left. Example of an axial tube connector joining two vertically oriented Cotrel-Dubousset Horizon rods with the coupling device.

SCOLIOSIS

Adolescent Idiopathic Scoliosis

The prototype Cotrel-Dubousset instrumentation system was developed for scoliosis, specifically adolescent idiopathic scoliosis (22). The surgical management of adolescent idiopathic scoliosis with the segmental hook-screw-rod Cotrel-Dubousset system has been investigated extensively. Most of the current technical advances in pediatric segmental spinal instrumentation have been in care of patients with adolescent idiopathic scoliosis. Thus it is essential that this patient population be covered extensively in the discussion of Cotrel-Dubousset instrumentation. The most common classification of adolescent idiopathic scoliosis has been the King method (38). Although the landmark article by King et al. has imparted scoliosis surgeons with valuable information (67,68), the study has been found to have poor reliability (18,43).

A new surgical classification of adolescent idiopathic scoliosis is being developed for uniform preoperative assessment of curve patterns and postoperative grading results (45). This two-dimensional treatment-based comprehensive system begins by separating the spine into three regions—proximal thoracic (PT), main thoracic (MT), and thoracolumbar/lumbar (TL/L). The major (largest) curve is documented and always is considered surgically structural, necessitating instrumentation and fusion. The minor (lesser) curves are then analyzed with respect to their structural characteristics. Structural criteria in the coronal and sagittal planes have been developed to differentiate minor curves that should be considered for inclusion in the instrumentation and fusion along with the major curve.

Structural characteristics in the coronal plane include inflexibility on side bending 25 degrees or more in the PT, MT, TL/L region. In the sagittal plane, hyperkyphosis of +20 degrees or more in the PT region (T2–5) and the thoracolumbar junction (T10–L2) also is a structural characteristic that necessitates inclusion in instrumentation and fusion of the major curve (Table 1). The basic premise is that major and structural minor curves are included in the instrumentation and fusion, whereas nonstructural minor curves are excluded from instrumentation and fusion if at all possible. A template can be made by means of determining the regions that are structural as opposed to nonstructural, and six curve types are produced: type 1, main thoracic (MT); type 2, double thoracic (DT); type 3, double major (DM); type 4, triple major (TM); type 5, thoracolumbar/lumbar (TL/L), and type 6, thoracolumbar/lumbar–main thoracic (TL/L–MT). These six curve types cover the entire spectrum of basic curve patterns of adolescent idiopathic scoliosis (Table 2) (45).

My colleagues and I have developed a lumbar spine modifier and sagittal thoracic modifier. Because the lumbar spine is the foundation of the spine, and because the resultant position of the lumbar spine is critical to the long-term success of fusion for scoliosis, the design of a lumbar spine modifier in types A,

TABLE 2. CURVE TYPES

Type	Proximal Thoracic	Main Thoracic	Thoracolumbar/ Lumbar	Curve Type
1	NS	S(M)	NS	Main thoracic
2	S	S(M)	NS	Double thoracic
3	NS	S(M)	S	Double major
4	S	S(M)	S	Triple major
5	NS	NS	S(M)	Thoracolumbar/ lumbar
6	NS	S	S(M)	Thoracolumbar/ lumbar–main thoracic

Surgical structural criteria for minor curves. Proximal thoracic—side-bending Cobb angle ≥25 degrees; T2–5 kyphosis ≥ +20 degrees. Main thoracic—side-bending Cobb angle ≥25 degrees; T10–L2 kyphosis ≥ +20 degrees. Thoracolumbar/lumbar—T10–L2 kyphosis ≥ +20 degrees. M, major (largest curve); NS, surgical nonstructural; S, surgical strucural.

B, and C has been based on the position of the center sacral vertical line (CSVL) in relation to the apex of the lumbar curve. In the type A lumbar modifier, the CSVL falls between the lumbar pedicles up to the stable vertebra and demonstrates minimal to no curvature or rotation to the lumbar spine (Fig. 14). In the type B lumbar modifier, the CSVL falls on the apex of the lumbar curve whether the apex is a body or a disc (Fig. 15). Thus the lumbar curve demonstrates mild to moderate curvature and rotation. For the type C lumbar modifier, the CSVL is completely medial to the apex of the lumbar curve whether the apex is a body or a disc (Fig. 16). These lumbar curve patterns (A to B to C) demonstrate greater curvature and usually also rotation. The ABC lumbar modifier terminology can be used to assess the position of the lumbar curve preoperatively and to grade the position of the lumbar curve postoperatively (37,44,66,78). The goal is for the distance between the apex of the lumbar spine and the CSVL to be as small as possible after surgical treatment.

Last, a sagittal thoracic modifier (−, N, +) is based on the T5–12 sagittal Cobb angle measurement. When this measurement is less than 10 degrees, a minus sign (−) or hypokyphotic modifier is produced; for a +10 to +40 degree measurement, N or normal kyphosis is present; and when the measurement is greater than 40 degrees, a plus sign (+) or hyperkyphotic measurement is present. The goal of instrumentation and fusion in the management of thoracic adolescent idiopathic scoliosis is to improve kyphosis for a patient with hypokyphosis (−), maintain the normal kyphotic modifier (N), and to reduce kyphosis for a patient with hyperkyphosis (+) (11,29,57,65,72).

Complete curve classification thus combines the curve type (1 through 6), the lumbar spine modifier (A, B, C), and the sagittal thoracic modifier (−, N, +). Thus curve classification have various permutations, such as: 1A−, 1AN, 1A+, 1B− through 6C+. Each of these permutations has classification and treatment implications (45). A one-page information sheet lists all necessary requirements for proper curve classification (Fig. 17).

For the six curve types, generalizations can be made regarding which regions of the spine should be included in the instrumen-

TABLE 1. RADIOGRAPHIC SURGICAL STRUCTURAL CRITERIA

Section of Spine	Coronal, Side Bend (Degrees)	Sagittal, Upright (Degrees)
Proximal thoracic	≥25	T2–5≥ +20
Main thoracic	≥25	T10–L2≥ +20
Thoracolumbar/lumbar	≥25	T10–L2≥ +20

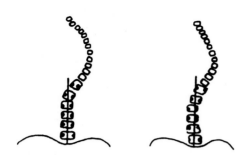

Lumbar Modifier A

- <u>CSVL</u> falls between lumbar pedicles up to stable vertebra

- Must have a thoracic apex

- If in doubt as to whether CSVL touches medial aspect of lumbar apical pedicle – <u>CHOOSE TYPE B</u>

- Includes King types III, IV, and V

CSVL between pedicles up to stable vertebra, no to minimal scoliosis and rotation to L-spine

FIGURE 14. Schematic of lumbar modifier A.

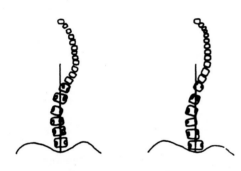

Lumbar Modifier B

- <u>CSVL</u> falls between medial border of lumbar concave pedicle and lateral margin of apical vertebral body or bodies (if apex is a disc)

- Must have a thoracic apex

- If in doubt as to whether CSVL touches lateral margin of apical vertebral body(ies) – <u>CHOOSE TYPE B</u>

- Includes King types II, III, V

CSVL touches apical vertebral body(ies) or pedicles, minimal to moderate L-spine rotation

FIGURE 15. Schematic of lumbar modifier B.

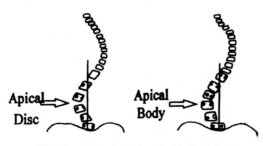

Apical → Disc

Apical → Body

Lumbar Modifier C

- <u>CSVL</u> falls lateral to lateral aspect of lumbar apical vertebral body or bodies (if apex is a disc)

- May have a thoracic, thoracolumbar and/or lumbar apex

- If in doubt as to whether CSVL actually touches lateral aspect of vertebral body(ies) – <u>CHOOSE TYPE B</u>

- Includes King types I, II, V, Double Major, Triple Major thoracolumbar and lumbar curves

CSVL does not touch apical vertebral body or the bodies immediately above and below the apical disc

FIGURE 16. Schematic of lumbar modifier C.

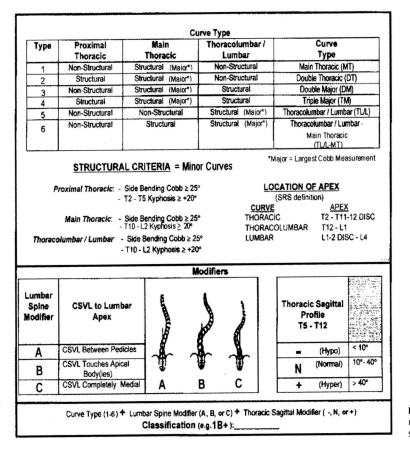

STRUCTURAL CRITERIA = Minor Curves

			Curve Type	
Type	Proximal Thoracic	Main Thoracic	Thoracolumbar / Lumbar	Curve Type
1	Non-Structural	Structural (Major*)	Non-Structural	Main Thoracic (MT)
2	Structural	Structural (Major*)	Non-Structural	Double Thoracic (DT)
3	Non-Structural	Structural (Major*)	Structural	Double Major (DM)
4	Structural	Structural (Major*)	Structural	Triple Major (TM)
5	Non-Structural	Non-Structural	Structural (Major*)	Thoracolumbar / Lumbar (TL/L)
6	Non-Structural	Structural	Structural (Major*)	Thoracolumbar / Lumbar - Main Thoracic (TL/L-MT)

*Major = Largest Cobb Measurement

Proximal Thoracic: - Side Bending Cobb ≥ 25°
- T2 - T5 Kyphosis ≥ +20°

Main Thoracic: - Side Bending Cobb ≥ 25°
- T10 - L2 Kyphosis ≥ 20°

Thoracolumbar / Lumbar - Side Bending Cobb ≥ 25°
- T10 - L2 Kyphosis ≥ +20°

LOCATION OF APEX
(SRS definition)

CURVE	APEX
THORACIC	T2 - T11-12 DISC
THORACOLUMBAR	T12 - L1
LUMBAR	L1-2 DISC - L4

Modifiers

Lumbar Spine Modifier	CSVL to Lumbar Apex
A	CSVL Between Pedicles
B	CSVL Touches Apical Body(ies)
C	CSVL Completely Medial

	Thoracic Sagittal Profile T5 - T12	
−	(Hypo)	< 10°
N	(Normal)	10° - 40°
+	(Hyper)	> 40°

Curve Type (1-6) **+** Lumbar Spine Modifier (A, B, or C) **+** Thoracic Sagittal Modifier (-, N, or +)

Classification (e.g.1B+): _____

FIGURE 17. One-page information sheet that contains all necessary items for proper curve classification with the new system.

tation and fusion (Table 3). A simple explanation is that for an MT type 1 curve, only the MT region should be instrumented and fused. For a DT type 2 curve, both the PT and main thoracic regions should be instrumented and fused. For a DM type 3 curve, the MT and TL/L regions should be instrumented and fused. For a TM type 4 curve, the PT, MT, and TL/L regions all should be instrumented and fused. For a TL/L type 5 curve, only the TL/L region should be instrumented and fused. For

TL/L-MT type 6 curves, both the MT and TL/L regions should be instrumented and fused.

The lumbar and sagittal plane modifiers also help direct treatment by directing techniques used to perform the instrumented correction. For MT type 1 curves with an A lumbar modifier, the goal is complete correction of the MT curve and a horizontal lowest instrumented vertebra whether instrumentation is anterior or posterior. For a type B modifier, the lowest instrumented vertebra can be made almost completely horizontal from the anterior approach. From a posterior approach, it may be wise to leave mild residual tilt to the lowest instrumented vertebra (stable vertebra) to accommodate the small lumbar curve below. This is even more important with a MT type 1 curve with a lumbar C modifier, in which with both anterior and posterior techniques, residual tilt should be maintained in the lowest instrumented vertebra to accommodate the lumbar curve below because it completely crosses the midline in its preoperative position.

The effect of spinal instrumentation in the sagittal plane has important considerations for placement of Cotrel-Dubousset instrumentation (6,11,46,52,65,70). The importance of the sagittal plane in both the evaluation and management of adolescent idiopathic scoliosis truly began with the advent of the Cotrel-

TABLE 3. TREATMENT OPTIONS AS DESIGNATED BY CURVE TYPE

Curve Type	Structural Region	Regions for Arthrodesis	Approach
1 MT	MT	MT	PSF or ASF
2 DT	PT, MT	PT, MT	PSF or ASF
3 DM	MT, TL/L	MT-TL/L	PSF
4 TM	PT, MT, TL/L	PT, MT, TL/L	PSF
5 TL/L	TL/L	TL/L	ASF or PSF
6 TL/L–MT	TL/L, MT	TL/L, MT	PSF

ASF, anterior spinal fusion; DM, double major; DT, double thoracic; MT, main thoracic; PSF, posterior spinal fusion; PT, proximal thoracic; TL/L, thoracolumbar/lumbar; TM, triple major.

Dubousset system. The treatment implications of the sagittal thoracic modifier are based on instrumented techniques of sagittal plane correction and maintenance. For a hypokyphotic ($-$) sagittal modifier, techniques to improve thoracic kyphosis with posterior rod rotation or posterior translation, as opposed to anterior convex compression techniques, should be performed. For patients with a normal kyphotic (N) sagittal modifier, thoracic kyphosis should be maintained in this normal range. For those with a hyperkyphotic ($+$) sagittal modifier, techniques to remove thoracic kyphosis should be performed. This usually entails application of posterior convex compression forces before any concave distraction forces. This situation is quite amenable to use of rod-dominoes to specifically treat different regions of the spine on alternating rods in a biomechanically directed manner. Surgeons must remember that posterior distraction forces (away from the apex) produce relative or absolute kyphosis, whereas posterior compression forces (toward the apex) produce relative or absolute lordosis.

Two other important principles specific to segmental instrumentation must be observed. First, forces should be placed on the spine that close open discs and open closed discs during the instrumentation sequence. A force that opens an already opened disc space has the possibility to produce imbalance. Second, it is always unwise to stop the proximal or distal extent of the instrumentation and fusion at posterior aspect of the apex of a coronal or sagittal curve. There is high risk of producing coronal imbalance when the procedure stops at the apex of a coronal curve (12) and of junctional kyphosis when the procedure stops at the apex of thoracic or thoracolumbar kyphosis.

If these principles of curve identification, selection of fusion level, and instrumentation technique are observed, results with the Cotrel-Dubousset system are quite gratifying. My center has had experience with more than 700 Cotrel-Dubousset instrumentation constructs for adolescent idiopathic scoliosis over more than 15 years. Numerous other operations have been performed to manage other disorders (see later). Our results with the original Cotrel-Dubousset system for adolescent idiopathic scoliosis have been published in both a 2-year follow-up (46) and 5- to 10-year follow-up (51) studies. As have other surgeons, we have found approximately 50% to 60% correction in Cobb angle, minimal late loss of correction, normalized sagittal contour both in the thoracic region, and postoperative maintenance or enhancement of TL/L lordosis (46). The pseudarthrosis rate has been quite low, less than 1%. The neurologic injury rate among patients with adolescent idiopathic scoliosis treated with Cotrel-Dubousset equipment has been zero at my institution (13,43). We attribute these results to a combination of using the pliable rod that is more forgiving, exact hook placement techniques (4), avoidance of pure distraction of the concave apex and relying more on translational type of forces, and the use of motor and somatosensory potentials and the intraoperative wake-up test of Stagnara as the standard of care for evaluation of neurologic function during these procedures (9,32,63,75).

Specific Curve Patterns

Curve Type 1: Main Thoracic

The MT curve pattern is the most commonly encountered surgical curve type in adolescent idiopathic scoliosis. Approximately 40% of operative curves are MT type 1. In this curve pattern, the PT and TL/L regions are nonstructural and can be left uninstrumented and unfused. Careful review of long-cassette coronal and lateral radiographs and of side-bending and push-prone radiographs is necessary to confirm this assessment (81). A helpful guide is the structural characteristics in the coronal and sagittal planes that has been developed and tested retrospectively and is being subjected to prospective evaluation (45).

A MT curve can have a lumbar modifier A, B, or even C position to the lumbar curve, listed in decreasing frequency. It also can have a thoracic sagittal plane that is either normal kyphosis (N), hypokyphosis ($-$), or hyperkyphosis ($+$), again, listed in decreasing frequency. The goals are to maximize spontaneous correction of the lumbar curve, avoid lumbar instrumentation and fusion, and restore a more normalized thoracic sagittal alignment (see earlier) (49). Basic fusion levels for the MT curve pattern extend proximally from neutral vertebra (usually T4 or T5) to the stable vertebra distally (between T11 and L4). The stable vertebra, predicted with the CSVL should be documented. For a pure thoracic overhang curve (lumbar A modifier), instrumentation and fusion usually can stop one or occasionally two levels short of stable in a posterior approach and usually one to three levels short of stable in an anterior approach (Fig. 18) (49). For the type B modifier, instrumentation and fusion usually must extend to the stable vertebra one level proximal. The level is similar for the posterior approach to a curve with a lumbar C modifier (Figs. 19, 20). With anterior instrumentation and fusion, the fusion levels extend from end vertebra to end vertebra (7).

The 1AN curve pattern is the most common curve pattern in adolescent idiopathic scoliosis. This is similar to a true King III curve pattern (38). The goal should be a horizontal position of the lowest instrumented vertebra and consideration of maintaining an adequate position of the lowest instrumented vertebra when the procedure stops short of the stable vertebra (49). This curve pattern can be managed with Cotrel-Dubousset instrumentation traditionally by a posterior approach with either hooks or pedicle screws at the distal end. I am more inclined to use the anterior approach for patients who have a hypokyphotic or frankly lordotic sagittal plane ($-$ sagittal modifier) alignment and a posterior approach for patients who have a hyperkyphotic ($+$) sagittal plane modifier (7). Either anterior or posterior instrumentation is acceptable for patients with normal thoracic sagittal kyphosis (N).

The King II curve pattern is the most troublesome since the advent of Cotrel-Dubousset instrumentation with regard to postoperative decompensation (12,48,55,56,58,66,79). This curve pattern is analogous to a type 1C curve in which both thoracic and lumbar curves completely cross the midline with a thoracic Cobb angle greater than the lumbar Cobb angle. Almost invariably the percentage thoracic side-bending correction is less than the percentage lumbar side bending correction. Nevertheless, exactly how far the lumbar apex deviates from the midline has never been explicitly detailed (43). However, the lumbar C modifier dictates that the apex of the lumbar spine, whether the apex is a body or a disc, completely deviate from the vertically directed CSVL. To explicitly determine guidelines for successful selective thoracic fusion of a true King II curve (new type 1C),

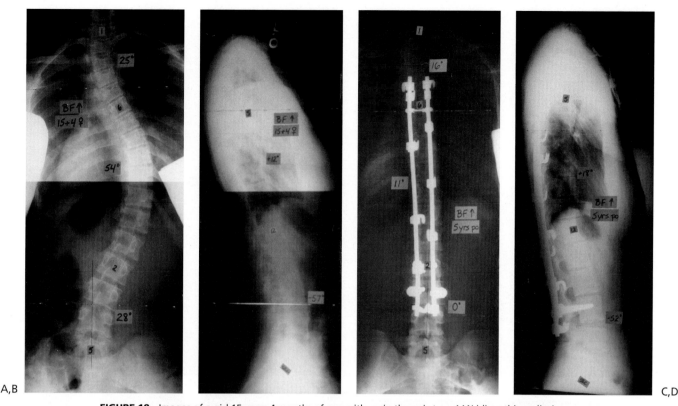

FIGURE 18. Images of a girl 15 years 4 months of age with main thoracic type 1AN idiopathic scoliosis. **A:** Upright frontal radiograph shows 54-degree right thoracic scoliosis. **B:** Sagittal plane image shows mild thoracic hypokyphosis between T5 and T12 (+12 degrees). Left side-bending radiograph shows nonstructural regions to the proximal thoracic and lumbar spine. Right side-bending radiograph shows correction of main thoracic curve to 25 degrees. **C:** Frontal view obtained 5 years after posterior Cotrel-Dubousset instrumentation from T5 to L3 shows maintenance of excellent coronal alignment. **D:** Lateral view obtained 5 years postoperatively shows maintenance of sagittal contour. An ideal result would have been a slightly more lordotic thoracolumbar junction; however, the unfused lower lumbar discs are in good alignment.

my colleagues and I developed ratio criteria for thoracic to lumbar (T:L) Cobb measurements, apical vertebral translation, and apical vertebral rotation (48). We found that selective thoracic fusion can be performed when the thoracic to lumbar (T:L) Cobb and apical vertebral translation ratios are greater than 1.2 and the T:L apical vertebral rotation is greater than 1.0 (48). There also can be no thoracolumbar junctional kyphosis and a maximal lumbar Cobb measurement of 60 degrees on the upright radiograph. These criteria were based solely on upright anteroposterior and lateral long-cassette spinal radiographs. The appearance of the thoracic region should be more prominent than the appearance of the lumbar region. Thus for a true King II curve or new 1C curve pattern, selective thoracic fusion is indicated, and the approach can be either posterior or anterior (44).

If the 1C curve pattern is managed with posterior instrumentation and fusion, the area involved usually extends from the neutral vertebra proximally (T4, T5) to the stable vertebra distally at the thoracolumbar junction (usually T12 or L1) (Fig. 20). My colleagues and I use hooks proximally and screws distally as spinal anchors. A claw construct (pedicle–transverse process

pedicle-supralaminar) is placed proximally, and a supralaminar-infralaminar claw rather than pedicle screws is used as a distal anchor. Apical hooks or wires can be used for correction of apical translational. A full 90-degree rod rotation maneuver is contraindicated because it carries a high risk of decompensation (12). Hooks are seated on a left-sided concave correcting rod from distal to proximal, and modest correction should be obtained. The goal is to obtain approximately 40% instrumented correction in the thoracic region to allow the lumbar region to correct spontaneously. Another way of looking at this is that the lowest instrumented vertebra should have residual tilt to accommodate the lumbar curve below. In my experience, the more horizontal is the lowest instrumented vertebra when the procedure stops at the thoracolumbar junction, the higher is the risk of postoperative decompensation of the lumbar curve.

An alternative way to manage these curve patterns is with anterior thoracic instrumentation and fusion (7,80). The thoracic spine is instrumented from upper- to lower-end vertebrae, usually from T4 or T5 down to T11 or T12. Anterior convex compression forces provide correction of scoliosis in the coronal plane and produces kyphosis in the apical thoracic region in

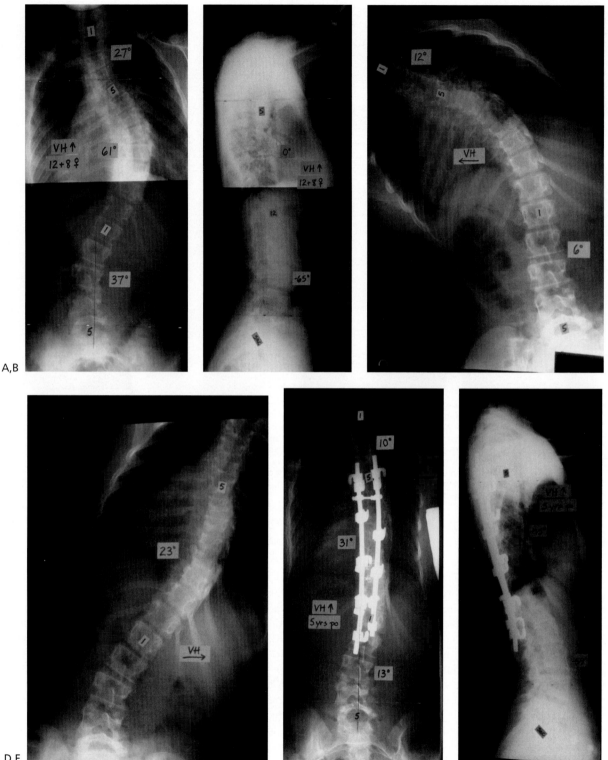

FIGURE 19. Images of a girl 12 years 8 months of age with main thoracic idiopathic scoliosis with hypokyphosis in the sagittal plane—a type 1B curve pattern. The center sacral vertical line touches the apical lumbar pedicle at L4 (lumbar B modifier). **A:** Standing frontal radiograph shows a 27-degree proximal thoracic, 61-degree main thoracic, and 37-degree lumbar curve. **B:** Upright lateral preoperative radiograph shows severe hypokyphosis of 0 between T5 and T12. **C:** Left side-bending radiograph shows nonstructural regions to the proximal thoracic (12 degrees) and lumbar (6 degrees) spine. **D:** Right side-bending radiograph shows a residual 23-degree main thoracic curve. Posterior Cotrel-Dubousset Horizon instrumentation was performed with a 90-degree rod rotation maneuver and thoracoplasty with the intent to improve thoracic kyphosis and to correct scoliosis. **E:** Frontal radiograph obtained 5 years postoperatively shows balanced correction in the coronal plane. **F:** Lateral postoperative view shows a more normalized thoracic sagittal contour measuring +15 degrees with harmonious thoracic, thoraco-lumbar, and lumbar sagittal alignment.

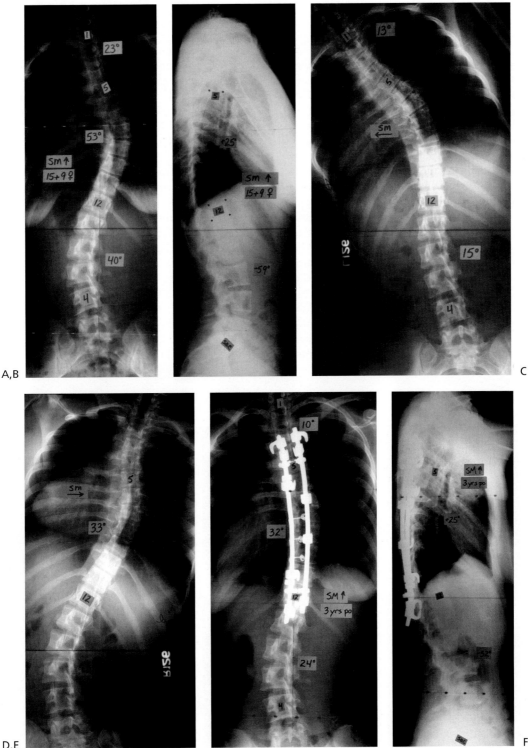

A,B

C

D,E

F

FIGURE 20. **A:** Images of a girl 15 years 9 months of age with 53-degree right thoracic, 40-degree left lumbar idiopathic scoliosis. The curve type most closely resembles a true King II curve because the apex of the lumbar curve is completely off the midline. In the new classification, this is a 1CN curve, because the center sacral vertical line (CSVL) does not touch the apex of the lumbar spine (apical bodies because the apex is a disc). **B:** Sagittal view shows a hint of a thoracolumbar junctional kyphosis but not enough to make it truly structural. The T5–12 sagittal alignment is within the normal range (+25 degrees). **C:** Left side-bending radiograph shows a nonstructural proximal thoracic (13 degrees) and lumbar curve bending out to 15 degrees. **D:** Right side-bending radiograph shows a more structural thoracic curve, as would be expected, bending out only to 33 degrees. Posterior fusion was performed with Cotrel-Dubousset instrumentation consisting of hooks, three apical Wisconsin wires, and rods from T4 to T12. Thoracic scoliosis was intentionally undercorrected to maintain overall coronal balance with residual lumbar curve below. **E:** Radiograph obtained 3 years postoperatively shows excellent coronal balance with a residual 32-degree thoracic and 24-degree lumbar curve. Lumbar spine position is now a B pattern, because the CSVL touches the apex of the lumbar curve, indicating true spontaneous apical correction to the lumbar curve. **F:** Postoperative lateral radiograph shows maintenance of sagittal alignment. This case shows the importance of both proper selection of curves for selective thoracic fusion and of limiting correction of the main thoracic curve to allow the lumbar spine to accommodate below.

the sagittal plane. Thus this operation is ideal for patients with hypokyphosis (sagittal modifier −) in thoracic sagittal alignment. In a comparison of posterior versus anterior instrumentation techniques for these 1C curve types (true King II curves), the anterior route was found to have thoracic instrumented correction and lumbar spontaneous correction superior to those obtained with the posterior approach (44). It appears that the anterior route allows slightly better instrumented correction and lower risk of decompensation of the lumbar curve. This may be because there are more distal levels to accommodate the instrumented correction performed by the anterior route and because the correction is done from an anterior convex compression route that potentially pulls up the lower thoracic region and translates the lumbar spine toward the apex. However, with either of the anterior or posterior techniques, I still recommend leaving residual tilt to the lowest instrumented vertebra to allow accommodation of the lumbar curve below.

Proper selection and operative management of a 1C (true King II) adolescent idiopathic scoliosis curve pattern can prove difficult with posterior segmental spinal instrumentation systems such as Cotrel-Dubousset. The surgeon must pay strict attention

to proper selection of a curve pattern that allows selective thoracic fusion and must use posterior (or anterior) instrumentation techniques that provide adequate thoracic correction without overcorrection. This allows appropriate spontaneous correction of the lumbar curve and maintenance of overall spinal balance.

Curve Type 2: Double Thoracic

DT type 2 curves (King type V) (38) are present when both the PT and MT regions are structural and must be included in the instrumentation and fusion. Radiographs show the PT region to be structural when there is a positive T1 tilt with the left first rib higher than the right (38,85). On opposite side bending, a residual PT curvature of 25 degrees or more also indicates a structural PT region. In the sagittal plane, hyperkyphosis (T2–5 +20 degrees or more) also renders that region structural. The patient usually has an elevated shoulder preoperatively and increased fullness to the left trapezial region (42,57). The surgeon must also be mindful, however, of the structural radiographic components of the PT curve even when the shoulders are level or the right shoulder is slightly high preoperatively (52). As with MT curves, the DT curve pattern can occur with an A, B, or

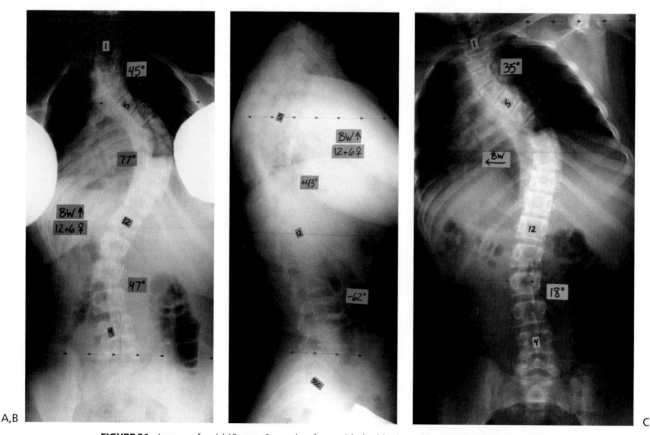

FIGURE 21. Images of a girl 12 years 6 months of age with double thoracic type 2B+ idiopathic scoliosis. **A:** Upright coronal view shows 45-degree proximal thoracic (PT), 77-degree main thoracic (MT), 47-degree compensatory left lumbar scoliosis. The center sacral vertical line touches the apical pedicle at L2; thus the lumbar modifier is B. **B:** Sagittal view shows thoracic hyperkyphosis measuring +43 degrees between T5 and T12 (+ sagittal modifier). **C:** Left side-bending radiograph shows the structural PT region bending out to only 35 degrees. The lumbar curve is nonstructural, bending out to 18 degrees. *(Figure continues.)*

C lumbar pattern and a −, N, or + sagittal thoracic modifier (Fig. 21).

Once the DT curve pattern is identified, there are several ways of surgically correcting it with segmental instrumentation such as Cotrel-Dubousset. Invariably, both the PT and MT curves are instrumented and fused through the posterior route (45). The instrumentation sequence depends on the sagittal plane alignment in both the PT and the MT regions. If the PT region is hyperkyphotic or normally kyphotic, convex compression in that region should be performed before any concave distraction. Conversely, when the MT region is hypokyphotic, concave distraction and posterior translational forces should be applied before any convex compression to improve thoracic kyphosis (85). In the rare instances in which a rod rotation maneuver is performed to manage the MT curve, a rod extension device such as a domino must be added before left upper thoracic convex compression is performed. The right-sided rod provides concave distraction to the upper thoracic curve and convex compression to the MT curve (52). Regardless of the instrumentation sequences performed, the goals of managing DT curves are to correct coronal and sagittal malalignment and to produce level shoulders with the best possible lumbar curve position (Fig. 22).

Curve Type 3: Double Major

When both the thoracic and lumbar curves are structural, the curve pattern is defined as DM. The typical pattern is a right thoracic, left TL/L curve in which the thoracic curve is nearly equal to the lumbar curve in Cobb measurement. A DM curve pattern has similar thoracic to lumbar structural characteristics as well, including Cobb magnitude, apical vertebral rotation, and apical vertebral translation (Fig. 23) (48). The lumbar curve often is more flexible than the thoracic on side bending. This indicates that the more rigid thoracic rib cage limits the flexibility of the thoracic curve. The TL/L component side bends 25 degrees or more and often has grade II residual Nash-Moe rotation or more at the apex on side bending. If kyphosis of the thoracolumbar junctional exists (T10–L2 sagittal Cobb angle + 20 degrees or more), these curve patterns must be considered DM type 3. In this circumstance, the TL/L region is structural because of the kyphosis, and the instrumentation and fusion must extend into the mid to lower lumbar spine to avoid stopping at the apex of the lumbar curve in the sagittal plane. The clinical appearance of the patient usually is fairly well-balanced coronal alignment in which the thoracic and lumbar prominences and trunk shifts offset each other. These patients often the least-

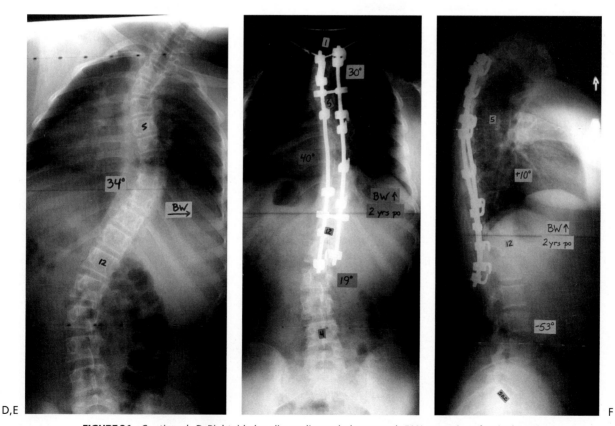

FIGURE 21. *Continued.* **D:** Right side-bending radiograph shows nearly 50% correction of main thoracic (MT) curve to 34 degrees. Posterior instrumentation and fusion from T2 to L1 with convex compression forces were performed over the MT region not only to correct scoliosis but also to remove some kyphosis. Posterior convex compression removes kyphosis in the sagittal plane. **E:** Coronal radiograph obtained 2 years postoperatively shows excellent spinal and shoulder balance. **F:** Postoperative lateral view shows removal of thoracic kyphosis by means of posterior convex compression instrumentation.

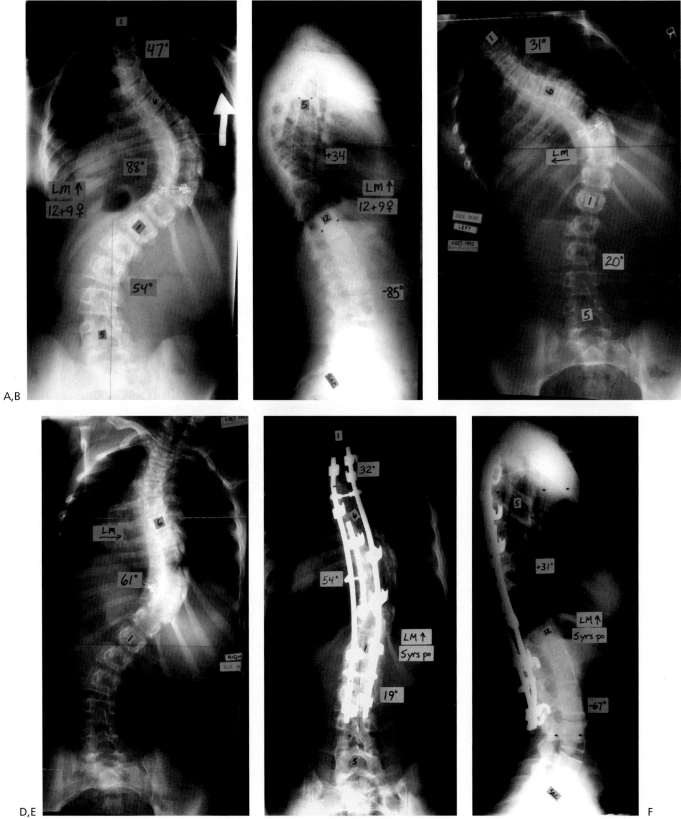

A,B

C

D,E

F

FIGURE 22. **A–F** *(Figure continues.)*

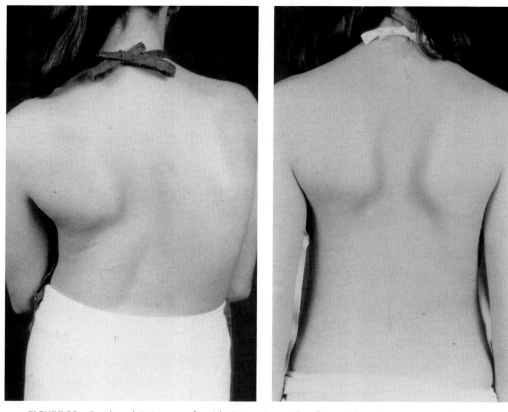

G

H

FIGURE 22. *Continued.* **A:** Images of a girl 12 years 9 months of age with 47-degree proximal thoracic (PT), 88-degree main thoracic (MT), and 54-degree lumbar scoliosis. The MT region is the most structural curve. **B:** Preoperative sagittal radiograph shows no abnormalities and excellent lumbar lordosis. **C:** Left side-bending radiograph shows PT region to be structural with a residual 31-degree curve and the lumbar region to be nonstructural (20 degrees). **D:** Right side-bending radiograph shows correction of the MT curve to only 61 degrees. Thus the classification is 2BN with the stable vertebra being L3. Anterior release and fusion of the MT curve was performed from T8 to L2 and was followed by posterior instrumentation and fusion with Cotrel-Dubousset instrumentation from T3 to L3, which was the stable vertebra preoperatively. **E:** Coronal radiograph obtained 5 years postoperatively shows excellent balance to spine. **F:** Postoperative lateral view shows maintenance of harmonious lumbar lordosis and overall global sagittal alignment. **G:** Preoperative clinical photograph shows marked trunk shift and asymmetry. **H:** Postoperative clinical photograph shows dramatic correction of deformity.

deformed appearance at upright examination because of the balancing effect of the two curves. However on forward bending, the thoracic and lumbar prominences are visible and may be almost symmetric according at scoliometer evaluation.

Many DM curve patterns can be corrected with a 90-degree rod rotation maneuver with a left-sided rod (thoracic concave–lumbar convex). This maneuver translates the apex of the thoracic and lumbar curves toward the midline for improved coronal correction, simultaneously improves thoracic kyphosis, and improves lumbar lordosis (49). Although hooks are well established in the lumbar spine, the placement of convex TL/L pedicle screws appears to provide superior three-column attachment to the spine (3,30,76) and appears to be a safe technique when performed by an experienced surgeon (14,53). This becomes important not only to provide a horizontal and central orientation to the lowest instrumented vertebra in the coronal plane but also to maximize instrumented thoracolumbar and lumbar lordosis in the sagittal plane.

Most DM type 3 curves occur with a type C lumbar modifier

because the apex of the TL/L spine is completely off the CSVL. There are occasions when the thoracic curve is quite large (more than 75 degrees), when a lumbar type B or even type A modifier is present and the TL/L region is structural because of inflexibility on side bending, or when there is thoracolumbar junctional kyphosis. The thoracic sagittal plane modifier dictates which instrumentation sequence is performed first in the thoracic region—concave distraction, translation, or derotation as opposed to convex compression and translation as the initial force application (73).

Curve Type 4: Triple Major

In these curve types, all three regions of the spine—PT, MT, and TL/L—are surgically structural. The MT curve usually is the major (largest) curve, although occasionally the TL/L curve is larger. Although triple major is a rare curve type, it is encountered and necessitate long instrumentation and fusion to cover all three structural regions of the spine. Initial anterior release and fusion sometimes is performed on either the thoracic or

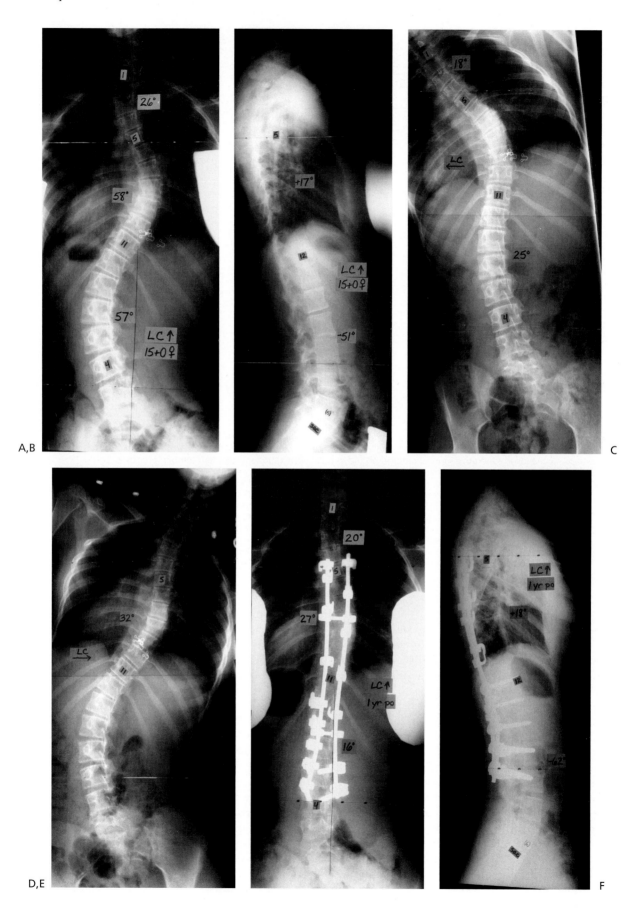

A,B

C

D,E

F

TL/L component because of the large curve size (more than 80 degrees), curve rigidity (more than 50 degrees residual side-bending curve), or hyperkyphosis in the thoracic, thoracolumbar, or lumbar sagittal plane.

A variety of constructs can be used to correct TM curve patterns with Cotrel-Dubousset instrumentation. If the thoracic and lumbar curves in the coronal and sagittal planes are amenable to a 90-degree rod rotation maneuver, this maneuver can be performed with a left-sided rod connecting the MT and TL/L regions. After this step, a domino can be applied to the upper end of the rod to connect to a second rod that attaches to the left (convex) portion of the PT curve. Convex compression forces can then be applied to this portion of the spine. A single correcting rod can be placed from the upper thoracic region (T2 or T3) down to the lowest instrumented vertebra, which is usually L3 or L4 in these TM curve patterns (Fig. 24).

A single rod can attach from the PT region to the lumbar region with appropriate cantilever, translational, and compression-distraction maneuvers for curve correction. It is imperative that sagittal plane alignment, especially in the TL/L region, be optimized in these long instrumentations and fusions. The thoracolumbar region should remain neutral to slightly lordotic while the lumbar region should have increasing lordosis from proximal to distal to optimize sagittal contour and balance (16,41,78). I prefer pedicle screws in the TL/L spine for superior correction in both the coronal and sagittal planes and to minimize postoperative loss of correction and pseudarthrosis.

Curve Type 5: Thoracolumbar/Lumbar

In this curve pattern, the TL/L curve is the major (largest) curve, having nonstructural PT and MT regions. A thoracolumbar curve exists when the apex is located in the body of T12 through the body of L1. A lumbar curve exists when the apex is located from the L1–2 disc to the L4 vertebral body. In these curve patterns that have varying degrees of curvature present in the MT region, it usually means the MT region does not have to be included in instrumentation and fusion of the TL/L curve. All of these curves have a lumbar type C modifier because any TL/L curve that requires surgical correction be completely deviated from the CSVL. The sagittal plane usually is fairly normal in these curve types but may have mild kyphosis in the thoracolumbar junction with or without hypolordosis of the proximal lumbar region.

A common instrumentation strategy for these curve patterns has been anterior instrumentation and fusion that covers the measured Cobb levels of the curve (Fig. 25) (36,59,77). The anterior Cotrel-Dubousset Horizon construct has provided excellent results in curve correction, maintenance of correction, and minimal pseudarthrosis (77). It is essential to maintain optimal TL/L sagittal alignment with these anterior convex compressive instrumentation constructs. Our preferred technique is to place structural grafts or cages into the anterior aspect of all disc spaces below T12 before insertion of the instrumentation (77). In this respect, the anterior half of the disc is held open in segmental lordosis before application of cantilever and rotational correcting forces with rod placement and convex compression forces that follow to optimize coronal correction. With this technique, I can obtain adequate coronal curve correction while maintaining or even occasionally increasing TL/L lordosis. Autogenous bone from an ipsilateral rib excised during the anterior exposure is used for placing bone graft both within structural cages and around the cages against adjacent vertebral end plates that have been mildly ablated to increase vascularity. The goals are horizontal and central orientation of the lowest instrumented vertebra in the coronal plane and maximal alignment in the sagittal plane.

A posterior approach to these curves can be used, most recently posterior transpedicular instrumentation and fusion. Often the lowest level of instrumentation is one level more distal with posterior rather than anterior techniques (7). However, this is certainly a matter of surgeon selection and opinion. Most scoliosis surgeons agree that posterior placement of hooks into the lumbar spine does not allow enough correction to equate with anterior techniques or posterior transpedicular techniques.

Curve Type 6: Thoracolumbar/Lumbar—Main Thoracic

In this curve pattern, the TL/L region is the major (largest) curve because it is larger than the MT curve. However, the MT curve is surgically structural in either the coronal plane (more than 25 degrees on side bending) or the sagittal plane (T10–L2, Cobb angle greater than +20 degrees) or both. Most of these curve patterns require posterior instrumentation and fusion that covers the MT and TL/L region. The instrumentation techniques used can be quite similar to those for DM curves; however, because the TL/L curve is inherently a larger curve, rod rotation maneuvers do not work as well in more equally matched thoracic and

FIGURE 23. Images of a 15-year-old girl with progressive double major (DM) idiopathic scoliosis. This is classified as a type 3CN curve pattern with the thoracic curve being the major curve. **A:** Upright coronal view shows 58-degree right thoracic with 57-degree left lumbar scoliosis. **B:** Sagittal view shows normalized thoracic (+ 17 degrees) region without thoracolumbar junctional kyphosis. **C:** Left side-bending radiograph shows the proximal thoracic region is nonstructural (18 degrees) and the lumbar region is structural, bending out to 25 degrees. **D:** Right side-bending radiograph shows the main thoracic curve bends out to 32 degrees. This is considered a DM curve (type 3CN) according to the objective structural criteria and because of the equal structural appearance to both the thoracic and lumbar regions. It would be extremely difficult to perform selective fusion on this curve type and obtain adequate radiographic and clinical results. Posterior instrumentation and fusion was performed from T5 to L4 with Cotrel-Dubousset Horizon instrumentation. Hooks were placed in the thoracic spine. Thoracolumbar and lumbar pedicle screws were used for both correction of scoliosis and maintenance of lumbar lordosis. **E:** Radiograph obtained 1 year postoperatively shows excellent correction with horizontal and central lowest instrumented vertebra (L4). **F:** Sagittal view shows normalized and harmonious thoracic and thoracolumbar and lumbar sagittal alignment, which is imperative in this long fusion.

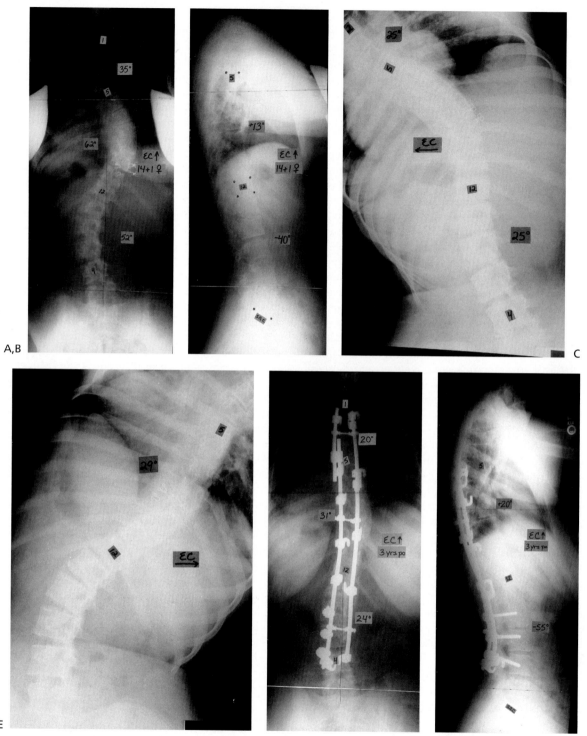

A,B

C

D,E

F

FIGURE 24. Images of a girl 14 years 1 month of age with triple major adolescent idiopathic scoliosis. The curve type classification is 4CN. **A:** Upright coronal view shows 35-degree proximal thoracic, 62-degree main thoracic (MT), and 52-degree left lumbar scoliosis. **B:** Sagittal view shows mild hypokyphosis with +13 degrees of kyphosis between T5 and T12. **C:** Left side-bending radiograph shows both proximal thoracic (25 degrees) and lumbar (25 degrees) regions are structural according to the radiographic criteria. **D:** Right side-bending view shows the MT region is more structural, bending out to 29 degrees. According to the radiographic criteria, all three regions of the spine are structural and should be considered for surgical fusion (classification 4CN). Long posterior Cotrel-Dubousset instrumentation was performed from T2 to L4. A rod rotation maneuver was performed over the thoracic and lumbar regions with a left concave rod between T5 and L4. An axial extension device (domino) was placed to correct the proximal left thoracic region with the short separate rod from T2 through T5. A long rod was placed on the right side of the spine to span the entire length of the construct from T2 to L4. **E:** Coronal radiograph obtained 3 years postoperatively shows good correction with adequate balance. **F:** Lateral radiograph shows harmonious sagittal contour throughout. The rod rotation maneuver slightly increased thoracic kyphosis (+7 degrees) and improved lumbar lordosis (−15 degrees), which should benefit the distal unfused lumbar spine in the long term.

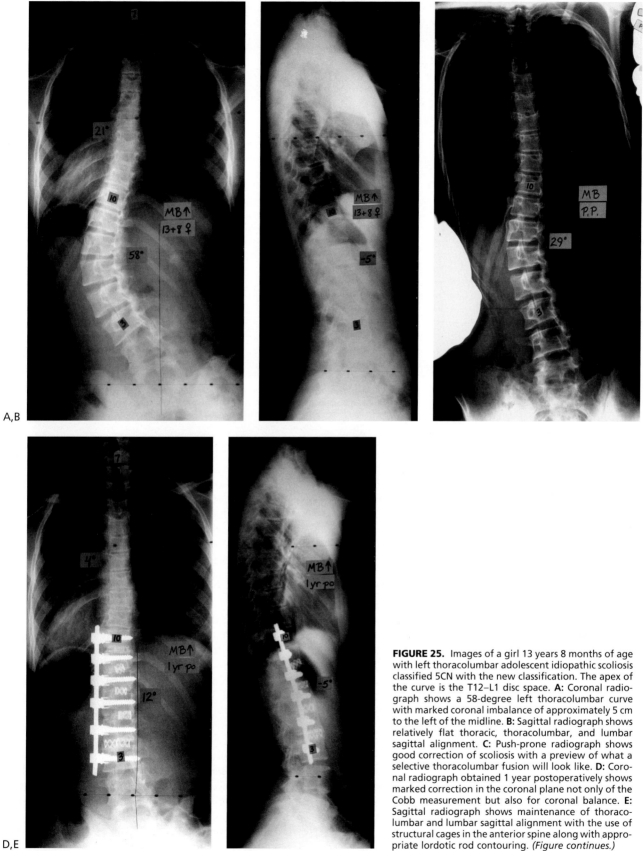

A,B

C

D,E

FIGURE 25. Images of a girl 13 years 8 months of age with left thoracolumbar adolescent idiopathic scoliosis classified 5CN with the new classification. The apex of the curve is the T12–L1 disc space. **A:** Coronal radiograph shows a 58-degree left thoracolumbar curve with marked coronal imbalance of approximately 5 cm to the left of the midline. **B:** Sagittal radiograph shows relatively flat thoracic, thoracolumbar, and lumbar sagittal alignment. **C:** Push-prone radiograph shows good correction of scoliosis with a preview of what a selective thoracolumbar fusion will look like. **D:** Coronal radiograph obtained 1 year postoperatively shows marked correction in the coronal plane not only of the Cobb measurement but also for coronal balance. **E:** Sagittal radiograph shows maintenance of thoracolumbar and lumbar sagittal alignment with the use of structural cages in the anterior spine along with appropriate lordotic rod contouring. *(Figure continues.)*

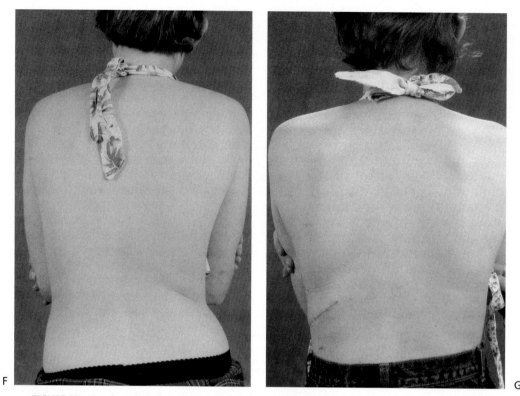

FIGURE 25. *Continued.* **F:** Upright clinical view shows marked trunk shift to the left and coronal imbalance. Anterior single Cotrel-Dubousset Horizon rod instrumentation and fusion from T10 to L3 were performed. **G:** Postoperative clinical standing view shows marked improvement in trunk shift and overall alignment.

lumbar curve patterns. I prefer convex pedicle screws placed in the TL/L region even extending into the lower thoracic region to gain purchase well above the apex of the TL/L curve (Fig. 26). Standard hook constructs are used in the thoracic region. Preliminary anterior release and fusion of the TL/L component sometimes is needed because of increased curve magnitude, rigidity, kyphosis, or risk of crankshaft phenomenon (73). In extremely rare instances, an anterior-only procedure may be performed on the TL/L region in which the structural MT region corrects spontaneously and balances into an acceptable position. As always, TL/L sagittal alignment is paramount in these fusions that extend into the mid and lower lumbar spine.

Results of Cotrel-Dubousset Instrumentation for Adolescent Idiopathic Scoliosis

Since 1985, surgeons at my institution have performed more than 700 Cotrel-Dubousset instrumentation procedures for the management of adolescent idiopathic scoliosis. Before 1996, all these operations were performed with a posterior approach and the original Cotrel-Dubousset system. Since 1996, we have used the Cotrel-Dubousset Horizon system with a posterior or an anterior approach for correction of isolated MT, thoracolumbar, and lumbar curves (82).

Over the last 15 years, our correction techniques have changed from primarily rod rotation techniques to more rod translational techniques. The newer techniques entail cantilever

insertion and application of mild compression and distraction forces on vertebral segments. The force applied is based on the angulation of the discs and on the alignment of the coronal and sagittal planes. The effect of these posterior techniques on three-dimensional correction of the deformity is unclear (39,40,83).

Through the years, our coronal results using Cotrel-Dubousset implants has averaged approximately 50% to 60% curve correction. Even with segmental spinal instrumentation, there is still a few degrees' loss of correction as the spinal settles. There appears to be less settling with the use of segmental pedicle screw instrumentation. We have reported our results with the original Cotrel-Dubousset system in the management of adolescent idiopathic scoliosis with 2-year (46) and with 5- and 10-year follow-up results (51). None of our patients has had pseudarthrosis, broken rods, or loss of correction in either the coronal or sagittal planes with use of the original Cotrel-Dubousset system. Our results with the newer Cotrel-Dubousset Horizon system mimic those of the original system.

In the sagittal plane, the results of segmental spinal instrumentation with systems such as the Cotrel-Dubousset have been even more impressive, especially in the TL/L region (11). In the MT region, production of kyphosis in patients with hypokyphosis or lordosis is possible but often is difficult. On average, thoracic sagittal alignment is minimally changed with posterior Cotrel-Dubousset instrumentation. In the TL/L spine, however, we can maintain or even enhance lordosis over the instrumented regions by means of a combination of proper intraoperative posi-

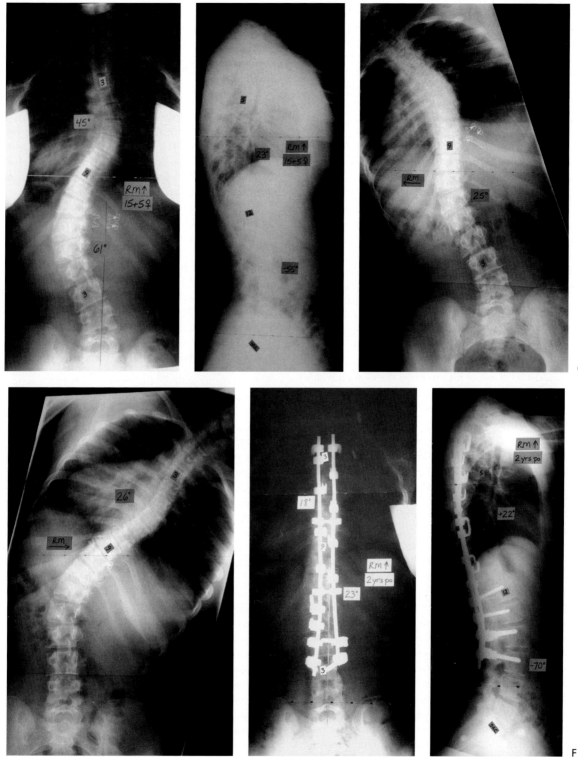

FIGURE 26. Images of a girl 15 years 5 months of age with progressive adolescent idiopathic scoliosis. **A:** Upright coronal view shows a 45-degree main thoracic (MT), 61-degree thoracolumbar (TL) curve pattern. **B:** Sagittal view shows normalized thoracic kyphosis and lumbar lordosis. **C:** Left side-bending view shows proximal thoracic curve is nonstructural, whereas the TL curve bends out to 25 degrees. **D:** Right side-bending view shows MT curve structural bending out to 26 degrees. The curve pattern is 6CN, the major (largest) curve being the TL curve; however, the MT curve is structural according to the objective criteria (>25 degrees on side bending). Posterior Cotrel-Dubousset Horizon instrumentation was performed from T3–L3. **E:** Coronal view obtained 2 years postoperative shows excellent correction with good position of the lowest instrumented vertebra (L3). **F:** Sagittal view obtained 3 years postoperatively shows improved thoracolumbar and lumbar lordosis with the use of pedicle screws between T12 and L3.

tioning of the patient, use of convex compression forces in the TL/L spine before concave distraction forces, application of multisegmental pedicle screw constructs, and appropriate rod bending and cantilever insertion (76). As other authors have shown (19,24,26,49,87), axial plane derotation has been minimal with posterior Cotrel-Dubousset implants. However, my colleagues and I believe use of anterior instrumentation techniques has improved apical derotation both radiographically and clinically.

Complications

At my institution the complication rate of Cotrel-Dubousset instrumentation for adolescent idiopathic scoliosis has been extremely low. The most concerning complication is spinal cord injury. At my institution there have been no major or minor neurologic deficits among patients with adolescent idiopathic scoliosis population treated by means of anterior or posterior segmental spinal instrumentation with the Cotrel-Dubousset or any other system. A few cases of early hook dislodgment have necessitated revision with transpedicular instrumentation. A common feature of these cases has been correction of TL/L kyphosis by means of posterior segmental instrumentation with hooks alone. We definitely advocate the use of transpedicular screws for distal fixation in the care of patients with any form of kyphosis in the TL/L spine for improved three-column support of the vertebrae during healing.

In more than 700 Cotrel-Dubousset consecutive operations for adolescent idiopathic scoliosis at my institution there have been 5 known cases of pseudarthrosis necessitating revision instrumentation and fusion (less than 1%). This compares quite favorably with results of other series in which Cotrel-Dubousset equipment was used. Early in our experience, there were several cases of postoperative coronal decompensation in false DM curves that were managed with selective thoracic fusion (46). Lessons learned in these cases, including appropriate identification of curve patterns that can undergo successful selective thoracic fusion and the ability to judge the appropriate amount of thoracic curve correction to allow spinal balance with a spontaneously corrected lumbar region below, have almost eliminated this difficulty. Since 1990, no instance of postoperative imbalance necessitating revision instrumentation and fusion has occurred when the Cotrel-Dubousset system has been used. However, many of these curve patterns that carry risk of postoperative decompensation (true King II, new types 1B and 1C) have been managed with anterior thoracic instrumentation, which has been shown to lessen the risk of decompensation with improved lumbar spontaneous curve correction as described elsewhere (7).

With use of the old Cotrel-Dubousset system, implant prominence was more than occasionally a problem. Certain implants were suspect, including convex thoracic pedicle hooks or DTT devices placed in the main or upper thoracic region. Although use of the lower-profile Cotrel-Dubousset Horizon system has lessened this problem, we still occasionally see a prominent implant on extremely thin female patients in long-term follow-up evaluations. This occurs because of muscle hypotrophy after successful spinal fusion over the instrumented regions. Although this is rarely a serious enough problem to manage surgically, we did remove implants from one patient 3 years postoperatively because of pain and prominence of the Cotrel-Dubousset Horizon system. The patient was found to have successful fusion and did well after implant removal.

We always use autogenous bone for fusion in the care of patients with adolescent idiopathic scoliosis. Approximately one half of these patients have undergone iliac crest bone grafting, and the other half have undergone convex rib thoracoplasty. We are careful to check the results of preoperative pulmonary function tests of patients on whom we are considering performing thoracoplasty (31). A decline in pulmonary function in the early postoperative period is normal after thoracoplasty (averaging 15%), but this improves to the preoperative baseline within 2 years of the operation for most patients (50,81).

Among patients with adolescent idiopathic scoliosis, the rate of implant-related complications of anterior or posterior Cotrel-Dubousset instrumentation should be only 1% or 2% in both the short and the long term. However, this figure is based on many factors, including appropriate patient selection, use of instrumentation techniques with the appropriate number of force applicators placed by means of mechanically appropriate techniques, and strict attention to frontal and sagittal balance, specifically sagittal plane alignment in the TL/L region.

Nonidiopathic Syndrome Scoliosis

Many patients with developmental and genetic syndromes such as neurofibromatosis (34,69), Marfan syndrome (Fig. 27), and Friedreich ataxia have scoliotic spinal deformities that necessitate surgical intervention. These deformities are quite amenable to management with Cotrel-Dubousset spinal instrumentation. Most patients with these syndromes are treated with posterior instrumentation with or without concomitant anterior fusion. Similar principles of instrumentation must be observed. These include secure segmental instrumentation with strong proximal and distal foundations; use of multiple implants, including distal segmental screw fixation and often extending more proximally; and appropriate application of compression, distraction, and translation forces in the sagittal and coronal planes. The operative goals are similar. These include optimizing frontal balance with ideal positioning of the lowest instrumented vertebra when instrumenting to L2 and below; techniques to obtain horizontal, central, and neutral orientation of the lowest segment on the pelvis; and in the sagittal plane, obtaining normalized thoracic, thoracolumbar, and lumbar regional alignment and maintaining global spinal balance.

Unique to these syndrome cases is that often there are greater degrees of sagittal and coronal plane malalignment, including hyperkyphosis in the thoracic, thoracolumbar, and lumbar regions; severe thoracic lordosis; large curve magnitudes with Cobb measurements greater than 100 degrees; vertebral dysplasia, as in neurofibromatosis (69) (Fig. 28); and often greater degrees of spinal osteoporosis among these usually less active children. Instrumentation techniques used to counteract these difficulties include more frequent use of anterior discectomy and fusion to obtain both increased curve flexibility and promote spinal fusion; use of more complex instrumentation techniques with increased use of dominoes, pedicle screws, and sublaminar or Wisconsin wires; and the use of additional external support with postoperative bracing after difficult reconstructions (Fig. 29).

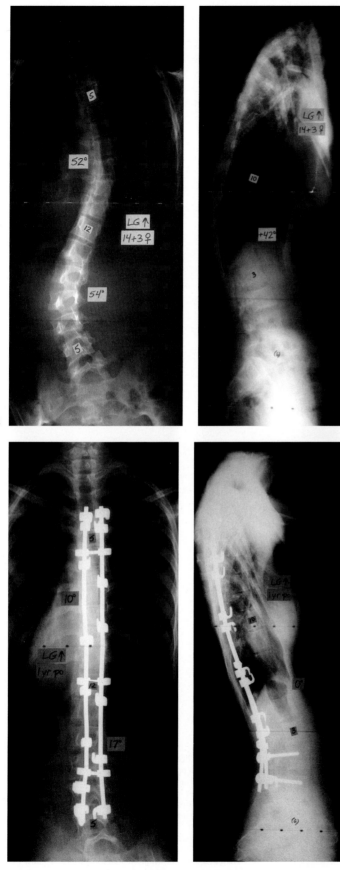

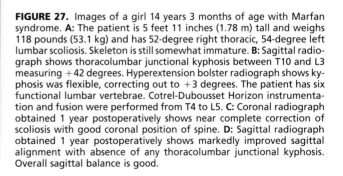

FIGURE 27. Images of a girl 14 years 3 months of age with Marfan syndrome. **A:** The patient is 5 feet 11 inches (1.78 m) tall and weighs 118 pounds (53.1 kg) and has 52-degree right thoracic, 54-degree left lumbar scoliosis. Skeleton is still somewhat immature. **B:** Sagittal radiograph shows thoracolumbar junctional kyphosis between T10 and L3 measuring +42 degrees. Hyperextension bolster radiograph shows kyphosis was flexible, correcting out to +3 degrees. The patient has six functional lumbar vertebrae. Cotrel-Dubousset Horizon instrumentation and fusion were performed from T4 to L5. **C:** Coronal radiograph obtained 1 year postoperatively shows near complete correction of scoliosis with good coronal position of spine. **D:** Sagittal radiograph obtained 1 year postoperatively shows markedly improved sagittal alignment with absence of any thoracolumbar junctional kyphosis. Overall sagittal balance is good.

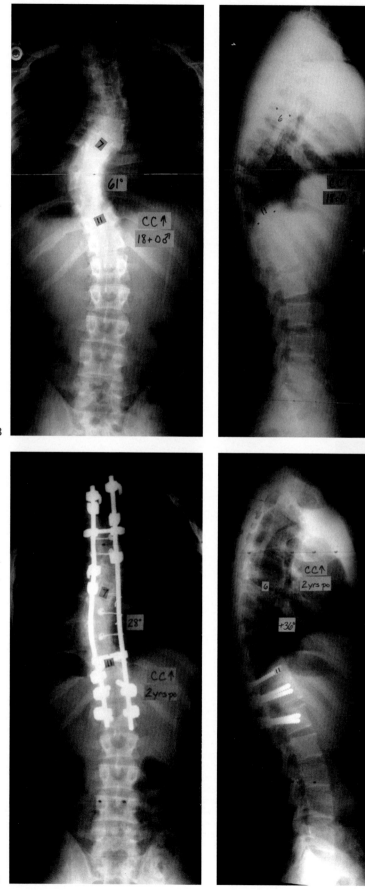

A,B

C,D

FIGURE 28. Images of an 18-year-old man with a confirmed diagnosis of neurofibromatosis with multiple café-au-lait spots. **A:** Frontal radiograph shows a short apex curve of 61 degrees between T7 and T11. **B:** Sagittal view shows similar but sharply angulated kyphosis over the same regions measuring +65 degrees. Combined anterior and posterior fusion was performed. The anterior entailed left thoracotomy and anterior spinal fusion from T6 through T12. The posterior approach entailed Cotrel-Dubousset Horizon instrumentation from T2 through L1. **C:** Coronal radiograph obtained 2 years postoperatively shows good sagittal balance and alignment. **D:** Sagittal view 2 years postoperatively shows decreased thoracic kyphosis to 36 degrees with good sagittal alignment.

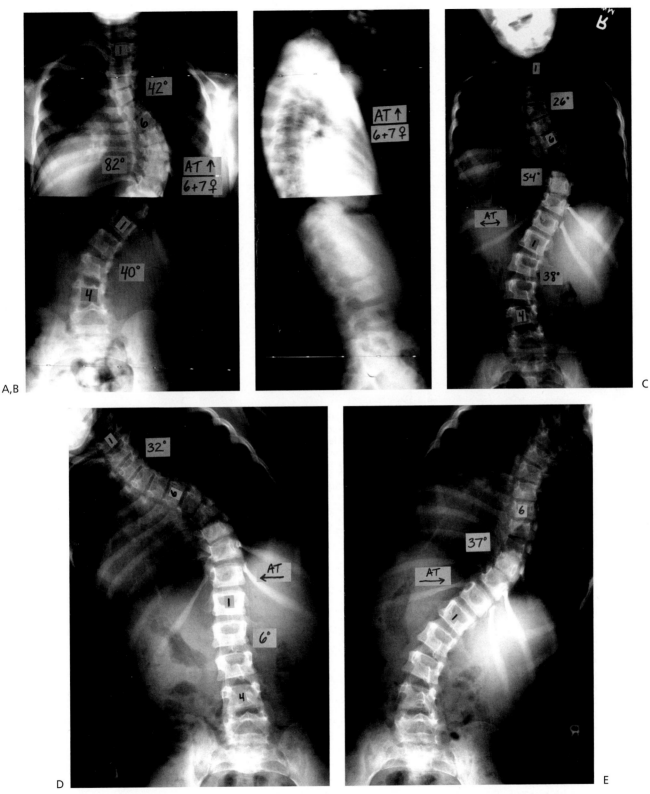

FIGURE 29. Images of a girl 6 years 7 months of age. **A:** Initial image shows 42-degree proximal thoracic (PT), 82-degree main thoracic (MT), 40-degree lumbar progressive scoliosis. Because hyperlaxity was found at the clinical examination and because of the large juvenile curvature, the patient underwent a genetics consultation, which revealed Marfan syndrome. **B:** Initial sagittal radiograph shows no unusual findings. **C:** Supine coronal view shows spontaneous correction of all three of curves as anticipated. **D:** Left side-bending, PT curve shows structural bending out to only 32 degrees. Lumbar spine was still quite flexible, bending out to 6 degrees. **E:** Right side-bending shows MT curve corrected to only 37 degrees. *(Figure continues.)*

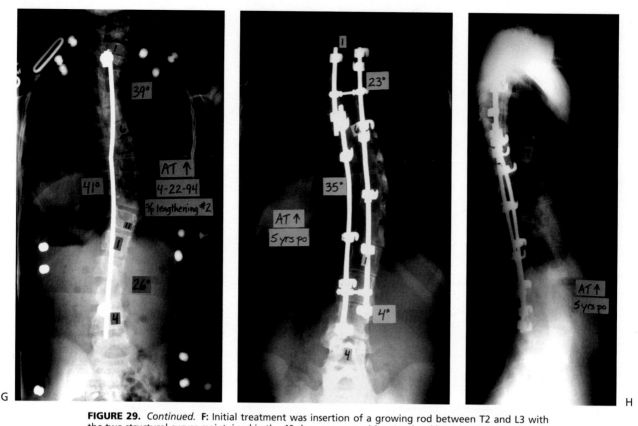

F,G   H

FIGURE 29. *Continued.* **F:** Initial treatment was insertion of a growing rod between T2 and L3 with the two structural curves maintained in the 40-degree range with several rod lengthenings. By the age of 10 years, the patient had undergone three rod lengthenings and had continued apical progression. Definitive spinal fusion with instrumentation included anterior release and fusion from T5 through T12 and same-day posterior instrumentation and fusion from T2 through L3 by means of pediatric Cotrel-Dubousset instrumentation. **G:** Coronal radiograph obtained 5 years postoperatively shows realignment in the frontal plane. Three rods were placed. The first was placed from T5 through L3 with a 90-degree rod rotation maneuver performed for improvement in both thoracic and lumbar sagittal alignment. A short compression rod was placed between T2 and T5 on the left side. A long rod spanned the entire fusion levels from T2 through L3 on the right side. **H:** Sagittal view obtained 5 years postoperatively shows relatively flat regional alignment with good overall balance.

Special consideration should be given to patients with spinal canal anomalies associated with scoliosis. These include syringomyelia (2,15), Arnold-Chiari malformation, and tethered spinal cord (28), among others. These patients often have atypical curve patterns, such as left thoracic curves, hyperkyphosis in the thoracic sagittal region, marked spinal imbalance, and increased spinal rigidity (Fig. 30). A complete history interview and thorough physical examination must be performed for any patient being prepared for an operation to correct a spinal deformity. Clinical indicators of an intraspinal anomaly include history of any type of neurologic symptoms in the upper or lower extremities, back or extremity pain out of proportion to typical overuse syndromes, asymmetric abdominal reflexes, spinal rigidity, any subtle neurologic finding in the upper or lower extremities, or juvenile onset of scoliosis (28,54). All these features warrant total-spine magnetic resonance imaging from occiput to the sacrum to evaluate the spinal canal. If an anomaly is located, consul-

tation with a neurosurgeon is appropriate for prognostic information and any potential surgical treatment. My colleagues and I have not found large curve size (greater than 70 degrees) by itself to be a sign of spinal canal anomaly (62).

The management of scoliosis in the presence of intraspinal anomalies with or without corrective neurosurgical procedures can be quite challenging. These patients often have progressively large, stiff, and kyphotic curves that prove a great surgical challenge (69). Many patients need anterior spinal fusion because of previous posterior laminectomy by the neurosurgical team. This renders the posterior-only approach prone to pseudarthrosis. These patients often have associated thoracic hyperkyphosis that necessitates convex compression instrumentation for simultaneous correction of the scoliosis and resolution of the hyperkyphosis before any concave distraction techniques can be performed. This also is quite important for the status of the spinal canal. In the care of these patients, the goal is to avoid any

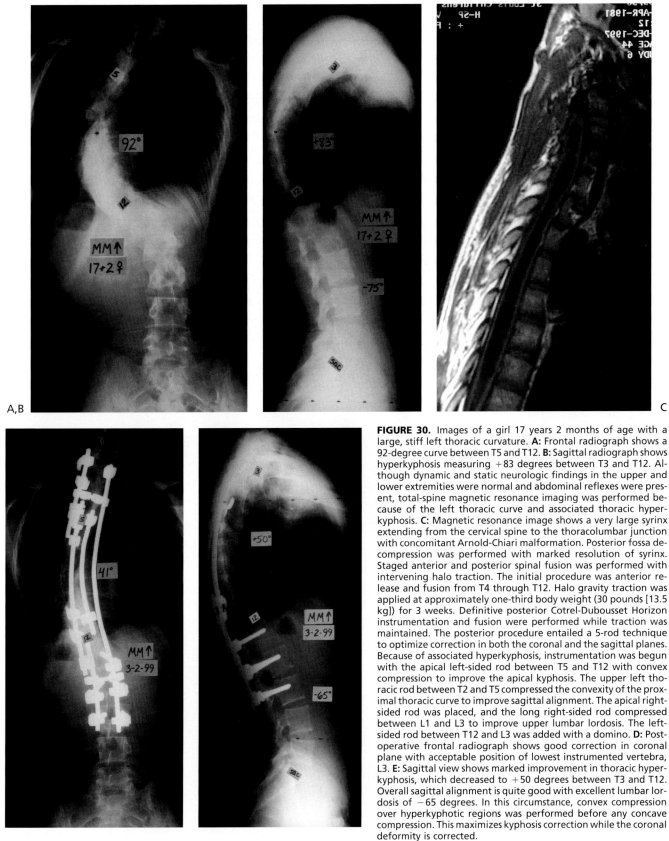

A,B

C

D,E

FIGURE 30. Images of a girl 17 years 2 months of age with a large, stiff left thoracic curvature. **A:** Frontal radiograph shows a 92-degree curve between T5 and T12. **B:** Sagittal radiograph shows hyperkyphosis measuring +83 degrees between T3 and T12. Although dynamic and static neurologic findings in the upper and lower extremities were normal and abdominal reflexes were present, total-spine magnetic resonance imaging was performed because of the left thoracic curve and associated thoracic hyperkyphosis. **C:** Magnetic resonance image shows a very large syrinx extending from the cervical spine to the thoracolumbar junction with concomitant Arnold-Chiari malformation. Posterior fossa decompression was performed with marked resolution of syrinx. Staged anterior and posterior spinal fusion was performed with intervening halo traction. The initial procedure was anterior release and fusion from T4 through T12. Halo gravity traction was applied at approximately one-third body weight (30 pounds [13.5 kg]) for 3 weeks. Definitive posterior Cotrel-Dubousset Horizon instrumentation and fusion were performed while traction was maintained. The posterior procedure entailed a 5-rod technique to optimize correction in both the coronal and the sagittal planes. Because of associated hyperkyphosis, instrumentation was begun with the apical left-sided rod between T5 and T12 with convex compression to improve the apical kyphosis. The upper left thoracic rod between T2 and T5 compressed the convexity of the proximal thoracic curve to improve sagittal alignment. The apical right-sided rod was placed, and the long right-sided rod compressed between L1 and L3 to improve upper lumbar lordosis. The left-sided rod between T12 and L3 was added with a domino. **D:** Postoperative frontal radiograph shows good correction in coronal plane with acceptable position of lowest instrumented vertebra, L3. **E:** Sagittal view shows marked improvement in thoracic hyperkyphosis, which decreased to +50 degrees between T3 and T12. Overall sagittal alignment is quite good with excellent lumbar lordosis of −65 degrees. In this circumstance, convex compression over hyperkyphotic regions was performed before any concave compression. This maximizes kyphosis correction while the coronal deformity is corrected.

type of lengthening of the spinal column (canal) with distractive techniques. It is strongly recommended that the posterior column be shortened with convex compression techniques as the initial force in operations on patients with any type of intraspinal anomaly, even if the anomalies have been addressed in previous surgical procedures.

A helpful technique in convex compression instrumentation is the use of dominoes for initial placement of a short thoracic convex rod with compression forces. Another technique is secondary extension with both proximal and distal and dominoes after the corrective maneuvers in the MT region. These techniques are especially helpful in operations on larger curves when application of a single rod from the upper thoracic region to the lower lumbar region is difficult. The tendency is for the proximal or distal implant to pull off the spine during compression on the center of the construct, which tends to elevate the proximal and distal ends of the rod secondarily. In this manner, the convex regions of the MT, PT, and TL/L spine all are approached and instrumented first, before instrumentation is placed in a distractive mode in the corresponding concave regions of the curves. With these techniques, my colleagues and I have not encountered any type of neurologic deficit in operations on patients who have undergone previous operations for

anomalies of the spinal canal (84). We also strongly recommend spinal cord monitoring with both somatosensory evoked potentials and motor evoked potentials and the use of frequent wake-up tests (84).

Neuromuscular Scoliosis

Neuromuscular disorders with associated spinal deformity that necessitate surgical correction include cerebral palsy, Duchenne muscular dystrophy, and spinal muscular atrophy, to name a few. These patients can be separated into those who can walk and those who cannot, that is, those who need spinal instrumentation that stops short of the pelvis or extends to the pelvis (1). Cotrel-Dubousset instrumentation certainly is versatile enough to manage these often complex spinal deformities in a technically feasible manner.

Patients with ambulatory cerebral palsy often have neuromuscular scoliosis that necessitates operative intervention. Most of these patients can be treated successfully with a posterior Cotrel-Dubousset system. The surgeon must be careful to pick the appropriate proximal and distal instrumentation and fusion levels. It usually is best not to "cheat" to try to save levels in operations on these patients (Fig. 31). The lowest instrumented

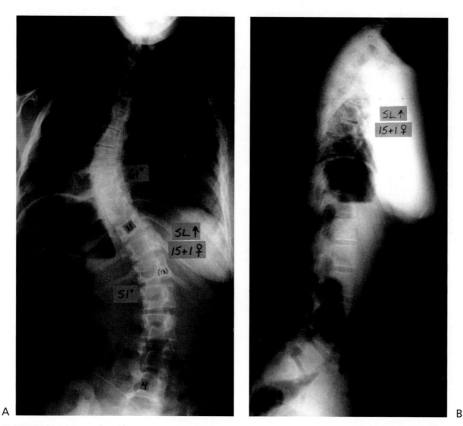

FIGURE 31. Images of a girl 15 years 1 month of age with ambulatory cerebral palsy and spastic diplegia. **A:** Initial image shows 61-degree left thoracic, 51-degree right lumbar scoliosis. **B:** Regional sagittal alignment was unremarkable; however, the global sagittal alignment was somewhat anterior owing to diplegia. *(Figure continues.)*

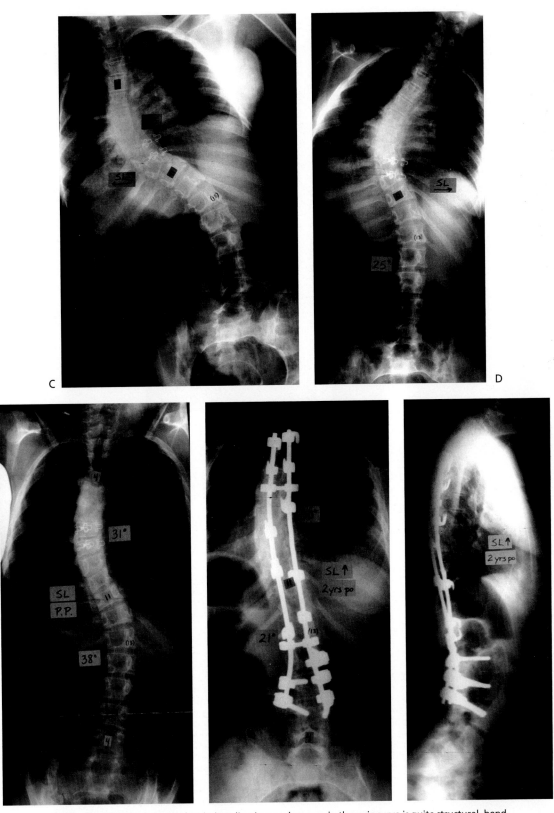

FIGURE 31. *Continued.* **C:** Left side-bending image shows main thoracic curve is quite structural, bending out to only 53 degrees. **D:** Right side-bending view shows lumbar curve is more flexible, bending out to 25 degrees. **E:** Push-prone radiograph shows good alignment and balance between T3 and L3 with correction of both the left thoracic and right lumbar regions. Posterior Cotrel-Dubousset Horizon instrumentation and fusion were performed between T3 and L3. **F:** Coronal radiograph obtained 2 years postoperatively shows good coronal balance and position of L3. **G:** Lateral radiograph obtained 2 years postoperatively shows normalized regional thoracic kyphosis and lumbar lordosis with continued anterior sagittal balance due to diplegia. Ambulatory status was not affected by the posterior fusion.

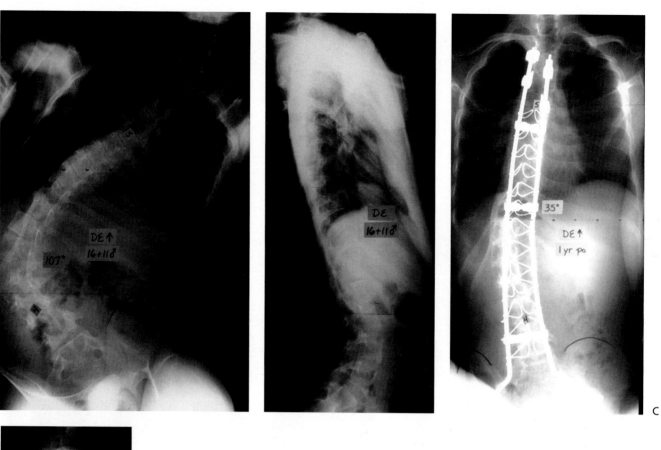

A,B

C

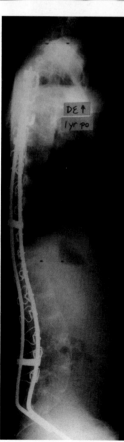

D

FIGURE 32. Images of a boy 16 years 11 months of age with spastic quadriplegic cerebral palsy. The parents stated that the sitting position was deteriorating badly even with wheelchair modifications. The patient's health was fairly good, and there was no history of serious respiratory illnesses such as pneumonia. **A:** Sitting upright frontal view shows a 107-degree left lumbar neuromuscular scoliosis with marked pelvic obliquity. Right rib cage almost touches the right ilium. **B:** Sagittal radiograph shows flat thoracic kyphosis. Same-day anterior and posterior spinal fusion were performed. Through a thoracoabdominal approach, anterior release and fusion were performed between T10 and the sacrum. Autogenous rib graft and structural tricortical allograft iliac wedges were placed in the lower lumbar disc spaces. The patient was placed in a halo with right-sided ipsilateral femoral traction. Fifteen pounds (6.6 kg) were placed on the skull and 20 lb (9 kg) on the right femur. This provided excellent coronal correction of pelvic obliquity during the posterior procedure. **C:** Posterior instrumentation and fusion extended from T3 to the sacrum. Cotrel-Dubousset Horizon rods, bilateral claws at the proximal end of fusion, multiple 16-gauge sublaminar wires, and three cross-links were used. The graft comprised autogenous local bone and fresh frozen femoral head allograft with demineralized bone matrix mixed in. Coronal radiograph obtained 1 year postoperatively shows marked improvement in coronal alignment and near complete horizontalization of pelvic obliquity. **D:** Sagittal postoperative radiograph shows excellent sitting posture.

vertebra should be the true stable vertebra with the expectation that the lower fusion mass is completely centered over the pelvis (38). Previously described principles of strong proximal and distal foundations with intermediate hook, wire, or screw fixation points provide adequate fixation. Sublaminar wires often are helpful to patients with neuromuscular scoliosis. It is reasonable to use sublaminar stainless steel wires with the traditional knurled Cotrel-Dubousset rod. My colleagues and I have not found that to be a problem, and wire breakage due to friction against the knurls has not occurred. This cannot be said of sublaminar cables. Friction against the knurls slowly fractures individual parts of the cable and causes total cable failure.

In the care of patients with neuromuscular scoliosis who cannot walk, instrumentation and fusion invariably have to be extended to the pelvis (Fig. 32) (1). There are two common means of gaining sacral pelvic fixation for patients with neuromuscular scoliosis—a standard Galveston bend of the distal rods seating into the distal ilium (1) or use of iliac screws that line up with the vertically directed rods extending from the sacrum to the upper thoracic region. I have had extensive experience in both of these techniques. For iliac wing screw fixation, I use Liberty iliac screws that have an offset connector to attach to the medialized longitudinal Cotrel-Dubousset rod to capture the entire spine above with hooks, wires, or screws (Fig. 33). Although not absolutely mandatory, I most often use bilateral S1 pedicle

screws to help support the iliac wing screws. I prefer this bilateral-S1, bilateral iliac screw construct for posterior-only operations on patients with spastic neuromuscular disorders when strong lumbosacral fixation is needed for successful arthrodesis. Certainly, however, a traditional Galveston bend in a Cotrel-Dubousset or Cotrel-Dubousset Horizon rod provides adequate bilateral purchase into the iliac wings and can be successful in operations on patients with flaccid neuromuscular disorders such as Duchenne muscular dystrophy (1).

Juvenile Scoliosis

The traditional Cotrel-Dubousset 7-mm knurled rod and the newer 5.5-mm Cotrel-Dubousset Horizon rod systems accommodate patients from adolescence through adulthood. Because the rod has a low profile, some older and larger children can undergo instrumentation with the Cotrel-Dubousset Horizon system. For most children, however, this system becomes too bulky for posterior use in the spine. In the past, a pediatric Cotrel-Dubousset system based on a 5-mm knurled rod was used in operations on these smaller patients. My colleagues and I have not used this system, which is similar to the 7-mm rod system, recently because of the shortcomings described earlier. We await the development of a pediatric Cotrel-Dubousset Horizon system to accommodate smaller persons with all the advantages of the Horizon system.

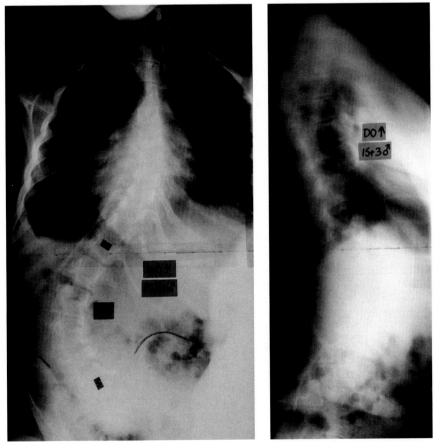

FIGURE 33. Images of a boy 15 years 3 months of age with a spastic quadriplegic cerebral palsy. **A:** Initial image shows progressive lumbar scoliosis measuring 64 degrees and a fair amount of trunk shift and pelvic obliquity. **B:** Sagittal view shows lumbar hyperlordosis. A posterior-only procedure was performed from T2 to the sacrum. *(Figure continues.)*

A,B

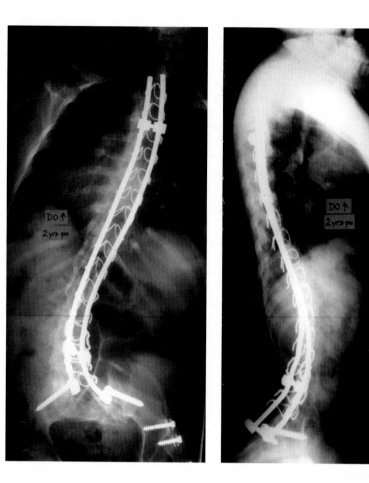

C,D

FIGURE 33. *Continued.* **C:** Radiograph obtained 2 year postoperatively shows maintenance of alignment with level pelvis. Cotrel-Dubousset Horizon rods and bilateral Liberty iliac screws were placed for sacropelvic fixation. **D:** Postoperative lateral view shows improved alignment with lessened lumbar hyperlordosis. The Liberty iliac screws were used instead of the Galveston technique to gain better purchase on iliac wings in this posterior-only procedure.

KYPHOSIS

Most types of pediatric kyphosis can be managed with Cotrel-Dubousset instrumentation (20,70). The most common diagnoses are Scheuermann kyphosis, postlaminectomy kyphosis, congenital kyphosis, and syndrome kyphosis (Fig. 34). Operations for kyphosis are inherently more challenging than operations for scoliosis and have much higher implant and neurologic complication rates. Operations for kyphosis invariably require combined anterior release and fusion with posterior instrumentation and fusion. With the advent of strong bilateral pedicle screw fixation, posterior-only techniques sometimes can be used.

Scheuermann kyphosis is the prototypical pediatric kyphotic deformity necessitating instrumentation and fusion (Fig. 35). My best results have been achieved with same-day anterior release and fusion of the MT kyphotic deformity coupled with posterior instrumentation and fusion extending from T2 or T3 down to the "stable" vertebra in the sagittal plane. Which is the stable vertebra is determined by means of drawing a vertical line from the back edge of the sacrum and picking the most proximal lumbar vertebra most closely bisected by this line. The first disc, which is in slight lordosis, invariably lies directly above this vertebra. This is a safe place to stop the distal level of instrumentation and fusion in the surgical management of kyphosis.

Traditional Cotrel-Dubousset constructs for posterior instrumentation of Scheuermann kyphosis include six pairs of single-level, bilateral, pedicle, transverse process claws from T2 to T6 or T3 to T7 (70). These are all closed hooks that are all seated in compression. At the distal end, either hooks or, preferably, pedicle screws are used with six points of fixation—most commonly three pairs of pedicle screws at a minimum at the lowest three levels of the instrumentation and fusion. Cantilever correction of the instrumentation is achieved by means of tunneling the rod into the proximal hooks and lowering both rods simultaneously into the distal screws, which are captured with appropriate set bolts. The entire construct is seated in compression, and thorough posterior fusion over the instrumented levels is performed with iliac crest bone grafting.

It has become possible to perform these operations with a posterior-only approach with multilevel pedicle screw fixation and apical wedge osteotomies to shorten the posterior column. The instrumentation hinges on the middle column and causes minimal gaping of the anterior column. This operation surgery is performed through a posterior approach with meticulous dissection to the tips of the transverse processes of each level to be instrumented for thorough anatomic landmark localization and careful bilateral pedicle screw placement. Smith-Peterson osteotomy is performed at several apical levels as needed for shortening of the posterior column and correction of kyphosis. Cantilever

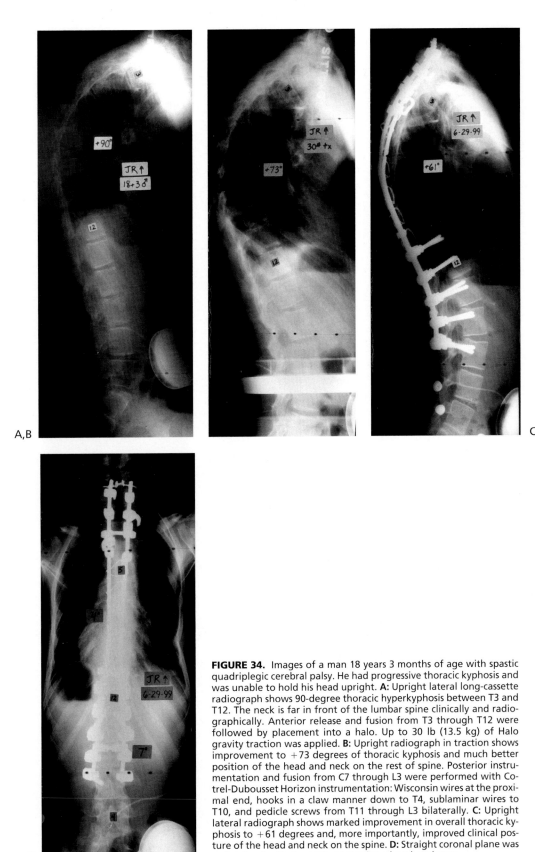

A,B

C

D

FIGURE 34. Images of a man 18 years 3 months of age with spastic quadriplegic cerebral palsy. He had progressive thoracic kyphosis and was unable to hold his head upright. **A:** Upright lateral long-cassette radiograph shows 90-degree thoracic hyperkyphosis between T3 and T12. The neck is far in front of the lumbar spine clinically and radiographically. Anterior release and fusion from T3 through T12 were followed by placement into a halo. Up to 30 lb (13.5 kg) of Halo gravity traction was applied. **B:** Upright radiograph in traction shows improvement to +73 degrees of thoracic kyphosis and much better position of the head and neck on the rest of spine. Posterior instrumentation and fusion from C7 through L3 were performed with Cotrel-Dubousset Horizon instrumentation: Wisconsin wires at the proximal end, hooks in a claw manner down to T4, sublaminar wires to T10, and pedicle screws from T11 through L3 bilaterally. **C:** Upright lateral radiograph shows marked improvement in overall thoracic kyphosis to +61 degrees and, more importantly, improved clinical posture of the head and neck on the spine. **D:** Straight coronal plane was maintained with the instrumentation placed as shown.

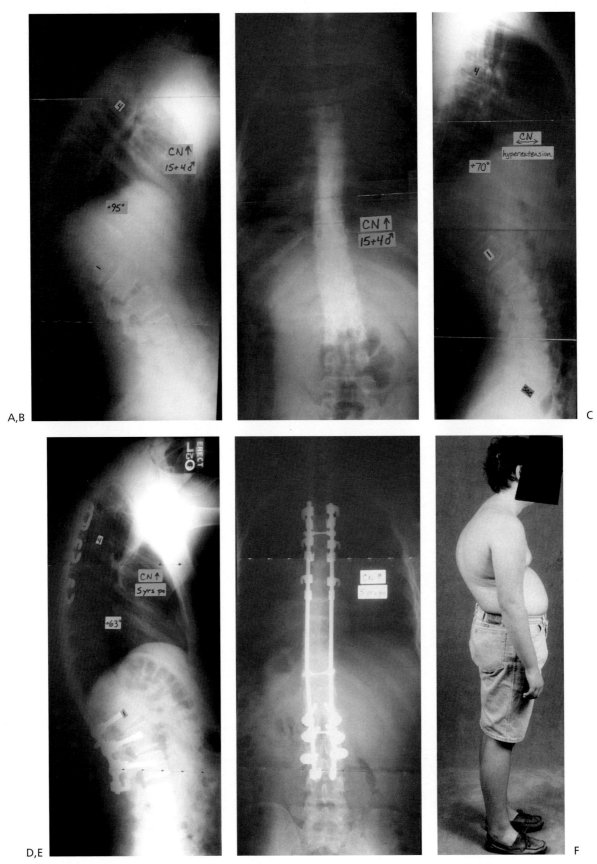

A,B

C

D,E

F

FIGURE 35. **A–F** *(Figure continues.)*

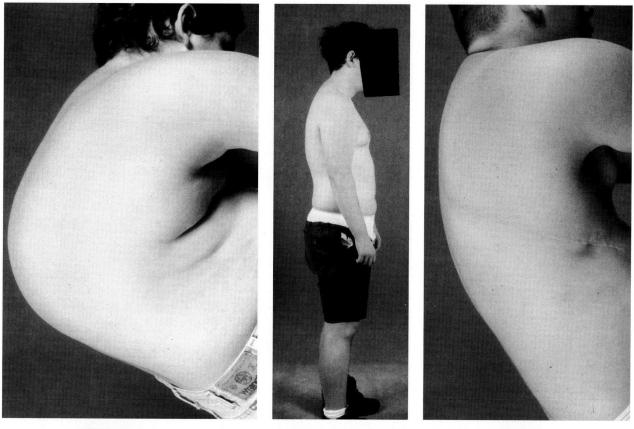

G,H

I

FIGURE 35. *Continued.* Images of a boy 15 years 4 months of age, 76 inches (1.9 m) tall, and weighing close to 300 lb (135 kg). He had painful Scheuermann kyphosis. **A:** Upright sagittal radiograph shows 95-degree thoracic kyphosis between T4–L1. **B:** Upright coronal view shows no unusual findings. **C:** Hyperextension radiograph over a bolster placed at the apex of the thoracic region shows modest correction to only 70 degrees. Findings at total-spine magnetic resonance imaging were unremarkable. Same-day anterior and posterior spinal fusion was performed anteriorly through a single thoracotomy. Disc excision and fusion from T5 through L1 also were performed. Posterior Cotrel-Dubousset instrumentation and fusion were performed from T3 through L3. **D:** Sagittal radiograph obtained 5 years postoperatively shows improvement of thoracic kyphosis to +63 degrees. Overall alignment is quite good. **E:** Coronal view 5 years postoperatively is maintained with an instrumentation construct consisting of six pairs of single-level claws between T3 and T7 and three pairs of bilateral pedicle screws between L1 and L3 with bilateral infralaminar hooks on L3. Thus there are a total of 12 fixation points above and eight fixation points below kyphosis with the two rods joined with three device for transverse traction cross-links. **F:** Preoperative clinical view shows marked kyphosis and resultant poor sagittal posture. **G:** Forward-bending view shows accentuation of the large kyphotic apex. **H:** Postoperative upright view shows a more normalized sagittal contour and posture. **I:** Forward radiograph shows marked diminution of thoracic hump. Five years after the operation the patient was pain free and had good alignment.

correction with rods occurs by means of seating the rods into the proximal screws and lowering the rods into the more distal instrumentation. Bilateral multilevel compression forces are applied to complete the correction. Although certainly not mainstream, these techniques certainly can be adequately performed with current Cotrel-Dubousset Horizon tools and implants (Fig. 36).

Postlaminectomy kyphosis poses additional problems because of lack of posterior column bone and because kyphotic deformities often are large. Anterior fusion is an absolute requirement in operations on these patients and is the cornerstone of any

surgical treatment. Posterior implants must be applied with secure proximal and distal foundations (Fig. 37). Depending on the amount of previous laminectomy, pedicle hooks can be placed in laminectomy sites if the facet joints are still intact. We prefer to keep hooks off the apex, because posterior cantilever correction tends to translate these hooks anteriorly, crack the superior facet, and plunge the hook into the spinal canal. The other instrumentation option is pedicle screw fixation, which avoids any type of canal intrusion with proper placement (4). Instrumentation principles are similar to those described for Scheuermann kyphosis.

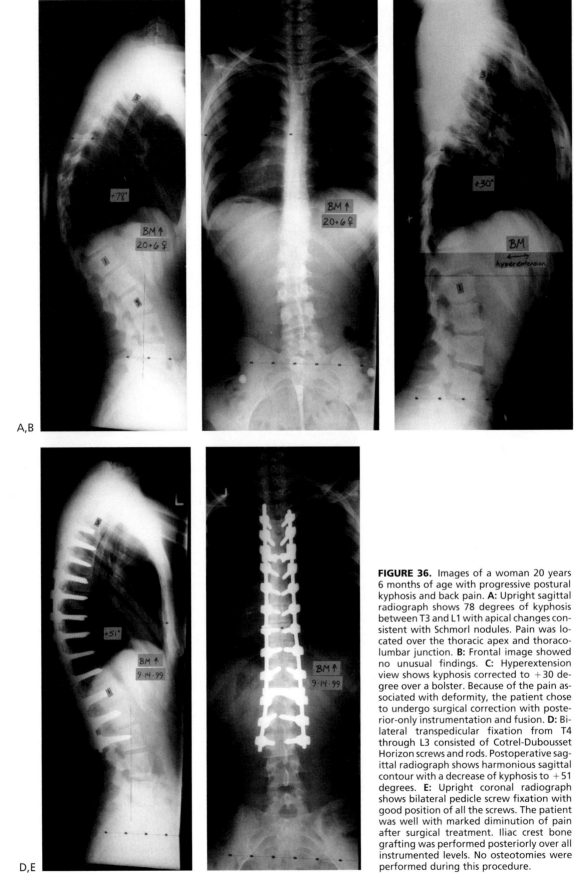

A,B

C

D,E

FIGURE 36. Images of a woman 20 years 6 months of age with progressive postural kyphosis and back pain. **A:** Upright sagittal radiograph shows 78 degrees of kyphosis between T3 and L1 with apical changes consistent with Schmorl nodules. Pain was located over the thoracic apex and thoracolumbar junction. **B:** Frontal image showed no unusual findings. **C:** Hyperextension view shows kyphosis corrected to +30 degree over a bolster. Because of the pain associated with deformity, the patient chose to undergo surgical correction with posterior-only instrumentation and fusion. **D:** Bilateral transpedicular fixation from T4 through L3 consisted of Cotrel-Dubousset Horizon screws and rods. Postoperative sagittal radiograph shows harmonious sagittal contour with a decrease of kyphosis to +51 degrees. **E:** Upright coronal radiograph shows bilateral pedicle screw fixation with good position of all the screws. The patient was well with marked diminution of pain after surgical treatment. Iliac crest bone grafting was performed posteriorly over all instrumented levels. No osteotomies were performed during this procedure.

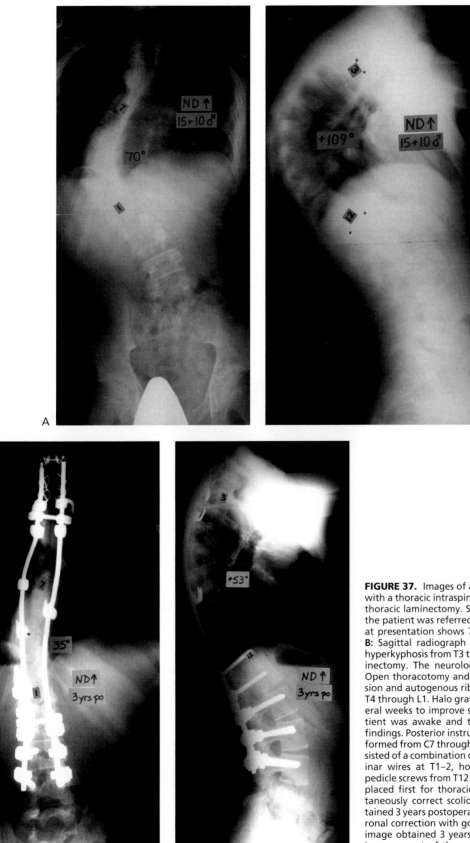

FIGURE 37. Images of a boy 15 years 10 months of age with a thoracic intraspinal tumor necessitating posterior thoracic laminectomy. Spinal deformity developed, and the patient was referred to us for further care. **A:** Image at presentation shows 70-degree left thoracic scoliosis. **B:** Sagittal radiograph shows 109 degrees of thoracic hyperkyphosis from T3 through T12 due to previous laminectomy. The neurologic findings were not unusual. Open thoracotomy and anterior release with spinal fusion and autogenous rib grafting were performed from T4 through L1. Halo gravity traction was applied for several weeks to improve sagittal alignment while the patient was awake and to carefully monitor neurologic findings. Posterior instrumentation and fusion were performed from C7 through L4. The posterior construct consisted of a combination of Wisconsin wires at C7, sublaminar wires at T1–2, hooks in the thoracic spine, and pedicle screws from T12 through L4. A left-sided rod was placed first for thoracic convex compression to simultaneously correct scoliosis and kyphosis. **C:** Image obtained 3 years postoperatively shows maintenance of coronal correction with good balance of spine. **D:** Sagittal image obtained 3 years postoperatively shows marked improvement of thoracic kyphosis with good regional and global sagittal alignment.

SPONDYLOLISTHESIS

Three types of instrumentation can be performed for pediatric spondylolysis or spondylolisthesis (10). In operations on patients with bilateral pars defects at L4 and above and chronic pain refractory to conservative treatment, bilateral pars instrumentation can be performed. Prerequisites for this procedure are bilateral pars defects of a chronic nature with L2–3 spondylolisthesis with an intact disc at the level immediately below the spondylolytic level (L4–5 for pars defects at L4). Although there are many techniques to stabilize the pars with instrumented fusion, the most common current technique is a pedicle screw infralaminar hook-rod construct with compression of the pars after bone grafting. This appears to be a stronger construct than traditional Bucks wiring or wiring of the posterior elements to a pedicle screw. This type of pedicle screw hook-rod construct should minimize any type of injury to adjacent facet joints or ligaments (10).

Low-grade, low dysplasia spondylolisthesis at L5–S1 occasionally necessitates surgical intervention. The goal is to treat just the L5–S1 segment with either posterior-only or combined anterior and posterior fusion with posterior instrumentation. Pedicle screw constructs are invariably used in these cases. At my institution the results have been superior to those obtained with uninstrumented fusion and cast immobilization. However, pedicle screw placement must be precise. A variety of screw diameters (5.0 mm, 5.5 mm, and so on) must be available for instrumentation of an L5 pediatric pedicle with spondylolisthesis. These pedicles often are quite sclerotic, small, and medially based. They provide a challenge to the surgeon trying to obtain proper screw placement. Placement becomes much easier if Gill laminectomy has been performed and direct visualization of the medial pedicle wall can be obtained.

Surgical management of high-grade dysplastic isthmic spondylolisthesis at L5–S1 is challenging, and there are several noteworthy points for use of Cotrel-Dubousset instrumentation (Fig. 38) (60). The first decision to be made is whether instrumentation extends to L4 or can stop at L5. I base this decision on the position of the L4 segment in relation to L5, the degree of retrolisthesis present, and whether disc degeneration to L4–5 is present at magnetic resonance imaging (I have found the last to be rare). The angulatory relation of L5 to the sacrum (the slip

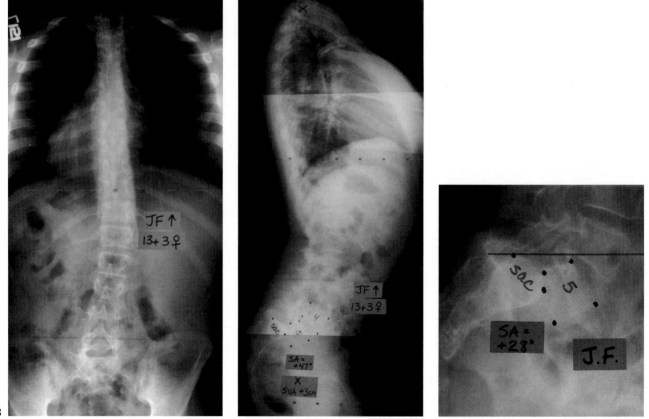

A,B   C

FIGURE 38. Images of a girl 13 years 3 months of age with lumbosacral back pain, bilateral posterior thigh and calf pain, and difficulty with forward bending. **A:** Long-cassette posteroanterior radiograph shows mild thoracolumbar scoliosis. **B:** Long-cassette lateral radiograph of the entire spine shows high-grade spondylolisthesis of L5 on the sacrum. There was approximately 80% slip with a slip angle of +47 degrees. Overall sagittal alignment was 3 cm in front of the sacrum. **C:** Supine spot lateral radiograph shows spondylolisthesis deformity. In the supine position, the slip is approximately 60%, and the slip angle is reduced to +28 degrees. *(Figure continues.)*

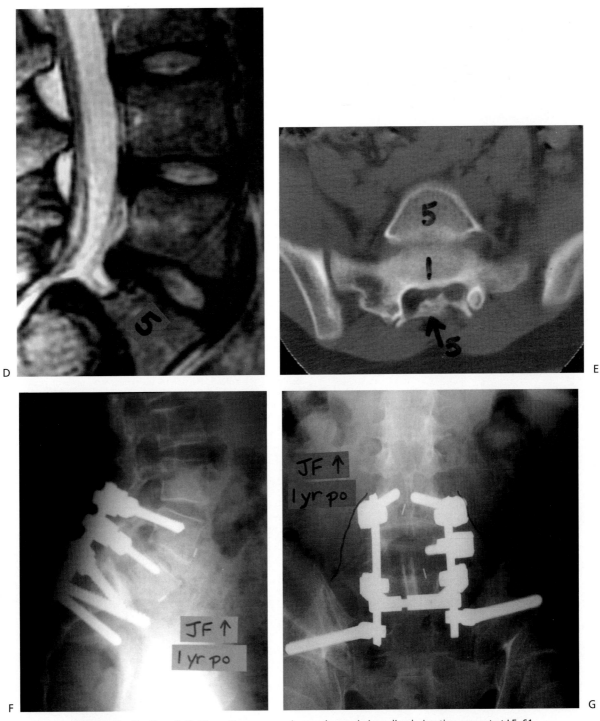

FIGURE 38. *Continued.* **D:** Magnetic resonance image shows obvious disc desiccation present at L5–S1 with the apparent pincer effect of the spinal canal behind the back edge of the sacrum and lumbosacral disc to the front edge of the L5 posterior element. **E:** Axial computed tomographic scan through the L5–S1 region shows the dysplastic posterior arch of L5, which has subluxed anteriorly into the spinal canal and caused severe canal stenosis at the L5–S1 level. A two-stage 2-day operation was performed. The initial approach was posterior, and it revealed wide L5 and S1 decompressions. Pedicle screws were placed at L4, L5, S1, and both iliac wings. Partial reduction of L4 and L5 onto the sacrum was performed. Posterolateral fusion also was performed. One week later an anterior fibular dowel graft was placed from the L5 body into the sacrum. The patient used a brace for 3 months and did quite well. **F:** Lateral radiographs obtained 1 year postoperatively show reduction of spondylolisthesis to grade II with an improved slip angle. **G:** Ferguson posteroanterior view 1 year postoperatively shows bilateral posterolateral fusions (outlined in *black*) present from L4 to the sacrum.

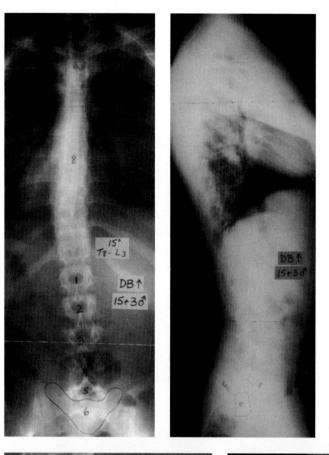

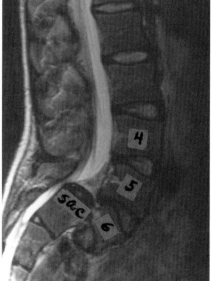

A,B

FIGURE 39. Images of a boy 15 years 3 months of age with lumbosacral back pain, bilateral lower extremity radicular pain, and numbness to the dorsal aspects of both feet. **A:** Upright anteroposterior view shows six lumbar vertebrae with a Napoleon hat sign at L6. Slight thoracolumbar scoliosis also is present. **B:** Upright long-cassette lateral view shows, although it is difficult to see, spondyloptosis of the L6 body on the sacrum. **C:** Sagittal magnetic resonance image shows alignment of L4, L5, and L6 on the sacrum. Complete spondyloptosis of the L6 vertebra is present. There was a pincer effect between the back of the lumbosacral disc and the back edge of the L5 and L6 posterior elements. Thus, the patient appeared to have grade IV spondylolisthesis of L5 at the sacrum. Same-day anterior and posterior L6 vertebrectomy were performed. Through an anterior approach, the L6 vertebral body was removed, and the base of the pedicles was taken down. Both L6 nerve roots were identified. The posterior elements of L6 and the remainder of the L6 pedicles were excised through a posterior approach. L5 was repositioned on the sacrum and held with bilateral pedicle screws at L5–S1 and iliac wing screws bilaterally. Soft posterior lumbar interbody fusion was performed. One week later, anterior structural grafting of a new L5–S1 disc space was performed to improve healing. **D:** Lateral view obtained 2 years postoperatively shows solid arthrodesis of L5 onto the sacrum with L6 completely excised. **E:** Ferguson posteroanterior view obtained 2 years postoperatively shows solid posterolateral fusion from L5 to the sacrum. Pain had completely resolved. Partial L5 weakness was present postoperatively that was worse than it had been before the operation. However, strength returned to baseline by 3 months postoperatively and had continued to improve up to 1 after the operation. At that time the patient was fully active.

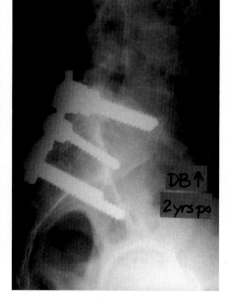

C,D

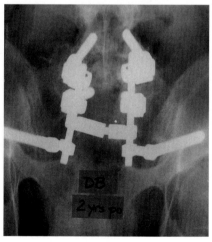

E

angle) is evaluated. The more kyphotic the lumbosacral the relation, the more likely it is that instrumentation and fusion are needed to L4. Thus pedicle screw fixation is obtained optionally at L4, definitively at L5, and bilaterally at S1. In instrumented reduction of these high-grade slips, I always use bilateral iliac wing screw fixation for a second point of lumbosacral fixation (60). The rationale is to obtain equal moment arms of fixation above and below the spondylolytic level, which is between the L5 and S1 screws. Thus for a construct of L4 to the sacrum, there are construct, four points of fixation above (bilateral L4 and L5 screws) and four points of fixation below (bilateral S1 and iliac wing screws) the slipped L5–S1 segment.

A variety of Cotrel-Dubousset Horizon compatible screws can be used, including fixed or multiaxial Cotrel-Dubousset Horizon screws, Danek variable angle screws, and Liberty iliac wing screws. All these screws attach to the 5.5-mm diameter Cotrel-Dubousset Horizon rod with appropriate connectors, and a cross-link is added. Correction occurs by means of intraoperative positioning of the hips and extension (after appropriate decompression), cantilever translation of the anterior sacral-pelvic unit to meet the slipped L4 and L5 segments, and posterior translation of the L5 segment to meet the sacrum. I strongly advocate circumferential L5–S1 fusion for these difficult operations either posteriorly by means of reach-around interbody fusion or by means of formal anterior fusion (60).

A similar construct is used to manage lumbosacral spondyloptosis with L5 spondylectomy as advocated by Gaines and Nichols (25). After anterior and posterior L5 resection, bilateral screws are placed in the L4 segment, the S1 segment, and the iliac wings. If a gap is present in the L4-sacrum disc space anteriorly, anterior interbody fusion should be considered to aid in definitive stabilization (Fig. 39).

MISCELLANEOUS SURGICAL INDICATIONS

Cotrel-Dubousset instrumentation can be used to manage surgical pediatric spinal problems such as tumor, infection, or trauma (Fig. 40). In these cases, posterior Cotrel-Dubousset instrumentation is used as a stabilization device to allow spinal healing after ablative tumor excision, débridement for infection, or trauma realignments, as for burst injuries (Fig. 41) (20). For the lumbar region, I prefer pedicle screw instrumentation for these reconstructions, commonly with hooks in the thoracic region. These procedures usually are performed with a fairly straight coronal plane to obtain or maintain sagittal alignment during instrumentation and fusion. Appropriate anterior column support is needed when the anterior column is rendered unstable, as in corpectomy for tumor, infection, or trauma with compromise of the spinal canal.

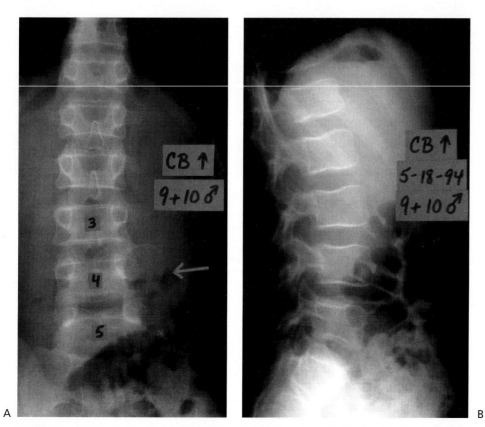

FIGURE 40. Images of a boy 9 years 10 months of age with a 6-month history of right anterior thigh pain. **A:** Upright coronal lumbar radiograph shows an expansile lesion of the right transverse process at L4. **B:** Lateral radiograph shows no unusual findings. *(Figure continues.)*

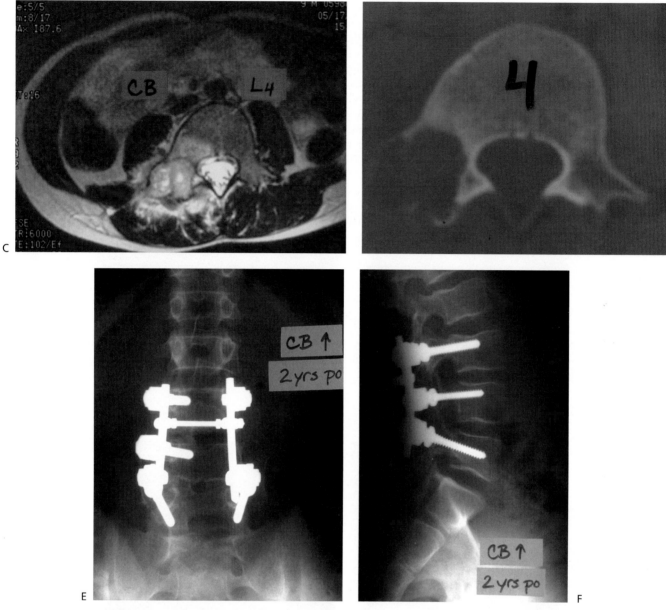

FIGURE 40. *Continued.* **C:** Magnetic resonance image shows a lesion radiating from the pedicle into the transverse process and posterior arch at L4. **D:** Computed tomographic scan shows a thin bony rim around a suspected aneurysmal bone cyst. A biopsy was performed, and the results confirmed the presence of advanced bone cancer. Wide posterolateral excision, instrumentation, and fusion were performed because the L3–4 and L4–5 facet joints had been violated unilaterally above and below for complete excision of the tumor. Posterior instrumentation and fusion from L3 to L5 with bilateral pedicle screws and Cotrel-Dubousset rods and insertion of a device for transverse traction cross-link thus were performed. **E:** Coronal view obtained 2 years postoperatively shows solid arthrodesis from L3 through L5. **F:** Lateral radiographs obtained 2 years postoperatively show good alignment over instrumented and noninstrumented levels. Pain and neurologic weakness completely resolved soon after surgical treatment.

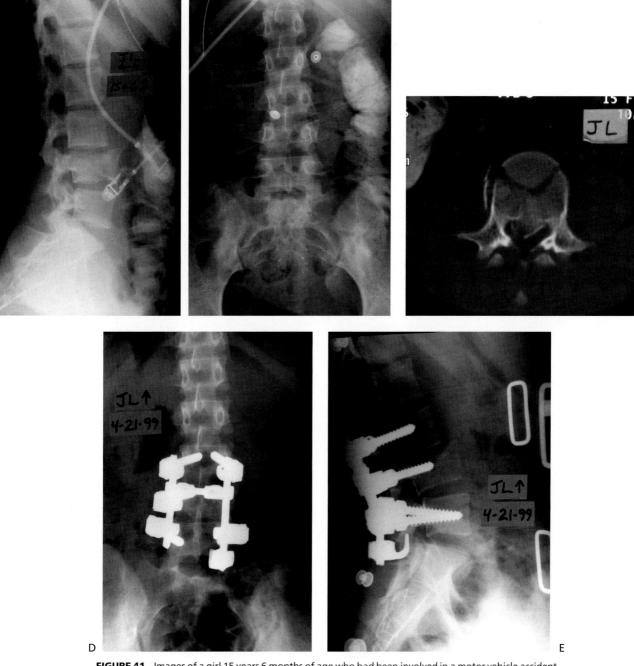

FIGURE 41. Images of a girl 15 years 6 months of age who had been involved in a motor vehicle accident in which she had ejected from the vehicle and sustained an L4 burst fracture. The neurologic findings were normal. **A:** Lateral radiograph shows anterior and middle column involvement of L4 and loss of lordosis between L3 and L5. **B:** Anteroposterior (AP) radiograph shows widened interpedicular distance at L4. **C:** Computed tomographic scan shows approximately 60% canal compromise by retropulsed fragment and shows the body comminution and split of the fracture pattern. Both nonoperative and operative management of fractures were discussed with the patient and her parents. They chose an operative approach. Posterior L3–L5 postural reduction was performed with posterior instrumentation and fusion with Cotrel-Dubousset Horizon rods and variable angle screws and an offset infralaminar hook at L5. Screws were placed bilaterally at L3, left at L4, and bilaterally at L5. Postural reduction and lordosis were placed into instrumentation. **D:** Follow-up AP radiograph shows instrumentation construct. **E:** Lateral radiograph shows improved lordosis and healing of the fracture site. A brace was worn for 6 months after the operation to protect the instrumentation during healing.

SUMMARY

All surgeons who operate on the spines of children are indebted to the tireless efforts of Yves Cotrel and Jean Dubousset for the techniques, implants, and introduction to segmental spinal instrumentation. The original Cotrel-Dubousset system revolutionized spinal surgery as the third generation of spinal implants, following Harrington's rod, and Luque's segmental wiring principles. All pediatric spinal surgeons have learned the importance of three-dimensional analysis and correction of deformities.

Although still not in widespread use, specific advances with the Cotrel-Dubousset Horizon system have improved our technical abilities to instrument the spine efficiently with increased versatility, removability, and a low-profile system. It was the first, and truly remains a universal spinal system with application to the entire thoracic and lumbar spine in the anterior and posterior aspects. Although instrumentation-related complications always are possible, they can be minimized with strict attention to patient selection; preoperative planning; avoidance of overcorrection in the coronal and sagittal planes; consideration of anterior fusion of large curves, especially with associated kyphotic malalignment; application of secure multisegment hook, rod, and screw anchors; and attainment of idealized frontal and sagittal alignment from a segmental, a regional, and a global perspective. Last and most important, adequate arthrodesis must be performed over the instrumented levels to maintain long-term instrumented spinal alignment.

REFERENCES

1. Allen Jr BL, Ferguson RL (1984): The Galveston technique of pelvic fixation with L-rod instrumentation of the spine. *Spine* 9:388–394.
2. Aria S, Ohtsuka Y, Moriya H, et al. (1993): Scoliosis associated with syringomyelia. *Spine* 18:1591–1592.
3. Barr SJ, Schuette AM, Emans JB (1997): Lumbar pedicle screws versus hooks: results in double major curves in adolescent idiopathic scoliosis. *Spine* 22:1369–1379.
4. Been HD, Kalkman CJ, Traast HS (1994): Neurologic injury after insertion of laminar hooks during Cotrel-Dubousset instrumentation. *Spine* 19:1402–1405.
5. Bergoin M, Bollini G, Hornung H, et al. (1988): Is the Cotrel-Dubousset really universal in the surgical treatment of idiopathic scoliosis? *J Pediatr Orthop* 8:45–48.
6. Bernhardt M, Bridwell KH (1989): Segmental analysis of the sagittal plane alignment of the normal thoracic and lumbar spines and thoracolumbar junction. *Spine* 14:717–721.
7. Betz RR, Harms J, Clements DH, et al. (1999): Comparison of anterior and posterior instrumentation for correction of adolescent idiopathic scoliosis. *Spine* 24:225–239.
8. Birch JG, Herring JA, Roach JW, et al. (1988): Cotrel-Dubousset instrumentation in idiopathic scoliosis: a preliminary report. *Clin Orthop* 227:24–29.
9. Booke JS, Banta JV, Bunke FJ, et al. (1993): Somatosensory evoked potential monitoring during Cotrel-Dubousset instrumentation: report of a case. *Spine* 18:518.
10. Boos N, Marchesi D, Aebi M (1991): Treatment of spondylolysis and spondylolisthesis with Cotrel-Dubousset instrumentation: a preliminary report. *J Spine Disord* 4:472–479.
11. Bridwell KH, Betz R, Capelli AM, et al. (1990): Sagittal plane analysis in idiopathic scoliosis patients treated with Cotrel-Dubousset instrumentation. *Spine* 15:921–926.
12. Bridwell KH, McAllister JW, Betz RR, et al. (1991): Coronal decompensation produced by Cotrel-Dubousset "derotation" maneuver for idiopathic right thoracic scoliosis. *Spine* 16:769–777.
13. Bridwell KH, Lenke LG, Baldus C, et al. (1998): Major intraoperative neurologic deficits in pediatric and adult spinal deformity patients: incidence and etiology at one institution. *Spine* 23:324–331.
14. Brown CA, Lenke LG, Bridwell KH, et al. (1998): Complications of pediatric thoracolumbar and lumbar pedicle screws. *Spine* 23:1566–1571.
15. Charry O, Koop S, Winter R, et al. (1994): Syringomyelia and scoliosis: a review of twenty-five pediatric patients. *J Pediatr Orthop* 14:309–317.
16. Connolly PJ, von Schroeder HP, Johnson GE, et al. (1995): Adolescent idiopathic scoliosis:long-term effect of instrumentation extending to the lumbar spine. *J Bone Joint Surg Am* 77:1210–1216.
17. Cotrel Y, Dubousset J, Guillaumat M (1988): New universal instrumentation in spinal surgery. *Clin Orthop* 227:10–23.
18. Cummings RJ, Loveless FA, Campbell J, et al. (1998): Interobserver reliability and intraobserver reproducibility of the system of King et al for the classification of adolescent idiopathic scoliosis. *J Bone Joint Surg Am* 80:1107–1111.
19. Cundy P, Patterson D, Hillier T, et al. (1990): Cotrel-Dubousset instrumentation and vertebral rotation in adolescent idiopathic scoliosis. *J Bone Joint Surg Br* 72:670–674.
20. Denis F (1983): The three column spine and its significance in the classification of acute thoracolumbar spinal injuries. *Spine* 8:817–831.
21. Denis F (1988): Cotrel-Dubousset instrumentation in the treatment of idiopathic scoliosis. *Orthop Clin North Am* 19:291–311.
22. Dubousset J, Cotrel Y (1991): Application technique of Cotrel-Dubousset instrumentation for scoliosis deformities. *Clin Orthop* 164:103–110.
23. Dubousset J, Herring JA, Shufflebarger H (1989): The crankshaft phenomenon. *J Pediatr Orthop* 9:541–550.
24. Ecker M, Betz R, Trent P, et al. (1988): Computer tomography evaluation of Cotrel-Dubousset instrumentation in idiopathic scoliosis. *Spine* 13:1141–1144.
25. Gaines RW, Nichols WK (1985): Treatment of spondyloptosis by two-stage L5 vertebrectomy and reduction of L4 onto S1. *Spine* 10:680–686.
26. Gray JM, Smith BW, Ashley RK, et al. (1991): Derotational analysis of Cotrel-Dubousset instrumentation in idiopathic scoliosis. *Spine* 16:S391–393.
27. Guidera KJ, Hooten J, Weatherly W, et al. (1993): Cotrel-Dubousset instrumentation: results in 52 patients. *Spine* 18:427–431.
28. Gupta P, Lenke LG, Bridwell KH (1998): Incidence of neural axis abnormalities in infantile and juvenile patients with spinal deformity: is a magnetic resonance image screening necessary? *Spine* 23:206–210.
29. Halm H, Castro WH, Jerosch J, et al. (1995): Sagittal plane correction in "King-classified" idiopathic scoliosis patients treated with Cotrel-Dubousset instrumentation. *Acta Orthop Belg* 61:294–301.
30. Hamill CL, Lenke LG, Bridwell KH, et al. (1996): The use of pedicle screws to improve correction in the lumbar spine of adolescent idiopathic scoliosis: is it warranted? *Spine* 21:1241–1249.
31. Harvey Jr CJ, Betz RR, Clements DH, et al. (1993): Are there indications for partial rib resection in patients with adolescent idiopathic scoliosis treated with Cotrel-Dubousset instrumentation? *Spine* 18:1593–1598.
32. Hicks RG, Burke DJ, Stephen JP (1991): Monitoring spinal cord function during scoliosis surgery with Cotrel-Dubousset instrumentation. *Med J Aust* 154:82–86.
33. Hirabayashi S, Kumano K, Kuroki T (1991): Cotrel-Dubousset pedicle screw system for various spinal disorders: merits and problems. *Spine* 16:1298–1304.
34. Holt RT, Johnson JR (1989): Cotrel-Dubousset instrumentation in neurofibromatosis spine curves: a preliminary report. *Clin Orthop* 245:19–23.
35. Johnston C, Ashman R, Sherman MC, et al. (1987): Mechanical consequences of rod contouring and residue scoliosis in sublaminar segmental instrumentation. *J Orthop Res* 5:206–216.

36. Johnston BS, Herring JA, Johnson CE, et al. (1994): Treatment of adolescent idiopathic scolisis using Texas Scottish Rite Hospital instrumentation. *Orthop Trans* 19:1598–1665.

37. Kalen V, Conklin M (1990): The behavior of the unfused lumbar curve following selective thoracic fusion for idiopathic scoliosis. *Spine* 15:271–274.

38. King HA, Moe JH, Bradford DS, et al. (1983): The selection of fusion levels in thoracic idiopathic scoliosis. *J Bone Joint Surg Am* 65: 1302–1313.

39. Labelle H, Dansereau J, Bellefleur C, et al. (1995): Preoperative three-dimensional correction of idiopathic scoliosis with the Cotrel-Dubousset procedure. *Spine* 20:1406–1409.

40. Labelle H, Dansereau J, Bellefleur C, et al. (1995): Comparison between preoperative and postoperative three-dimensional reconstructions of idiopathic scoliosis with the Cotrel-Dubousset procedure. *Spine* 20:2487–2492.

41. Lagrone M, Bradford D, Moe J, et al. (1988): Treatment of symptomatic flat back after spinal fusion. *J Bone Joint Surg Am* 70:569–580.

42. Lee CK, Denis F, Winter RB, et al. (1993): Analysis of the upper thoracic curve in surgically treated idiopathic scoliosis: a new concept of the double thoracic curve pattern. *Spine* 18:1599–1608.

43. Lenke LG, Betz RR, Bridwell KH, et al. (1998): Intraobserver and interobserver reliability of the classification of thoracic adolescent idiopathic scoliosis. *J Bone Joint Surg Am* 80:1097–1106.

44. Lenke LG, Betz RR, Bridwell KH, et al. (1999): Spontaneous lumbar curve coronal correction after selective anterior or posterior thoracic fusion in adolescent idiopathic scoliosis. *Spine* 24:1663–1671.

45. Lenke LG, Betz RR, Harms J, et al. A new and reliable 3-dimensional classification of adolescent idiopathic scoliosis. *J Bone Joint Surg.* Submitted.

46. Lenke LG, Bridwell KH, Baldus C, et al. (1992): Cotrel-Dubousset instrumentation for adolescent idiopathic scoliosis. *J Bone Joint Surg Am* 74:1056–1067.

47. Lenke LG, Bridwell KH, Baldus C, et al. (1992): Analysis of pulmonary function and axis rotation in adolescent and young adult idiopathic scoliosis patients treated with Cotrel-Dubousset instrumentation. *J Spinal Disord* 5:16–25.

48. Lenke LG, Bridwell KH, Baldus C, et al. (1992): Preventing decompensation in King type II curves treated with Cotrel-Dubousset instrumentation: strict guidelines for selective thoracic fusion. *Spine* 17: S274–S281.

49. Lenke LG, Bridwell KH, Baldus C, et al. (1993): Ability of Cotrel-Dubousset instrumentation to preserve distal lumbar motion segments in adolescent idiopathic scoliosis. *J Spinal Disord* 6:339–350.

50. Lenke LG, Bridwell KH, Blanke K, et al. (1995): Analysis of pulmonary function and chest cage dimension changes following thoracoplasty in idiopathic scoliosis. *Spine* 20:1343–1350.

51. Lenke LG, Bridwell KH, Blanke K, et al. (1998): Radiographic results of arthrodesis with Cotrel-Dubousset instrumentation for the treatment of adolescent idiopathic scoliosis: a five- to ten-year follow-up study. *J Bone Joint Surg Am* 80:807–814.

52. Lenke LG, Bridwell KH, O'Brien MF, et al. (1994): Recognition and treatment of the proximal thoracic curve in adolescent idiopathic scoliosis treated with Cotrel-Dubousset instrumentation. *Spine* 19: 1589–1597.

53. Lenke LG, Padberg AM, Russo MH, et al. (1995): Triggered EMG threshold for accuracy of pedicle screw placement: an animal model and clinical correlation. *Spine* 20:1585–1591.

54. Lewonowski K, King JD, Nelson MD (1992): Routine use of magnetic resonance imaging in idiopathic scoliosis patients less than eleven years of age. *Spine* 17:S109–S116.

55. Lonstein JE (1992): Decompensation with Cotrel Dubousset instrumentation: a multicenter study [abstract]. *Orthop Trans* 16:158.

56. McCall RE, Bronson W (1992): Criteria for selective fusion in idiopathic scoliosis using Cotrel-Dubousset instrumentation. *J Pediatr Orthop* 12:475–479.

57. Marsicano JG, Lenke LG, Bridwell KH, et al. (1998): The lordotic effect of the OSI frame on operative adolescent idiopathic scoliosis patients. *Spine* 23:1341–1348.

58. Mason DE, Carango P (1991): Spinal decompensation in Cotrel-Dubousset instrumentation. *Spine* 16:S394–S403.

59. Moe JH, Purcell GA, Bradford DS (1983): Zielke instrumentation (VDS) for the correction of spinal curvature. *Clin Orthop* 180: 133–153.

60. Molinari RW, Bridwell KH, Lenke LG, et al. (1998): Complications in the surgical treatment of pediatric high-grade isthmic dysplastic spondylolisthesis: a comparison of three surgical approaches. *Spine* 24: 1701–1711.

61. Moore MR, Boynham GC, Brown CW, et al. (1991): Analysis of factors related to truncal decompensation following Cotrel-Dubousset instrumentation. *J Spinal Disord* 4:188–192.

62. O'Brien MF, Lenke LG, Bridwell KH, et al. (1994): Preoperative spinal investigation in adolescent idiopathic scoliosis curves greater than or equal to 70°. *Spine* 19:1606–1610.

63. Padberg AM, Wilson-Holden TJ, Lenke LG, et al. (1998): Somatosensory- and motor-evoked potential monitoring without a wake-up test during idiopathic scoliosis surgery: an accepted standard of care. *Spine* 23:1392–1400.

64. Puno RM, Grossfeld SL, Johnson JR, et al. (1992): Cotrel-Dubousset instrumentation in idiopathic scoliosis. *Spine* 17:S258–S262.

65. Raso VJ, Russell GG, Hill DL, et al. (1991): Thoracic lordosis in idiopathic scoliosis. *J Pediatr Orthop* 11:599–602.

66. Richards BS (1992): Lumbar curve response in type II idiopathic scoliosis after posterior instrumentation of the thoracic curve. *Spine* 17: S282–S286.

67. Richards BS, Birch JG, Herring JA, et al. (1989): Frontal plane and sagittal plane balance following Cotrel-Dubousset instrumentation for idiopathic scoliosis. *Spine* 14:733–737.

68. Roye DP, Farcy JP, Rickert JB (1992): Results of spinal instrumentation of adolescent idiopathic scoliosis by King type. *Spine* 17: S270–S273.

69. Shufflebarger HL (1989): Cotrel-Dubousset instrumentation in neurofibromatosis spinal problems. *Clin Orthop* 245:24–28.

70. Shufflebarger HL (1994): Cotrel-Dubousset spinal instrumentation. In: Weinstein SL, ed. *The pediatric spine: principles and practice.* New York: Raven Press, pp. 1545–1583.

71. Shufflebarger HL (1994): Theory and mechanisms of posterior derotation spinal systems. In: Weinstein SL, ed. *The pediatric spine: principles and practice.* New York: Raven Press, pp. 1515–1543.

72. Shufflebarger HL, Clark CE (1990): Fusion levels and hook patterns in thoracic scoliosis with Cotrel-Dubousset instrumentation. *Spine* 15: 916–920.

73. Shufflebarger H, Clark C (1991): Prevention of the crankshaft phenomenon. *Spine* 16:S409–S411.

74. Shufflebarger H, King W (1987): Composite measurement of scoliosis. *Spine* 12:228–232.

75. Stephen JP, Sullivan MR, Hicks RG, et al. (1996): Cotrel-Dubousset instrumentation in children using simultaneous motor and somatosensory evoked potential monitoring. *Spine* 21:2450–2457.

76. Suk SI, Lee CK, Min HJ, et al. (1994): Comparison of Cotrel-Dubousset pedicle screws and hooks in the treatment of idiopathic scoliosis. *Int Orthop* 18:341–346.

77. Sweet FA, Lenke LG, Bridwell KH, et al. (1999): Maintaining lumbar lordosis with anterior single solid-rod instrumentation in thoracolumbar and lumbar adolescent idiopathic scoliosis. *Spine* 24:1655–1662.

78. Takahashi S, Delecrin J, Passuti N (1997): Changes in the unfused lumbar spine in patients with idiopathic scoliosis: a 5- to 9-year assessment after Cotrel-Dubousset instrumentation. *Spine* 22:517–523.

79. Thompson JP, Transfeldt EE, Bradford DS, et al. (1990): Decompensation after Cotrel-Dubousset instrumentation of idiopathic scoliosis. *Spine* 15:927–931.

80. Turi M, Johnston CE, Richards BS (1993): Anterior correction of idiopathic scoliosis using TSRH instrumentation. *Spine* 18:417–422.

81. Vedantam R, Lenke LG, Bridwell KH, et al. (2000): Comparison of push-prone and side bending radiographs for predicting postoperative

coronal alignment in thoracolumbar and lumbar adolescent idiopathic scoliosis. *Spine* 25:76–81.

82. Vedantam R, Lenke LG, Bridwell KH, et al. (2000): A prospective evaluation of pulmonary function in patients with adolescent idiopathic scoliosis relative to the surgical approach used for spinal arthrodesis. *Spine* 25:82–90.

83. Willers U, Transfeldt EE, Hedlund R (1996): The segmental effect of Cotrel-Dubousset instrumentation on vertebral rotation, rib hump and the thoracic cage in idiopathic scoliosis. *Eur Spine J* 5:387–393.

84. Wilson-Holden TJ, Padberg AM, Lenke LG, et al. (1999): Efficacy of intraoperative monitoring for pediatric patients with spinal cord pathology undergoing spinal deformity surgery. *Spine* 24:1685–1692.

85. Winter RB (1989): The idiopathic double thoracic curve pattern: its recognition and surgical management. *Spine* 14:1287–1292.

86. Wojcik A, Webb J, Burwell R (1990): Harrington-Luque and Cotrel-Dubousset instrumentation for idiopathic thoracic scoliosis. *Spine* 15: 424–431.

87. Wood KB, Transfeldt EE, Ogilvie JW, et al. (1991): Rotational changes of the vertebral-pelvic axis following Cotrel-Dubousset instrumentation. *Spine* 16:S404–S408.

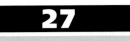

MOSS MIAMI SPINAL INSTRUMENTATION

HARRY L. SHUFFLEBARGER

The origin of all current multiple hook-screw-rod systems is the implant design of Yves Cotrel combined with the concept of approaching scoliotic deformities with an awareness of the three-dimensional nature of these deformities described by Dubousset and coworkers (7). This resulted in the development of the Cotrel-Dubousset spinal system, introduced in Europe in 1982, and first presented to the United States in 1984. Use of the Cotrel-Dubousset system rapidly spread across the United States and the rest of the world. Cotrel et al. (6) described the universal nature of the device. I have extensive experience with the device and have developed a large body of information regarding application of the system (16,17,23,26). Many devices were subsequently developed, all variations on the design, theory, and mechanisms of implementation of the Cotrel-Dubousset system (1,2,12).

Development of the Moss Miami system was the result of my collaboration with Jurgen Harms and Lutz Biederman, both of Germany. Design criteria were developed in mid 1992 and were followed by prototype development in late 1992. The first operations were performed in Germany in early 1993 and in the United States in mid 1993. The design criteria included many facets considered to represent marked improvement over existing devices.

The design criteria encompassed several areas. A closure mechanism (method of fixing the spinal anchor to the longitudinal member or rod) was designed that is easily placed and easily removed and supplied excellent fixation without the possibility of spontaneous disassembly (22). No preloading of the rod with blockers, connectors, or any other device was necessary. A construct with a considerably lower profile than that of existing devices was needed. Basing the system on a 5-mm rod met the size requirements. A small number of implants and instruments, so there would be low hospital inventories, was another criterion. Ability to use the device from both anterior and posterior approaches was desired. All of these objectives were achieved with the initial prototypes. After more than 6 years of use of the device, there has been little change or addition to either instruments or implants. This attests to the validity of the design

criteria and to the effectiveness of the system in all varieties of pathologic conditions of the spine.

DESIGN RATIONALE AND IMPLANT DESCRIPTION

Closure Mechanism

Existing spinal systems have similar spinal anchors (hooks or screws) and similar longitudinal members (rods). The primary differences between existing devices are the closure mechanisms. The closure mechanism is the method by which the spinal anchor attaches to the longitudinal member. The Cotrel-Dubousset closure mechanism was to break off the metallurgically hardset screw into the relatively soft rod, or *penetration*. This method precludes adjustability and nondestructive removal of the device.

Another method of function of closure devices is friction between spinal anchor and rod. With the Moss Miami system, friction is achieved with a dual, self-locking closure system. The elements of the closure device with an implant are illustrated in Fig. 1. All implant bodies are identical with a posterior open design. The upright portion of the implant is threaded on both the inner and outer surfaces. The devices for closure are the inner nut (innie) and outer screw (outie). The innie is placed first, being cannulated for a hex-ended inserter and holder. The hex fitting also is used for the tightening instruments. The innie has a smooth, flat surface, so the rod is forced into the implant and a large surface area exists for development of friction for a secure closure.

The outie is placed after the innie is placed, but before any tightening of the innie is done. Should the innie be tightened before the outie is placed, the uprights of the implant body may open slightly, making placement of the outie impossible. The outie converts the open implant to a functionally closed implant. The outie provides additional points of contact with the rod, generating more friction. The outie prevents the body of the implant from opening when the innie is tightened. Open implants with a single inner screw must have very thick walls in the upright portion to prevent opening of the uprights with tightening of the set screw. Any opening of the uprights would cause unloading of the device and carry risk of spontaneous disassembly. The outie prevents any opening and provides addi-

H. L. Shufflebarger: Division of Spinal Surgery, Department of Orthopedic Surgery, Miami Childrens Hospital, Miami, Florida 33155.

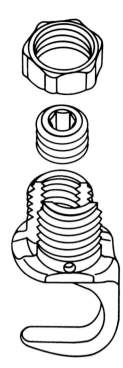

FIGURE 1. The Moss Miami common implant design and closure mechanism features an open-body implant threaded on both the inner and outer surfaces. The closure device consists of an inner screw (innie) and outer nut (outie). The innie is placed first to hold the rod, followed by placement of the outie, which converts the open implant to a functionally closed implant

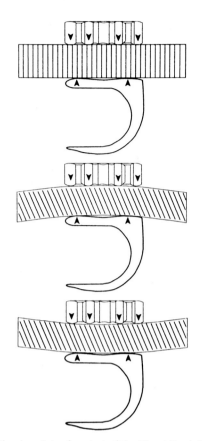

FIGURE 2. The six points of contact of the Moss Miami closure mechanism. These are provided by the innie and outie in conjunction with the bottom surface of the implant. Any physiologic bend in the rod is assured of a secure closure mechanism.

tional friction, increasing the security of the closure. The six points of contact of the closure mechanism with the rod and spinal anchor are illustrated in Fig. 2. A unique instrument (Fig. 3) was developed with the initial instruments that allows quick placement of the closure device. A second instrument to prevent cross-threading of the closure elements is available, but it is rarely needed.

After the closure device is placed, loading sequences can be performed (distraction or compression). The innie is used for maintaining the spinal anchor position during loading maneuvers. The final tightening is made by means of tightening the outie and retightening the innie. This last innie tightening opens the uprights of the implant body very slightly; this prevents the outie from spontaneous loosening or displacement.

In cyclical testing in excess of 5.5 million cycles, no loosening of the closure mechanism has occurred (22). In more than 6 years use of the device and more than 1,000 operations, no spontaneous loosening or disassembly has occurred. Removal is simple and rapid.

The closure mechanism is identical for all implants. All implants are posterior open. No preloading of the rod is needed for any Moss Miami construct. The system is easy to learn and implement for both the instrument nurse and the surgeon.

Implants

The rod diameter is the primary determinant of implant size and thus construct height and prominence. A secondary deter-

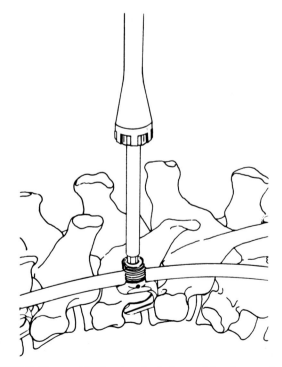

FIGURE 3. The combination inserter instrument for placement of the innie and outie assures easy placement and alignment of the closure components.

minant of prominence is the closure mechanism (see earlier) that presents the lowest profile available.

A 5-mm rod was chosen as the basis of the Moss Miami system. Several factors contributed to this choice. These include mechanical testing with various rod diameters and metallurgic treatments. Elasticity and bending characteristics also were evaluated (W. Matthis, personal communication) (18). The Moss Miami 5-mm rod allows more than 5.5 million cycles before fatigue failure, sufficient to attain fusion. The elasticity is such that a large deformation is needed to produce plastic deformation. The elasticity is an asset during rod placement in the surgical procedure. The stiffness, however, is sufficient to correct most large and stiff deformities. The rod may appear to deform during placement in some instances. There is some memory in the rod, and it usually tends to return to the bend placed in the rod. A titanium set is available for the Moss Miami system. All implants are titanium. The titanium rod is 5.5 mm in diameter. The slightly larger diameter in titanium is needed to attain adequate yield strength.

Two additional rod diameters have become available. A 4-mm rod with correspondingly smaller implants is available for small or asthenic patients and for anterior approaches to the thoracic spine. I have used the 5-mm rod system without difficulty in operations on patients with weights as low as 15 kg. A 6.0-mm rod set also is available. This was supplied to accommodate large patients or very stiff deformities. I have found the 5-mm rod system adequate for these situations.

The five basic Moss Miami hooks are pedicle, lamina, thinblade lamina, reduced distance lamina, and angled lamina (Fig. 4). Specialty hooks include oblique-blade hooks (for supralaminar positioning in the upper thoracic spine), offset body hooks (to align with pedicle screws), and extended body hooks. A transverse-process hook for construction of single-level pedicle-transverse claws also is offered. The axial connectors and transverse connectors are shown in Fig. 4, as are monoaxial and polyaxial screws. The Kostuik sacral connector, staple, and washer complete the Moss Miami implants (J. Kostuik, personal communication). These components are all that are necessary for any spinal instrumentation.

Screws are available in monoaxial and polyaxial versions with diameters of 5, 6, and 7 mm; larger screws are available on special request. The polyaxial screw is an important advance in screw technology. The ease of rod insertion and the load-sharing ability of the screw are unique. Figure 5 shows the load-sharing features of the polyaxial screw. The ideal relation of rod to screw is perpendicular. With monoaxial screws, precise rod bend is mandatory to attain this relation. In the absence of an exact perpendicular relation of rod to screw (because the screw is fixed in bone and should not move), placement of the closure device can only produce poor closure mechanics or movement of the screw in the bone (loosening of the screw). The ability of the head of the polyaxial screw to rotate in any direction ensures that the relation of the rod to screw will always be perpendicular and prevent transfer of stress to the screw-bone interface.

When forces are applied to the screw (distraction or compression) the rod moves within the body of the screw. With a monoaxial screw and any bend in the rod, movement of the rod within the screw alters the relation. This can only transfer the force to the bone-screw interface and loosen or produce inadequate loading of the screw. The head of the polyaxial screw moves with the rod, preventing transferring the force to the screw-bone interface, another load-sharing feature.

The correction method advocated with Moss Miami is not a rod rotation maneuver as with the Cotrel-Dubousset device. Translation and cantilever mechanics are advocated instead. A complete explanation is presented in Chapter 25. To facilitate the translation maneuver, translation implants (Fig. 6) were developed in 1997. Screws with the same flange, reduction screws, are available. Reduction screws are useful in bringing the screw to the rod, as in reduction of a spondylolisthesis.

The flanged implants are threaded on the inside of the flange or tab. A stress riser is present at the base of the tab. The tab is broken after use, resulting in a normal Moss Miami implant. The flanged implants are used in a like manner. The rod is inserted into the posterior portion of the tab. The outie is placed to prevent the flange from opening. A key is available to place just posteriorly to the implant and anteriorly to the rod to prevent opening of the flange. The key is removed after the outie is placed (Fig. 7). With the outie in place, the innie is placed in the inner threaded portion of the tab. The innie is then advanced down the shaft of the tab, taking the rod with it. Eventually the threads of the implant body are entered by the innie. At this point, the outie can be placed on the threads of the body of the implant and the tabs removed. These devices greatly facilitate rod placement. They function as instruments and implants. The need for rod-approximation instruments is greatly reduced or eliminated. Slow correction of any deformity—scoliosis, kyphosis, or spondylolisthesis—is possible.

Moss Miami screws may be placed either anteriorly in the vertebral body or posteriorly in the pedicle. The 4-mm device is particularly useful for anterior procedures in the thoracic spine. The 5-mm screws are useful in anterior operations in the lower thoracic spine and lumbar spine.

An axial connector is used in difficult rod alignment situations and for extension of constructs. An axial connector with both 5-mm and 7-mm canals allows connection to 7-mm rod systems. Distraction and compression can be applied through the axial connectors. The transverse connector consists of a 2.0-mm rod and hooks with set screws. Two types of hooks are available. A hook with a slotted shoe can be placed with the transverse rod in place. The transverse connector can be placed in either compression or distraction directions. Kostuik has developed an axial connector for use with a transverse sacral bar. This connect the bar to proximal instrumentation (J. Kostuik, personal communication).

Washers are useful for adjusting the anterior-posterior position of pedicle screws. Each washer position the screw 3 mm more posterior. A maximum of three washers is recommended. Staples are available for use with vertebral body screws to distribute the load of the screw over a greater surface area (Fig. 4).

The description of the Moss Miami implant system explains and affirms the initial design criteria. Little deviation from the initial criteria has occurred. Constructs are very low profile. The closure mechanism is secure, easily placed, easily adjusted, and easily removed. It requires no preloading of the rod. The number of implants and instruments probably is the lowest required with

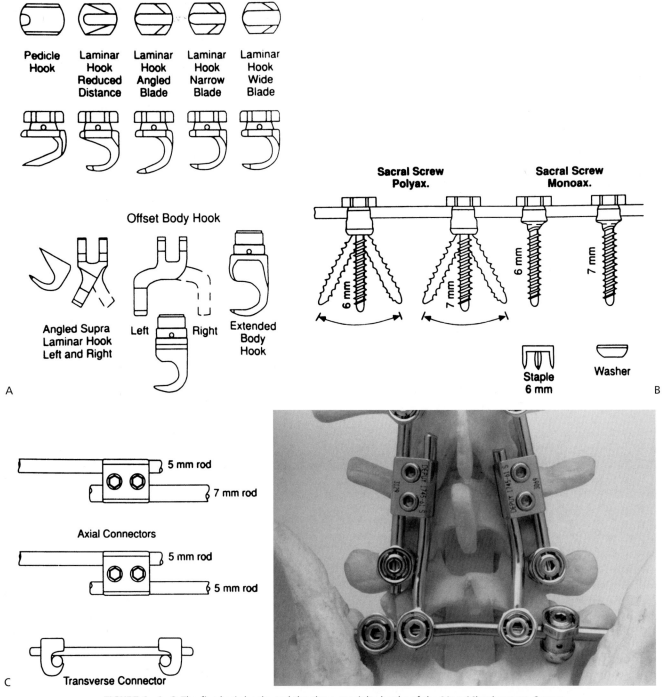

FIGURE 4. **A–C:** The five basic hooks and the three specialty hooks of the Moss Miami system. Screws are polyaxial and monoaxial. Staples are provided for anterior use. Washers are useful in the posterior aspect to equalize the heights of the screws. **D:** Kostuik axial connector designed for connection of a transverse sacral bar with proximal instrumentation. The transverse bar is fixed to the ilium and crosses proximally to the sacroiliac joint. The transverse bar is secured to the sacrum by bicortical screws. The axial connector is medial to the sacral screws to afford a connection to proximal instrumentation.

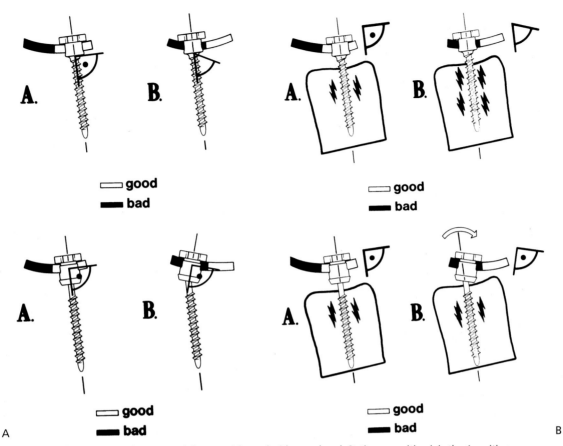

FIGURE 5. **A, B:** *Top,* monoaxial screw with a rod with some bend. Optimum position is in the *A* position. As the rod is moved through the screw (as distraction or compression is applied in correcting spinal problems), the rod and screw no longer have a perpendicular relation. This mechanical situation can only transfer stress and load to the screw-bone interface and dispose to screw loosening. *Bottom,* improved situation with polyaxial screws. Screw head accommodates the bend in the rod and negates the transfer of stress to the bone-screw interface.

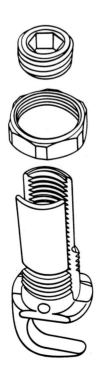

FIGURE 6. The translation hook features an extension of the implant body. The extended portion of the flange is threaded to accommodate the innie. The outer portion is smooth. Implementation of the device eliminates many instruments. A key is supplied at the base of the flange to prevent the flange from opening.

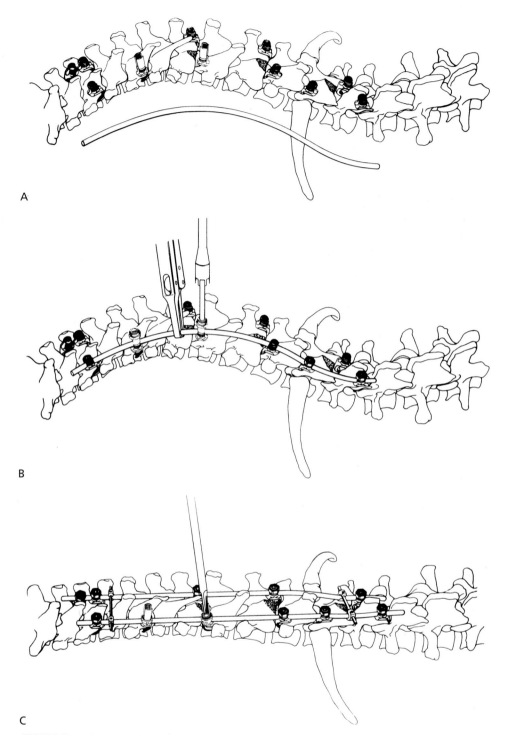

A

B

C

FIGURE 7. A–C: Progressive and segmental correction of scoliosis with a translation hook. After the rod is inserted into the translation implant, the outie is placed and then the innie. The innie is used to pull the spine to the rod and spinal anchors. After completion of the correction, the tabs on the translation implants are broken and removed.

any current device. Anterior or posterior use is possible. Addition of the flanged implants is an important advance that facilitates the rod placement stage of the surgical procedure.

INDICATIONS FOR MOSS MIAMI SPINAL INSTRUMENTATION

The Moss Miami system can be used successfully to manage any spinal condition in which instrumentation is indicated. It can be used from either the anterior or posterior approach or a combination. Spinal anchors can be hooks, screws, or a combination of hooks and screws. The diagnostic conditions include deformity, degenerative disease, trauma, and spinal reconstruction.

Deformity

Long-segment deformity is best represented by adolescent idiopathic scoliosis and Scheuermann kyphosis. Adolescent idiopathic scoliosis is the prototype in discussions of long-segment constructs for deformity. The mechanics of correction with the Moss Miami system are translation with posterior angulation (usually with distraction direction forces and the concave rod placed first) and cantilever with anterior angulation and translation (usually with compression direction forces and the convex rod placed first). A complete discussion on the mechanics of scoliosis correction is contained in Chapter 25.

Bone anchors can be hooks or screws or a combination of these (see Chapter 24). Excellent results in the management of adolescent deformity are obtained with the posterior approach (18,19,24). Any curve size and pattern can be easily approached with the device. Use of translation implants greatly facilitates rod placement and correction of the deformity. Figure 7 shows the sequence of steps in correction of an idiopathic curve with translation implants. Figure 8 depicts a similar curve managed with the translation technique and implants. Figure 9 depicts an adolescent thoracolumbar curve managed with screws as the bone anchor but still according to the convex-first rod placement principle with compression forces. Figure 10 represents a double curve in which a combination of thoracic hooks and lumbar screws are used to attain excellent correction. It is my scientifically unsupported opinion that screws are superior in correction of both the coronal and sagittal planes in the lumbar spine.

Use of biplanar fluoroscopy and stimulus-evoked electromyography of the screws (5) almost ensures adequate placement of pedicle screws in scoliosis. Screw placement adds a small amount of time to the surgical procedure, but is worth the added correction and stability. One distal level frequently can be saved with screws. Akbarnia et al. (1) and Suk et al. (27) reported excellent results with posterior placement of screws to manage adolescent idiopathic scoliosis. With the Moss Miami system, use of a polyaxial screw greatly facilitates rod placement.

Betz et al. (3) reported on the use of anterior instrumentation for the management of thoracic idiopathic scoliosis. The primary

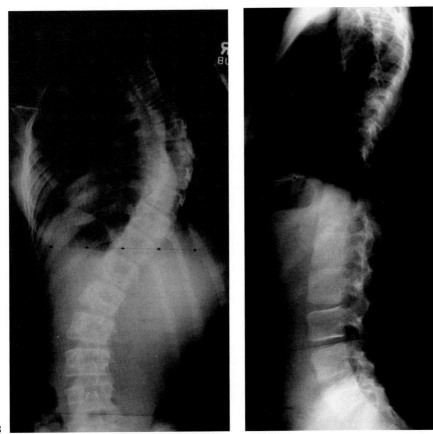

FIGURE 8. A, B: Preoperative radiographs show marked thoracic scoliosis, King type 3. After surgery with translation maneuvers, near complete correction of the scoliosis is evident. In the sagittal plane, hypokyphosis has been restored to a normal sagittal contour. *(Figure continues.)*

A,B

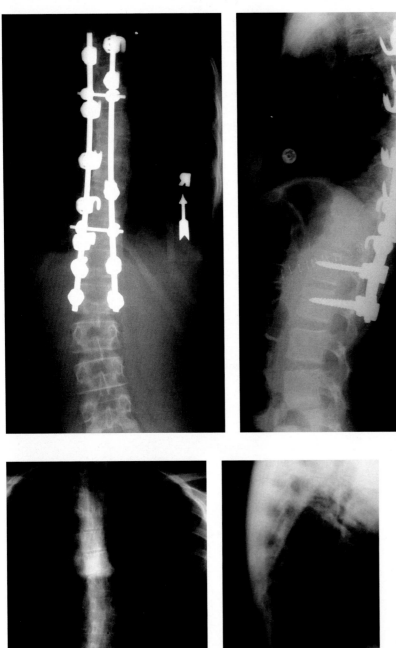

C,D

FIGURE 8. *Continued.* **C, D:** Preoperative radiographs show marked thoracic scoliosis, King type 3. After surgery with translation maneuvers, near complete correction of the scoliosis is evident. In the sagittal plane, hypokyphosis has been restored to a normal sagittal contour.

A,B

FIGURE 9. **A, B:** Thoracolumbar scoliosis with marked decompensation to the left in the coronal plane. The upper lumbar kyphosis common to this curve pattern is evident. Only screws are used with the posterior approach. Complete correction of scoliosis has been achieved, particularly in terms of vertebral rotation. Lateral radiograph shows restoration of lumbar lordosis. *(Figure continues.)*

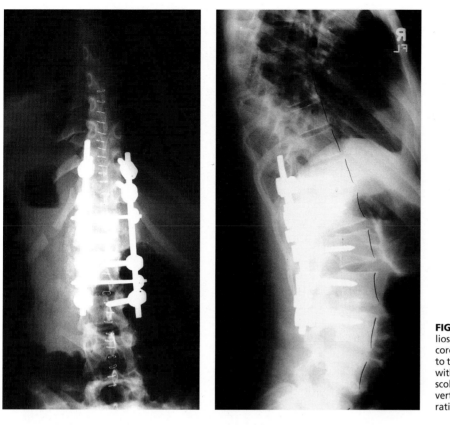

C,D

FIGURE 9. *Continued.* **C, D:** Thoracolumbar scoliosis with marked decompensation to the left in the coronal plane. The upper lumbar kyphosis common to this curve pattern is evident. Only screws are used with the posterior approach. Complete correction of scoliosis has been achieved, particularly in terms of vertebral rotation. Lateral radiograph shows restoration of lumbar lordosis.

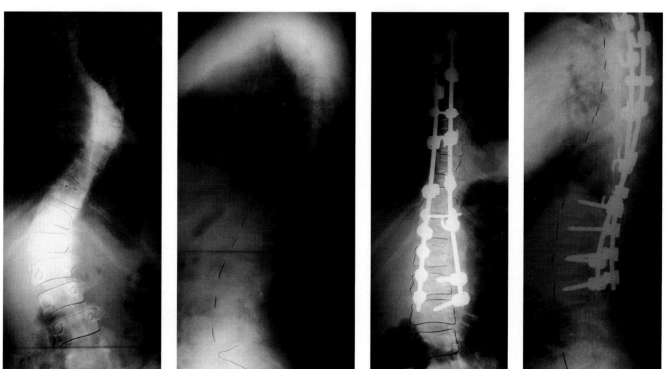

A,B   C,D

FIGURE 10. A–D: Double structural idiopathic curve. A combination of thoracic hooks and lumbar screws is used to effect near complete correction of the deformity from the posterior only approach. A concave thoracic and convex lumbar first approach was used.

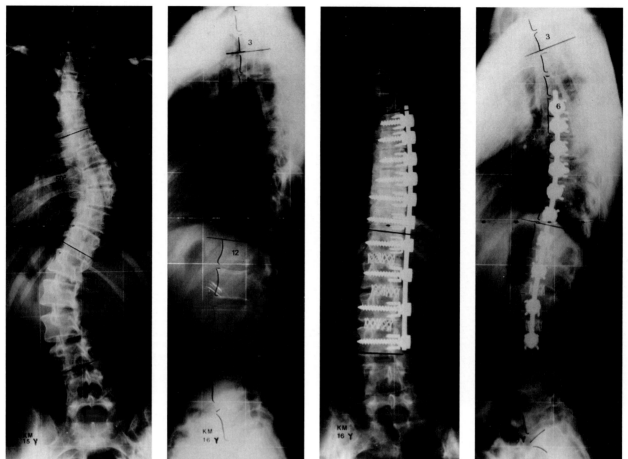

A,B

C,D

FIGURE 11. A–D: Double structural idiopathic deformity managed with an anterior-only approach. Complete correction of right thoracic and left lumbar curves is evident. Structural interbody grafts are present at and distal to the thoracolumbar junction. These grafts serve to produce and maintain lumbar lordosis.

advantage was saving two distal levels, usually stopping at T12. Use of a 4-mm solid-rod system reportedly alleviates some of the problems initially encountered, particularly rod breakage and excessive kyphosis. The kyphosis is relieved with structural interbody grafts (3,13). Figure 11 shows anterior Moss Miami instrumentation in the management of idiopathic scoliosis.

Scoliosis of other causes is likewise well suited to Moss Miami instrumentation, as are paralytic and congenital deformities. The 5-mm system has been used without difficulty or prominence in the care of children weighing as little as 15 kg. The principles of implant placement for idiopathic scoliosis are appropriate for nonidiopathic deformity. Figure 12 shows management of nonidiopathic deformity by means of Moss Miami instrumentation.

Moss Miami instrumentation also is well suited for use in the management of adult scoliosis when surgery is indicated. Selective thoracic fusion in the care of an adult usually can be approached with the same principles as the operation on an adolescent, except preliminary anterior release may be needed more frequently.

For adults who need fusion well into the lumbar spine, an anterior procedure in the lumbar segments has been routine for the past several years. This also is applicable to some adolescent and paralytic deformities that necessitate fusion to the distal lumbar spine or sacrum. Lee et al. (13) found that discectomy with morselized graft produces the most unstable situation possible. Addition of structural interbody graft increases the stability of the spine and the construct to that before discectomy. For this reason, when an anterior procedure is performed on a child or an adult, structural grafts are used at the distal levels. This unloads the posterior device, and prevents distal failure. Figure 13 shows an adult idiopathic deformity managed with structural grafts in the distal lumbar spine. In this instance, a three-stage procedure usually is needed: posterior release, anterior discectomy, and structural graft followed by posterior instrumentation and fusion. Only with this sequence can maximum lordosis be attained and maintained (19,21).

Kyphosis of any cause is well managed with the Moss Miami system. An anterior procedure is needed to manage most problems in kyphosis. The three-stage approach described earlier sometimes is needed. This is particularly true when there have been previous operations or when the fusion extends well into the lumbar spine. Figure 14 shows postlaminectomy kyphosis

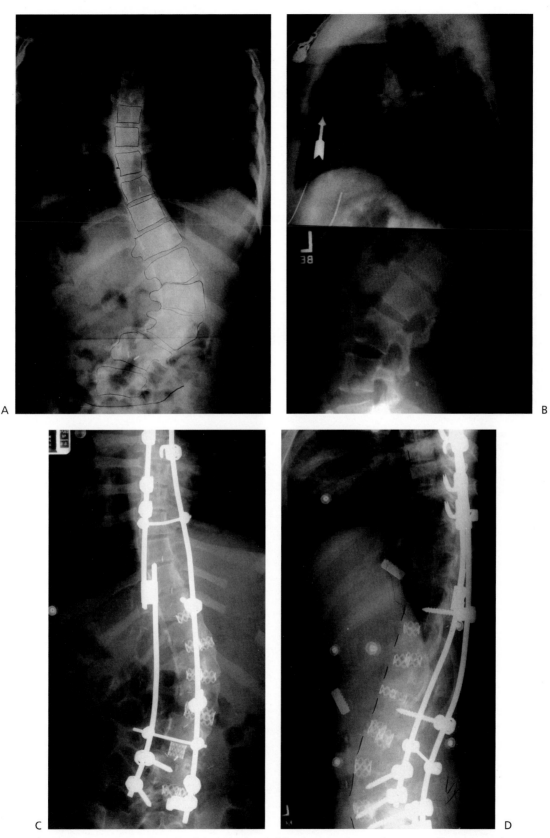

FIGURE 12. A–D: Nonidiopathic deformity after multilaminectomy for arteriovenous malformation and subsequent progressive deformity. Preoperative radiographs show marked coronal plane deformity and a paucity of posterior elements. Lateral view shows global thoracic kyphosis. After surgery, coronal and sagittal balance was restored with marked correction of the coronal and sagittal deformities.

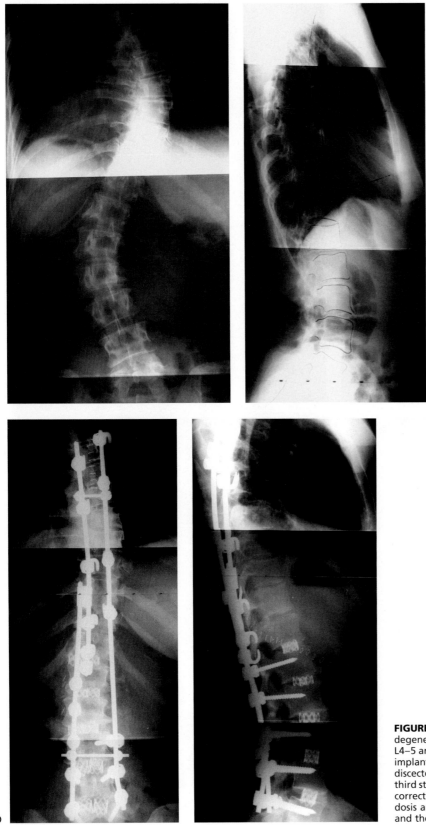

A,B

C,D

FIGURE 13. A–D: Idiopathic deformity in an adult with distal degenerative disease. Discography showed a positive curve at L4–5 and a negative curve at L5–S. Posterior wide release and implant placement were followed by the anterior procedure, discectomy, and placement of a structural anterior device. The third stage was posterior placement of the rod. Near complete correction of the coronal deformity and excellent lumbar lordosis are evident. Anterior distraction produced the lordosis, and the structural grafts maintained the lordosis.

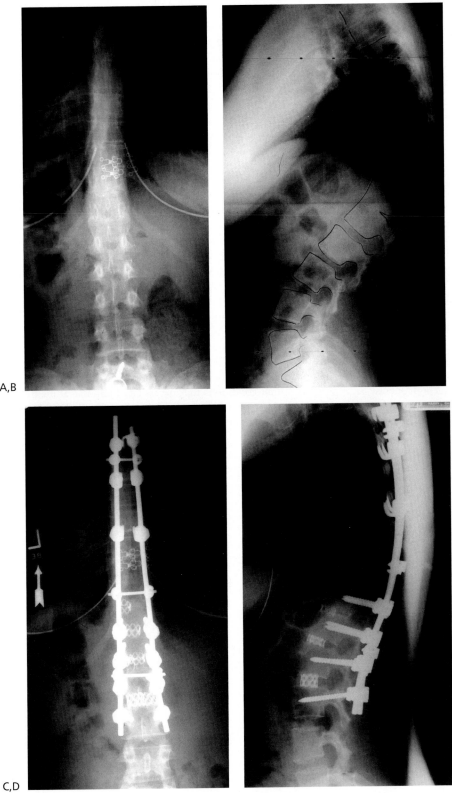

A,B

C,D

FIGURE 14. A–D: Increased thoracic kyphosis caused by multilevel anterior unsegmented bars. A three-stage procedure was used to correct the deformity. Posterior release and screw and hook placement were followed by anterior osteotomies and cage placement. The result was correction of the deformity. The third stage was posterior placement of the tension band, or rod.

managed with a same-day three-stage procedure. The result was spectacular correction of a marked kyphotic deformity.

Moss Miami instrumentation can be used in the surgical management of deformity of any cause and form in the care of adolescents and children. The low profile is ideally suited to this population. Excellent results—no failure or loss of correction at 2 years—have been reported for the management of idiopathic disease (18,24).

Spondylolisthesis

Degenerative conditions usually are not a facet of the surgical management of adolescent or pediatric spinal disorders. Spondylolisthesis is a reasonable adolescent analogue to adult degenerative disease that necessitates short-segment instrumentation. For the past several years I have routinely used instrumented reduction with structural anterior support provided by the posterior approach.

In situ fusion of high dysplastic spondylolisthesis (14) carries several risk factors. Several authors have reported continued progression of the deformity (slip angle and translation) in as many as one third of patients treated with in situ fusion (4,8,10). Schoenecker et al. (15) reported a 6% incidence of cauda equina syndrome among patients with high-grade spondylolisthesis undergoing in situ fusion. In addition, in situ fusion does nothing to correct the sagittal plane deformity, which frequently causes problems later in life.

Harms et al. (9) reported excellent results (a success rate more

than 98%) in the care of patients undergoing instrumented reduction with structural anterior graft as a posterior lumbar interbody fusion. I also have reported excellent results without neurologic complications in a consecutive series of 18 patients high dysplastic spondylolisthesis (20). The procedure is shown in Fig. 15. The elements are (a) a Gill procedure with exposure of both L5 and S1 roots following the L5 roots laterally beyond the alar transverse ligament; (b) application of temporary distraction; (c) lumbosacral discectomy and excision of the sacral dome if indicated; (d) removal of cartilage end plates; (e) anterior decortication and grafting; (f) placement of structural interbody graft; (g) release of distraction; (h) placement of screws in L5 and the sacrum; (i) placement of rods from L5 to the sacrum and application of compression forces; and (j) posterolateral graft and fusion. The integrity of the L5 root is ensured by means of continual inspection throughout the procedure and by means of direct stimulation of the root. Initial stimulation thresholds are high (more than 5 mAmp). These should gradually decrease during the procedure. Any increase should alert the surgeon to possible L5 root neurapraxia. Figure 16 shows a radiographic example of the procedure in the management of high dysplastic spondylolisthesis.

Moss Miami instrumentation in conjunction with use of a Harms cage is an excellent and safe method of reduction of high-grade spondylolisthesis and maintenance of the corrected position. Other conditions that necessitate lumbosacral instrumentation can be approached in a like manner. At the lumbosacral junction, anterior column support is recommended when

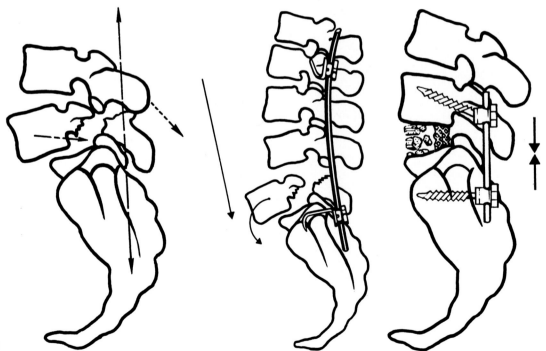

FIGURE 15. A: High dysplastic spondylolisthesis and the direction of forces necessary to reduce the deformity. **B:** Temporary distraction with partial reduction. This is necessary to remove the disc and sacral dome and place the structural interbody graft from the posterior approach. **C:** Completed procedure with the structural interbody graft and the morselized autograft in the anterior portion of the interspace. Single level instrumentation and reduction of spondylolisthesis are evident.

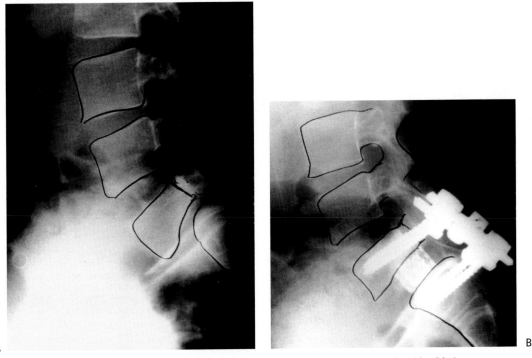

FIGURE 16. A, B: Reduction achieved with the technique illustrated in Fig. 15. Considerable improvement in slip angle, sacral inclination, and the percentage displacement is evident.

any appreciable change in sagittal plane alignment occurs. Figure 17 shows the anterior column deficit produced with correction of lumbosacral kyphosis.

With reference to sacral fixation, several possibilities exist with Moss Miami instrumentation. Figure 18 shows use of bilateral bicortical screws, which is the preferred method. The possibility of using the Roger Jackson (11) method of intrasacral rod placement is quite easily met with Moss Miami instrumentation. Figure 19 shows the intrasacral method of fixation advocated by Roger Jackson.

Reconstruction

Reconstruction after failed surgery, instrumentation or noninstrumentation, is easily accomplished with the Moss Miami system. The variety of implants and connectors and the ability to provide anterior column support, usually in the three-stage procedure (19,21) affords a versatile approach to reconstruction. Categories that necessitate reconstructive procedures include tumors, pseudoarthrosis, implant failure, imbalance, and postlaminectomy deformities. Figure 20 shows reconstruction of lumbar

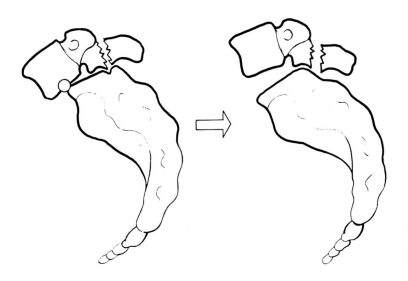

FIGURE 17. Anterior column deficit produced by reduction of spondylolisthesis. Unless the space in front is filled with a structural graft, all loads are transferred to the posterior device.

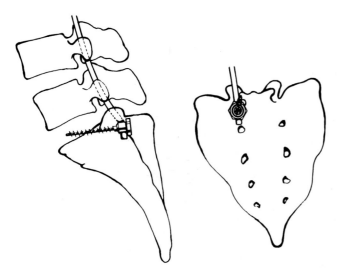

FIGURE 18. S1 screw. The end plate is engaged by the screw. This provides bicortical fixation.

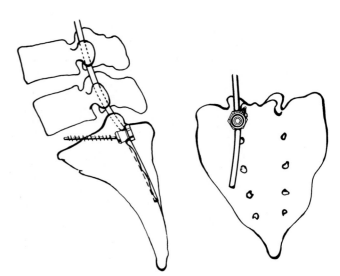

FIGURE 19. Roger Jackson intrasacral rod technique. The rod passes through the screw to a position anterior to the posterior cortex of the sacrum. The cantilever pull-out forces on the screw are converted to anteriorly directed forces on the screw.

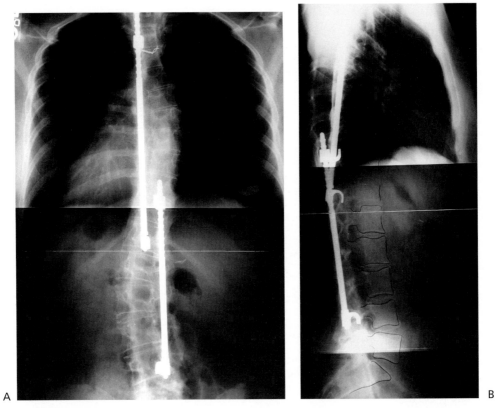

A   B

FIGURE 20. A, B: Lumbar flat-back syndrome caused by Harrington distraction instrumentation. The only lordosis is between L4 and the sacrum. These two levels were degenerated and painful at discography. *(Figure continues.)*

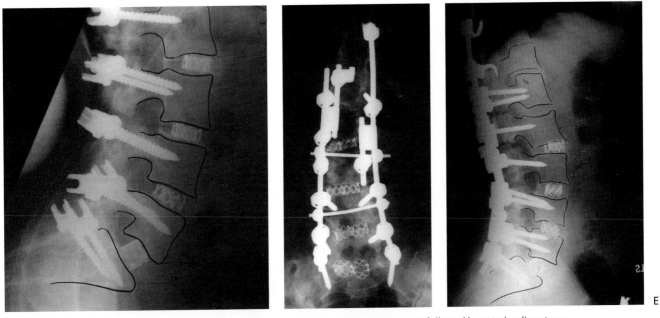

C,D

E

FIGURE 20. *Continued.* **C:** Posterior osteotomies and screw placement followed by anterior discectomy and structural grafting have been done. Production of lordosis with anterior structural grafts is evident. No rods have been placed. **D, E:** The third stage is rod placement, which provides a posterior tension band.

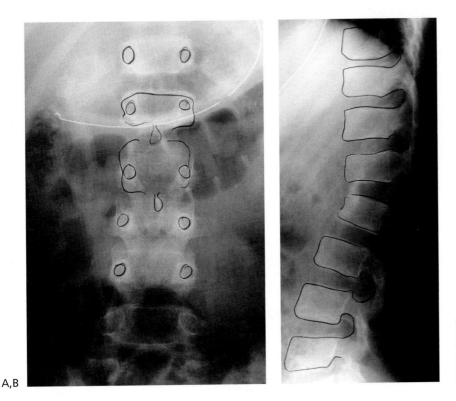

A,B

FIGURE 21. A, B: Flexion distraction injury at the L1–2 level in a 10-year-old child. Three-dimensional computed tomographic reconstruction shows the posterior ligamentous injury that allows facet dislocation. Bony injury is present at the posterior attachment of the end plate and anulus. *(Figure continues.)*

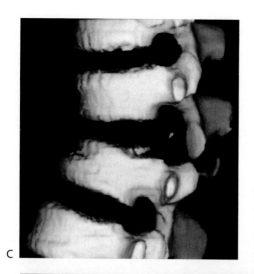

FIGURE 21. *Continued.* **C:** Flexion distraction injury at the L1–2 level in a 10-year-old child. Three-dimensional computed tomographic reconstruction shows the posterior ligamentous injury that allows facet dislocation. Bony injury is present at the posterior attachment of the end plate and anulus. **D, E:** Single-level reduction has been achieved with a pedicle screw system. No immobilization was used.

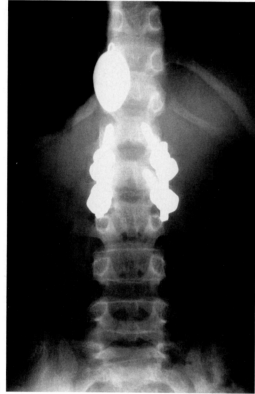

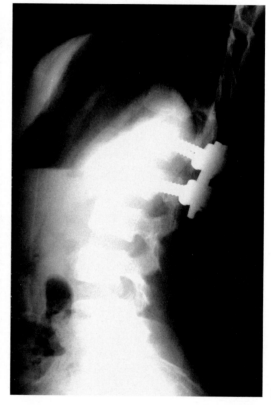

flat-back syndrome. Excellent realignment was achieved with the three-stage procedure.

Trauma

Spinal trauma is relatively uncommon among children and adolescents. The use of pedicle fixation and the possibility of anterior column reconstruction when indicated are similar to those of all other posterior multiple hook-screw-rod systems. The polyaxial screw affords a substantial advantage to this system. The ability to mix hooks and screws easily is another advantage. Figure 21

shows a flexion distraction injury fixed with monosegmental instrumentation and fusion.

SUMMARY

Moss Miami spinal instrumentation can be used to manage any problem for which spinal instrumentation is indicated. Application can be either anterior or posterior. The posterior open implant design greatly simplifies the entire surgical procedure, as does introduction of translation implants. The security of the closure mechanism affords patient and surgeon a measure of security not previously available. Polyaxial screws, which have load-sharing features, offer additional advantages and additional simplification of surgical techniques. The results are excellent with implementation of the system in primary operations and in reconstructive procedures. A flexible, elastic 5-mm rod can be used to attain correction of most deformities and to maintain the correction until arthrodesis is complete.

REFERENCES

1. Akbarnia B, Asher M, Hess F, et al. (1996): Safety of pedicle screws in pediatric patients with scoliosis and kyphosis. Presented at the 31st Annual Meeting of the Scoliosis Research Society, Ottawa, Ontario, Canada, September 25–28, 1994.
2. Asher M (1996): Isola spinal instrumentation for scoliosis. In: Bridwell K, DeWald R, eds. *The textbook of spinal surgery.* Philadelphia: Lippincott-Raven, pp. 569–610.
3. Betz R, Harms J, Clements D, et al. (1999): Comparison of anterior and posterior instrumentation for correction of adolescent thoracic idiopathic scoliosis. *Spine* 24:225–231.
4. Boxall D, Bradford D, Winter R, et al. (1979): Management of severe spondylolisthesis in children and adolescents. *J Bone Joint Surg Am* 61:479–489.
5. Calancie B, Madsen P, Lebwohl N (1994): Stimulus evoked EMG monitoring during transpedicular lumbosacral spine instrumentation. *Spine* 19:2780–2785.
6. Cotrel Y, Dubousset J, Guillaumat M (1988): New universal instrumentation in spinal surgery. *Clin Orthop* 227:10–32.
7. Graf H, Hecquet J, Dubousset J. (1983): 3-Dimensional approach to spinal deformity: application to the study of the prognosis of pediatric scoliosis. *Rev Chir Orthop Reparatrice Appar Mot* 69:407–418.
8. Hanley E, Levy J (1989): Surgical treatment of isthmic lumbosacral spondylolisthesis: analysis of variables influencing results. *Spine* 14:48–57.
9. Harms J, Jeszenszky D, Stoltze D, et al. (1997): True spondylolisthesis reduction and monosegmental fusion in spondylolisthesis. In: Bridwell K, DeWald R, eds. *The textbook of spinal surgery.* Philadelphia: Lippincott-Raven, pp. 1337–1347.
10. Hensinger R, Lang J, MacEwen G (1976): Surgical management of spondylolisthesis in children and adolescents. *Spine* 1:207–218.
11. Jackson R (1997): Insertion of intra-sacral rods for sacral fixation and spinal correction with in situ rod contouring techniques. In: Bridwell K, DeWald R, eds. *The textbook of spinal surgery.* Philadelphia: Lippincott-Raven, pp. 2187–2209.
12. Johnson C, Ashman R, Richards S, et al. (1996): TSRH Universal Spine Instrumentation. In: Bridwell K, DeWald R eds. *The textbook of spinal surgery.* Philadelphia: Lippincott-Raven, pp. 535–568.
13. Lee J, Milne E, Shufflebarger H, et al. (1998): Anterior column support in long segment kyphosis constructs [abstract]. *Orthop Trans* 22:640.
14. Marchetti P, Bartolozzi P (1997): Classification of spondylolisthesis as a guideline for treatment. In: Bridwell K, DeWald R, eds. *The textbook of spinal surgery.* Philadelphia: Lippincott-Raven, pp. 1211–1254.
15. Schoenecker P, Cole H, Herring J, et al. (1990): Cauda equina syndrome following in situ arthrodesis of severe spondylolisthesis of the lumbosacral junction. *J Bone Joint Surg Am* 72:369–379.
16. Shufflebarger H (1994): Cotrel-Dubousset spinal instrumentation. In: Weinstein S, ed. *The pediatric spine.* New York: Raven Press, pp. 1545–1583.
17. Shufflebarger H (1994): Theories and mechanisms of posterior derotation spinal systems. In: Weinstein S, ed. *The pediatric spine.* New York: Raven Press, pp. 1515–1544.
18. Shufflebarger H (1996): Moss Miami instrumentation. In: Bridwell K, DeWald R, eds. *The textbook of spinal surgery.* Philadelphia: Lippincott-Raven, pp. 675–694.
19. Shufflebarger H (1998): Complex revision spinal surgery: posterior-anterior-posterior sequence [abstract]. *Orthop Trans* 22:642.
20. Shufflebarger H (1998): High grade isthmic dysplastic spondylolisthesis: monosegmental surgical treatment. Presented at the 33rd Annual Meeting of the Scoliosis Research Society, New York, September 16–20, 1998.
21. Shufflebarger H (1999): Posterior-anterior-posterior sequence in revision spinal surgery. In: Marguiles J, ed. *Revision spine surgery.* St Louis: Mosby, pp. 175–187.
22. Shufflebarger H, Biederman L, Matthis W (1995): Comparison of closure mechanisms on non-threaded rod systems. Presented at the 30th Annual Meeting of the Scoliosis Research Society, Asheville, North Carolina, 13–16, 1995.
23. Shufflebarger H, Clark C (1990): Fusion levels and hook patterns in thoracic idiopathic scoliosis with Cotrel-Dubousset instrumentation. *Spine* 15:916–928.
24. Shufflebarger H, Clark C (1996). Cantilever and translation mechanics with a 5mm rod system. Results in adolescent idiopathic scoliosis. Presented at the 31st Annual Meeting of the Scoliosis Research Society, Ottawa, Ontario, Canada, September 25–28, 1994.
25. Shufflebarger H, Clark C (1998): Effect of wide posterior release on correction in adolescent idiopathic scoliosis. *J Pediatr Orthop* 7:117–124.
26. Shufflebarger H, Ellis R, Clark C (1989): Cotrel-Dubousset instrumentation in adolescent idiopathic scoliosis [abstract]. *Orthop Trans* 13:79.
27. Suk S, Kim J, Kim W, et al. (1997): Preservation of distal lumbar motion segments with segmental pedicle screw fixation in King type 1 adolescent idiopathic scoliosis. Presented at the 32nd Annual Meeting of the Scoliosis Research Society, St. Louis, September 25–27, 1997.

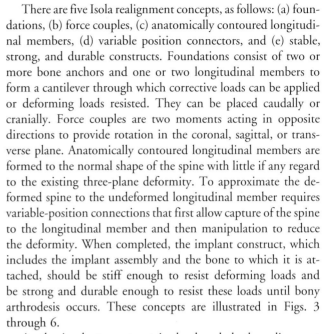

FIGURE 3. Cantilever foundations. Model shows placement of proximal and distal multiple hook, transversely connected, rod foundations **(A)** with force couple deformity reduction **(B)**.

A,B

There are five Isola realignment concepts, as follows: (a) foundations, (b) force couples, (c) anatomically contoured longitudinal members, (d) variable position connectors, and (e) stable, strong, and durable constructs. Foundations consist of two or more bone anchors and one or two longitudinal members to form a cantilever through which corrective loads can be applied or deforming loads resisted. They can be placed caudally or cranially. Force couples are two moments acting in opposite directions to provide rotation in the coronal, sagittal, or transverse plane. Anatomically contoured longitudinal members are formed to the normal shape of the spine with little if any regard to the existing three-plane deformity. To approximate the deformed spine to the undeformed longitudinal member requires variable-position connections that first allow capture of the spine to the longitudinal member and then manipulation to reduce the deformity. When completed, the implant construct, which includes the implant assembly and the bone to which it is attached, should be stiff enough to resist deforming loads and be strong and durable enough to resist these loads until bony arthrodesis occurs. These concepts are illustrated in Figs. 3 through 6.

As the implant construct is developed, both realignment and mechanical stabilization are accomplished. Realignment may necessitate destabilization through rib osteotomy (86), facet joint resection (108), osteotomy (45,73), discectomy (67), or even corpectomy (32,33). Achieving biologic stability through ample arthrodesis involves attention to detail, including selection of the arthrodesis site—anterior, posterior, or combined; preparation of the arthrodesis bed; graft selection; and graft placement.

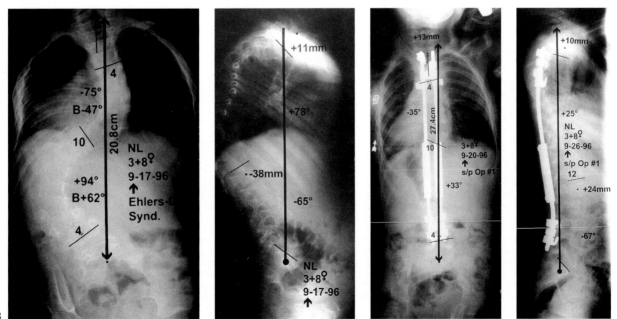

A,B

C,D

FIGURE 4. Girl 3 year 8 months of age with Ehler-Danlos syndrome and progressive scoliosis. Standing preoperative posteroanterior **(A)** and lateral **(B)** radiographs. **C, D:** Corresponding postoperative views after sequential anterior thoracolumbar anulotomy and posterior cantilever correction instrumentation.

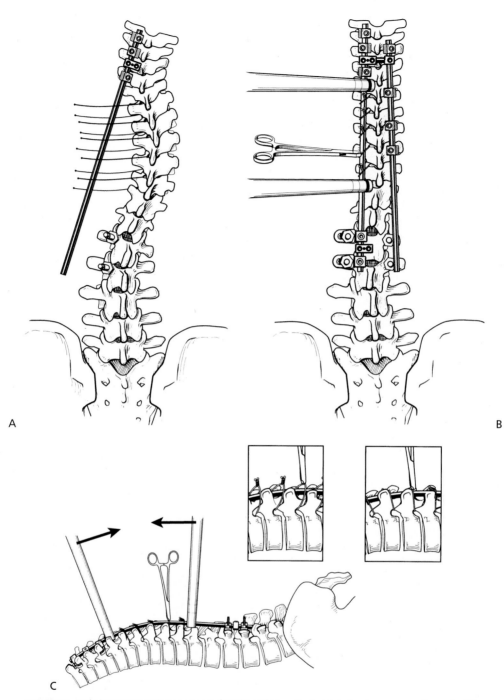

FIGURE 5. Isola instrumentation sequence for idiopathic scoliosis, triple torsion curve pattern. **A:** After insertion of left anchors and initial placement of the left rod, rod orientation into the global parasagittal plane is achieved by means of rotation as necessary and secured with an upper instrumented vertebra, transverse process, lamina claw foundation. Flexion at the upper instrumented vertebra usually is necessary and can be achieved by means of rotating the rod into position while gently holding the upper transverse process lamina claw into position with the compressor instrument. When lateral displacement of the facet hook is a concern, as it is with the T2 convex foundation in double thoracic scoliosis, the hook should be placed under the lamina. As the caudal end of the left rod is brought to the lumbar pedicle screw anchor, angular position of the T2 coronal plane is improved. The lower thoracic curve apex and periapex are translated medially and posteriorly by the apex and periapical anchors. **B:** Initial placement of the right side rod. In these constructs in which the rod initially may be lateral to the pedicle screw lower anchors, it is best to use anchors with shorter (half length) posts. As the right side rod is brought to the lower anchors, a medially and anteriorly directed load is applied to the lower thoracic apex. Finally, caudal convex compression followed by caudal concave distraction loads are applied to level in the coronal plane, lower end vertebra. **C:** In situ benders can be used to deform the rod within its elastic deformation range and loosen the subpars wires (*insert, left*) so that they can be tightened without injury to the knots (*insert, right*). (*Figure continues.*)

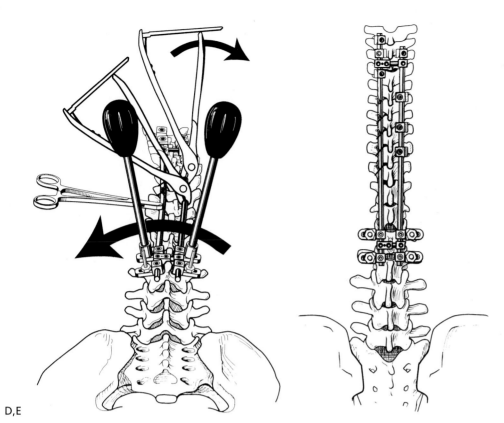

FIGURE 5. *Continued.* **D:** Transverse plane angular correction of thoracolumbar/lumbar curve is accomplished by means of corrective rotation load on the pedicle screws with countertorsional load resistance in the upper portion of the construct. **E:** Completed construct.

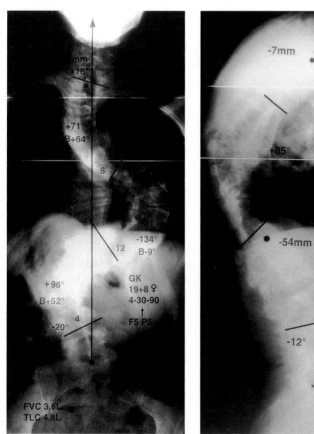

FIGURE 6. Preoperative standing posteroanterior **(A)** and lateral **(B)** radiographs of a woman 18 years 8 months of age show triple curve pattern. *(Figure continues.)*

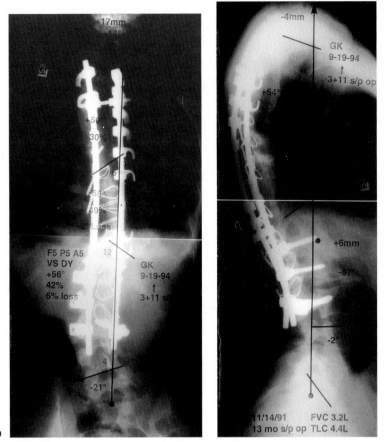

C,D

FIGURE 6. *Continued.* Standing posteroanterior **(C)** and lateral **(D)** radiographs obtained 3 years 11 months after the operation.

COMPONENTS

There are seven Isola design principles, as follows: minimal internal and external profile; simplicity; versatility; dimension standardization with Harrington rod since 1985 (71), variable screw placement since 1987 (113), and Kaneda smooth rod since 1993 (61); stable, strong, and durable components, connections, and constructs; user-friendly instrumentation; and cost-effectiveness. Examples of the four categories of components—longitudinal members, anchors, connectors, and accessories—are shown in Fig. 7.

The system is based on 6.35-mm (¼-inch) and 4.76-mm (³⁄₁₆-inch) smooth rod longitudinal members. The clinical utility of the stainless steel versions of these rods has been amply demonstrated with Harrington and Luque instrumentation. Hybrid longitudinal members incorporate features of a hole or plate in continuity with the rod or rods of varying diameter, the so-called plate-rod combination and rod-rod combination. In addition, the system is compatible with the Variable Screw Placement plate.

To achieve the Isola principles in design, the variable-throat-height hook series was developed to accommodate posterior anatomic elements of different thickness and orientation, thus eliminating anatomic specific constraints, such as transverse processes, laminae, facets, pedicle, thoracic, and lumbar. With the use of hooks of minimum throat diameter, the potential danger of

mixing hooks and sublaminar wires has been avoided (103). The 9.5-mm throat height hook is the same as the Harrington 1253 hook, and the 6.35-mm throat matches that of the pediatric Harrington hook. There are five throat heights in the 6.35-mm rod compatible series (5 to 11 mm in 1.5-mm increments) and five in the 4.76-mm rod series (3.5 to 9.5 mm in 1.5-mm increments). To limit hook-blade profile in the spinal canal, blade width was reduced from the 9.0 mm of the standard Harrington 1253 hook to 7.0 mm in the 6.35-mm rod line and from 7.0 mm to 5.0 mm in the 4.76-mm rod series. Five-millimeter wide hook blades are available in the 6.35-mm rod series and are especially useful for supralaminar placement and lumbar sublaminar placement.

Wire and cable anchors include single 16-gauge beaded end, double 16-gauge looped on one end and beaded on the other end, Drummond-style button wires (56), and Songer-style cables (110). Although problems have been reported with use of sublaminar wires (55,122), they can be used safely (44,123) and remain useful because they lend themselves to segmental placement, are variable-position connections, and are inexpensive (84,85). Screw anchors can be placed in almost any bony anatomic site that accommodates the screw, such as the vertebral bodies through the pedicles posteriorly, the vertebral bodies anteriorly, the sacrum, and the ilium.

Thoracolumbar and lumbar pedicle screws have become much better accepted since the mid 1990s. They can be used

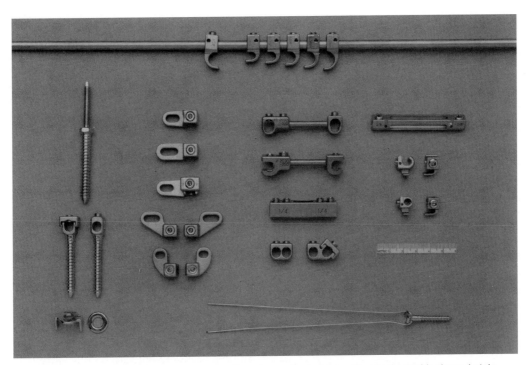

FIGURE 7. Sample implant components. *Top,* drop-entry hook position and variable-throat-height hooks. *Left column,* screws with anterior washers and staples. *Second column from left,* regular, extended, open, offset, and minioffset slotted connectors. *Second column from right,* closed and open drop-entry transverse, tandem, closed bypass, and open-closed bypass connector. *Far right column,* pediatric components include telescoping connector, open top-entry hook, closed side set-screw hooks, and screw-wire anchor combination.

safely in pediatric operations (2,34), and use of constructs containing them provide better correction of deformity (27,63, 70,74,80,105). In addition, the crankshaft phenomenon can probably be prevented both experimentally (79) and clinically (36). This is probably partly because pedicle screws have been shown experimentally to increase the torsional rigidity of scoliosis constructs (126) and are more stable than hooks (77).

The hook and screw anchor to longitudinal member connection is based on the V-groove hollow-ground (VHG) connection. As the set screw is tightened the rod is pushed into a spine slightly smaller in diameter than the rod (V-groove), and a recess (hollow-ground) is placed in the center of the connector body to accommodate three-point contact in the sagittal plane. The connection may be open body or closed body. The open connection is closed with a sliding cap, a designed initiated by Dr. Robert W. Gaines, Jr. This provides for rod capture with subsequent freedom of manipulation on the rod until the set screw is tightened.

Incorporated into the closed-body hooks is a drop-entry feature, which is analogous to the nose of a Concord jet during take-off and landing. With the set screw in the loosened position, the hook body assumes a 10-degree angle to the longitudinal rod. This, coupled with the built-in 5-degree blade angle relative to the body and the slightly shortened hook blade, allows safe placement of the hook over the lamina or transverse process while it is on the longitudinal rod. During tightening of the set screws, the hook body becomes parallel to the rod and in the process tightens the hook blade into the bone.

The slotted-style rod to screw connector provides six degrees of freedom of motion and manipulation, as follows: vertical, mediolateral, and anteroposterior translation and coronal, transverse, and sagittal angulation. Adjustment of anteroposterior translation and sagittal angulation is accomplished with flat washers and opposing 15-degree taper washers.

Iliac and variable screw placement screws are connected to eye-rod holes and plate-rod combination slots by means of stable and strong bolt connections. Wires are twisted to form their own connections. Cables are secured with crimps.

The rod to rod connectors allow transverse, side by side (bypass), and end to end (tandem) connection of the rods. The threaded transverse and bypass connectors have largely been supplanted by closed VHG connection-based components because they add strength and decrease the profile. From time to time, however, the threaded versions are useful because of their versatility.

The accessories include washers 3.0 and 5.0 mm thick to provide variable-position sagittal translation. This allows placement of screws into maximum torque, which provides maximum strength (129). Space for bone graft material also is provided. The 15-degree wedge washers provide up to 15 degrees sagittal plane angular position variability. The 9.53-mm (3/8-inch) acorn nut is for completion of eye-rod-screw and plate-rod-screw connections. The 7.94-mm (5/16-inch) long, 4-mm-thick hex nut completes split and slotted bolt connections.

The implant components discussed are compatible with the 6.35-mm rod. Most of these components are available in 4.76-

mm compatible versions. There also are special 4.76-mm components for especially small children. Almost all the components are available in titanium as well as steel.

MECHANICS

The mechanical characteristics of the Isola spinal implant system have been extensively studied (41,42,117). The comparative flexion-compression load stiffness and strength of longitudinal member to bone screw connection subconstructs (42) and constructs (50) have shown Isola constructs to be slightly greater in stiffness than most other constructs tested and usually much stronger. Since the latest published studies, additional refinement of the screws has occurred and resulted in further increases in strength and durability (B.W. Cunningham, personal communication, 1995).

With few exceptions, transverse connection should be used. It increases torsional and lateral bending stiffness but not axial compression or flexion-extension stiffness. However, transverse connection does adversely affect the endurance limit of the longitudinal members (111). Therefore I recommend the transverse connectors be placed at the end of constructs. For one and two motion constructs, one transverse connection usually is adequate, but for three or more motion segments, I recommend use of two transverse connectors. Three transverse connections are seldom, if ever, needed.

BIOMECHANICS

My colleagues and I have conducted experiments to study the biologic characteristics of stable, strong, and durable posterior spinal instrumentation constructs with and without fusion (19,49,51,79,109). Adult mongrels and juvenile Walker hounds have been used. For the worst-case scenario, human-size spinal implants were used, although mature dogs are one-half to one-fourth human body weight and one-tenth human spine axial load. The studies were based on the premise that axial flexion-compression is the most important spinal instrumentation and fusion loading mode. The general hypothesis was that potentially harmful effects of posterior spinal implant constructs of adequate stiffness and strength to stabilize the spine during arthrodesis are measurable but acceptably small. In general, L3 and L5 were instrumented, L4 was as spanned vertebra, and L2 and L6 were adjacent vertebrae. The effects of stress shielding and stress concentration on bone mineral density and fusion and on underlying and adjacent vertebral body stiffness were studied at intervals ranging from 3 months to 12 months postoperatively.

Instrumentation without fusion resulted in an approximately 20% decrease in bone mineral density in the stress-shielded (L4) vertebra at 3 months; this percentage had not increased up to 6 months postoperatively. Low-torque nut tightening caused loosening of implant interconnections in some specimens. High-torque connection tightening at 6.4 Nmm did not allow any clinical loosening at 9 months. However, with high-torque nut tightening, 20 of 56 connections had some loosening at the

implant-bone interface by 9 months postoperatively in unfused spines. In specimens in which either the bone-implant interface loosened or the implant-bone interface loosened, the bone mineral density of the stress-shielded (L4) vertebra returned to nearly normal within 9 months. In specimens with secure implant-implant interconnections and implant-bone interface, an approximately 20% reduction in stress-shielded vertebra persisted but did not worsen after 3 months (51). With the addition of facet fusion, the stress-shielded (L4) vertebra still lost about 18% of bone mineral density after 3 months; this percentage did not increase over the following 3 months (49).

Posterior facet arthrodesis produced an increase in two-motion-segment stiffness from 368 Nmm to 1,349 Nmm for 4.76-mm rod constructs and to 799 Nmm for 6.35-mm rod constructs at 6 months. Both were significantly increased from the control values. Stiffness in the 6.35-mm specimens was significantly less than in the 4.76-mm specimens. In a subsequent experiment in which extraarticular and facet intraarticular arthrodesis was performed, the comparative stiffness at 12 months was 1,594 Nmm for 4.76-mm rod specimens and 1,244 Nmm for 6.35-mm rod specimens; the value among the controls was 376 Nmm. Differences in fusion stiffness between the two rod size specimens did not vary, and the increase in specimen stiffness caused by retained implants was about 15% for the 4.76-mm rod group and 22% for the 6.35-mm rod group. The axial compression stiffness of the bypassed vertebral bone was 3,161 Nmm compared with 4,394 Nmm for sham and control vertebra at the same level (19). This 28% decrease in bone mineral density was comparable with the 20% decrease in bone mineral density mentioned earlier.

These observations support the hypothesis that potentially harmful biologic side effects of use of a posterior spinal implant construct of adequate stiffness and strength to stabilize the spine during arthrodesis are measurable but are acceptably small.

INSTRUMENTS

The instruments, like the components, can be categorized as anchor related, longitudinal member related, and connector related, although there is some overlap. Anchor-related instruments include the pedicle probe, ball tip sounder, pedicle markers, iliac markers and sacral sounders, and taps. Also in this category are hook starters, hook holders, the hook driver, and open hook holders. Anchor-related instruments are supplemented by the wire retriever and end cutters.

Longitudinal member instruments are a tabletop rod cutter, variable radius benders (22), rod holders, and a pusher. The tabletop rod cutter provides shear cuts and allows easy sizing of rods. Longer rods can be cut and the remaining portion saved for future use. The variable radius benders work on a four-point principle to provide the capability to form anatomically correct bends, including Luque-Galveston constructs, and avoid kinking and excessive marking of the rod.

Connector-related instruments include cannulated locking wrenches, an open hook cap remover, a set-screw wrench, a connector drift, distractors and compressor, approximators, a transverse connector-rod tightener, and open-end wrenches.

Three instruments can be used to obtain needed measurements: calibrated 3.2-mm (⅛-inch) Steinmann pin (iliac markers and sacral sounders), a goniometer, and a divider.

TECHNIQUES

Intraoperative techniques other than implants have been described in detail (21). Because implant techniques have been described in a number of publications (1,8–12,14,18,23,24, 30,87,118), only a few points are made herein.

Anchors usually are placed before any decompression or destabilization is performed. Pedicle screw anchors are placed by means of the anatomic method; fluoroscopic control is not necessary (31,112). Although several authors have reported frequent (60) and even unusual (72) complications of pedicle screw placement, there has been sufficient experience to support the contention that the screws can be used safely and effectively (2,27, 31,34,70,74,80,105).

My approach involves the following. Posterior elements are thoroughly exposed so that there can be no doubt about the location of the important anatomic landmarks, including the superior facet process, transverse process, accessory process, pars interarticularis and its lateral edge, and the lamina. Ideally placed lower thoracic (Fig. 8A) and midlumbar (Fig. 8B) pedicle markers are shown as references.

In the lumbar spine the entry site of the pedicle as viewed posteriorly is approximately at a point joining the cephalocaudal middle of the transverse process and the mediolateral space defined by vertical lines along the lateral pars interarticularis edge medially and the accessory process laterally. This entry site also can be viewed as the junction of the superior facet process, transverse process, and pars interarticularis. In the thoracic spine, this entry site is vertically located at the upper edge of the transverse process, which is at just the lowest edge of the inferior facet process and mediolaterally one third of the width of the facet joint laterally to medially.

A rongeur or gouge is used to remove a portion of the outer cortex at the entry site. An awl and small oval curettes are helpful instruments for further defining the site of entry into the pedicle. The pediatric Variable Screw Placement pedicle probe is used to pass through the pedicle and into the vertebral body. Its angled tip follows the cancellous tube of bone. If the probe ever exits sharply, it is assured that it is out of the pedicle. If this occurs, the ball-tip probe is used to determine which was exited, and the angled tip of the variable screw placement probe is redirected to pick up the cancellous bone of the pedicle center. In the sagittal plane, the pedicle probe is directed perpendicularly to an imaginary line joining similar points on the posterior edges of the adjacent vertebra on the inferior edge of the laminae. This places the probe in a position perpendicular to the anticipated passage line of the longitudinal member and parallel to the superior end plate of the vertebral body. The large cephalocaudal diameter of the pedicle makes it possible to adjust the angular position of the sagittal plane so that the screws are almost always within a few degrees of perpendicular to the passage line of the longitudinal member.

The position of the screw in the transverse plane can be adjusted somewhat according to the desired use. If prevention of anterior translation is a prime consideration, the transverse plane angle of the screw in relation to the midsagittal plane can be increased by means of starting the entry point somewhat laterally and directing the probe medially (26). To gain additional pullout strength of the triangulated screws (26), it is desirable for the pedicle screw to approach as closely as possible the anterior wall of the vertebral body (92,130). This is done by palpating the bottom of the hole with the ball-tip probe and advancing the tap 5 mm farther before again palpating the bottom of the hole. In this manner it is possible to exit the anterior vertebral body by no more than 5 mm, which is believed to be safe in the lumbar spine (25).

Until considerable experience is gained, it is recommended that as each pedicle entry site is made, bone wax be placed and a blunt pedicle marker inserted. When all the markers are placed, intraoperative posteroanterior and lateral radiographs are obtained to confirm positioning. With experience, this step is seldom necessary, and screws can be placed at pedicle probing to increase the efficiency of the operation. However, if there is any doubt that the medullary canal of the pedicle has been properly probed, pedicle screw placement is not done at that site.

The adequacy of pedicle screw placement is best determined at pedicle probing and screw site preparation. When the patient is incompletely pharmacologically paralyzed, unwanted stimuli of nerves usually can be detected. Low-voltage stimulation during pedicle probe placement also can be helpful (39,102). Although I advocate use of biplanar radiographs, I recognize that these images do not show the full extent of screw perforation of the cortical cortex (81). However, cortical penetration of 4 mm is almost always tolerated (81), and even up to 6 mm may be tolerated (107). If there is doubt about screw placement in the postoperative period, computed tomographic evaluation probably is best (81).

Screw fixation at the S1 pedicle differs somewhat from that at other levels. Except in operations on patients with high-grade spondylolisthesis, the vertebral pedicle screw sites, beginning proximal to distal, are located first to help confirm the mediolateral location of the S1 entry site. The S1 pedicle screw is not medial to the pedicle screw placement sites. The technique is described and illustrated elsewhere (12,15).

The strongest anchor in the pelvis lies between the iliac cortical tables (4,40,90). The iliac posts and screw placement sites are prepared with a technique similar to that used for placement of pedicle screws. A probe is used to locate and develop the intracortical passage line, which begins at the posterosuperior iliac spine and extends just cephalad (about 5 to 10 mm) to the sciatic notch. In children, this length usually is 6 cm; in adults it is 8 cm. This technique makes placement of 6.35-mm posts or screws possible in all but the smallest patients. My colleagues and my technique is described and illustrated elsewhere (11,15,24,30). We recommend that the sacroiliac joint not be distorted through distraction or rotation during placement of the construct.

Hook and wire anchor placement, preparation of the longitudinal member, and construct assembly are illustrated elsewhere (11,30). New since the mid 1990s are the closed drop-entry transverse connectors. Because they encircle the rod, the closed

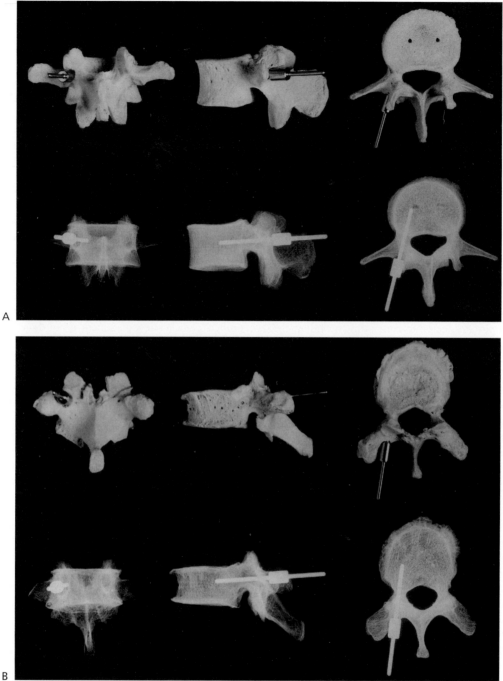

FIGURE 8. Pedicle markers in position for midlumbar **(A)** and low thoracic **(B)** vertebrae. At placement only the posterior coronal view is directly visible (*top left*). Visualizing the remaining position requires thorough knowledge of vertebral segment anatomy. Radiographs show ideally placed markers.

connections are twice as strong as the threaded rod connectors (W.L. Carson, personal communication, 1998). In addition, they have been helpful in allowing sequential application of corrective loads. The placement technique is shown in Fig. 9. The open drop-entry, threaded transverse connector, or modular cross connector, can be kept in reserve for the few instances in which the closed drop-entry transverse connector cannot be used.

Several precautions must be taken to assure optimum use of the implants. First, before screws are placed, the surgeon must confirm that the sagittal orientation of the pedicle screws is as perpendicular as possible to the desired longitudinal rod position after correction has been made. If needed, opposing tapered washers can be used to correct up to 15 degrees' lack of perpendicularity between the screw anchor and the longitudinal members. Second, it is essential that rods extend 3 to 5 mm out of the end of the VHG connector; if they do not, the VHG mechanism will not be effective. Third, routine bending of the longitudinal member when both ends are already affixed to the spine

is not generally recommended. In situ bowing is very helpful in approximating the rod and spine as the variable position connectors (such as wires) are further tightened (Fig. 5B,C). When only one end is affixed, in situ bending may be helpful. Fourth, set screws should be completely tightened before the nuts to ensure three-point rod capture by the VHG mechanism. Set screws are tightened to approximately 6.8 Nm (60 in-lb), whereas the connector nut torque is 11.3 Nm (100 in-lb). Set screw and nut tightness should be rechecked before closure. If additional tightening is achieved, the tightness should be rechecked again. Fifth, it is very important that the 3.18-mm ($\frac{1}{8}$-inch) set screw driver be completely engaged in the set screw before torque is applied. Sixth, thoracic foundations for resisting flexion load, such as staggered claws and sublaminar hooks or wires or claws at the upper vertebra and sublaminar wires at each segment below, should be fully segmental. Use of spinous process wires alone at the top of a construct should be avoided (127). Seventh, adjacent mobile motion segments should be protected by means of assuring normal anatomic alignment and preserving dorsal

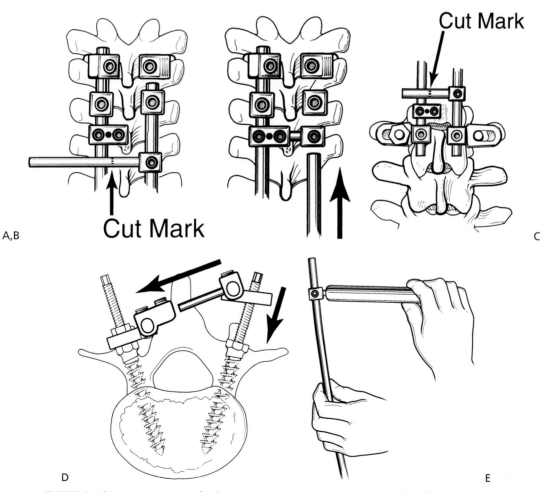

FIGURE 9. Placement sequence of a drop-entry transverse connector includes identification of the cut line at the cephalic connection **(A)**, completion of the cephalic transverse connection **(B)**, placement of a cut mark for the caudal connection **(C)**, and making the caudal connection **(D)**. If a coronal plane bend is necessary to accommodate rods not completely parallel, the rod portion of the connector can be prebent by means of securing the V-groove hollow-round connection securely on a 6.35-mm ($\frac{1}{4}$-inch) rod **(E)**.

stabilizing structures such as ligaments, facets, and deep back muscles.

During closure, the erector spinae fascia is secured to the spinous process and transverse connectors with interrupted permanent sutures to close the dead space and restore lordosis to the erector spinae fascia in the lumbar spine (115). The fascia is closed with a running absorbable stitch to obtain hemostatic closure. Closed suction in the subcutaneous layer is used if hemostatic closure is not possible or if there is concern about hematoma formation.

CLINICAL APPLICATIONS

Idiopathic Scoliosis

The most common angular deformity, scoliosis, is a three-dimensional deformity (48,52,54,57,98,100,114) that can be visualized as imperfect geometric torsion (18,20). As the result of the torsion, the apex vertebra is translated medially to laterally and angulated (rotated) in the transverse plane. Anteroposterior translation of a lesser degree also is common, usually anteriorly with thoracic curves and posteriorly with lumbar curves. The principal end vertebra deformity is coronal plane angulation. Because the end vertebra also can have abnormal sagittal plane angulation or transverse plane angulation, the end vertebra with the coronal plane deformity may not be the end vertebra with the sagittal and transverse plane deformity. The apex and end vertebrae have undergone cephalic to caudal vertical axis negative translation, or spinal shortening.

The philosophical starting point in classifying these deformities is that they represent a spectrum of one, two, three, or even four torsions. The goal during surgery is to provide as much correction as possible while preserving as many motion segments as possible. This was a major point of the study in which King et al. (78) described the selection of fusion levels for thoracic idiopathic scoliosis with Harrington instrumentation. These concepts have been validated (89). Following their lead, we continue to evolve toward a torsional classification in which compensatory curves that can be excluded are identified (18).

Selection of the end vertebra depends largely on the configuration of the deformity when gravity loaded, that is, during standing. Selection is influenced by the extent of correction to be obtained and the relative extent and stiffness of compensatory curves. An important goal is to provide overall coronal and sagittal spinal balance at T1 and the end instrumented vertebrae in relation to the midsacral gravity reference line.

The cranial end vertebra selected for instrumentation usually is the centered vertebra, defined as the first vertebra at or above the upper end vertebra that is midway between the sides of the rib cage. The logic behind this selection is that the spine is normally aligned in the midsagittal plane of the body, and this centralized vertebra is stabilized by the rib cage into the midsagittal plane. It usually is one or two levels above the coronal plane end vertebra. The exceptions to this are high thoracic scoliosis and compensatory thoracic curves in which the upper instrumented level typically may be the upper end vertebra. If upper thoracic hypokyphosis or hyperkyphosis exists, the upper end vertebra may be more than two levels above the coronal plane

end vertebra. In no case is T1 primarily instrumented in idiopathic scoliosis.

Selection of the caudal end vertebra for instrumentation is different for single curves, single curves with large compensatory curves, and double curves. For single curves, the caudal end vertebra instrumented should meet the following criteria: In the coronal plane, it should not be cephalic to the lower end vertebra or caudal to the stable vertebra. It usually is one vertebra below the lower end vertebra, which usually is one or two vertebrae above the stable vertebra. In the sagittal plane, the lower instrumented vertebra should have normal intersegmental alignment below it. In the transverse plane, the lower instrumented vertebra should be neutral (0 degrees rotation). The vertebra selected for caudal instrumentation of double thoracic curves usually is one vertebra below the lower end vertebra.

The most difficult selection of the caudal end vertebra for instrumentation involves thoracic curves with large compensatory thoracolumbar or lumbar curves. Although no criteria suggested by various investigators are absolute, they do provide a good framework for decision making in this difficult area (78,83,88). Selective exclusion of the compensatory thoracolumbar or lumbar curve usually is indicated if the following criteria are met: In the coronal plane, the T1 to midsacral gravity-reference-line mediolateral translation should be no more than 1 cm toward the side of the compensatory curve. The inflection vertebra (where the curves change direction) never should be below the stable vertebra. The thoracic/lumbar-thoracolumbar Cobb ratio and apex global translation ratio both should be greater than 1.2. The flexibility index should be greater than approximately 25 to 30. The thoracic Cobb angle should be less than 80 degrees. The lumbar/thoracolumbar Cobb angle should be less than approximately 45 degrees. In the sagittal plane, there should be normal intersegmental angular alignment below the lowest instrumented vertebra and no thoracolumbar kyphosis, as would be evidenced by T12 global extension greater than 18 degrees, L1 posterior offset greater than −12 mm, or T11–L2 kyphosis greater than 5 degrees. In the transverse plane, the thoracic/lumbar-thoracolumbar apex transverse angulation ratio should be greater than 1.2, and the end instrumented vertebra (usually inflection or one below) should have no transverse plane rotation toward the major curve convexity (18).

Some surgeons advocate selective anterior instrumentation and fusion for these predominant thoracic curves as well as some single thoracic curves. My colleagues and I have not taken this approach for several reasons, including the generally satisfactory results of posterior surgery and the problem of lower thoracic hyperkyphosis, both within and below the instrumented level that is being reported in preliminary studies of anterior instrumentation (29).

If these criteria are not met, the lumbar/thoracolumbar curve usually should be included selectively, although it almost always is possible to stop one level above the lower end vertebra if this vertebra becomes horizontal on bending, if its transverse plane angulation is approximately 10 degrees or less, and if the sagittal plane intersegmental angle is normal below the vertebra selected for instrumentation. This is best done with pedicle screw anchors in the lumbar spine (27,70,105).

For true double thoracic/thoracolumbar-lumbar curves, the

lowest instrumented vertebra usually is the lower end vertebra, but not lower than L4. The surgeon should be aware of the possible sacralization of L5, which would leave only one motion segment after fusion to L4. In the care of patients who need fusion to L4, the indications for surgery may have to be modified, or sequential anterior thoracolumbar/lumbar discectomy and arthrodesis may be necessary to allow the added correction necessary to save an additional distal motion segment (16). Because of the likelihood that fusion to L4 accelerates adjacent segment degeneration (46) and restricts spinal motion (124), I avoid fusion to L4, or its equivalent, if at all possible.

Selective exclusion of compensatory thoracic scoliosis is indicated if the thoracic curve bends to about 20 degrees or less and there will be no residual hyperkyphosis above the projected anterior fusion (68,69). These curves are probably best managed anteriorly if normal sagittal plane alignment can be restored and maintained. However, after a minimum of 2 years of follow-up evaluation, correction of deformity and maintenance of correction, as well as the patient's perception of the outcome, are equivalent between those treated with posterior and those treated with anterior surgery (37).

The instrumentation sequence for idiopathic scoliosis typi-

cally begins with apex corrective force application to a concave longitudinal member for inducing kyphosis and reducing lordosis. To reduce kyphosis and increase lordosis, instrumentation should begin with the convex longitudinal member. Many of these concepts as well as the results of the first 7 years of use of these principles have been published in the peer-reviewed literature (18,35). It will be helpful to examine the cases of patients from this published series and those of recently treated patients who illustrate continued evolutionary features in the application of these principles. The instrumentation sequences have been continuously updated and reported (11,15,24,30).

Single Torsion Thoracic

An example of a midthoracic apex curve is shown in Fig. 10. Selection of the instrumentation levels for the low thoracic curve (Fig. 11), is somewhat different and is influenced by two factors. First, the hyperkyphosis and resulting T12 hyperextension preclude anterior instrumentation and fusion. Second, the lack of rotation at the lower end vertebra, L2, makes it possible to instrument that vertebra using pedicle screw anchors, which makes coronal plane leveling possible.

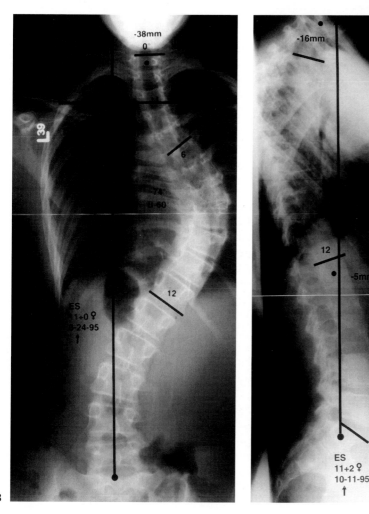

A,B

FIGURE 10. Images an 11-year-old girl with thoracic scoliosis. **A:** Standing preoperative posteroanterior (PA) radiograph shows the concept of the centered vertebra. **B:** Standing preoperative lateral radiograph. *(Figure continues.)*

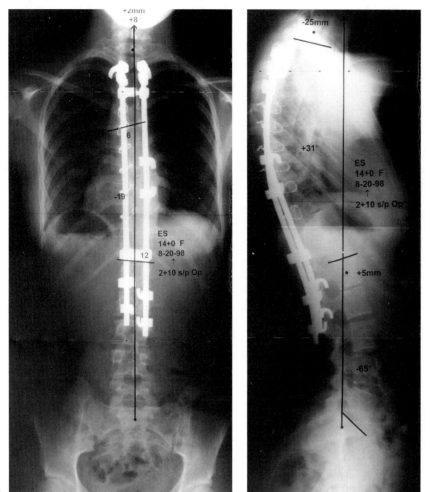

FIGURE 10. *Continued.* Standing PA **(C)** and lateral **(D)** radiographs 2 years 10 months after the operation show the instrumentation pattern, which includes a convex apex periapical transverse process intersegmental claw. The concave ribs were treated by means of osteotomy and are shown well healed.

Selection of thoracic concave anchors is based on curve size and stiffness. Open concave facet hooks are used in curves that will be easily reduced to less than 20 degrees, whereas single subpars wires are used in larger and stiffer curves. Both provide some angular correction in the transverse plane (hooks about 40% and wires about 20%), whereas sublaminar wires provide no correction in the transverse plane (65,125). The thoracic convex anchors usually are periapical transverse process intersegmental claws and are used to provide a cantilever apex curve correction (Fig. 5B).

Double Torsion Thoracic Predominant

Characteristics of this deformity are detailed earlier. The critical issue is selection of the lower instrumented vertebra and the anchorage for it. The lower instrumented vertebra is almost always T12, but it may be T11 or L1. It is the stable vertebra, is neutral (not rotated), cannot be above the lower end vertebra of the thoracic curve, and there cannot be thoracolumbar kyphosis. I prefer a pedicle screw for anchorage at this site because pedicle screws (35) control the position of the lower instrumented vertebra more securely than do hooks (101). A typical patient is shown in Fig. 12.

Double Torsion Thoracic and Thoracolumbar/Lumbar Similar

The thoracolumbar/lumbar lower end vertebra usually is L3, but occasionally is L2 or L4. If the thoracolumbar/lumbar curve is quite flexible, including lower motion segment concave disc opening on convex bending, the torsional instrumentation sequence allows saving of one additional motion segment distally with the instrumentation ending in the vertebra above the lower end vertebra. A typical patient is shown in Fig. 13. If these criteria are not met, thoracolumbar/lumbar anterior discectomy and fusion may allow the added correction necessary to save a motion segment (16). A somewhat unusual double thoracic–thoracolumbar/lumbar similar curve pattern is that in which the thoracolumbar/lumbar curve occurs primarily in the sagittal plane (24).

Double Torsion, Thoracolumbar/Lumbar Predominant

A posterior approach can be used with pedicle screw anchorage at the lower end. This operation almost always preserves three

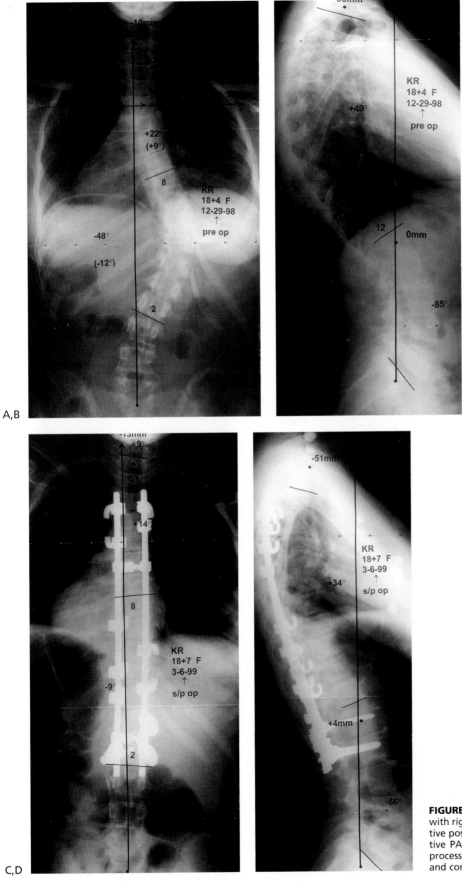

FIGURE 11. Images of a woman 18 years 4 months of age with right, low apex, thoracic idiopathic scoliosis. Preoperative posteroanterior (PA) **(A)** and lateral **(B)** and postoperative PA **(C)** and lateral **(D)** radiographs show a transverse process intersegmental claw, minioffset slotted connectors, and concave open facet hooks.

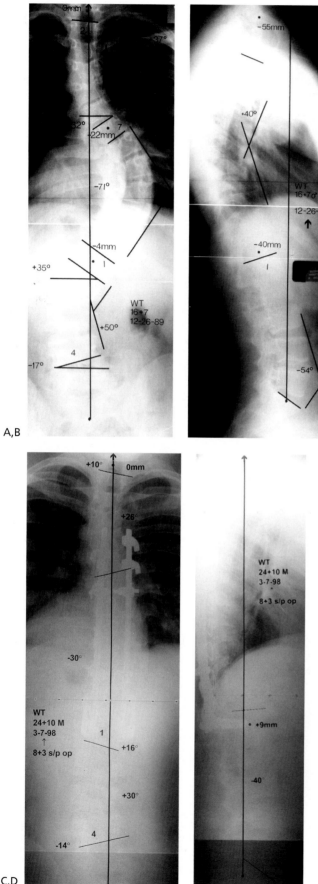

A,B

C,D

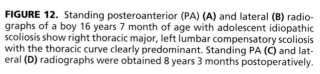

FIGURE 12. Standing posteroanterior (PA) **(A)** and lateral **(B)** radiographs of a boy 16 years 7 month of age with adolescent idiopathic scoliosis show right thoracic major, left lumbar compensatory scoliosis with the thoracic curve clearly predominant. Standing PA **(C)** and lateral **(D)** radiographs were obtained 8 years 3 months postoperatively.

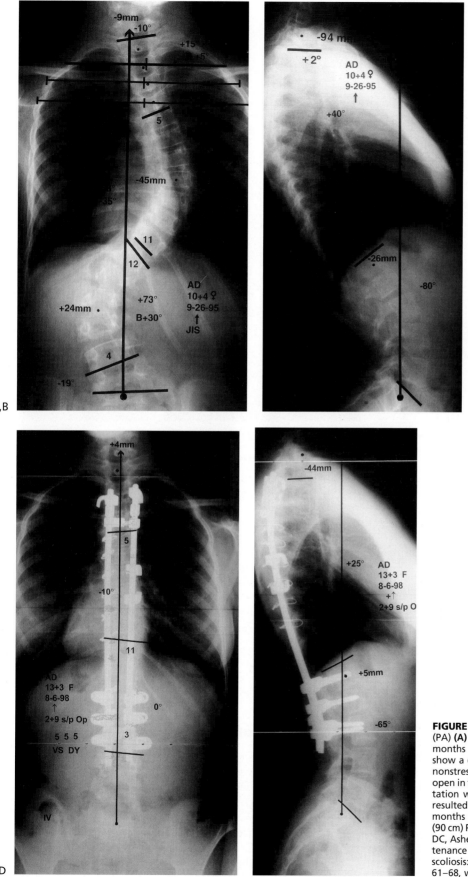

A,B

C,D

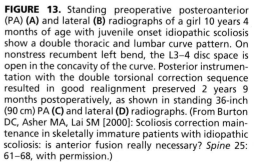

FIGURE 13. Standing preoperative posteroanterior (PA) **(A)** and lateral **(B)** radiographs of a girl 10 years 4 months of age with juvenile onset idiopathic scoliosis show a double thoracic and lumbar curve pattern. On nonstress recumbent left bend, the L3–4 disc space is open in the concavity of the curve. Posterior instrumentation with the double torsional correction sequence resulted in good realignment preserved 2 years 9 months postoperatively, as shown in standing 36-inch (90 cm) PA **(C)** and lateral **(D)** radiographs. (From Burton DC, Asher MA, Lai SM [2000]: Scoliosis correction maintenance in skeletally immature patients with idiopathic scoliosis: is anterior fusion really necessary? *Spine* 25: 61–68, with permission.)

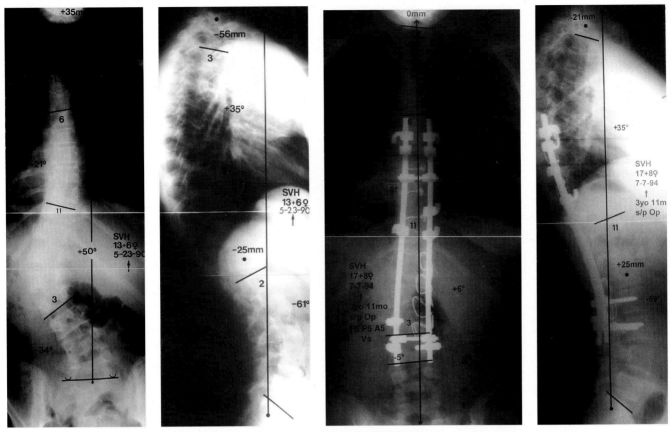

FIGURE 14. Standing preoperative posteroanterior (PA) **(A)** and lateral **(B)** radiographs of a girl 13 years 6 month of age with adolescent idiopathic scoliosis show a left lumbar major and right thoracic compensatory curve pattern. Three years 11 months postoperatively, coronal plane **(C)** and sagittal plane **(D)** alignment remains unchanged. At a follow-up evaluation 6 years 3 months after the operation the patient had no pain, was fully functional, and was very satisfied with the outcome.

distal motion segments (Fig. 14). Both process and patient-based outcomes are very good with this approach (121). If necessary, sequential anterior discectomy and fusion can be performed to provide mobility (16). When the thoracic curve is adequately flexible, to approximately 20 degrees or less on recumbent non-stress side bending, and hyperkyphosis does not extend above the anticipated level of anterior instrumentation, these curves can be instrumented anteriorly (16). An example is shown in Fig. 15.

Single Torsion Thoracolumbar/Lumbar

Unless hyperkyphosis is expected above the projected anterior instrumentation level, it is probably best that patients with single torsion thoracolumbar/lumbar curves undergo anterior instrumentation. Great care must be taken, however, to restore and preserve sagittal alignment. Single thoracolumbar/lumbar curves usually are best instrumented from end vertebra to end vertebra or from one below the upper end vertebra to the lower end vertebra. If the lower end vertebra is L4 and the lumbar spine is normally segmented, thorough anterior discectomy and fusion to L2–3 and posterior torsional instrumentation to the midthoracic spine should be considered (16).

Double Thoracic Torsion

Exact definition of the double thoracic torsion curve pattern is difficult because of the disassociation between the T1 tilt and shoulder height (82). The criteria are T1 tilt toward the high thoracic curve concavity of more than 5 degrees and convex rib elevation. A recent example is shown in Fig. 16.

Triple Torsion

See Principles and Figs. 5 and 6.

Neuromuscular Angular Deformity

Included in this category are a large number of very different disease processes and deformity patterns that strongly influence the indications for surgery and the selection of instrumented vertebrae. For example, patients with cerebral palsy and progressive scoliosis, even in the absence of pelvic obliquity, usually need instrumentation and fusion to the pelvis to prevent additional pelvic deformity below a lumbar lower instrumented vertebra. On the other hand, for a patient with myelomeningocele and moderate pelvic obliquity it is probably better to perform

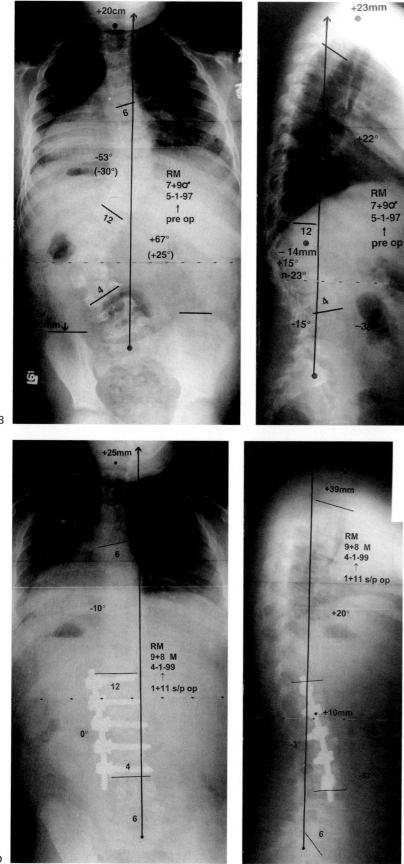

A,B

C,D

FIGURE 15. A boy 7 years 9 months of age with obesity (height 51.5 inches [1.3 m], weight 103 pounds [46.4 kg]) was found to have scoliosis as a result of an examination by the school nurse because the boy reported back pain. Preoperative posteroanterior (PA) **(A)** radiograph shows left lumbar major, right thoracic compensatory scoliosis with correction of the thoracic compensatory scoliosis from 53 to 30 degrees on recumbent nonstress bend radiograph. A standing lateral **(B)** radiograph shows thoracolumbar junction kyphosis without hyperkyphosis above. Treatment consisted of end vertebra to end vertebra anterior instrumentation with 360-degree discectomy and structural allograft bone grafting. Standing PA **(C)** and lateral **(D)** radiographs obtained 1 year, 11 months postoperatively show good realignment. At that time, the patient was fully functional, had no pain, and he and his parents were very satisfied with the outcome. Because of the large amount of growth remaining and the possibility of gradual loss of correction, the patient will be examined once a year until fully grown.

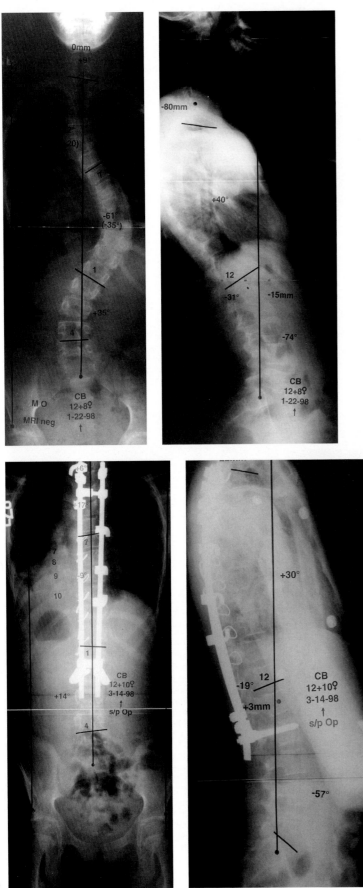

A,B

C,D

FIGURE 16. Preoperative posteroanterior (PA) **(A)** and lateral **(B)** radiographs and postoperative PA **(C)** and lateral **(D)** radiographs of a girl 12 years 10 months of age with double thoracic scoliosis show an instrumentation construct for double thoracic scoliosis with concave rib osteotomies and minioffset slotted connectors.

instrumentation into the lumbar spine to preserve pelvic mobility and reduce the likelihood of sitting-surface pressure ulcers on the insensate skin. For patients with profound retardation, surgery may not be indicated even in the presence of large deformities. For patients with Duchenne muscular dystrophy, surgery is indicated before the deformity becomes a functional concern.

The guidelines for instrumentation in the care of many patients with neuromyopathy who can walk are similar to those for the treatment of those with idiopathic scoliosis. Due concern must be given to the likelihood that a patient with neuropathy has hyperkyphosis and thus needs longer fusion. Pedicle screw anchors in the lower lumbar spine may help preserve distal motion segments (120).

In the correction of pelvic obliquity it usually is best that the end vertebra corrective load be applied first (125) (Fig. 17). In

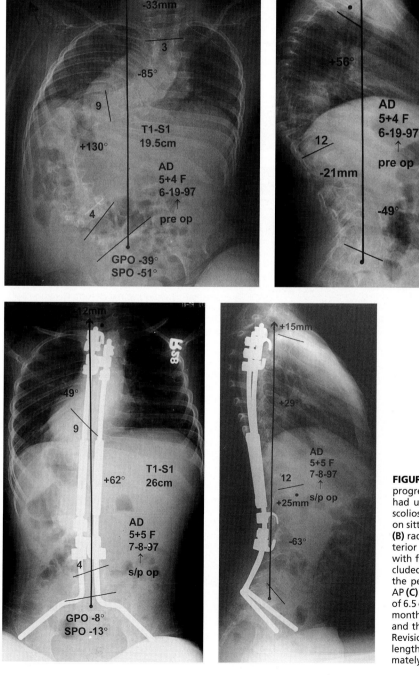

FIGURE 17. Images of a girl 5 years 4 months of age with progressive myopathic scoliosis due to Ullrich syndrome who had undergone sequential casting that did not control the scoliosis. Because of the magnitude of the deformity as shown on sitting 36-inch (90 cm) anteroposterior (AP) **(A)** and lateral **(B)** radiographs, anterior convex anulotomy followed by posterior proximal and distal cantilever foundation placement with force couple correction was planned. The pelvis was included in the distal foundation because of the magnitude of the pelvic deformity. Postoperative radiographs show good AP **(C)** and lateral **(D)** correction and a T1–S1 spine length gain of 6.5 cm. The instrumentation construct is lengthened every 6 months. Extensive anterior hip releases have been performed, and the patient has undertaken brace therapeutic standing. Revision to include fusion will be planned when no further lengthening can be gained or when she reaches approximately 8 years of age.

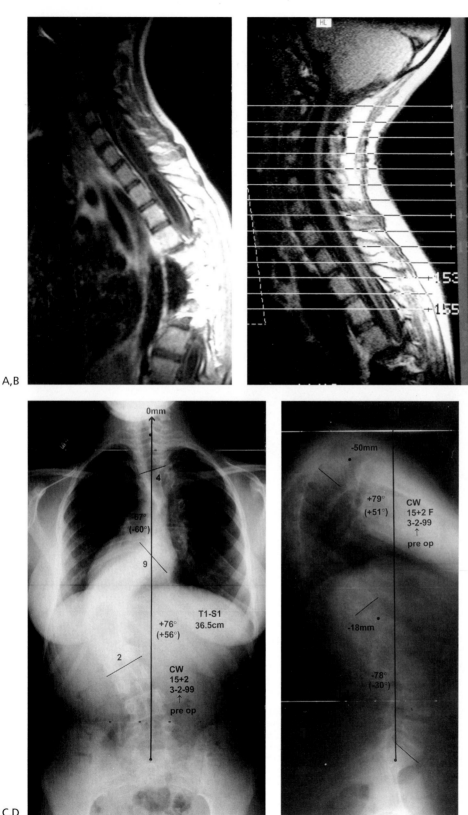

A,B

C,D

FIGURE 18. A girl 15 years 2 months of age was first evaluated at 12 years 6 months of age because scoliosis had been detected during a school screening. The patient had no symptoms, and the neurologic findings, including four-quadrant abdominal cutaneous reflexes, were normal. Standing spinal deformity radiographs showed 45-degree right thoracic and 48-degree left thoracolumbar scoliosis and thoracic hyperkyphosis of 54 degrees. For the indication of a scoliosis deformity configuration atypical of idiopathic scoliosis, occiput to sacrum screening magnetic resonance imaging (MRI) was performed. The images showed a Chiari I malformation **(A)** and a large syrinx that involved almost the entire length of the spinal column. When the patient was 13 years 5 months of age, foramen magnum decompression, fourth ventricle to subarachnoid shunt, and placement of a muscle pledget adjacent to the obex was performed without complication. The patient then could not be reached for 18 months. When contacted, she was found to have no symptoms and had normal neurologic findings except that only the right lower quadrant abdominal cutaneous reflex was weak. **B:** Magnetic resonance image shows marked decrease in the syrinx. Because of the findings on preoperative standing posteroanterior (PA) **(C)** and lateral **(D)** radiographs, an operation consisting of proximal and distal cantilever foundations with biplanar force couple reduction was planned. *(Figure continues.)*

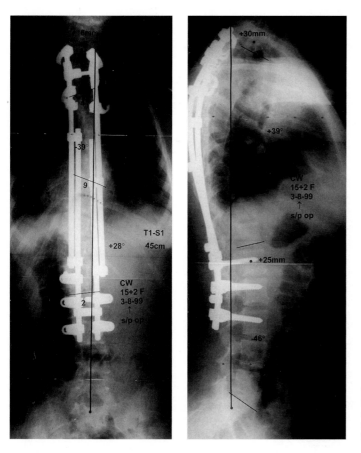

E,F

FIGURE 18. *Continued.* Postoperative radiographs showed good PA **(E)** and lateral **(F)** correction and a T1 to S1 length gain of 8.5 cm. The operation was performed through the posterior-only approach with somatosensory evoked potential monitoring. There were no complications.

the presence of pelvic extension with associated hyperlordosis, apex loading of the concave side first is recommended. Even though the patient can walk, spinal deformity extending into the pelvis necessitates instrumentation and arthrodesis to the pelvis, best done with intrailiac Galveston-type posts.

Other Types of Scoliosis

The Isola spinal implant system is useful in the management of the full range of types of scoliosis of known causation. A particularly interesting recent application is illustrated in Fig. 18. A patient with normal neurologic but phenotypically atypical scoliosis was found to have an unanticipated Chiari I malformation and syringomyelia. The Isola system also is useful in the treatment of children less than approximately 8 years of age (116), who need subfascial rodding and periodic lengthening (3) (Figs. 4 and 17).

Scheuermann Hyperkyphosis

This is another example of a deformity ideally suited to application of the end vertebra load first (8,118). An example is shown

in Fig. 19. Transverse process–facet hook claws are as strong as transverse process–pedicle hook claws (38) and are currently the upper foundation of choice. Multiple (four to six) long (92,130), triangulated (26) pedicle screws have proved to be an ideal lower foundation.

Spondylolisthesis

Spondylolisthesis is one of the most controversial areas in spinal deformity surgery. I usually do not attempt reduction if anteroposterior translation is less than 50%, provided that sagittal plane lumbosacral angulation is nearly normal. If instability cannot be documented on motion radiographs, I generally perform posterolateral arthrodesis without decompression and without instrumentation.

In the care of patients 10 years or younger with deformities of 50% or more, I do not use instrumentation or anterior fusion but have performed posterolateral arthrodesis supplemented by sagittal plane angular realignment with a bilateral pantaloon hyperextension cast and bed rest for 4 months. The patient then becomes mobile with a Norton-Brown brace.

In the care of older patients with anteroposterior translation greater than 50%, instrumentation with reduction of lumbosacral kyphosis and posterolateral fusion generally provides some

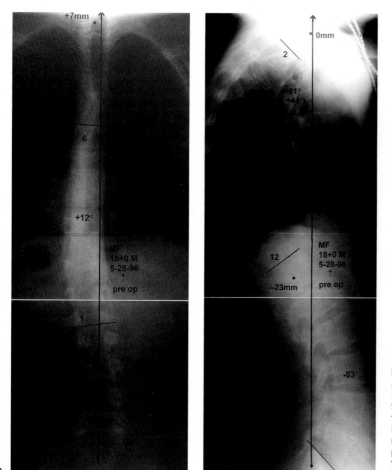

A,B

FIGURE 19. Standing preoperative posteroanterior (PA) **(A)** and lateral **(B)** radiographs of an 18-year-old man with increasing upper back pain show the poor trunk appearance of Scheuermann hyperkyphosis. Treatment consisted of sequential-anterior T4–T10 discectomy and fusion followed by T3–L3 instrumentation and fusion and reduction with an upper thoracic hook-rod cantilever foundation, captured upper lumbar pedicle screw posts, and manipulation into extension with continued anterior loading of the rod at the distal end and tightening of the pedicle screw nuts. *(Figure continues.)*

reduction and a stable fusion. If decompression is needed, transdiscal L5–S1 fusion is added. Translational reduction of one Myerding grade usually can be accomplished with a decrease in thoracolumbar kyphosis. Thus in addition to some deformity improvement, the increase in deformity associated with noninstrumented fusion is avoided (12). An example is shown in Fig. 20. If anteroposterior translation is 100% or greater, I use the Gaines approach (62) of staged anterior corpectomy followed by posterior instrumentation with sagittal plane correction of the angular position and anteroposterior translation correction as possible.

Trauma

The most common fracture of the thoracolumbar spine that necessitates surgical treatment is a burst fracture, usually Denis type B (53). Management of this condition is controversial and is beyond the scope of this chapter. My goal in management of these fractures is to instrument one vertebra above and one below the fractured vertebra, thus involving only two motion segments. I have used anulotactic reduction techniques that usually are successful in indirect decompression of the canal and in restoration of sagittal plane alignment and vertical axis height. Realignment is assessed with intraoperative lateral radiographs, which

often provide an idea of the adequacy of decompression. If there is doubt, intraoperative myelography is performed. Although relatively contraindicated if blood is evident during the lumbar puncture, imaging probably is safe if a water-soluble contrast agent is used, especially if the blood in the spinal fluid clears. When the original sagittal plane angular deformity is greater than approximately 10 degrees, anterior column restoration through a posterolateral transpedicular and peripedicular approach, including removal of the damaged disc and thorough bone grafting, is necessary to achieve long-term stabilization and prevent implant fatigue (59). It is important to use screws as large as is safely possible, transverse connections, and postoperative hyperextension bracing at all times for 6 to 8 months postoperatively when the patient is out of bed (Fig. 21).

Two-motion-segment posterior constructs for the management of burst fractures are heavily loaded, and implant failure has been documented (5,93). There are many alternatives for strengthening the construct, including use of stronger implant anchors, extension of the instrumentation by one or two motion segments (with planned eventual shortening in some), and addition of anterior structural bone grafting (5,91,128). The most common posttraumatic deformity is hyperkyphosis, a deformity well suited to simultaneous or sequential-simultaneous realignment (17) (Fig. 22).

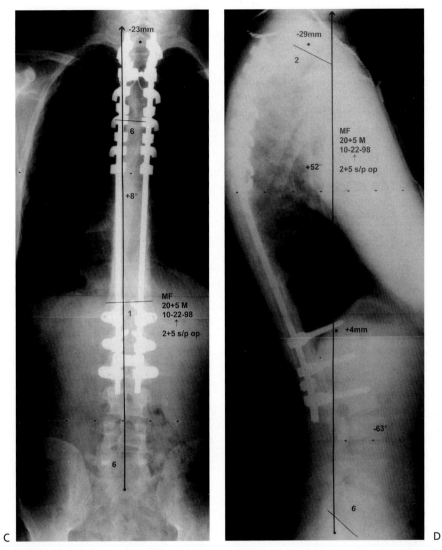

FIGURE 19. *Continued.* PA **(C)** and lateral **(D)** images show that spinal alignment 2 years 5 months postoperatively is well maintained. The patient was satisfied with the outcome and would definitely undergo the same treatment for the same problem. He self-rated his function as normal, pain as none to mild and manageable, and trunk appearance as very good.

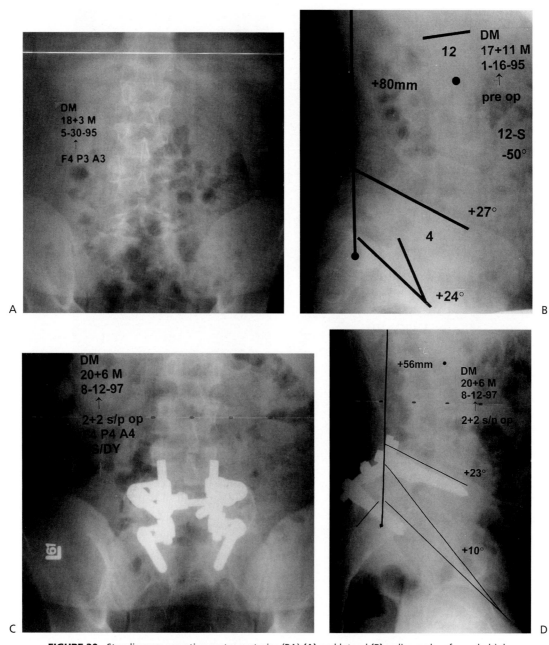

FIGURE 20. Standing preoperative posteroanterior (PA) **(A)** and lateral **(B)** radiographs of a male high school football player 18 years 4 months of age with progressive low back pain and dysplastic grade IV spondylolisthesis, class I. Treatment consisted of partial reduction with L4 to sacrum instrumentation and posterolateral intraarticular and extraarticular arthrodesis with iliac crest autograft and no decompression. PA **(C)** and lateral **(D)** radiographs obtained 2 years 2 months after the operation show spondylolisthesis maintained at grade III. The fusions appears well healed. The patient was satisfied with the outcome and would definitely undergo the same treatment again. At the follow-up evaluation the patient did report mild low back and posterior thigh pain, but he was taking no medication.

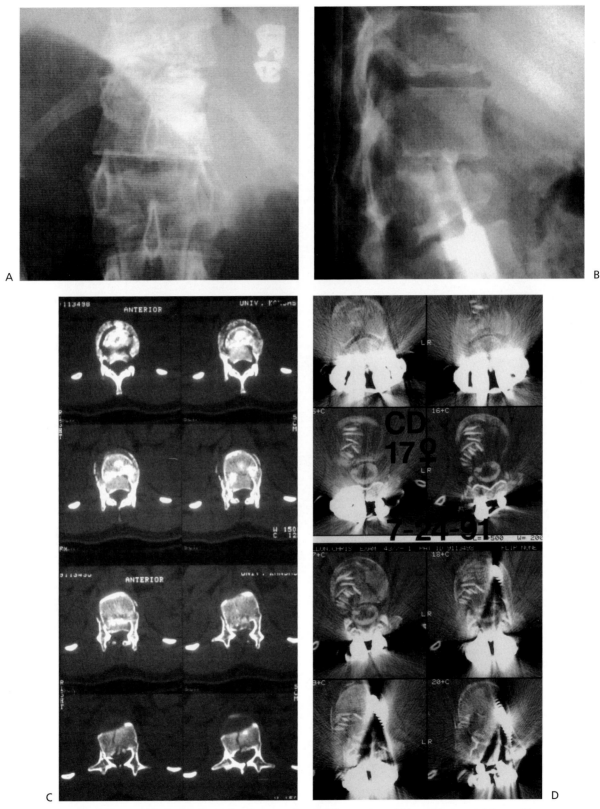

FIGURE 21. A girl 17 years 2 months of age was involved in a motor vehicle accident, sustaining an L1 burst fracture. Anteroposterior (AP) **(A)** and lateral radiographs **(B)** and a computed tomography (CT) scan **(C)** show an L1 burst fracture with more than 50% canal intrusion. The patient was unable to void, and perineal sensation was diminished. Treatment consisted of instrumented realignment with both direct decompression and transpedicular decompression with biologic stabilization through the transpedicular body and T12–L1 disc grafting. **D:** Postoperative myelographic CT scan shows open spinal canal. *(Figure continues.)*

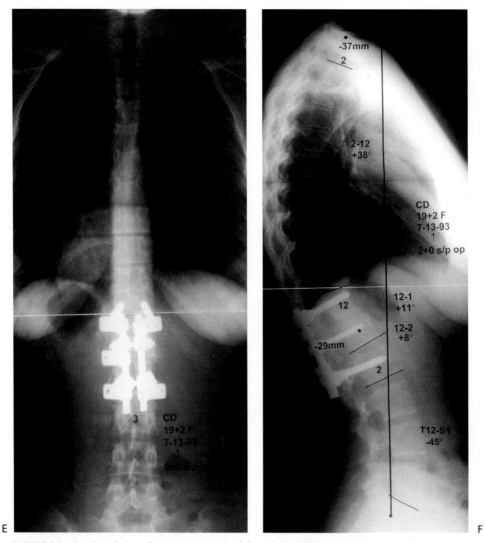

FIGURE 21. *Continued.* Standing posteroanterior **(E)** and lateral **(F)** radiographs obtained 2 years postoperatively show good healing and acceptable alignment of the fracture site. The patient still needed intermittent catheterization. She rated her outcome as very satisfactory and for the same condition would definitely undergo the same treatment.

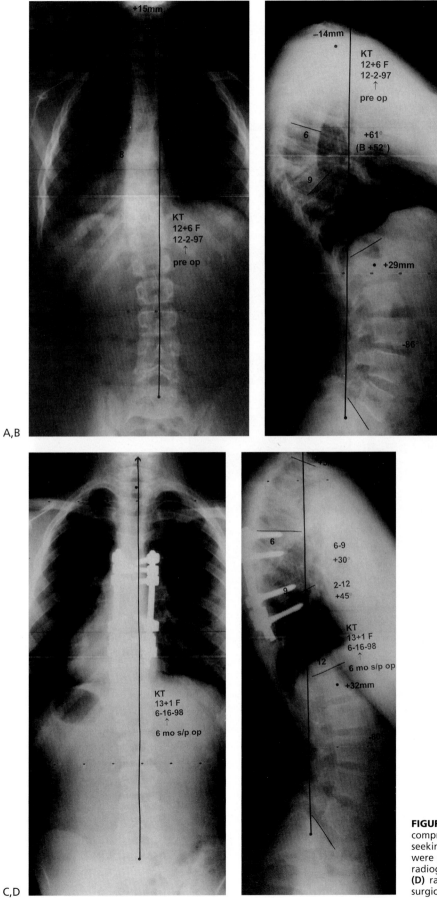

A,B

C,D

FIGURE 22. A boy 12 years 7 months of age sustained a T8 compression fracture in a sledding accident 12 months before seeking evaluation of spinal deformity. The neurologic findings were normal. Standing posteroanterior (PA) **(A)** and lateral **(B)** radiographs show preoperative appearance. PA **(C)** and lateral **(D)** radiographs show postoperative sequential-simultaneous surgical realignment.

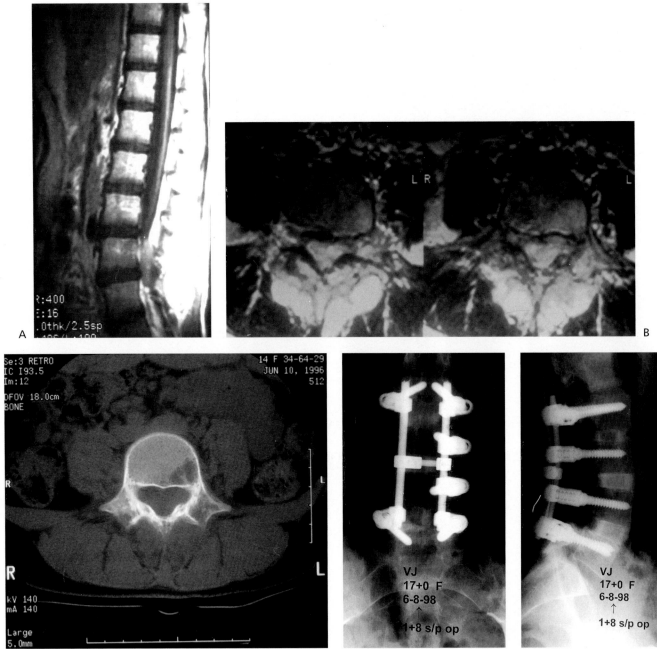

FIGURE 23. Images of a girl 15 years 4 months of age with Ewing sarcoma involving the soft tissues and posterior elements of L3–4 (left greater than right). Pretreatment sagittal plane reconstruction **(A)** and axial **(B)** magnetic resonance images and L4 computed tomographic image **(C)** show preoperative findings. Treatment consisted of tumor debulking and posterior stabilization followed in a staged manner by anterior structural interbody grafts. After chemotherapy and radiation therapy, the patients was disease free 1 year 8 months postoperatively. Standing anteroposterior **(C)** and lateral **(D)** radiographs show the intact titanium implant construct and some incorporation of the femoral ring structural interbody grafts. (Courtesy of Kim Templeton, MD.)

Tumor

Pedicle screw anchors are valuable in stabilizing the spines of patients with tumors (Fig. 23).

COMPLICATIONS

The complications in series of patients who underwent posterior instrumentation for idiopathic scoliosis (35) or for neuromuscular scoliosis (127) are consistent with findings in other series. The incidence of delayed deep wound infection is 1.2%. There have been few reports of late pain of unknown causation at the operative site. Six years of follow-up study at my institution suggests that the frequency of need for implant removal because of late pain at the operative site presumed to be due to implant irritation is statistically similar to that for Harrington, Cotrel-Dubousset, and Isola instrumentation (47). My thesis is that unexplained late pain at the operative site is caused by fretting corrosion at the connections and that this phenomenon can be decreased if the strongest connections possible are provided.

SUMMARY

The Isola spinal implant system is based on the work of Harrington and Steffee. I acknowledge my debt to the many researchers who have preceded me in the quest for an ideal spinal implant system (7,48,56,58,66,76,85,94,104). The importance of patient selection must be consistently emphasized. A studied attempt must be made to apply corrective and to resist deforming translational (vertical, anteroposterior, and mediolateral) forces and angular (coronal, sagittal, and transverse plane) moments, thereby providing three-dimensional spinal realignment and controlling all six degrees of freedom of spinal motion. Five basic instrumentation concepts aid this effort: development of foundations, provision for force couples, anatomic contouring of the longitudinal members, development of variable position connections that make longitudinal member to anchor capture as easy as possible, and the use of stable, strong, and durable constructs.

ACKNOWLEDGMENTS

I fully acknowledge my co-contributors, Walter E. Strippgen, Charles F. Heinig, MD, and William L. Carson, PhD, as well as many, many others who have contributed to the growth and development of the Isola spinal implant system, to name but two, Arthur D. Steffee, MD, and Terry Stahurski, MS. I also thank Jan Brunks, academic secretary; Barbara Funk, MA, editor; Michael Collins, illustrator; and the Department of Photography and Graphics at the University of Kansas Medical Center. The studies were funded in part by an educational grant from DePuy AcroMed.

REFERENCES

1. Akbarnia BA, Asher MA (1998): Isola instrumentation for fractures. In: McCarthy RE, ed. *Spinal instrumentation techniques.* Rosemont, IL: Scoliosis Research Society.

2. Akbarnia BA, Asher MA, Hess WF, et al. (1998–99): Safety of the pedicle screw in pediatric patients with scoliosis and kyphosis. *Orthop Trans* 22:252–253.

3. Akbarnia BA, McCarthy RE (1998): Pediatric Isola instrumentation without fusion for the treatment of progressive early onset scoliosis. In: McCarthy RE, ed. *Spinal instrumentation techniques.* Rosemont, IL: Scoliosis Research Society.

4. Allen BL, Ferguson RL (1982): The Galveston technique for L rod instrumentation of the scoliosis spine. *Spine* 7:276–284.

5. Alvine GV, Swaim JM, Asher MA (1997): The safety and efficacy of variable screw placement (VSP) and Isola spine implant systems for the surgical treatment of thoracolumbar burst fractures. *J Bone Joint Surg Br* 79[Suppl III]:306.

6. American Society for Testing Materials (ASTM) (1999): *Standard terminology relating to spinal implants.* Standard F1582–98. Philadelphia: American Society for Testing Materials.

7. Armstrong GWD, Connock SHG (1975): A transverse loading system applied to a modified Harrington instrumentation. *Clin Orthop* 108:70–75.

8. Asher M (1994): Isola hyperkyphosis instrumentation. In: Brown CW, ed. *Spinal instrumentation techniques.* Rosemont, IL: Scoliosis Research Society.

9. Asher M (1994): Isola instrumentation for degenerative disc disease. In: Brown CW, ed. *Spinal instrumentation techniques.* Rosemont, IL: Scoliosis Research Society.

10. Asher M (1994) Isola instrumentation for fractures. In: Brown CW, ed. *Spinal instrumentation techniques.* Rosemont, IL: Scoliosis Research Society.

11. Asher M (1994): Isola instrumentation for scoliosis. In: Brown CW, ed. *Spinal instrumentation techniques.* Rosemont, IL: Scoliosis Research Society.

12. Asher M (1994): Isola instrumentation for spondylolisthesis. In: Brown CW, ed. *Spinal instrumentation techniques.* Rosemont, IL: Scoliosis Research Society.

13. Asher MA (1995): The three planar evaluation of spinal position and deformity possible from biplanar radiographs. In: D'Amico M, Mewrolli A, Santambrogio GC, eds. *Three dimensional analysis of spine deformities.* Amsterdam: IOS Press, pp. 179–184.

14. Asher MA (1996): Anterior segmental instrumentation of thoracolumbar and lumbar scoliosis utilizing Isola spinal instrumentation. In: Brown CW, ed. *Spinal instrumentation techniques.* Rosemont, IL: Scoliosis Research Society.

15. Asher MA (1996): Isola spinal instrumentation system for scoliosis. In: Bridwell KH, Dewald RL, eds. *The textbook of spinal surgery.* Philadelphia: JB Lippincott, pp. 569–609.

16. Asher MA (1998): Anterior surgery for thoracolumbar and lumbar idiopathic scoliosis. *State Art Rev* 12:701–711.

17. Asher MA (1999): Salvage of severe flexion deformities of the thoracolumbar spine. In: Margulies JY, Aebi M, Farcy JPC, eds. *Revision spine surgery.* St Louis: Mosby, pp. 156–166.

18. Asher MA, Burton DC (1999): A concept of idiopathic scoliosis deformities as imperfect torsion(s). *Clin Orthop* 364:11–25.

19. Asher MA, Carson WL, Hardacker JW, et al. (1995): The effects of implant size and time on facet plus posterior fusion, underlying anterior column and adjacent disc stiffness of the canine lumbar spine. Presented at the Annual Meeting North American Spine Society Washington DC, October 18–21, 1995.

20. Asher MA, Cook LT (1995): The transverse plane evolution of the most common adolescent idiopathic scoliosis deformities: a cross-sectional study of 181 patients. *Spine* 20:1386–1391.

21. Asher MA, Fox DK (1995): Anesthesia for patients undergoing surgery for thoracolumbosacral spine deformity. In: Porter S, ed. *Anesthesia for surgery of the spine.* New York: McGraw-Hill, pp. 171–198.

22. Asher MA, Strippgen WE, Heinig CF, et al. (1991): *Spinal rod and plate bending technique.* Rosemont, IL: American Academy of Orthopaedic Surgeons, VT-210015.

23. Asher MA, Strippgen WE, Heinig CF, et al. (1992): Isola spinal implant system: principles, design, and applications. In: An HS, Cotler JM eds. *Spinal instrumentation.* Baltimore: Williams & Wilkins, pp. 325–351.

24. Asher MA, Strippgen WE, Heinig CF, et al. (1994): Isola spinal instrumentation: emphasizing application during the first two decades of life. In: Weinstein SL ed. *The pediatric spine: principles and practice.* New York: Raven Press, pp. 1619–1658.

25. Asprinio D, Curcin A (1995): Retroperitoneal structures at risk with lumbar pedicle screws: an anatomic and radiographic assessment. Paper no. 16. Presented at the 30th Annual Meeting of the Scoliosis Research Society, Asheville, North Carolina, September 13–16, 1995.

26. Barber JW, Boden SD, Ganey T, et al. (1998): Biomechanical study of lumbar pedicle screws: does convergence affect axial pullout strength? *J Spinal Disord* 11:215–220.

27. Barr SJ, Schuette AM, Eamns JB (1997): Lumbar pedicle screws versus hooks: results in double major curves in adolescent idiopathic scoliosis. *Spine* 122:1369–1379.

28. Bernhardt M, Bridwell KH (1989): Segmental analysis of the sagittal plane alignment of the normal thoracic and lumbar spines and thoracolumbar junction. *Spine* 14:717–721.

29. Betz RR, Harms J, Clements DH, et al. (1999): Comparison of anterior and posterior instrumentation for correction of adolescent thoracic idiopathic scoliosis. *Spine* 24:225–239.

30. Boachie-Adjei O, Asher MA (1998): Isola instrumentation for scoliosis. In: McCarthy RE ed. *Spinal instrumentation techniques.* Rosemont, IL: Scoliosis Research Society.

31. Boachie-Adjei O, Bansal M, Girardi FP, et al. (1998): Safety and efficacy of pedicle screw placement for adult spinal deformity utilizing free hand pedicle probing anatomic technique. Paper no. 58. Presented at the 33rd Annual Meeting of the Scoliosis Research Society, New York, NY, September 16–20, 1998.

32. Boachie-Adjei O, Bradford DS (1991): Vertebral column resection and arthrodesis for complex spinal deformities. *J Spinal Disord* 4: 193–202.

33. Bradford DS, Tribus CB (1997): Vertebral column resection for the treatment of rigid coronal decompression. *Spine* 22:1590–1599.

34. Brown CA, Leneke LG, Bridwell KH, et al. (1998): Complications of pediatric thoracolumbar and lumbar pedicle screws. *Spine* 23: 1566–1571.

35. Burton DC, Asher MA, Lai SM (1999): The selection of fusion levels using torsional correction techniques in the surgical treatment of idiopathic scoliosis. *Spine* 24:1728–1739.

36. Burton DC, Asher MA, Lai SM (2000): Scoliosis correction maintenance in skeletally immature patients with idiopathic scoliosis: is anterior fusion really necessary? *Spine* 25:61–68.

37. Burton DC, Asher MA, Lai SM (1999): A comparison of anterior vs posterior instrumented fusion for the treatment of thoracolumbar and lumbar idiopathic scoliosis. Paper no. 16. Presented at the 34th Annual Meeting of the Scoliosis Research Society, San Diego, California, September 23–25, 1999.

38. Butler T, Asher M, Jayaraman G, et al. (1994): The strength and stability of some dorsal thoracic anchor and anchor sites in osteoporotic spine. *Spine* 19:1956–1962.

39. Calancie B, Madsen P, Lebwohl N (1994): Stimulus-evoked EMG-monitoring during transpedicular lumbosacral spine instrumentation: initial clinical results. *Spine* 19:2780–2786.

40. Camp JF, Caudle R, Ashman RD, et al. (1990): Immediate complications of Cotrel-Dubousset instrumentation to the sacro-pelvis: a clinical and biomechanical study. *Spine* 15:932–941.

41. Carson WL, Duffield RC, Arendt M, et al. (1990): Internal forces and moments in transpedicular spine instrumentation: the effect of pedicle screw angle and transfixation—the 4R-4bar linkage concept. *Spine* 15:893–901.

42. Carson WL, Redman RS, Richards KO (1992): Bending stiffness and strength of VSP, Isola, CD, TSRH, and Luque longitudinal member to bone screw connection subconstructs. *Orthop Trans* 16:143–144.

43. Chapman T (1988): Harrington rods with sublaminar wires in the treatment of idiopathic scoliosis. *Orthop Trans* 12:270.

44. Cheung KMC, Luik KDK (1997): Prediction of correction of scoliosis with use of the fulcrum bending radiograph. *J Bone Joint Surg Am* 79:1144–1150.

45. Chewning SJ, Heinig CF (1994): Osteotomy. In: Weinstein SL, ed.

The pediatric spine: principles and practice. New York: Raven Press, pp. 1443–1458.

46. Cochran T, Irstam L, Nachemson A (1983): A long-term anatomical and functional changes in patients with adolescent idiopathic scoliosis treated by Harrington rod fusion. *Spine* 8:576–583.

47. Cook S, Asher M, Lai SM, et al. (2000): Reoperation after primary posterior instrumentation and fusion for idiopathic scoliosis: toward defining late operative site pain of unknown cause. *Spine* 25:463–468.

48. Cotrel Y, Dubousset J (1985): New segmental posterior instrumentation of the spine. *Orthop Trans* 9:118.

49. Craven TG, Asher MA, Carson WL, et al. (1994): The effects of implant stiffness on the bypassed bone mineral density and facet fusion stiffness of the canine spine. *Spine* 19:1664–1673.

50. Cunningham BW, Sefter JC, Shono Y, et al. (1993): Static and cyclical biomechanical analysis of pedicle screw constructs. *Spine* 18: 1677–1688.

51. Dalenberg D, Asher M, Jayaraman G, et al. (1993): The effect of a stiff spinal implant and its loosening on bone mineral content in canines. *Spine* 18:1862–1866.

52. Deacon P, Dickson RA (1987): Vertebral shape in the median sagittal plane in idiopathic thoracic scoliosis: a study of true lateral radiographs in 150 patients. *Orthopedics* 10:893–895.

53. Denis F (1983): The three column spine and its significance in the classification of acute thoracolumbar spine injuries. *Spine* 8:817–831.

54. DeSmet AA, Tarlton MA, Berridge AS, et al. (1983): The top view of analysis of scoliosis progression. *Radiology* 147:369–372.

55. Dove J (1989): Segmental wiring for spinal deformity: a morbidity report. *Spine* 14:229–231.

56. Drummond D, Guadagni J, Keene JS, et al. (1984): Interspinous process segmental spinal instrumentation. *J Pediatr Orthop* 4: 397–404.

57. Dubousset J (1994): Three-dimensional analysis of the scoliosis deformity. In: Weinstein SL, ed. *The pediatric spine: principles and practice.* New York: Raven Press, pp. 479–496.

58. Dwyer AF, Newton NC, Sherwood AA (1969): An anterior approach to scoliosis: a preliminary report. *Clin Orthop* 62:192–202.

59. Ebelke DK, Asher MA, Neff JR, et al. (1991): Survivorship analysis of VSP spine instrumentation in the treatment of thoracolumbar and lumbar burst fractures. *Spine* 16:428–439.

60. Esses SI, Sachs BL, Dreyzin V (1993): Complications associated with the technique of pedicle screw fixation: a selected survey of ABS members. *Spine* 18:2231–2239.

61. Gaines RW, Kaneda K (1996): Kaneda SR instrumentation. In: Brown CW, ed. *Spinal instrumentation techniques.* Rosemont, IL: Scoliosis Research Society.

62. Gaines RW Jr, Nichols WK (1991): Treatment of lumbosacral spondyloptosis by spondylectomy and reduction. In: Bridwell KH, DeWald RL, eds. *The textbook of spinal surgery.* Philadelphia: J.B. Lippincott.

63. Girardi FP, Boachie-Adjei O, Burke S, et al. (1998): A comparative study of two segmental instrumentation systems in the surgical treatment of adolescent idiopathic scoliosis. Paper no. 71. Presented at the 33rd Annual Meeting of the Scoliosis Research Society, New York, NY, September 16–20, 1998

64. Girardi FP, Boachie-Adjei O, Rawling BA (2000): Safety of sublaminar wires with Isola instrumentation for the treatment of idiopathic scoliosis. *Spine* 25:691–695.

65. Gondo H (1996): Evaluation of spine and thoracic cage configuration change following Isola spinal instrumentation of adolescent idiopathic scoliosis [in Japanese; tables and abstract in English]. *J Jpn Scoliosis Soc* 11:75–84.

66. Hack HP, Zielke K, Harms J (1985): Spinal instrumentation and monitoring. In: Bradford DS, ed. *The pediatric spine.* New York: Thieme, pp. 491–517.

67. Haher TR, Felmy W, Baruch H, et al. (1989): The contribution of the three columns of the spine to rotational stability: a biomechanical model. *Spine* 14:663–669.

68. Hall JE (1994): Anterior surgery in the treatment of idiopathic scoliosis. *J Bone Joint Surg Br* 76[Suppl I]:3.

69. Hall JE, Millis MB, Snyder BD (1997): Short segment anterior instru-

mentation for thoracolumbar scoliosis. In: Bridwell KH, DeWald RL, eds. *The textbook of spinal surgery.* Philadelphia: JB Lippincott, pp. 565–674.

70. Hamill CL, Lenke LB, Bridwell KH, et al. (1996): The use of pedicle screw fixation to improve correction in the lumbar spine of patients with idiopathic scoliosis: is it warranted? *Spine* 21:1241–1249.

71. Harrington PR (1962): Treatment of scoliosis: correction and internal fixation by spine instrumentation. *J Bone Joint Surg Am* 44:591–610.

72. Heini P, Scholl E, Syler D, et al. (1998): Fatal cardiac tamponade associated with posterior spinal instrumentation: a case report. *Spine* 23:2226–2230.

73. Heinig CF (1984): Eggshell procedure in segmental spinal instrumentation. In: Luque E, ed. *Segmental spinal instrumentation.* Thorofare, NJ: Slack, pp. 221–234.

74. Ibrahim K, Bueche MJ (1996): The effect of using lumbar pedicle screws on fusion extension, curve correction and spinal balance in adolescent idiopathic scoliosis instrumentation. Paper no. 81. Presented at the 31st Annual Meeting of the Scoliosis Research Society, Ottawa, Ontario, Canada, September 25–28, 1996.

75. Jackson RP, McManus AC (1994): Radiographic analysis of sagittal plane alignment and balance in standing volunteers and patients with low back pain matched for age, sex, and size: a prospective controlled clinical study. *Spine* 19:1611–1618.

76. Jacobs RR, Schlaepfer F, Mathys R Jr, et al. (1984): A locking hook spinal rod system for stabilization of fracture-dislocations and correction of deformities of the dorsolumbar spine: a biomechanical evaluation. *Clin Orthop* 189:168–177.

77. King AG, Tahmoush KM, Thomas KA (1997): Biomechanical testing of pedicle screws versus lamina hooks as distal anchors for scoliosis instrumentation. Paper no. 40. Presented at 32nd Annual Meeting of the Scoliosis Research Society, St. Louis, MO, September 25–27, 1997.

78. King HA, Moe JH, Bradford DS, et al. (1983): The selection of fusion levels in thoracic idiopathic scoliosis. *J Bone Joint Surg Am* 65:1302–1313.

79. Kioschos HC, Asher MA, Lark RG, et al. (1996): Overpowering the crankshaft phenomenon: the effect of posterior spinal fusion with and without stiff internal fixation on anterior spinal column growth in immature canines. *Spine* 21:1168–1173.

80. Kling TF, Puschak T, Montgomery SJ, et al. (1997): Isola instrumentation in the surgical treatment of adolescent idiopathic scoliosis. Paper no. 80. Presented at the 32nd Annual Meeting of the Scoliosis Research Society, St. Louis, MO, September 25–27, 1997.

81. Laine T, Makitalo K, Schlenzka D, et al. (1997): Accuracy of pedicle screw insertion: a prospective CT study in 30 low back patients. *Eur Spine J* 6:402–405.

82. Lee CK, Denis F, Winter RB, et al. (1993): Analysis of the upper thoracic curve in surgically treated idiopathic scoliosis: a new concept of the double thoracic curve pattern. *Spine* 18:1599–1608.

83. Lenke LG, Bridwell KH, Baldus C, et al. (1992): Preventing decompensation in King type II curves treated with Cotrel-Dubousset instrumentation. *Spine* 17:S274–S281.

84. Luque ER (1992): *Segmental spinal instrumentation.* Thorofare, NJ: Slack.

85. Luque ER, Cardosa A (1977): Treatment correction of scoliosis with rigid internal fixation: a preliminary report. *Orthop Trans* 1:136–137.

86. Mann DC, Nash CL, Wilham MR, et al. (1989): Evaluation of the role of concave rib osteotomies in the correction of thoracic scoliosis. *Spine* 14:491–495.

87. Margulies JY, Karlin LI, Asher MA (1998): Sequences of surgical techniques for anterior segmental instrumentation of thoracolumbar and lumbar scoliosis based on the anterior Isola spinal system. In: McCarthy RE, ed. *Spinal instrumentation techniques.* Rosemont, IL: Scoliosis Research Society.

88. McCall RE, Bronson W (1992): Criteria for selective fusion in idiopathic scoliosis using Cotrel-Dubousset instrumentation. *J Pediatr Orthop* 12:475–479.

89. McCance SE, Denis F, Lonstein JE, et al. (1998): Coronal and sagittal balance in surgically treated adolescent idiopathic scoliosis with the King II curve pattern: a review of 67 consecutive cases having selective thoracic arthrodesis. *Spine* 19:2063–2073.

90. McCord DH, Cunningham BW, Shono YU, et al. (1992): Biomechanical analysis of lumbosacral fixation. *Spine* 17:S235–S243.

91. McCormack T, Karaikovic E, Gaines RW (1994): The load sharing classification of spine fractures. *Spine* 19:1741–1744.

92. McKinley TO, McLain RF, Yerby SA, et al. (1999): Characteristics of pedicle screw loading. *Spine* 24:18–25.

93. McLain RF, Sparling E, Benson DR (1993): Early failure of short segment pedicle instrumentation for thoracolumbar fractures. *J Bone Joint Surg Am* 75:162–167.

94. Moe JH, Winter RB, Bradford DS, et al. (1978): *Scoliosis and other spinal deformities.* Philadelphia: WB Saunders.

95. Nachemson A (1989): Lumbar discography: where are we today? [Editorial.] *Spine* 14:555–557.

96. North American Spine Society (1988): Position statement on discography. *Spine* 13:1343.

97. Pehrsson K, Larsson S, Oden A, et al. (1992): Long-term follow-up of patients with untreated scoliosis: a study of mortality, causes of death, and symptoms. *Spine* 17:1091–1096.

98. Perdriolle R (1979): *La scoliose.* Paris: Maloine.

99. Polly DW, Sturm PF (1998): Traction versus supine side bending: which technique best determines curve flexibility? *Spine* 23:804–808.

100. Raso VJ, Gillespie R, McNeice GM (1980): Determination of the maximum plane of deformity in idiopathic scoliosis. *Orthop Trans* 4:23.

101. Richards BS (1992): Lumbar curve response in type II idiopathic scoliosis after posterior instrumentation of the thoracic spine. *Spine* 17:S282–S286.

102. Rose RD, Welch WC, Belzer JR, et al. (1997): Persistently electrified pedicle stimulation instruments in spinal instrumentation: technique and protocol development. *Spine* 22:334–343.

103. Rossier AB, Cochran TP (1984): The treatment of spinal fractures with Harrington compression rods and segmental sublaminar wiring: a dangerous combination. *Spine* 9:796–799.

104. Roy-Camille R, Saillant G, Mazel C (1986): Internal fixation of the lumbar spine with pedicle screw plating. *Clin Orthop* 203:7–17.

105. Sato S, Asher MA (1997): Comparison of lamina hook to pedicle screw anchors for correction of double structural adolescent idiopathic scoliosis. In: Sevastk JA, Diab KM, eds. *Research into spinal deformities.* Amsterdam: IOS Press, pp. 437–438.

106. Schultz AB, Ashton-Miller JA (1991): Biomechanics of the human spine. In: Mow VC, Hayes WC, eds. *Basic orthopaedic biomechanics.* New York: Raven Press, pp. 337–374.

107. Schulze CJ, Munzinger E, Weber U (1998): Clinical relevance of accuracy of pedicle screw placement. *Spine* 23:2215–2221.

108. Shufflebarger HL, Clark CE (1998): Effect of wide posterior release on correction in adolescent idiopathic scoliosis. *J Pediatr Orthop B* 7:117–123.

109. Smith KR, Hunt TR, Asher MA, et al. (1991): The effect of a stiff spinal implant on the bone-mineral content of the lumbar spine in dogs. *J Bone Joint Surg Am* 73:115–123.

110. Songer MN, Spencer DL, Meyer PR, et al. (1991): The use of sublaminar cables to replace Luque wires. *Spine* 16:S418–S421.

111. Stambough JL, Sabri EH, Huston RL, et al. (1998): Effects of cross-linkage on fatigue life and failure modes of stainless steel posterior spinal constructs. *J Spinal Disord* 11:221–226.

112. Steffee AD (1989): The variable screw placement system with posterior lumbar interbody fusion. In: Lin PM, Gill K, eds. *Lumbar interbody fusion.* Rockville, MD: Aspen, pp. 81–93.

113. Steffee AD, Biscup RS, Sitkowski DJ (1986): Segmental spine plates with pedicle screw fixation: a new internal fixation device for disorders of the lumbar and thoracolumbar spine. *Clin Orthop* 203:45–53.

114. Stokes IAF (1994): Three dimensional terminology of spinal deformity: a report presented to the Scoliosis Research Society by the Scoliosis Research Society Working Group on 3-D Terminology of Spinal Deformity. *Spine* 19:236–248.

115. Tveit P, Daggfeldt K, Hetland S, et al. (1994): Erector spinae lever arm length variations with changes in spinal curvature. *Spine* 19:199–204.

116. Vanlommel E, Fabry G, Urlus M, et al. (1993): Harrington instrumentation without fusion for the treatment of scoliosis in young children. *J Pediatr Orthop B* 1:116–118.

117. Voth B, Duffield RC, Carson WL (1991): *Finite element analysis of internal forces and moments in bilevel and trilevel spine instrumentation: the effects of pedicle angle, transfixation, vertebra offset and variations in vertebra size* [thesis]. Columbia, MO: University of Missouri—Columbia.

118. Wagner TA, Asher M (1998): Isola hyperkyphosis instrumentation. In: McCarthy RE, ed. *Spinal instrumentation techniques.* Rosemont, IL: Scoliosis Research Society.

119. Weinstein SL, Dolan L, Spratt KF, et al. (1998): Natural history of idiopathic scoliosis: back pain at 50-year follow-up. Paper no. 4. Presented at the 33rd annual meeting of the Scoliosis Research Society, New York, NY, September 16–20, 1998.

120. Whitiker C, Burton DC Asher M (2000): Treatment of neuromuscular patients with posterior instrumentation and arthrodesis ending with lumbar pedicle screw anchorage. *Spine* 25:2312–2319.

121. White SF, Asher M, Lai SM, et al. (1999): Patients' perceptions of overall function, pain, and appearance following primary posterior instrumentation and fusion for idiopathic scoliosis (IS). *Spine* 24:1693–1699.

122. Wilber RG, Thompson GH, Shaffer JW, et al. (1984): Postoperative neurological deficits in segmental spinal instrumentation: a study using spinal cord monitoring. *J Bone Joint Surg Am* 66:1178–1187.

123. Winter RB, Anderson MB (1985): Spinal arthrodesis for spinal deformity using posterior instrumentation and sublaminar wiring: a preliminary report of 100 consecutive cases. *Int Orthop* 9:239–245.

124. Winter RB, Carr P, Matlson HL (1997): A study of functional spinal motion in women after instrumentation and fusion for deformity or trauma. *Spine* 22:1760–1764.

125. Wood KB, Olesweski JM, Schendel MJ, et al. (1997): Rotational changes of the vertebral pelvic axis after sublaminar instrumentation in adolescent idiopathic scoliosis. *Spine* 22:51–57.

126. Wood KB, Wentorf FA, Kim KT, et al. (1998): Torsional rigidity of scoliosis constructs. Paper 11. Presented at the 33rd Annual Meeting of the Scoliosis Research Society, New York, NY, September 16–20, 1998.

127. Yazici M, Asher MA, Hardacker JW (2000): Safety and efficacy of Isola-Galveston instrumentation and arthrodesis in the treatment of neuromuscular spinal deformities. *J Bone Joint Surg* 82A:524–543.

128. Yerby SA, Ehtsehami JR, McLain RF (1997): Offset laminar hooks decrease bending moments of pedicle screws during in situ contouring. *Spine* 22:376–381.

129. Zdeblick TA, Kunz DN, Cooke ME, et al. (1993): Pedicle screw pullout strength: correlation with insertional torque. *Spine* 18:1673–1676.

130. Zindrick MR, Wiltse LL, Widell EH, et al. (1986): A biomechanical study of intrapedicular screw fixation in the lumbar spine. *Clin Orthop* 203:99–112.

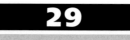

LUQUE ROD INSTRUMENTATION

RON L. FERGUSON

Luque rod instrumentation is a transverse loading spinal instrumentation using smooth rods and sublaminar wires to correct and stabilize the deformed spine (5).

The use of wires to fix the spine for both trauma and deformity originated in Texas in the late nineteenth century (27). In 1891, B. E. Hadra, a German immigrant physician and head surgeon at the Texas Medical College in Galveston, reported the use of "a figure-of-eight silver wire" around the spinous processes to stabilize a cervical spine injury (19). He subsequently used wiring of spinous processes to stabilize the spine in Pott's disease "to secure rest and prevent deformity" of the infected spine (19).

The first transverse loading system using smooth rods and spinous process wires for correction and fusion of the scoliotic spine was described by Resina and colleagues (50) in 1977. They reported 100 cases in which smooth elastic steel rods were attached to the spine by steel wire passed through the base of the spinous process. Forty-five percent correction was maintained at 2 years' follow-up, with a pseudarthrosis rate of 5% to 7%. They also mentioned using a distraction rod in conjunction with their smooth rod and wire constructs to give added correction. This was the first documentation of a combined transverse loading and axial distraction system.

The idea of segmental spinal instrumentation using smooth rods and sublaminar wires to treat spinal deformities was developed by Dr. Eduardo Luque of Mexico City (37–39). Luque, in conjunction with neurosurgeon Dr. Javier Verdura, used sublaminar fixation to methyl methacrylate in a C3 and C4 fracture in 1972. From this experience, Luque conceived the idea of using sublaminar wiring to fix spinal deformity rods to the spine. In 1973 and 1974, Luque began augmenting Harrington instrumentation with sublaminar wires. He noted that the combination of Harrington rods and sublaminar wires often fractured at the ratchet-shaft junction. He began using smooth rods that did not fracture as often but tended to migrate. While visiting Luque in 1976, Ben L. Allen, Jr. recommended that an "L" be placed into one end of the rod (6). With this, the L-shaped rod came into being.

Allen began using Luque instrumentation with sublaminar wires at the University of Texas Medical Branch in Galveston

that year. He subsequently helped refine the technique (6,22) and developed the intralaminar iliac pelvic fixation method known as the Galveston pelvic fixation technique (5).

Luque originated the term *segmental spinal instrumentation* (36). It has subsequently been applied to any spinal instrumentation with multiple fixation sites. Allen coined the term *Luque rod instrumentation* to differentiate the smooth L-shaped rod and sublaminar wire instrumentation system from other segmental instrumentation systems. Other pseudonyms in common use are *Harri-Luque* to describe the use of Harrington instrumentation combined with sublaminar wires. *Wisconsin fixation* (15,33) employs spinous process wires and buttons attached to smooth rods, Harrington rods, or both. The term Luque rod instrumentation has come to be synonymous with almost any system that uses sublaminar wires and smooth rods.

The purpose of this chapter is to describe the theory, technique, and results of Luque rod instrumentation in the treatment of deformities of the spine.

BIOMECHANICS

Mechanical testing of the segmentally wired Luque system in the spine has demonstrated three main characteristics (7,24,43,48). First, Luque rods correct the deformed spine by applying transverse forces (26,59). This occurs when the wires pull the spine to the concave rod or when the convex rod applies a three-point bending force to the spine (Fig. 1). The ability to apply these forces to the spine is affected by the stiffness of the rods and the quality of the bony tissues. The $\frac{3}{16}$-inch rods are elastic and conform to the scoliotic spine more than $\frac{1}{4}$-inch rods. White and Panjabi (59) calculated that transverse loading forces are most efficient in deformities of less than 53 degrees. The moment arm of any force is always perpendicular to the force applied. In transverse loading systems, the moment arm becomes smaller when the scoliotic deformity is more then 53 degrees and becomes larger as the degree of curvature decreases. The opposite occurs with systems using axial distraction as the correction mode.

Second, the Luque system is not stiff in axial loading (7,24,43,48). This has two effects. The instrumented segment is not stress bypassed. This is borne out in animal studies demonstrating less osteopenia in Luque instrumented spines than in axial distraction or combined instrumentations such as the

R. L. Ferguson: Chief of Staff, Shriners Hospital for Children, Spokane, Washington 99210.

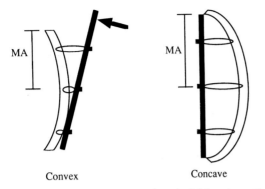

Convex   Concave

FIGURE 1. Transverse loading corrects the spinal deformity on the convex side by three-point bending forces. The concave rod corrects the lateral bend deformity by pulling the deformed spine to the rod. The moment arm *(MA)* increases as the spinal curvature decreases in magnitude, making this loading method more efficient as the spinal curvature is corrected.

Cotrel-Dubousset instrumentation (41). Second, this instrumentation is not useful when spinal collapse must be prevented, such as when a defect in the bony structure must be supported.

Third, the Luque system lacks torsion rigidity (8,21,43,46). This characteristic is theoretically detrimental to obtaining arthrodesis. Poor torsional stiffness may lead to loss of correction or decreased ability to obtain correction of the scoliotic curvature. Torsional stiffness and rotational correction are enhanced by coupling the rods into a single unit. This can be done with cross-links, rectangular rods, or the unit rod (13,14,40,46).

An alternative method of fixing smooth rods to the spine uses wires through metal buttons attached at the base of the spinous processes (17). Testing of this construct was carried out in Holstein calf spines. This method of fixation yielded about 80% of the failure strength of sublaminar wire.

McNeice (44) examined the failure mode and the ultimate strength of sublaminar fixation in human vertebrae. He tested single and double wires and Parham band pullout strengths of the human posterior arch. He found that double wires would fail by fracture of the pedicle 75% of the time and failed on average at 250 lb of load; single wires cut through the lamina 75% of the time and failed on average at 190 lb of load. Further increasing the width of the pullout device did not increase the load to failure above that of the double wires or change the failure mode. Thus, wider sublaminar implants do not impart a mechanical advantage.

Pelvic fixation with the Luque system provides secure attachment to the wings of the ilium using intralaminar pelvic placement of the rods. Jacobs (35) compared Harrington alar hooks and sacral bars and the Galveston technique of pelvic fixation. The Galveston technique of pelvic fixation failed at an average 82-Nm flexion load; the Harrington techniques failed at an average 33-Nm load.

ADVANTAGES AND DISADVANTAGES

Before a surgeon can decide which spinal instrumentation to use, he or she must consider the advantages and disadvantages

of the system's application to particular patients. The Luque system has numerous pros and cons. Understanding these enables the surgeon to make proper patient selection.

Advantages of the Luque system include early mobilization of the patient with minimal or no postoperative immobilization (1,2,4,5,21,28,34). This decreases postoperative medical complications. The Luque system also has the main advantage of multiple fixation sites that distribute the load more evenly per level and decrease the likelihood of bone implant failure. This makes their technique useful in osteopenic bone. The Luque system offers secure pelvic fixation with the Galveston technique (6). Sagittal contouring of the spine can be accomplished, in situ stabilization of the spine without correction is possible, and Luque rod instrumentation allows axial compression to occur along the instrumented portion of the spine. Luque rods also have the following advantages as a second-stage procedure after anterior release and fusion of the spine (21): no anterior instrumentation is necessary, the percentage correction of scoliosis and pelvic obliquity is the same as with anterior and posterior instrumentations, total operative time and blood loss are less when no anterior instrumentation is used, complications specific to anterior instrumentation are avoided, and the arthrodesis rates are similar. The small spine of a young child can be instrumented using sublaminar wires and rods after the spine attains its adult diameter at 6 years of age (18,51). Luque rods have been advocated for use as growing rods (38,42,51). However, multiple complications, including premature arthrodesis of the spine, loss of correction, and loss of fixation requiring reinstrumentation, make the efficacy of Luque instrumentation for use as a growing rod questionable (18). If necessary, revision surgery to repair pseudarthrosis or add levels to a previous fusion can be accomplished (22).

The Luque system also has several noteworthy disadvantages. First, it is invasive (6). Sublaminar wire passage requires opening the spinal canal at multiple levels, with instrumentation through the spinal canal at each level. Neurologic injury rates are between 0% (2,21,28) and 17% (60), averaging 1% to 2% (14,26). Luque rod instrumentation does not provide axial or torsional stability to the instrumented spine. If the rods and wires require removal, the wires must be withdrawn through the spinal canal. The wire tips cannot be controlled as they are being pulled through the fusion mass. I have had one neurologic injury with the removal of more than 1,000 wires. Luque rod instrumentation is also technically demanding, with a distinct learning curve (4,5). As surgeons gain more experience with the technique, the operative times, blood loss, and complications decrease. The disadvantages can be considerable, especially in surgeons who are unfamiliar with the procedure.

INDICATIONS

The primary indication for Luque rod instrumentation is correction and arthrodesis of neuromuscular spinal deformities (1,2,11,20,21,28,38,57) (Fig. 2). Patients with diseases such as cerebral palsy, myelomeningocele, muscular dystrophy, the spinal muscular atrophies, spinal cord injury, arthrogryposis, and poliomyelitis have similar bony anomalies and medical conditions. They frequently have osteopenic bone, often need anterior

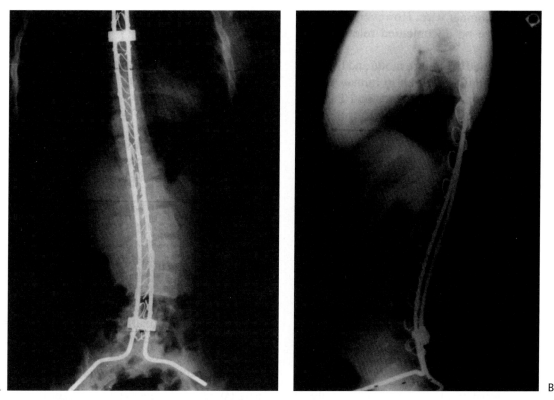

FIGURE 2. Anteroposterior **(A)** and lateral **(B)** radiographs of a cerebral palsy patient who underwent Luque instrumentation from T2 to the sacrum with $^3/_{16}$-inch rods that were cross-linked. The sagittal curvatures were well maintained.

surgery for release and fusion of the spine, and do not tolerate postoperative immobilization because of the negative effects on pulmonary function, the production of severe osteopenia, and the development of pressure sores under casts or braces. Many of these children have collapsing neuromuscular spinal deformities with resultant pelvic obliquity, requiring instrumentation to the pelvis (20).

Patients with osteopenic bone, as found in osteogenesis imperfecta, renal osteodystrophy, or severe osteomalacia or osteoporosis, benefit from the multiple fixation sites afforded by Luque rod instrumentation. Segmental instrumentation systems have been recommended in collagen diseases, such as Marfan syndrome (10) and neurofibromatosis (53).

Luque rod instrumentation has been reported in adult scoliosis (47) and adolescent idiopathic scoliosis (14,29,60) as well as spinal trauma (23).

PREOPERATIVE PLANNING

Correctability of the deformed spine must be evaluated preoperatively (6). Large residual postoperative spinal deformities predispose the patient to pseudarthrosis, instrumentation failure (31,58), and trunk decompensation. Herndon and associates (31) noted a significant increase in Luque rod fracture rates when the residual curvature averaged 44 degrees as compared with 32 degrees of residual curvature. Ashman and colleagues (7)

calculated that the endurance limit of 316L stainless-steel rods (the point below which rods theoretically will cycle indefinitely without fatigue failure) to be 37 degrees of curvature in the rod. The goal at surgery should be to correct curvatures into that range. Maximal forced bending radiographs are taken in all patients before surgery to evaluate curve correctability. If not attainable by bend films, anterior surgery should be considered when the spine does not correct to 50 degrees or less.

When fusions are carried to the pelvis with the Galveston technique, the patient should be examined for hip extension contracture. Myelodysplastic children with hip extension contractures sit by either flexing their spines or tilting their pelvises into flexion through the sacroiliac joints. When the spine is fused to the pelvis with the Galveston technique, neither the sacroiliac joint nor the spine can flex. The child may be unable to sit erect postoperatively, or if the legs are forced into a flexed sitting posture, the instrumentation may be fractured out of the wings of the ilium. The contracture should be resolved before or at the time of surgery on the spine.

The Galveston technique of pelvic fixation limits the amount of bone available for bone graft harvest from the ilia. The graft windows are small because they cannot include the area over the intralaminar segment of the pelvic fixation rods. Alternative sources for bone graft acquisition include the fibulae, thoracoplasty rib bone, or bank bone.

When Luque rod instrumentation is used in a myelodysplastic patient with an extensive open posterior laminar defect, fixa-

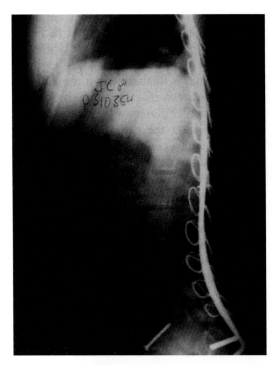

FIGURE 5. Lateral radiograph of a cerebral palsy patient who underwent fusion to the pelvis with Luque instrumentation. Note the maintenance of the sagittal contours of the spine.

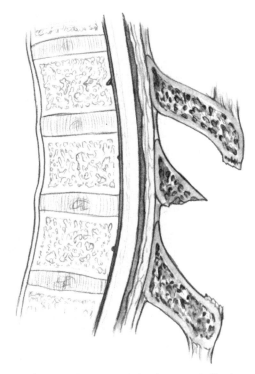

FIGURE 6. Thoracic spinous process has been vertically trimmed to expose ligamentum flavum.

lateral bend added to it. If the scoliosis is rigid and the spinal curvature short and sharp, some lateral bend should be added to the rods. The ³⁄₁₆-inch rods will need less lateral contouring than ¹⁄₄-inch rods because the ³⁄₁₆-inch rods are more elastic. The goal of Luque rod surgery is to have the rods opposed to the lamina after the wires are tightened. If the rods are displaced from the lamina at the completion of instrumentation, the construct is weakened. To judge the amount of lateral bend that must be added to the ³⁄₁₆-inch rods, the surgeon must apply a maximal manual bend to the exposed spine. The distance from the base of the spinous process to a line that would align the spine is measured. If this distance is greater than 2.5 cm, lateral curvature should be placed into the rod to bring it within this distance. The ¹⁄₄-inch rods must be contoured to lie within 1 to 1.5 cm of the spinous processes.

The sagittal and lateral curvatures placed in the rod should be gentle without acute angulations. French rod benders are ideally suited for this task. If used properly, these tools will not notch the rods. Notching greatly decreases the rod's fatigue strength.

Exposure of Neural Canal

The neural canal must be opened on each side lamina so that segmental wires can be affixed to the lamina. To expose the ligamentum flavum in the thoracic spine, the spinous processes must be removed. This is done with a rongeur held vertically to the spine to preserve the bases of the spinous processes (Fig. 6). This ridge is used by the convex rod to apply three-point bending forces to the scoliotic curvature. If this ridge of bone is not present, the rods may displace across the midline, with loss of corrective force. After the spinous process is removed, the ligamentum flavum lies exposed. The lumbar ligamentum flavum is exposed by removing the interspinous ligaments. The lumbar spinous processes are preserved unless they obstruct access to the ligamentum flavum. If the lumbar spine is very lordotic, exposure of the ligamentum flavum is facilitated by placing towel clips at the bases of adjacent spinous processes and pulling them apart. Once exposed, the ligamentum flavum is thinned with a rongeur until the midline raphe between its two halves is identified. A number 4 Penfield or similar dissector is used to separate the two halves and enter the neural canal (Fig. 7). This should be done with a cephalad-caudal motion and not by pushing the dissector in a purely anterior direction toward the spinal canal.

After all the ligamenta flava are exposed, appropriate-sized 45-degree Kerrison rongeurs are used to remove them at each level (Fig. 8). If epidural bleeding is encountered, Gelfoam soaked in thrombin solution should be inserted into the opening. The epidural vessels tend to be located in the lateral aspect of the neural canal and can be avoided to some extent by staying midline. A 5- to 8-mm midline hole in the ligamentum flavum is sufficient.

Wire Shaping

After all laminae to be instrumented have the neural canal exposed on each side, the wires can be passed. To shape a sublami-

without removing thei[...]
placed between the se[...]
the caudal extent of th[...]
double wire at the co[...]
by the next set of sing[...]
(Fig. 13). The other e[...]
spine and trimmed to f[...]
by a maximal manual [...]
wires adjacent to the e[...]
the straight end of the [...]
ened sequentially, with [...]
and a rod pusher use[...]
intercalary wire is cut a[...]
end double wires shoul[...]
being tied onto the ro[...]

The towel is remov[...]
spread carefully to avoi[...]
ina. The convex rod is [...]
Its end is oriented bel[...]
At the overlap of the [...]
double wires must be r[...]
rods to the lamina. The[...]
at the angle of the L in[...]
wires at that end is tigh[...]
pusher is used to push [...]
of the scoliotic curvatu[...]
force must be applied t[...]
correction of the spine[...]
below the L of the conc[...]

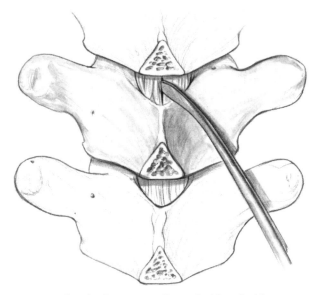

FIGURE 7. After the ligamentum flavum is thinned with a rongeur, the midline raphe is separated with a small dissector.

nar wire, a single 0.042-inch wire is folded double. The goal of wire shaping is to contour the wire so that it will pass through the spinal canal with the least depth of penetration. A loop at the end of the double wire is maintained so that a hook can be placed through it to retrieve the wire from the spinal canal once it appears around the lamina and is visible in the interlaminar space. A shallow curve is bent into the doubled end (61). The diameter of the curve should be slightly longer than the width of the lamina it is to be passed under. The two free ends of the wire should be separated to facilitate control of the wire. The wire must pass easily and never be forced. Damage to the spinal cord and nerve roots may be imparted by the wire. Force equals mass times acceleration. The surgeon cannot alter the mass of

the wire passed through the canal but can control the acceleration. Thus, one should pass the wire slowly and never apply an increasing load to the wire to get it past an obstruction. If the wire does not pass easily, it should be slowly removed, its shape in comparison to the anatomy reassessed, adjustments made, and then repassed. Because the lamina slopes from caudad to cephalad and the spinal canal is narrowest at the cephalic end of the lamina, the wire should be introduced under the caudal end of the lamina.

Wire Passage

There are three phases to passing a wire around a lamina. First, the wire is introduced into the spinal canal through the hole in the ligamentum flavum (Fig. 9). The ligamentum flavum can pose an impediment to wire introduced into the spinal canal. Although a hole is made in the ligamentum flavum, it still forms a pouch under the inferior edge of the lamina. One must introduce the wire just deeply enough into the spinal canal to bypass this pouch. If the wire catches in the pouch, it is removed and repassed.

Second, the wire is advanced forward until the curve of the wire meets the inferior lamina (Fig. 10). The tip of the wire is held against the anterior surface of the lamina at all times during the advancement.

Third, the wire is rolled around the edge of the lamina; the eye of the wire should protrude at its superior edge (Fig. 11). A hook or Kocher clamp is used to pull the wire from the hole until equal lengths of it are around the lamina. Constant posterior tension must be maintained on the wire to prevent it from dropping back into the neural canal and contusing the neural elements. Two double wires are passed around the most superior

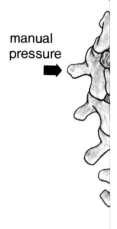

manual pressure

FIGURE 13. Concave tech[...]
of the L and at the oppo[...]
spine to reduce it to the [...]

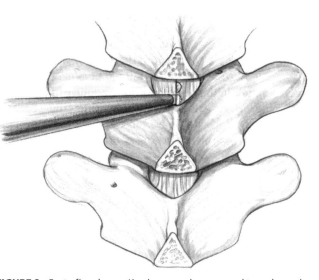

FIGURE 8. Forty-five-degree Kerrison punches are used to make a window in the ligamentum flavum.

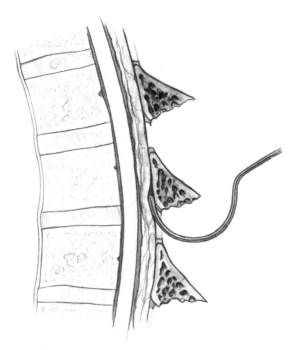

FIGURE 9. Wire introduced under the ligamentum flavum.

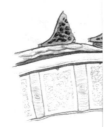

FIGURE 10. Wire advar
on the anterior lamina.

and inferior lamina in
These are not cut. T
wire passed around th
equal lengths, taking
neural canal while pul
is cut at its tip and
crimped onto the lar
from inadvertently be
A systematic crimpin

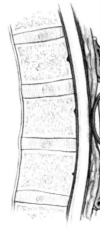

FIGURE 11. Loop of w
of the lamina.

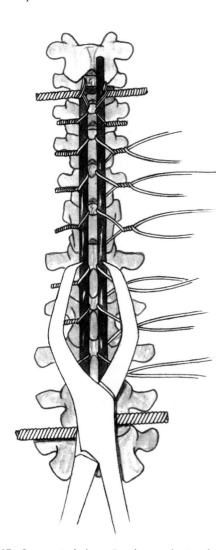

FIGURE 15. Concave technique. A rod approximator clamp is used to pull the two rods together. This brings the rods in contact with the lamina. Note that the concave wires are loose and will need to be tightened.

wire. Because correction with this technique depends on the rod creating a three-point bending force on the lamina of the deformed spine, the sagittal contour of the rod must allow contact force to be applied to the lamina (Fig. 16). One does not wish, however, to flatten all normal kyphosis or to increase existing hypokyphosis. The convex rod should not be allowed to cross the midline because the correcting force applied by this rod will be lost. A rod pusher is used to push the rod onto the lamina, and the wire is tightened to prevent the rod from crossing the midline. The wires are tightened sequentially until the end of the rod is reached (Fig. 17). The last set of double wires is not tightened until the concave rod is applied. The wires on the concave side are spread. The L of the concave rod is placed on top of the convex rod, and the double wire at the angle of the concave L is tightened. The second double wire is tightened around both rods where they overlap. The straight end of the concave rod is placed on top of the L of the convex rod and wired into place. A rod pusher reduces the convex L onto the

FIGURE 16. Convex technique. The rod is wired at its L. Force is placed on the rod to correct the deformity.

lamina, and the double wires are tightened. This derotates the convex rod. The single intercalary wires are tightened around the concave rod (Fig. 18). If necessary, a rod approximator clamp or rod pusher may be used to reduce the concave rod to the lamina while the wires are tightened. The rods are coupled using cross-links.

Kyphosis Correction

Kyphosis correction is similar to placing two convex rods. Because the overlap of the rods may be prominent in kyphotic patients, both L ends of the rods are placed in the low thoracic or lumbar area of the spine, where the prominent tips are covered by a larger muscle mass and lordosis is present. Two sets of double wires are placed at the cephalic and caudal extent of the spine to be instrumented. Single wires are placed on each side of the intercalary lamina. Both rods accomplish correction by three-point bending at the apex of the kyphosis and transverse loading of the wires at the ends of the kyphosis. The wire tightening is begun one level above the L on the first rod that is placed. The rod is progressively pushed onto the lamina with a rod pusher, and all the wires are tightened, including the cephalad double wire. When the second rod is placed onto the spine, the without removing their crimp on the lamina. The Luque rod is placed between the separated wires, with the L end located at the caudal extent of the spinal segment to be instrumented. The double wire at the corner of the L is tightened first, followed by the next set of single wires on the lamina adjacent to this (Fig. 13). The other end of the concave rod is placed onto the spine and trimmed to fit after the correct rod length is estimated by a maximal manual correction of the spine. The two single wires adjacent to the end double wire are then tightened about the straight end of the rod. The intercalary single wires are tightened sequentially, with manual corrections applied to the spine and a rod pusher used to reduce the rod to the spine. Each intercalary wire is cut after it is twisted to a length of 1 cm. The end double wires should be cut 2 cm in length to facilitate their being tied onto the rods.

The towel is removed from the convex wires, and they are spread carefully to avoid removing their crimps around the lamina. The convex rod is placed between the row of spread wires. Its end is oriented below the straight end of the concave rod. At the overlap of the L end of the rod and straight end, the double wires must be maneuvered so that they will secure both rods to the lamina. The L end of the convex rod is first tightened at the angle of the L in the rod. Next, the second set of double wires at that end is tightened where the two rods overlap. A rod pusher is used to push the rod progressively onto the convexity of the scoliotic curvature as the wires are tightened. Moderate force must be applied to the rod to obtain three-point bending correction of the spine. The straight end of the rod is placed below the L of the concave rod by using a rod pusher to derotate

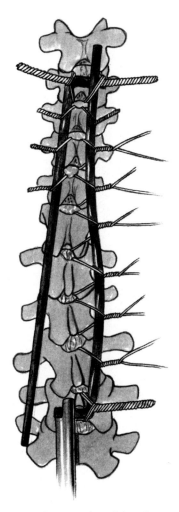

FIGURE 14. Concave technique. After all the wires on the concave rod are fastened, the convex rod is strained into place. Note the rod pusher levering the L on the concave rod to allow the convex rod's straight limb to be placed under it.

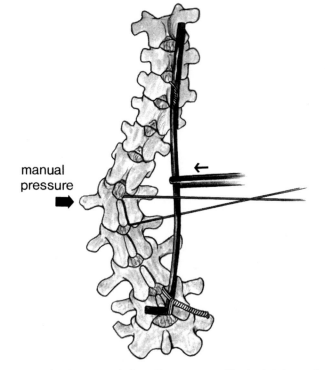

manual pressure

FIGURE 13. Concave technique. The concave rod is wired at the angle of the L and at the opposite end. Manual pressure is applied to the spine to reduce it to the rod as the wires are tightened.

the concave L off the lamina to allow the convex rod to be pushed under it (Fig. 14). This should be done as early in the tightening sequence as possible to allow mobility in the convex rod for this maneuver. All wires are tightened, including the double end wire. At this point, the rods may not be flush on the lamina.

Next, a rod clamp is used to approximate the concave rod to the convex rod at the apex of the curvature (Fig. 15). More correction of the scoliotic curvature is obtained with this maneuver, and the wires on the concave rod will require further tightening. The two rods should be "worked" onto the lamina using repeated passes of the rod clamps and rod pushers. After all wires are tightened, the two rods are cross-linked. A rod clamp is used to strain the rods together before the cross-links are applied.

Convex Technique

Preparation of the wires for rod placement is carried out as in the concave technique except on the convex side. The angle of the L is placed at the cephalic end and wired with the double

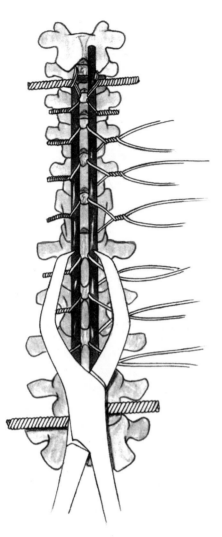

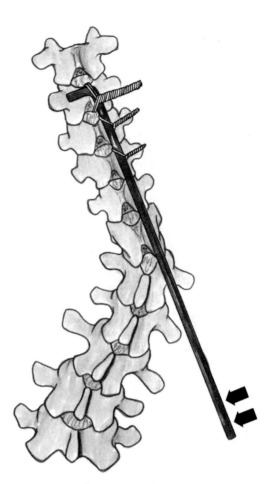

FIGURE 16. Convex technique. The rod is wired at its L. Force is placed on the rod to correct the deformity.

FIGURE 15. Concave technique. A rod approximator clamp is used to pull the two rods together. This brings the rods in contact with the lamina. Note that the concave wires are loose and will need to be tightened.

wire. Because correction with this technique depends on the rod creating a three-point bending force on the lamina of the deformed spine, the sagittal contour of the rod must allow contact force to be applied to the lamina (Fig. 16). One does not wish, however, to flatten all normal kyphosis or to increase existing hypokyphosis. The convex rod should not be allowed to cross the midline because the correcting force applied by this rod will be lost. A rod pusher is used to push the rod onto the lamina, and the wire is tightened to prevent the rod from crossing the midline. The wires are tightened sequentially until the end of the rod is reached (Fig. 17). The last set of double wires is not tightened until the concave rod is applied. The wires on the concave side are spread. The L of the concave rod is placed on top of the convex rod, and the double wire at the angle of the concave L is tightened. The second double wire is tightened around both rods where they overlap. The straight end of the concave rod is placed on top of the L of the convex rod and wired into place. A rod pusher reduces the convex L onto the

lamina, and the double wires are tightened. This derotates the convex rod. The single intercalary wires are tightened around the concave rod (Fig. 18). If necessary, a rod approximator clamp or rod pusher may be used to reduce the concave rod to the lamina while the wires are tightened. The rods are coupled using cross-links.

Kyphosis Correction

Kyphosis correction is similar to placing two convex rods. Because the overlap of the rods may be prominent in kyphotic patients, both L ends of the rods are placed in the low thoracic or lumbar area of the spine, where the prominent tips are covered by a larger muscle mass and lordosis is present. Two sets of double wires are placed at the cephalic and caudal extent of the spine to be instrumented. Single wires are placed on each side of the intercalary lamina. Both rods accomplish correction by three-point bending at the apex of the kyphosis and transverse loading of the wires at the ends of the kyphosis. The wire tightening is begun one level above the L on the first rod that is placed. The rod is progressively pushed onto the lamina with a rod pusher, and all the wires are tightened, including the cephalad double wire. When the second rod is placed onto the spine, the

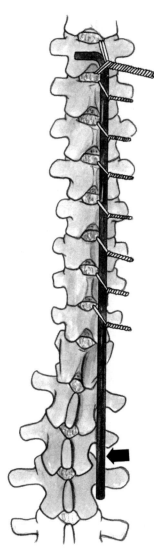

FIGURE 17. Convex technique. The wires are progressively tightened to the rod as the rod imparts a three-point bending force to the spine.

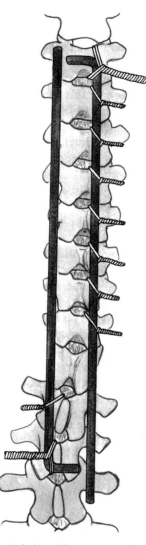

FIGURE 18. Convex technique. The concave rod is wired to the spine. If the concave rod is displaced from the lamina, the rod approximator clamp is applied, as in the concave technique.

two L's are crossed, and the double wires at the caudal end are tightened around both L's. The second rod is progressively strained onto the kyphotic spine, and the wires are tightened. The wires on the first rod are reexamined to see if they are loose; if so, they are retightened.

Wire Tightening

Wire tightening may be done with a pair of pliers. However, commercially available wire twisters make the task much simpler, more efficient, safer, and faster. To tighten the wire, the assistant should begin to twist the wire by hand. Most wire tighteners turn in a clockwise direction; the hand twists in the wire should be the same. This will remove the crimp on the lamina. The assistant should maintain upward tension on the wire to prevent it from protruding downward into the spinal canal. The surgeon applies the wire twister at the junctions of the twists in the wire.

The ends of the wires are snugged to the handles of the twister so that adjacent wires are not entangled as the wire is tightened. In the concave technique, the spine should be manually reduced to the rod, and the rod should be pushed to the spine using a rod pusher. When maximal manual correction is obtained, the wire is tightened to the rod. In the convex technique, the rod is pushed onto the spine with a rod pusher. Twisting of the wires should never be used to pull the rod to the lamina because this will excessively fatigue the wires. The wire twist end point is reached when the wires assume a 45-degree orientation to each other in the twisted segment or begin to change color from shiny to dull gray. The latter is a sign of excessive cold working of the metal, and further twisting will fatigue the wire. After the first pass of wire tightening, the concave rod may not lie on the lamina, especially at the apex of the curvature. This will be achieved after the convex rod is placed. After the wires are twisted, they may be cut 1 cm above the rod. (More than three twists must be left to prevent unraveling of the wire.)

After the rods are wired in place, the cut ends of the wires are bent down into the midline. This placement prevents them from blocking transverse process graft sites. The wires should be below the level of the remaining spinous processes if possible. The double end wires should be wired down, with a single wire passed around the rods to prevent them from protruding once the patient is standing and loading these wires.

Decortication of the transverse processes and facet joints may be used. Decortication of the lamina should be avoided because this weakens the site of sublaminar attachment. Copious amounts of bone graft are applied lateral to the rods. The wound is closed in a routine manner.

If wires break while being twisted into place, they must be removed. The wire should be cut opposite the side of the lamina from which it is to be removed as near the edge of the lamina as possible. A pair of pointed wire clippers is necessary to do this (Fig. 4). The wire must be slowly removed from the canal by rolling it out from under the lamina. The surgeon should endeavor to keep the now sharp tip of the wire on the anterior surface of the lamina until it can be delivered from the wound. A wire can be repassed to replace the removed one if indicated.

Postoperative Care

Postoperatively, patients may be mobilized as necessary. Immobilization postoperatively is at the surgeon's discretion. If 316L stainless-steel implants are used, immobilization may be a consideration. Even then, it may only be necessary to manage patients in part-time orthoses.

GALVESTON TECHNIQUE OF PELVIC FIXATION

The exposure of the pelvis is made through the midline incision used to expose the spine. The distal extent of the incision should be caudal to the posterosuperior iliac spine. It may be curved off the sacral prominence to prevent pressure on the incision postoperatively. The plane of dissection to the wings of the ilium is between the erector spinae fascia and the subcutaneous fat. The ilium is exposed from the posterosuperior iliac spine to the midportion of the iliac wing and to the sciatic notch. Depending on the diameter of the spinal rod to be used, an appropriate diameter drill bit is selected to develop the insertion hole for pelvic fixation into the wing of the ilium. The insertion point of the pelvic limb is at the posterosuperior iliac spine (Fig. 19). A notch, 8 to 10 mm in depth, is cut into the wing of the ilium at the posterosuperior iliac spine. The pelvic limb insertion hole is then placed under direct vision by drilling a hole with the appropriate-sized drill bit depending on rod size (³⁄₁₆ or ¼ inch).

The insertion hole is directed 1 to 1.5 cm above the sciatic notch and should fit between the cortices of the wing of the ilium in the transverse bar. If the insertion point is above the posterosuperior iliac spine, the rods may be directed through the membranous portion of the ilium, and the fixation is inadequate. A constant resistance of the bone to the drill will be noted. If this resistance is lost, the drill has penetrated the cortex of the ilium. If there is doubt about the positioning of the insertion hole, it should be explored with a smaller-diameter pin to ensure

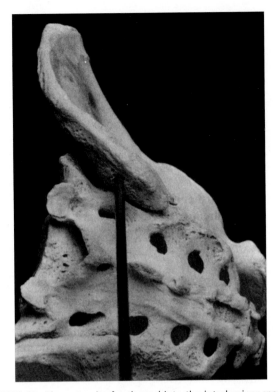

FIGURE 19. The entry site for the rod into the interlaminar space in the wing of the ilium. The entry point is at the level of the posterosuperior iliac spine and just posterior to the sacroiliac joint.

that all walls are intact. Six centimeters is the minimal intracortical distance that is necessary for the fixation to be stable, and this distance should be measured and noted for later use by measuring the probe placed into the insertion hole (6). After both of the pelvic insertion holes are drilled, Gelfoam may be packed into them, or guide pins may be inserted to stop blood loss.

The Galveston technique pelvic rod has two bends that create three sections of rod. The sections are called the pelvic, sacral, and spinal segments for the areas they overlie. Two bends must be made: one between the pelvic and sacral sections and one between the sacral and spinal sections.

The rods should be shaped so that they are compensated to the pelvis and not aligned along the spine. This allows the pelvis to be corrected to the spine when the rods are wired to the spine, thus correcting pelvic obliquity.

The initial bend in the rod is made with two sleeve benders. This bend separates the spinal and sacropelvic sections of the pelvic rod (Fig. 20). The length of rod needed for this bend is calculated by adding the intralaminar length of the pelvic insertion hole to the distance from the insertion point in the iliac wing to just lateral to the midline of the sacrum. This latter distance is usually 1.5 to 2 cm and represents the sacral portion of the rod. The rod is measured, and two sleeve benders are used to make the bend. The angle of the bend depends on the amount of pelvic obliquity the patient has. The degrees of the bend are calculated from the relationship of the pelvic guide pin, which is placed into the insertion hole to give a visual

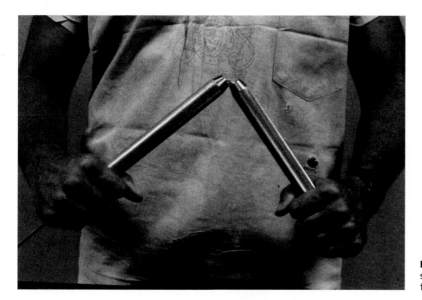

FIGURE 20. The first bend in the rod is made with two sleeve benders. This bend will separate the spinal segment from the sacropelvic segments.

reference to the angle and path of the hole. This angle ranges from 60 to 90 degrees. The second bend is used to make the rod lie on the sacrum. It is made by clamping the bent segment of the rod with the channeled vise grips and using a sleeve bender to produce a 45-degree bend at the junction between the sacral and pelvic segments of the rod (Fig. 21). The rods cannot be interchanged after the second bend is made (Fig. 22). After the pelvic, sacral, and spinal sections of the pelvic rod are shaped, the two-holed alignment tool is slipped onto the pelvic guide pin, and the pelvic section of the Luque rod is placed in the second hole. This holds the Luque rod in a constant relationship with the pelvis. Appropriate sagittal and lateral contouring of the rod can be carried out using French benders and rod benders (Fig. 23). The sagittal contours should be balanced with about equal amounts of kyphosis and lordosis. Lateral contouring may be necessary for rigid curves when ¼-inch rods are used or to allow three-point bending forces to occur between the convex rod and the spine. A second rod is then shaped for the opposite ilium in a similar manner.

Exposure of the interlaminar spaces and wires is carried out as previously described. Double wires are used at the cephalad lamina only. The concave lumbar curvature is usually instrumented first because this is the curvature that most affects the pelvic obliquity. The wires are spread on the concave side after the convex wires are covered with a towel.

The pelvic guide pin must be removed before inserting the rod into the pelvis. The concave pelvic rod is rotated so that the spinal segment is perpendicular to the patient's spine. The pelvic section is introduced into the iliac insertion hole and tapped into the wing of the ilium with a rod pusher and mallet (Fig. 24). Care must be taken not to torque the rod as it is driven into the insertion hole because the pelvic portion can be driven out of the pelvis and not down the predrilled hole, leading to poor fixation. The spinal section is rotated onto the spine between the spread wires as this is done. The length of the rod is estimated using manual reduction of the spine, and the rod is trimmed. The cephalad double wires are tightened first. The intercalary wires are tightened sequentially in a caudad to cepha-

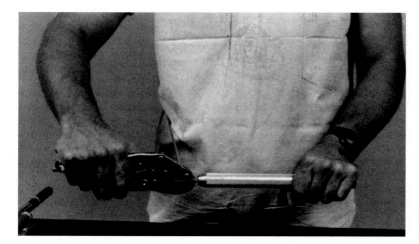

FIGURE 21. The second bend is made with the channeled vise grips and a sleeve bender. This will produce the sacral portion of the rod.

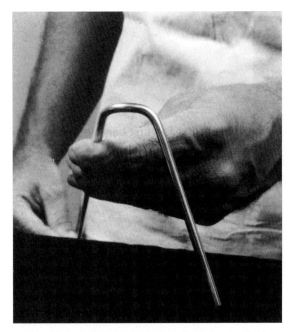

FIGURE 22. The completed pelvic rod configuration. Sagittal contouring of the rod has not been carried out.

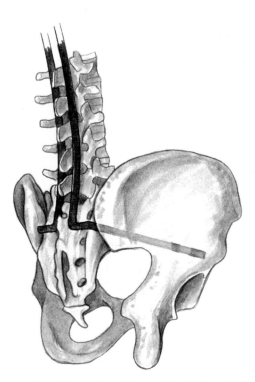

FIGURE 24. The pelvic portions of the rods should lie within 1.5 cm of the sciatic notch in the transverse bar.

lad direction with the rod reduced to the spine using manual force and rod pushers. The rod may not be completely reduced to the spine with the first pass of wire tightening. The convex rod is placed, and the wires are tightened sequentially. Final straining of the rods into apposition with the lamina is carried out using rod approximation clamps and further wire tightening. The rods are cross-linked at two levels, and the two superior double wires are wired to the rods. If bone graft is to be taken from the wings of the ilium, the surgeon must not expose the pelvic portion of the rods.

Inadequate compensation can be improved by small amounts of in situ bending of the rod. Excessive bending can pull the wires through the lamina. Large amounts of pelvic obliquity can be corrected by adding a hook to the rod entering the high pelvis. Distraction of this hook after initial wire tightening depresses the high side and helps level the pelvis. This should be carried out before cross-links are applied. Copious bone graft is applied lateral to the rods over the ala of the sacrum and continuing up the transverse processes. Decortication of the transverse processes and the facet joints is done at the surgeon's discretion.

Postoperatively, 45-degree oblique views of the pelvis in the

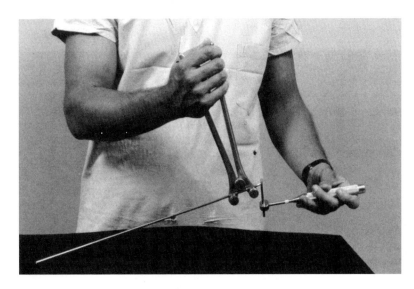

FIGURE 23. The two-holed pelvic alignment tool is used to align the rod for implant with the pelvic guide pin. French benders are used to place sagittal and lateral bend contours as needed.

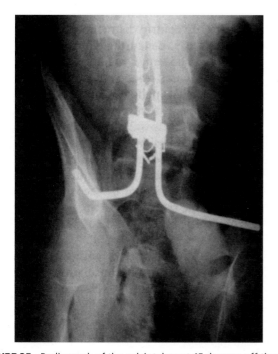

FIGURE 25. Radiograph of the pelvis taken at 45 degrees off the midline to delineate the wing of the ilium. Note that the pelvic segment of the pelvic fixation rod lies within the halo of bone representing the transverse bar of the ilium.

anteroposterior plane with 45-degree cephalad inclination of the x-ray tube in relation to the ilium delineates the individual wings of the ilium (Fig. 25). The placement of the rods into the intralaminar space can be judged by this technique (Fig. 26). Adequate placement renders postoperative immobilization unnecessary. However, if malalignment of the rods is found, immobilization should be considered.

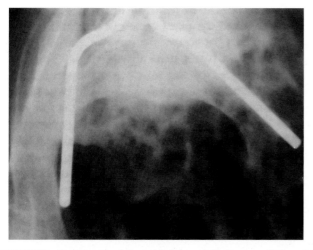

FIGURE 26. Radiograph of the pelvis taken at 45 degrees off the midline and at 45 degrees of cephalad inclination. This delineates the wing of the ilium. One can clearly see that the pelvic segment of the pelvic fixation rod lies outside the ilium.

Unit Rod

The unit rod is one continuous Luque rod connected at the top with the pelvic bends already placed in the ends. The advantage of this rod is that it is coupled by the rod being continuous and thus has more rotational stability. The disadvantages are that rigid curvatures with limited correctability may be difficult to instrument because it may be problematic positioning the rod on either side of the spinous processes. If the pelvic insertion holes are not aligned exactly, the rod may be difficult to insert into the pelvis.

When properly used, the results are excellent (13,14,40,45). The spine is prepared as above with wire passage and pelvic insertion hole. Both sets of wires must be separated. Simultaneously, one limb of the rod is inserted into the pelvis at a time. The rods are then "joysticked" to align the pelvis with the spine, and the wires are placed around the rods and sequentially tightened.

REVISION

Revision of Luque instrumentation, for either pseudoarthrosis or extension of the instrumentation, can be accomplished by attaching new rods to the original ones if they are to be left in place or by removing the old rods and wires and placing new ones (20). This decision should be made based on whether the old rods are intact or fractured. Fractured rods and wires should be removed and new rods and wires placed. After the rods are removed, the wires are exposed. The surgeon should not attempt to use the old wires. They are fatigued and will not tolerate retightening by twisting. The old wires are cut near the fusion mass and twisted or levered out of the bone. Because the surgeon cannot control the tip of the wire as it is pulled through the spinal canal, this must be done slowly. Renshaw and colleagues (49) found no protective fibrous tract formed around the intraspinal segments of the wires after 4 years in one patient. An alternative to removing the wires is to cut them and leave them buried in the bone. This may not be desirable if one is planning reinstrumentation or in an infected spine.

After the old hardware is removed, the fusion mass is stripped of soft tissue, and the pseudarthrosis is débrided. To replace the wires, one must create osseous bridges in the previous fusion mass. This can be accomplished in multiple ways. The holes for passage of wire between the bridges of bone need not enter the spinal canal but can be made between the diploe of the fusion mass and the outer cortex of the fusion. Using a rongeur, burr, or gouge, the surgeon makes holes in the cortex of the fusion mass about 2 cm apart down both sides of the fusion mass opposite each other. A tunnel for wire passage is made between the holes using a towel clip and curettes. This may be done across the midline if the fusion mass is abundant or along each side of the fusion mass. Care must be taken not to enter the spinal canal inadvertently. Single or double wires are passed through the hole on one side of the fusion mass and out the hole on the other side. There should be four wires above and below the pseudoarthrosis. A single ¼-inch rod or two ³⁄₁₆-inch rods can then be attached to the previous fusion mass and the

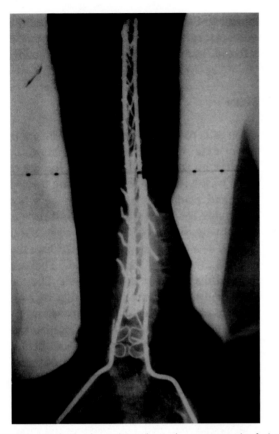

FIGURE 27. Cerebral palsy patient who underwent posterior fusion to L3 for a kyphoscoliosis. Her curvature subsequently progressed below the fused segment. She underwent anterior release and fusion to S1 and posterior extension of her spinal fusion to the sacrum. The wires are bent laterally where the two rods are tied together to leave the midline fusion mass clear for graft placement. Note that two sets of sublaminar wires were passed at L4 and L5.

area decorticated and grafted. The rods should have L's placed in them to prevent migration.

If the old rods are intact, as might occur when extending a fusion, the new wires may be passed around the old rods. This may require bone removal for access to the original rods. A new rod can be wired to the old rod (Fig. 27). Rigid rod couplers are now available with some spinal systems that will fit smooth rods. These couplers may be used to attach the old rods to the new rods without the use of wires. Difficulty may be encountered if the old rods are covered in bone. The fixation between the rods is much stiffer with couplers. A decision can be made at surgery about which technique to use.

A fusion may be extended by attaching the old rods to the new ones as previously described and then placing sublaminar wires to the new levels. The Galveston technique of pelvic fixation allows a lower lumbar spinal fusion to be extended into the pelvis. The pelvic rods are attached to the old fusion mass as previously described. If possible, sublaminar wires may be passed around previously unfused laminae. Attachment to the pelvis is as previously described.

ADJUNCTS TO LUQUE FIXATION

Luque fixation represents a pure transverse loading system to correct the deformed spine. In the past, smooth rods did not lend themselves to hook placement. However, numerous systems have now been developed with hooks that can be attached to smooth rods. The addition of hooks to the Luque rod converts this to a combined transverse-axial loading system. Mechanical benefits include application of a much more efficient correcting force and prevention of axial settling. Eccentric distraction on hooks used in pelvic fixation cases can further correct pelvic obliquity. Care must be taken not to flatten the lumbar lordosis. Sublaminar wires placed next to hooks stabilize them and prevent their pullout. Caution must be used when wiring rods next to intraspinal hooks; the hooks can be pushed into the spinal canal as the wire is tightened, causing compression of neural elements (52). When hooks and wires are combined, either the hooks should be placed into facet joints in the thoracic spine or the diameter of curvature of the hook should be essentially the same size as the laminar diameter for intraspinal placement. This will prevent protrusion of the hook into the neural canal when the wires are tightened.

Disadvantages of using hooks with this system do exist. Distraction hooks may cause stress bypass of the area needing arthrodesis. The Harri-Luque system has been reported to have a high neurologic complication rate (16,29,60). Whether this is secondary to overcorrection of the spine with this powerful tool or a result of poor technique is unclear.

Another technique to increase axial stability or provide an alternative method of gaining purchase to the spine with Luque instrumentation is the use of pedicle screws. These may be useful when the posterior elements are absent either secondary to surgery or congenitally. Because pedicle screws are located more laterally than hooks or wires, their lateral moment is greater. Theoretically, this gives pedicle screws an advantage in correcting lateral bends of the spine.

The Luque system has poor rotational stability. Improvements can be made with rigid cross-links placed between the rods. Derotation of the spine can be obtained once the Luque system is in place by using a rotating device called a pigtail and then cross-linking the rods rigidly. The derotation allows further correction to be obtained at the time of surgery and prevents loss of correction by rotation of the spine around the rods over time.

Cross-links improve the lateral bending stiffness of the rods (41). They also allow load sharing between the rods. This may be helpful when pelvic fixation is used. We routinely use cross-links and derotation on all Luque instrumentations that are amenable to this technique.

An alternative method of torsionally stiffening the rods is to use a continuous rod for the deformity instead of two separate rods. The unit rod (45) and rectangular rod (13) are two examples. These rod configurations can be used in spinal deformities that are supple preoperatively or that are made correctable by anterior release.

Songer and associates (54) advocated the use of cables instead of wires with the Luque system. The fatigue resistance of cables is much greater than that of monofilament wire. Gaines and Abernathie (26) recommended the use of Mersilene tapes to replace wires. They believe that these are safer and can be removed from the neural canal with less risk for neural damage than wires.

COMPLICATIONS

Complications have occurred in 27% (4) to 67% (55) of patients undergoing Luque instrumentation. Because many of the reports averaged the investigators' initial cases with their most recent cases, these figures do not take into account the learning curve that occurs with this technique (4). Also, most of the cases reported were in patients with neuromuscular spinal deformities who, historically, have the highest complication rates in spinal deformity surgery (1,2,8,11,28,32,39,45,55–57).

Neurologic injuries are the most feared complication with this technique and are reported to occur in up to 17% of cases (55). Most reported injuries were hyperalgesia that resolved in 7 to 28 days. The minority were major spinal cord injuries. Allen and Ferguson (3) surveyed a group of surgeons who trained in the Luque technique of spinal and pelvic instrumentation. In the 512 cases reported, the rate of major neurologic injury was 0.4%. At final follow-up in this group of patients, only one patient was left with a mild residual neurologic problem after a partial cord injury. There was a 2.6% rate of hyperalgesia; all cases resolved in the immediate postoperative period. Allen and Ferguson emphasized that the technique can be safe if the surgeon is properly trained.

Dove (16) pooled the morbidity reports from the British Scoliosis Society between 1983 and 1984. He reported a 1.4% neurologic injury rate overall in 1,121 patients. The only statistically significant finding in the report was the injury rate occurring in patients in whom the segmentally wired Harrington rods were used as compared with the Harrington distraction rods. Three major neurologic injuries occurred in the Harri-Luque group and only one in the Harrington distraction group. Report of morbidity and mortality statistics from the Scoliosis Research Society in 1990 (26) demonstrated 44 neurologic injuries in 5,269 spinal surgery patients (0.8%). Four of 355 patients (1.1%) who underwent Luque rodding had a neurologic injury. Most of these patients had neuromuscular spinal deformities. Six of 232 (2.6%) of the patients undergoing Harrington rod and sublaminar wire fixation developed neurologic complications. Most of these patients were in the idiopathic group. No breakdown of major or minor neurologic injuries was made. Whether this consistent increase in neurologic injury reported with the Harri-Luque technique from both North America and Britain is secondary to overcorrection from combined axial and transverse loading forces applied to the spine, to operator inexperience, or to some other factor is not clear (60).

Infection with the use of Luque instrumentation was reported to occur in up to 15% of cases (55). Most Luque rod procedures are done in patients with neuromuscular scoliosis, who have a higher infection rate (55). As experience has evolved, the treatment of choice for infected Luque instrumentation is to drain the wound and, if necessary, débride the wound but leave the graft and instrumentation in place. Prolonged antibiotic therapy is necessary (28). A high percentage of patients so treated have gone on to solid arthrodesis. If drainage persists, the hardware may be removed after arthrodesis has occurred (8). In 1990, the Scoliosis Research Society reported a 4% infection rate with the use of Luque instrumentation, whereas the entire population sample had an infection rate of 1% (29). The Luque patients included a higher percentage of neuromuscular patients (70%) than the series as a whole (18%). Neuromuscular patients, especially myelodysplastic patients, are know to have a higher postoperative infection rate.

Broken wires occurred in 13% of Luque rod cases in a large personal series using 316L stainless-steel wires. The wires that most often fatigue are the end wires at the L. Fracture of one or two proximal wires usually has minimal consequences (28). External support may be considered if this occurs early in the postoperative period. Whether Mersilene tapes fracture over time is not known because these are not visible on radiographs (23). The role of cables in preventing fatigue is theoretically good, but no long-term study is available at this time to validate this, and their expense is high.

Broken rods with Luque instrumentation are usually secondary to pseudarthrosis. Positive factors reported to prevent fracture of rods were use of newer metals (4), $\frac{1}{4}$-inch diameter rods (28,31), external immobilization (30), smaller residual curvatures of the spine (21,31), and anterior fusion in conjunction with posterior Luque instrumentation (31). Pseudarthrosis has been reported to occur in up to 14% of cases using Luque rods (55). A higher incidence of rod fracture was reported when $\frac{3}{16}$-inch 316L stainless-steel rods were used (28,31). Large residual spinal curvatures after instrumentation have been related to pseudarthrosis and rod fracture (31). Smooth rods with wire fixation have been noted to cycle for up to 4 years before fatiguing secondary to pseudarthrosis. Thus, prolonged follow-up is indicated. The Scoliosis Research Society morbidity and mortality report lists a 1% pseudarthrosis rate with Luque rods and a 7% rate for the entire population of cases (29). A 1.4% instrument failure rate (rods and wires) with Luque rods occurred, with an entire population failure rate of 1.8%. Thus, instrument failure is no greater in this system, even though 70% were used in neuromuscular cases with higher pseudarthrosis rates.

Prominent hardware from Luque rods presents a problem in up to 12% of cases (31). This complication may range from only a nuisance to penetration of the skin by the implant with subsequent infection, requiring removal of the instrumentation. The most common prominent piece of hardware is the end double wire. These may protrude when the hardware is loaded as the patient begins to ambulate. This complication is preventable by wiring the end double wires to the rods. The L on the rod may also become prominent and occasionally requires removal. Care should be taken at the time of implantation to trim this as short as possible to decrease the chance of prominence. The tip of the L may also be bent down before it is implanted to make it less prominent. In kyphotic patients, both L's may be placed at the caudal end of the instrumentation, where the soft tissues are thicker.

Reoperation has been reported to be necessary in up to 26% of cases (57). These operations are usually necessary to treat pseudarthrosis, infection, broken rods, or prominent hardware.

Medical complications, such as pulmonary compromise, urinary tract infections, and gastrointestinal problems, occur in up to 9% of cases (12) and are more common in patients with neuromuscular disorders. Many of these appear in the first day or two postoperatively and are not related to the hardware but rather to the surgical trauma and anesthesia. The ability to mobilize the patient out of bed immediately is helpful. Long-term pulmonary complications secondary to recumbency, immobilization restricting the abdominal or thoracic cage, and pressure sores caused by immobilization are eliminated.

Deaths have been reported in up to 2% of cases (12). These cases were usually secondary to pulmonary complications in the immediate postoperative period or secondary to later, unrelated complications.

Of note in Swank and colleagues' series (57) and in a large personal series is that two-stage anterior and posterior procedures have a much higher complication rate than single-stage anterior and posterior procedures. These complications are usually of a medical nature. Factors involved may be related to the larger curvatures involved in these procedures and the subsequent pulmonary deterioration that occurs secondary to the worsening scoliosis. Also, a large number of myelodysplastic and cerebral palsy patients have been included in the anterior and posterior fusion groups.

RESULTS

Luque instrumentation has proved to be as effective in correcting scoliotic curvatures and obtaining arthrodesis as other available instrumentation systems. Reports on the subject have largely dealt with neuromuscular scoliosis.

In 1982, Luque (39) reported on a mixed group of 65 patients with either idiopathic or neuromuscular scoliosis secondary to poliomyelitis that he treated surgically and followed for an average of 18 months. The average curvature in this group of patients was 69 degrees, and the average correction was 72%. No patients were immobilized postoperatively. He reported an average of 2% loss of correction during the follow-up period. The 65 patients underwent 78 operations related to their spines. Twelve patients had complications, including seven cases of hyperalgesia, two of which had muscle weakness. All the neurologic injuries resolved. Two patients became infected: one deep and one superficial. Two pseudarthroses were identified.

In 1982, Allen and Ferguson (2) reported on 10 cerebral palsy patients undergoing Luque instrumentation. The average curve measured 71 degrees, and the average correction was 60% at 2.7 years' follow-up. Correction was 25% greater per fused segment in those patients undergoing anterior release and fusion in conjunction with their Luque instrumentation as compared with those undergoing posterior fusion alone. All patients obtained arthrodesis in their spines. One infection required removal of one of the two rods, resulting in a loss of 18 degrees of correction. This was the sole patient judged to lose correction during the follow-up period. Three patients were placed in casts:

one for the previously mentioned infection and two others for short fusions that were noted to be progressing beyond the instrumented segments.

In 1983, Ferguson and Allen (21) reported their results of two-stage anterior release and fusion followed by posterior Luque instrumentation. Nine neuromuscular patients with an average preoperative curvature of 81 degrees were followed for 24 months. The average correction of the scoliotic deformity was 64%, and the average correction of the pelvic obliquity in five patients was 67%. Two patients in this series were rebulked for poor fusion mass by radiographic criteria. One patient had one pelvic rod displaced without consequence. No infections occurred.

In 1984, Allen and Ferguson (5) described 44 cases of pelvic fixation carried out using intralaminar iliac wing rod placement. They noted that achievement of stable pelvic fixation with their technique necessitated that the pelvic segment of the rod be 6 cm or longer, completely intraosseous through the iliac course, and within 1.5 cm of the sciatic notch. With these criteria, the lumbosacral fusion rate was 94%, with "wipering" of the rods averaging 1.4 mm.

In 1987, Herndon and associates (31) reported on 58 patients who had scoliosis or kyphosis of varying etiologies and were treated with Luque instrumentation. The average follow-up was 2 years. Nineteen percent had one or both rods break. The $\frac{3}{16}$-inch 316L stainless-steel rods were used in all the patients who fractured their rods. None of the patients with fractured rods had anterior procedures. All the fractured rods occurred in significantly greater curvatures (85 degrees) than in those that did not fracture (73 degrees). Extra bank bone was added to only one of the patients with a fractured rod. Seven of the fractured rods were in patients with pelvic fixation. None of the patients with fractured rods had postoperative immobilization. Infection was not associated with fracture of the rods in this series.

In 1988, Allen and Ferguson (4) reported their experience with Luque instrumentation in idiopathic scoliosis. Fifty-six patients were followed for an average of 3.9 years. The patients' ages ranged from 11 to 53 years. The percentage of correction correlated with the ages of the patient groups. The average correction ranged from 63% in the youngest age group to 40% in the group older than 35 years of age, with an overall average correction of 51%. There was one neurologic injury that resolved, three pseudarthroses, two regraftings for insufficient bone mass by radiographic criteria without loss of fixation, and four instances of implant prominence requiring surgery, with a total reoperation rate of 15%. No wound infections occurred. No immobilization was used postoperatively.

In 1988, Gersoff and Renshaw (28) described 33 cerebral palsy patients who underwent posterior Luque instrumentation for spinal deformity. The mean curve measured 65 degrees preoperatively and 30 degrees postoperatively, a 54% correction. The mean loss of correction at 40 months was 3 degrees. No pseudarthroses, rod failure, or neurologic deficits occurred. The authors stressed the use of $\frac{1}{4}$-inch rods and double wires throughout, and they did not use immobilization postoperatively.

In 1989, Boachie-Adjei and colleagues (11) reported on 46 patients with neuromuscular disorders who underwent Luque instrumentation for spinal deformities. The average follow-up was 3 years. Half were cerebral palsy patients, and half had other neuromuscular etiologies. The average curvature measured 74 degrees preoperatively and 39 degrees postoperatively, a 47% correction. Those patients undergoing anterior and posterior surgeries had better correction than did those undergoing posterior instrumentation alone. Pseudarthrosis occurred in 6.5%. No neurologic injuries secondary to the instrumentation were noted. The infection rate was 4.3%.

In 1989, Swank and associates (57) reported their experience treating severely involved nonambulatory cerebral palsy patients with Luque instrumentation. They compared posterior Luque rods alone to anterior Zielke and posterior Luque instrumentation in 31 patients. The authors concluded that Luque instrumentation alone in a severely involved cerebral palsy population led to a high pseudarthrosis rate (40%) and recommended circumferential arthrodesis for these patients. The average correction in the posterior group was 53%, compared with 63% in the circumferentially fused and instrumented group. They noted that patients who did not have pelvic fixation lost compensation postoperatively and recommended pelvic fixation in this patient population. One neurologic complication was noted in this group after Zielke instrumentation. The infection rate was 13%, and the overall pseudarthrosis rate was 19%.

In 1989, Stevens and Beard (55) reported on 76 consecutive cases of paralytic neuromuscular scoliosis in which Luque instrumentation was used to correct the spinal deformities. They reported an overall complication rate of 63%, the highest occurring in the myelodysplastic population (90%). Major neurologic complications occurred in 13% of patients. There was a 46% instrumentation complication rate, including five broken rods and three pseudarthroses. A 15% rate of infection occurred.

In 1990, Banta (8) reported on 50 patients with myelomeningocele who were treated with combined anterior and posterior fusions for severe spinal deformity. Twenty of these patients underwent Luque instrumentation as the posterior part of their procedures. The anterior procedures were a combination of Dwyer instrumentation and anterior fusions without instrumentation. Banta recommended the use of ¼-inch rods where possible, long fusions with fixation to the pelvis using the Galveston technique, and postoperative immobilization in bivalved total-contact polypropylene spinal orthoses. The pseudarthrosis rate for all 50 patients was 5.7%, and the infection rate was 8%.

In 1991, Gau and associates (27) reported on 68 neuromuscular patients treated with Luque-Galveston instrumentation. Twenty patients underwent anterior and posterior fusions. Instrumentation complications occurred in 21%, including four broken rods and no broken wires. Ten percent developed pseudarthroses. Three patients had minor transient neurologic complications. The average curve correction at 4 years was 55%.

In 1990, Maloney and coauthors (40) reported on 10 neuromuscular patients whose scoliosis was treated with the Luque unit rod. Nine of these patients underwent anterior and posterior procedures. An average scoliosis correction of 81% and pelvic obliquity correction of 82% were reported. Complications were related to the wound in two patients.

In 1996, Dias and colleagues (14) reported 31 cerebral palsy patients who underwent spinal fusion with the unit rod. An average 77% correction was achieved at 2.8 years' follow-up. The

pelvic obliquity was corrected by 82%. Twenty-four patients had a posterior fusion above, and seven had a combined anterior and posterior fusion. No instrument-related complications occurred.

In 1996, Brook and associates (12) reported on Duchenne muscular dystrophy patients whose spinal deformities were treated with Luque instrumentation. They reported a 60% correction of scoliosis and had no instrumentation failures or pseudarthroses when the instrumentation was taken to the pelvis with the Galveston technique and when Texas Scottish Rite Hospital cross-links were used to couple the rods.

In 1996, Bulman and coauthors (13) reported on 30 cerebral palsy patients; 15 patients were treated with Luque rod fixation, and 15 were treated with the unit rod. The percentages of correction with the Luque unit rod were significantly higher than with the plain Luque technique.

In 1998, Benson and coworkers (9) reported a recent series of 50 consecutive spinal fusions for neuromuscular scoliosis treated since 1990 with Luque instrumentation, with an average follow-up of 10 years. The average correction at follow-up was 65%. Instrument-related complications occurred in two patients. No neurologic deterioration was noted.

In summarizing these series, several trends are noted. Most authors describe their experience with Luque instrumentation treating neuromuscular scoliosis. Cerebral palsy and myelomeningocele were the predominant diagnoses in these groups. On average, the curvatures were between 70 and 80 degrees, and pelvic obliquity was associated with many of the deformities. Both two-stage anterior and posterior procedures and posterior procedures alone were reported. Correction in posterior procedures averaged about 50%, and correction in combined anterior and posterior cases averaged 60% to 65%. Anterior instrumentation did not increase the percentage of correction when used in combined anterior and posterior procedures. Of note was that the loss of correction in all reported series averaged only 1 to 3 degrees at follow-up.

Opinion was mixed about whether postoperative immobilization should be used. Consensus appeared to be that if $^3/_{16}$-inch 316L rods and wires are used, postoperative support of the spine should at least be considered.

Correction of pelvic obliquity and maintenance of this correction was well documented. Pelvic obliquity correction of 47% (11) to 82% (21) was reported with the use of the Galveston technique of pelvic instrumentation. Loss of correction in pelvic fixation cases without instrumentation failure was minimal. Unit rods tended to yield greater amounts of correction; however, the ability to place these rods is limited to more supple curvatures and may be the reason for the bias.

Average operative times were between 3.5 and 4.5 hours for a posterior procedure with iliac crest bone graft. If pelvic fixation or thoracoplasty were included, 1 hour could be added to the operative time. Average blood losses for a posterior procedure ranged from 1,500 to 2,000 mL. As the surgeons became more proficient with the technique, the average operative time and blood loss decreased (4).

SUMMARY

Luque instrumentation is a well-accepted treatment for neuromuscular spinal deformities. Its advocacy in cases of severe osteopenia and collagen diseases is documented. Its use in adolescent idiopathic scoliosis by a surgeon with limited experience is discouraged.

The Luque system and its techniques of application have improved in recent years. Many of its mechanical deficiencies have been eliminated. It is a universal instrumentation system that can be adapted to manage deformities and that can be used for revision surgery, pelvic fixation, and when osteopenia is present. Spinal surgeons must master Luque instrumentation if they are to deliver state-of-the-art care to all their scoliotic patients.

REFERENCES

1. Allen BL Jr, Ferguson RL (1979): The operative treatment of myelomeningocele spinal deformity—1979. *Orthop Clin North Am* 10: 845–862.
2. Allen BL Jr, Ferguson RL (1982): L-rod instrumentation for scoliosis in cerebral palsy. *J Pediatr Orthop* 2:87–96.
3. Allen BL Jr, Ferguson RL (1986): Neurologic injuries with the Galveston technique of L-rod instrumentation for scoliosis. *Spine* 11:14–17.
4. Allen BL Jr, Ferguson RL (1988): The Galveston experience with L-rod instrumentation for adolescent idiopathic scoliosis. *Clin Orthop* 229:59–69.
5. Allen BL Jr, Ferguson RL (1984): The Galveston technique of pelvic fixation with L rod instrumentation of the spine. *Spine* 9:388–394.
6. Allen BL Jr, Ferguson RL (1982): The Galveston technique for L rod instrumentation of the scoliotic spine. *Spine* 7:276–284.
7. Ashman RB, Birch JG, Bone LB, et al. (1988): Mechanical testing of spinal instrumentation. *Clin Orthop* 227:113–125.
8. Banta V (1990): Combined anterior and posterior fusion for spinal deformity in myelomeningocele. *Spine* 15:946–952.
9. Benson ER, Thomson JD, Smith BG, et al. (1998): Results and morbidity in a consecutive series of patients undergoing spinal fusion for neuromuscular scoliosis. *Spine* 23:2308–2317.
10. Birch JG, Herring JA (1987): Spinal deformity in Marfan syndrome. *J Pediatr Orthop* 7:546–552.
11. Boachie-Adjei O, Lonstein JE, Winter RB, et al. (1989): Management of neuromuscular spinal deformities with Luque segmental instrumentation. *J Bone Joint Surg Am* 71:548–562.
12. Brook PD, Kennedy JD, Stern LM, et al. (1996): Spinal fusion in Duchenne's muscular dystrophy. *J Pediatr Orthop* 16:324–331.
13. Bulman WA, Dormans JP, Ecker ML, et al. (1996): Posterior spinal fusion for scoliosis in patients with cerebral palsy: a comparison of Luque rod and Unit rod instrumentation. *J Pediatr Orthop* 16:314–323.
14. Dias RC, Miller F, Dabney K, et al. (1996): Surgical correction of spinal deformity using a unit rod in children with cerebral palsy. *J Pediatr Orthop* 16:734–740.
15. Dove J (1986): Internal fixation of the lumbar spine: the Hartshill rectangle. *Clin Orthop* 203:135–140.
16. Dove (1989): Segmental wiring for spinal deformity: a morbidity report. *Spine* 14:229–231.
17. Drummond D, Guadagni J, Keene HS, et al. (1984): Interspinous process segmental spinal instrumentation. *J Pediatr Orthop* 4:397–404.
18. Eberle CF (1988): Failure of fixation after segmental spinal instrumentation without arthrodesis in the management of paralytic scoliosis. *J Bone Joint Surg Am* 70:696–703.
19. Eggers GWN (1961): Berthold Earnest Hadra (1842–1903): biography. *Clin Orthop* 21:32–39.
20. Ferguson RL, Allen BL Jr (1988): Considerations in the treatment of cerebral palsy patients with spinal deformities. *Orthop Clin North Am* 19:419–425.
21. Ferguson RL, Allen BL Jr (1983): Staged correction of neuromuscular scoliosis. *J Pediatr Orthop* 3:555–562.
22. Ferguson RL, Allen BL Jr (1983): The technique of scoliosis revision surgery utilizing L-rod instrumentation. *J Pediatr Orthop* 3:563–571.
23. Ferguson RL, Allen BL Jr (1984): A mechanistic classification of thoracolumbar spine fractures. *Clin Orthop* 189:77–88.
24. Ferguson RL, Tencer AF, Woodard P, et al. (1988): Biomechanical comparisons of spinal fracture models and the stabilizing effects of posterior instrumentation. *Spine* 13:453–460.
25. Ferguson RL, Allen BL, Tencer AF (1990): Biomechanical principles of spinal correction. In: Cotler JM, Cotler HB, eds. *Spinal fusion.* New York: Springer-Verlag, pp. 45–60.
26. Gaines RW Jr, Abernathie DL (1986): Mersilene tapes as a substitute for wire in segmental spinal instrumentation for children. *Spine* 11: 907–913.
27. Gau YL, Lonstein JE, Winter RB, et al. (1991): Luque-Galveston procedure for correction and stabilization of neuromuscular scoliosis and pelvic obliquity: a review of 68 patients. *J Spinal Disord* 4:399–410.
28. Gersoff WK, Renshaw TS (1988): The treatment of scoliosis in cerebral palsy by posterior spinal fusion with Luque-rod segmental instrumentation. *J Bone Joint Surg Am* 70:41–44.
29. Ginsburg HH, Scoles PV (1991): *Scoliosis Research Society morbidity and mortality committee 1990 complication report.* Presented at: Scoliosis Research Society Meeting; September 14–17, 1991; Minneapolis, Minnesota.
30. Hadra BE (1891): Wiring of the vertebrae as a means of immobilization in fractures and Pott's disease of the spine. *Philadelphia Times and Register,* p. xxiii.
31. Herndon WA, Sullivan JA, Yngve DA, et al. (1987): Segmental spinal instrumentation with sublaminar wires: a critical appraisal. *J Bone Joint Surg Am* 69:851–859.
32. Herring JA, Wenger DR (1982): Segmental spinal instrumentation: a preliminary report of 40 consecutive cases. *Spine* 7:285–298.
33. Heydemann JS, Gillespie R (1987): Management of myelomeningocele kyphosis in the older child by kyphectomy and segmental spinal instrumentation. *Spine* 12:37–41.
34. Hielbronner DM, Sussman MD (1988): Early mobilization of adolescent scoliosis patients following Wisconsin interspinous segmental instrumentation as an adjunct to Harrington distraction instrumentation: preliminary report. *Clin Orthop* 229:52–58.
35. Jacobs RR (1982): Personal communication.
36. Kadic MA, Verbout AJ (1991): Treatment of severe kyphosis in myelomeningocele by segmental spinal instrumentation with Luque rods. *Acta Orthop Belg* 57:45–51.
37. Luque ER (1982): The anatomic basis and development of segmental spinal instrumentation. *Spine* 7:256–259.
38. Luque ER (1982): Paralytic scoliosis in growing children. *Clin Orthop* 163:202–209.
39. Luque ER (1982): Segmental spinal instrumentation for correction of scoliosis. *Clin Orthop* 163:192–198.
40. Maloney WJ, Rinsky LA, Gamble JG (1990): Simultaneous correction of pelvic obliquity, frontal plane, and sagittal plane deformities in neuromuscular scoliosis using a unit rod with segmental sublaminar wires: a preliminary report. *J Pediatr Orthop* 10:742–749.
41. McAfee PC, Farey ID, Sutterlin CE, et al. (1989): Device-related osteoporosis with spinal instrumentation. *Spine* 14:919–926.
42. McAfee PC, Lubicky JP, Werner FW (1983): The use of segmental spinal instrumentation to preserve longitudinal spinal growth: an experimental study. *J Bone Joint Surg Am* 65:935–942.
43. McCarthy RE, Bruffett WL, McCullough FL (1999): S rod fixation to the sacrum in patients with neuromuscular spinal deformities. *Clin Orthop* 364:26–31.
44. McNeice G (1983): *Biomechanics research of fracture fixation: application to the thoracolumbar spine.* Report to the University of Texas Medical Branch, Galveston, Texas.
45. Moseley CF, Mosca V, Lawton L, et al. (1985): The unit rod in segmental instrumentation of the spine for neuromuscular scoliosis. Presented at the Scoliosis Research Society, San Diego.
46. Nasca RJ, Hollis M, Lemosn JE, et al. (1985): Cyclic axial loading of spinal implants. *Spine* 10:792–798.
47. Nuber GW, Schafer MF (1986): Surgical management of adult scoliosis. *Clin Orthop* 208:228–237.
48. Panjabi MM, Abumi K, Duranceau J, et al. (1988): Biomechanical evaluation of spinal fixation devices. II. Stability provided by eight internal fixation devices. *Spine* 13:1135–1139.

49. Renshaw TS, Solga PM, Drennan JC, et al. (1991): Studies of an L-rod sublaminar sire spinal fusion. *J Pediatr Orthop* 11:226–229.

50. Resina J, Alves A, Ferreira (1977): Technique of correction and internal fixation for scoliosis. *J Bone Joint Surg Br* 59:159–165.

51. Rinsky LA, Gamble JG, Bleck EE (1985): Segmental instrumentation without fusion in children with progressive scoliosis. *J Pediatr Orthop* 5:687–690.

52. Rossier AB, Cochran TP (1984): The treatment of spinal fractures with Harrington compression rods and segmental sublaminar wiring: a dangerous combination. *Spine* 9:796–799.

53. Sirois JL, Drennan JC (1990): Dystrophic spinal deformity in neurofibromatosis. *J Pediatr Orthop* 10:522–526.

54. Songer MN, Spencer DL, Meyer PR, et al. (1991): The use of sublaminar cables to replace Luque wires. *Spine* 16[Suppl 8]:418–421.

55. Stevens DB, Beard C (1989): Segmental spinal instrumentation for neuromuscular spinal deformity. *Clin Orthop* 242:164–168.

56. Sullivan JA, Conner SB (1982): Comparison of Harrington instrumentation and segmental spinal instrumentation in the management of neuromuscular spinal deformity. *Spine* 7:299–304.

57. Swank SM, Cohen DS, Brown JC (1989): Spine fusion in cerebral palsy with L-rod segmental spinal instrumentation: a comparison of single and two-stage combined approach with Zielke instrumentation. *Spine* 14:750–759.

58. Weiler PJ, Medley JB, McNeice GM (1990): Numeric analysis of the load capacity of the human spine fitted with L-rod instrumentation. *Spine* 14:1285–1293.

59. White AA III, Panjabi MM (1976): The biomechanics of scoliosis. *Clin Orthop* 118:100–111.

60. Wilber RG, Thompson GH, Shaffer JW, et al. (1984): Postoperative neurological deficits in segmental spinal instrumentation. *J Bone Joint Surg Am* 66:1178–1187.

61. Zindrick MR, Knight GW, Bunch WH, et al. (1989): Factors influencing the penetration of wires into the neural canal during segmental wiring. *J Bone Joint Surg Am* 71:742–750.

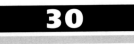

PEDICLE SCREW FIXATION

MICHAEL R. ZINDRICK
KAMAL I. IBRAHIM

The use of pedicle screws in pediatric and adolescent spinal surgery is a relatively recent development. In the adult spine, pedicle screw fixation has enjoyed widespread acceptance and use as a superior bone anchor in the lumbosacral and lower thoracic spine. Because of the reduced pedicle size in the immature spine, however, this tool has limited application. Pedicle screws are but one type of bone anchor used to attach posterior spinal instrumentation to the lumbosacral and lower thoracic spine and are offered as part of most state-of-the-art spinal internal fixation systems. The goals of this chapter are to familiarize the reader with the biomechanical advantages of screw anchor fixation and with the anatomy of the pedicle and surrounding structures and to demonstrate by way of case studies the use of pedicle screw fixation in a variety of conditions in children.

HISTORICAL PERSPECTIVE

The greatest advance in multisegmental fixation of the spine was made by Harrington (33,34). In addition to distraction rods, later advances in this system included compression rods, sacral bars, square-ended rods and hooks, and a variety of hook modifications (10,15,17,23,43,51,59,64,71,76). True segmental fixation of the spine was achieved with the use of segmental sublaminar wires as first described by Resina and Alves in 1977 (69) and then by Luque in 1982 (54).

The use of interpedicular screws has been the most recent major advance in internal fixation. By passing a screw through the pedicle from posterior to anterior to purchase the vertebral body, true three-dimensional grip of the vertebra can be achieved. The first reported use of a transpedicular screw was by Harrington and Tullos (35), who attempted the reduction of a spondylolisthesis in conjunction with a Harrington rod. Roy-Camille and colleagues (72) of France developed the first spinal fixation system to use the pedicle. Despite enthusiasm in Europe in the 1970s, it was not until the 1980s that this technique received widespread attention in North America. Steffee and coworkers (81) improved on the Roy-Camille plate by rigidly anchoring the screw to the plate independent of plate-bone

contact. Recently, there has been an explosion of systems developed that use the transpedicular screw as an anchor (15, 20–22,24,26,31,36,48,62,66,68,77,79,86,90). Many of these systems depend solely on transpedicular vertebral anchors; others incorporate hooks, sublaminar wire, and intraspinous wires in addition to transpedicular screws. This multitude of vertebral anchors gives these systems great versatility in dealing with a multitude of spinal disorders in all levels of the spine.

VERTEBRAL ANCHOR BIOMECHANICS

The Hook

Although the hook is strongest in resisting axial and extension loads, by the nature of its design and spinal laminar attachment, it is limited in its ability to resist flexion and torsional forces. Intact laminae are required for hook attachment, unless in a claw configuration, force application is unidirectional. To achieve rigidity and maximal correction with the Harrington rod distraction system, distractive forces must be applied over multiple noninvolved segments against intact ligamentous structures (ligamentotaxis), requiring either intact ligaments or the reconstruction of such. In the lumbar spine, this results in loss of lordosis and a flat back. Clearly, distraction systems have limited use in the lumbar spine, where short-segment fusion is needed most (11,14,43,44,67,87).

The Wire

Similar to the hook, the sublaminar wire requires intact laminae. By the nature of its insertion, the vertebral canal is violated. The ability to resist longitudinal forces is minimal, especially with a smooth rod. Modifications include pars wiring and Mersilene taping under the lamina (11,14,88).

The Screw

The attraction of pedicle screw system is that rigid fixation can be achieved over a short segment of the spine, limiting involvement of adjacent normal spinal segments. Laminae are not required to secure the vertebrae. Additionally, distraction is not a required component of construct stability of a pedicle

M. R. Zindrick and K. Ibrahim: Department Of Orthopaedics and Rehabilitation, Loyola University, Maywood, Illinois 60153.

screw–based system. The screw is inherently stable in its ability to resist load in all planes.

The strength of a construct using pedicular screw fixation depends on the strength of screw fixation in the pedicles. This is dependent on multiple factors, including insertion technique, screw design, and bone quality. The angle of insertion into the pedicle can effect superior facet impingement and availability of added vertebral body bone for thread purchase (52). The three-dimensional locking of adjacent pedicle screws with cross-links results in a combined pullout strength greater than that of either screw alone (13,73). This also stabilizes the construct, preventing collapse with lateral load (12).

Screw Fixation in the Sacrum

Screws can be inserted into the ala laterally, into the ala straight anteriorly, or into the vertebral body and sacral promontory medially. There are proponents of each direction of screw insertion. Anatomic and biomechanical studies have shown the best fixation to be in areas of greatest bone availability. The ala laterally and first sacral pedicle medially have the largest area for screw purchase. More distal sacral screw sites include the ala lateral to the S2 pedicle.

Finally, and of the utmost importance, it is essential to appreciate that an instrumentation system does not work in isolation but rather relies on the biologic system to share loads. The goal of a final construct should be the creation of a system that shares load between metal and biologic components. The posterior fixation device is much more likely to "survive" if there is an adequate anterior load path that acts to reduce the bending loads and motions the device is required to bear. Ultimately, however, all fixation devices are doomed to fail if biologic fusion is not achieved (3,18,19,56,61,80,82,89,94).

PEDICLE ANATOMY

An understanding of pedicle anatomy and morphology, especially of the immature pedicle, is necessary before a pedicle screw can be safely inserted. For obvious reasons, in children and adolescents, it is imperative that preoperative evaluation of the pedicle dimensions be carried out before pedicle screw insertion.

Although generally oval in shape, pedicle morphology varies throughout the spine. There is a considerable difference between thoracic, upper lumbar, and lower lumbar pedicles and their associated posterior landmarks.

The first published study concerning adult pedicle anatomy for screw insertion was by Saillant of France (74). Subsequent to this (a decade later), multiple authors studied pedicle morphology in somewhat greater detail (8,16,30,49,50,55,60, 63,78,93). For the most part, there is striking similarity in the data.

Reviewing computed tomography (CT) scans of more than 1,000 vertebrae in 203 children, Ferree (27–29) found that the pedicles of the lower lumbar spine (L4, L5, and S1) reached transverse extracortical pedicle diameters of 1 cm by the time the child was 7 years of age. In the upper lumbar spine (T12, L1, L2, and L3), pedicles did not reach similar size until the child was 12 years of age. The author concluded that pedicle

screw insertion, especially of the L5 and S1 vertebrae, is technically possible in young children.

Figures 1 to 5 represent the combined results of two pedicle morphology studies. The adult data are taken from Zindrick and colleagues (93); the other data shown are the results of a cadaveric study of immature spines (91,92). More than 11,500 measurements were acquired from 75 spines in patients aged 3 to 19 years. The immature spine was found to be proportionately smaller than the adult spine. The reduction in size, however, parallels that of the mature spine (Figs. 1, 2). Pedicles of the lower lumbar spine (L3 to L5) were noted to reach an average of 7 mm or greater in outer cortical dimension in the transverse plane by 9 to 11 years of age. In the sagittal plane, pedicle widths of greater than 7 mm were achieved by 6 to 8 years of age. In addition, transverse and sagittal angles do not appear to change with growth (Figs. 3, 4). Younger specimens demonstrated separation of the posterior elements from the vertebral body at the pedicle–vertebral body growth plate. The effect of a pedicle screw on the growing pedicle is not known. Studies have shown, however, the canal diameter is virtually unchanged after 4 years of age (65). This indicates that as the pedicle grows with age, the growth occurs lateral to the canal.

In general, pedicle morphology in children and adults follows similar trends. The pedicle isthmus width in the transverse (axial) plane is largest at L5; there is gradual narrowing in the upper lumbar spine, reaching a minimum in the midthoracic region (Fig. 1). It is this pedicle dimension that limits the screw diameter used in the pedicle. In the sagittal plane, the oval-shaped pedicle is broadest. Sagittal plane pedicle width is largest in the thoracolumbar region and smallest in the upper thoracic spine (Fig. 2). The angles between the pedicle and the vertebral body vary considerably throughout the spine. In the transverse plane, the pedicle angles from posterolateral to anteromedial at most levels, except in the region of the thoracolumbar junction (Fig. 3). Here, the pedicle angle may be neutral (parallel to the midline) or even reversed in angulation from that in other regions of the spine. It is imperative that the surgeon understand the pedicle angle in each particular patient to prevent canal penetration with an excessively medially angled screw or insertion tool. This knowledge is critical in the thoracolumbar region. In the sagittal plane, the pedicle is neutrally oriented in the lumbar spine (Fig. 4). Throughout most of the thoracic spine, the pedicle inclines in a cephalad direction.

The distance from the posterior elements and pedicle insertion zone posteriorly to the anterior cortex of the vertebral body is determined by vertebral body size and pedicle transverse angulation (Fig. 5). Generally, the longest path to the anterior cortex through the pedicle is along the pedicle axis at all levels. An exception to this rule is in the thoracolumbar region, where the posterolateral to anteromedial transverse planar angulation can decrease or even reverse (93). At all other levels, the distance to the anterior cortex is significantly longer along the pedicle axis than in a straight anterior direction. Knowledge of this additional distance affords the surgeon the option of safely inserting longer screws into the vertebra (beneficial in osteoporotic bone), minimizing or avoiding undesired anterior cortical penetration. In the immature spine, the distance to the anterior cortex increases with age as the size of the vertebral body increases.

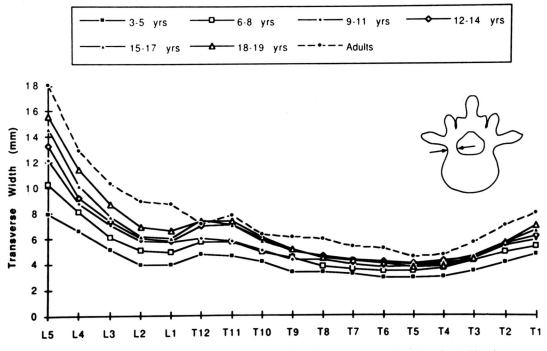

FIGURE 1. Mean adult and pediatric transverse pedicle isthmus width as a function of spinal level.

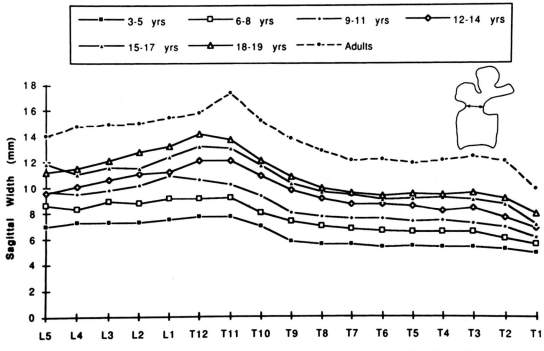

FIGURE 2. Mean adult and pediatric sagittal pedicle isthmus width as a function of spinal level.

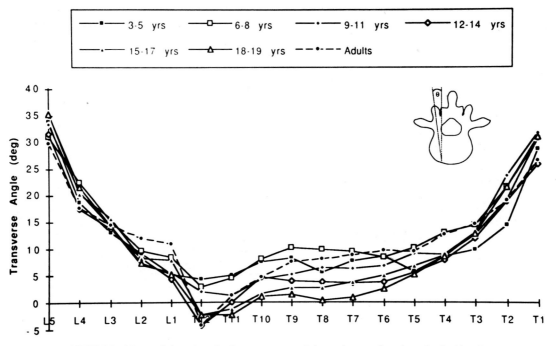

FIGURE 3. Mean adult and pediatric transverse pedicle angles as a function of spinal level.

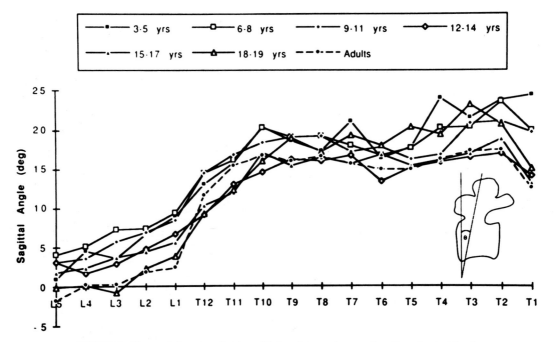

FIGURE 4. Mean adult and pediatric sagittal pedicle angles as a function of spinal level.

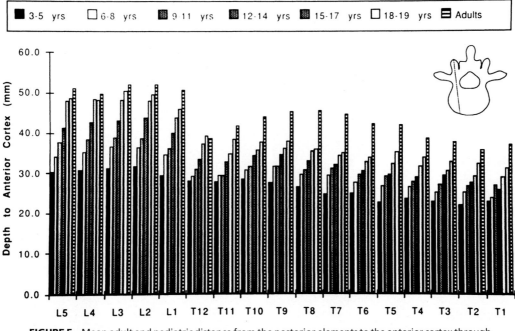

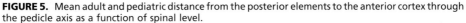

FIGURE 5. Mean adult and pediatric distance from the posterior elements to the anterior cortex through the pedicle axis as a function of spinal level.

The Sacrum

There are three places in the sacrum to insert screws for adequate purchase: medially into the S1 pedicle and body as close to the sacral end plate as possible, laterally into the sacral ala at the level of S1, and laterally into the ala at the level of S2. Additional caudal fixation sites include hook fixation into the S2 foramen and into the ilium using either rods or iliac screws (3,18,19, 56,61,80,82,89,94).

SURROUNDING STRUCTURES AT RISK DURING PEDICLE SCREW INSERTION

Many neighboring structures, although unseen during pedicle screw insertion, are at risk for injury. These structures include the dural sac and nerve roots medial, lateral, cephalad, and caudal to the pedicle and the great vessels anterior to the vertebral bodies and sacral ala. Their relationships can be appreciated by laboratory dissection and a thorough review of serial CT images of spinal levels, with particular attention to the regions lateral and anterior to the pedicles, vertebral bodies, and sacral ala (Fig. 6).

Penetration into the spinal canal at the time of pedicle screw insertion can cause significant injury to neural structures. Excessive medial angulation can cause pedicle splitting and medial pedicle cortical perforation. The exiting nerve root and ganglion are most at risk. Further medial angulation can result in penetration of the dural sac itself. Lateral screw placement can split the pedicle and the transverse process, resulting in injury to the nerve originating from the level above as it tracks lateral to the pedicle anterior to the transverse process. Cephalad or caudal screw misplacement can penetrate the foramen either above or below the pedicle, injuring the exiting nerve at that level.

The great vessels are anterior to the vertebral bodies in spinal levels above the bifurcation. At the level of the L3 and L4 vertebral bodies, the bifurcating common iliac artery and veins leave the midline, taking a lateral position, and lie directly anterior to the pedicles (58). In the sacral region, the great vessels—now the internal and external iliac artery and veins and their branches—lie laterally along the sacral ala. Medial and lateral "safe zones" for bicortical sacral screw insertion have been defined. These safe zones are areas of the sacrum that are free from close apposition of vital structures. Any penetration of the anterior cortex of the sacrum must be done with great care, and no probe, tap, or screw should penetrate more than a few millimeters beyond the most anterior aspect of the anterior sacral cortex. In the midline of the sacrum, a variable middle sacral artery can persist and lie directly anterior to the S1 vertebral body in the midline (57,58) (Fig. 7).

Surgical Planning (Anatomic Considerations)

Once the surgeon is armed with general anatomic principles, the specific anatomy of the individual patient's pedicles to be instrumented must be thoroughly evaluated and understood. Careful preoperative planning will eliminate most intraoperative problems. The dimensions of the pedicles planned for screw placement should be understood. Although preoperative plain radiographs can give a general idea of pedicle size, CT or magnetic resonance imaging will yield exact measurements of size and angle. Additionally, altered anatomy can be identified and appreciated preoperatively from these studies. Intraoperatively, radiographic assistance aids accurate screw placement. Biplanar or fluoroscopic views help to guide the surgeon.

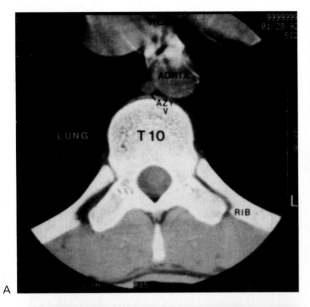

A

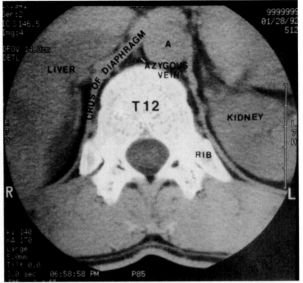

B

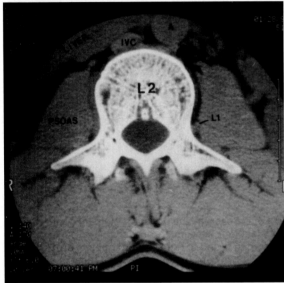

C

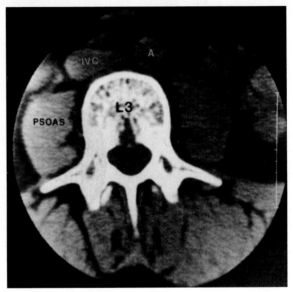

D

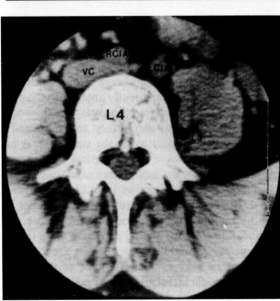

E

FIGURE 6. Axial computed tomography scan images of T10, T12, L2 to L5, and S1 and related structures (**A to G,** respectively). Note lateral structures in relationship to the pedicle. Also note anterior vascular structures lying in front of the vertebral bodies and sacral ala. *Azy V,* azygous vein; *A,* aorta; *IVC,* inferior vena cava; *VC,* vena cava; *RCIA* and *LCIA,* right and left common iliac artery; *RCIV* and *LCIV,* right and left common iliac vein; *As* and *Vs,* arteries and veins; nerve roots are also indicated where appropriate. *(Figure continues.)*

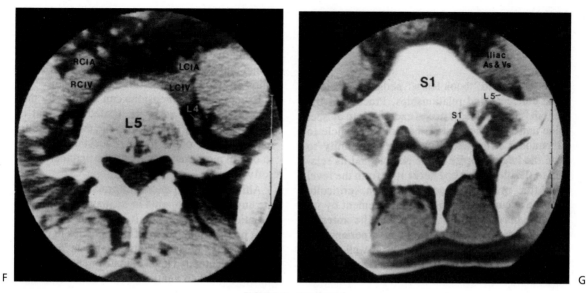

FIGURE 6. *Continued.*

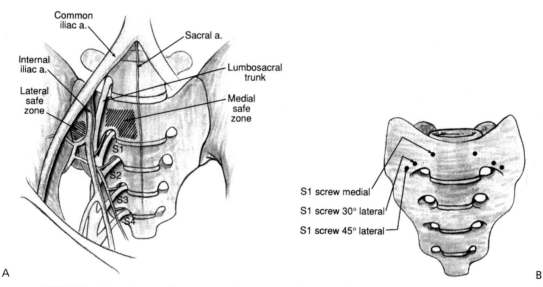

FIGURE 7. A: Anterior sacral anatomy and anterior sacral cortex safe zones. Medial safe zone is represented by left to right upward oblique cross-hatching and lateral safe zone by left to right downward oblique cross-hatching (57). **B:** Sacral anterior cortical penetration points for medial and lateral S1 screws (3). (Redrawn from Mirkovic S, Abitol JJ, Steinman J, et al. [1991]: Anatomic considerations for sacral screw placement. *Spine* 16:289–294, with permission.).

CLINICAL APPLICATION OF PEDICLE SCREWS IN CHILDREN

The use of pedicle screws in children is gaining popularity in spine fixation and deformity correction (1,5,32,39,40,42,45,53, 70,75,83,84). Pedicle screws enhance the ability to manipulate the vertebrae and achieve a greater degree of deformity correction. Anatomic studies proved the safety of pedicle screws insertion in pediatric spine, and recent clinical reviews support that conclusion (1,5,9,25,39,40,42).

PLANNING AND EXECUTION OF PEDICLE SCREWS IN SPECIFIC PEDIATRIC SPINAL CONDITIONS

Adolescent Idiopathic Scoliosis

When the fusion and instrumentation extend into the lumbar spine, pedicle screws are the best anchor for the construct. They allow better control on the vertebrae, which would achieve stronger fixation, and better correction, but at the same time would spare more lumbar vertebrae from being included in the

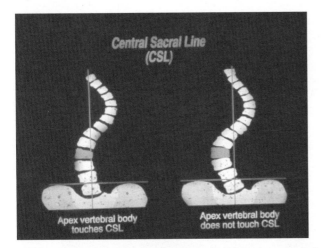

FIGURE 8. Type II curve, which is right thoracic. Left lumbar curve pattern is divided into two groups, A and B, depending on the lumbar curve mobility and severity. A type IIA lumbar curve is flexible, and the central sacral line intercepts lumbar apical vertebra; a type IIB lumbar curve is rigid and significant, and therefore, the central sacral line does not intercept lumbar apical vertebra. In type IIA curves, selective fusion of the thoracic spine is advised; in type IIB curves, the fusion and instrumentation should extend into the lumbar vertebrae to achieve coronal balance.

spine fusion than would hooks fixation (5,32,39,40,42,47, 53,75,83,84). In the curves of King Moe (46) types I, IIB (2–4,6,37,38,41) (Fig. 8), and IV (5,32,39,40,42,46,53,75, 83,84), the fusion and pedicle screw instrumentation extends to the most cephalad lumbar vertebra, which is fully mobile on the supine right and left side-bending radiographs (39,40,42) (see the case of type IIB curve later in Fig. 10). Instrumentation with the pedicle screws allows good grip on the terminal vertebrae to manipulate them into a horizontal position within the central sacral line, thus creating a balanced spine in the coronal plane; and by compressing them, appropriate lordosis in the sagittal plane is achieved (7,39,40,42).

The planning includes ensuring that an adequate number of hooks and wires for the thoracic curve are inserted; these are placed in divergent fashion on the concave side and convergent fashion on the convex side. Pedicle screws should be inserted on both sides—if technically possible—of the distal two or three lumbar vertebrae (40,42). The sequence of execution of correction during surgery is shown in Figure 9. Figure 10 shows a patient with a type IIB curve, which was corrected with this technique. Figure 11 shows a patient with a type I curve, and Figure 12 shows a patients with a type VI curve.

Spondylolisthesis

In cases of high-grade slip, when reduction is contemplated, the goals are to correct the kyphotic slip angle into lordosis, to have

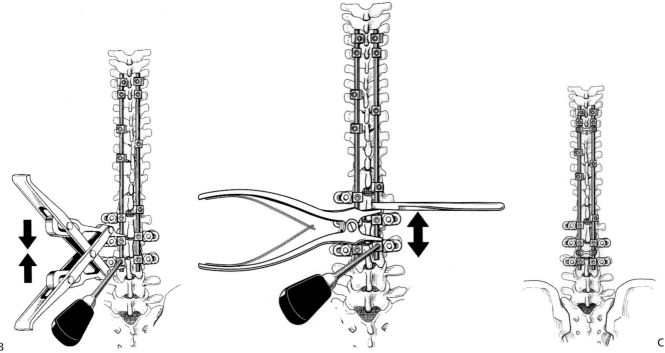

A,B   C

FIGURE 9. Execution during surgery: the two rods are bent according to the final sagittal correction. They are applied in the thoracic curve, the spine is translated to the rods, final correction is obtained for the thoracic curve, and its anchors are locked. Then, for the lumbar curve, the screws on the convex side are compressed against a fixed point on the rod, creating lumbar lordosis **(A)**. Finally, the screws on the concave side are distracted distally against a fixed instrument on the rod to rotate the lumbar vertebrae in the coronal plane into a horizontal position parallel to the pelvis, creating a balanced spine **(B, C)**.

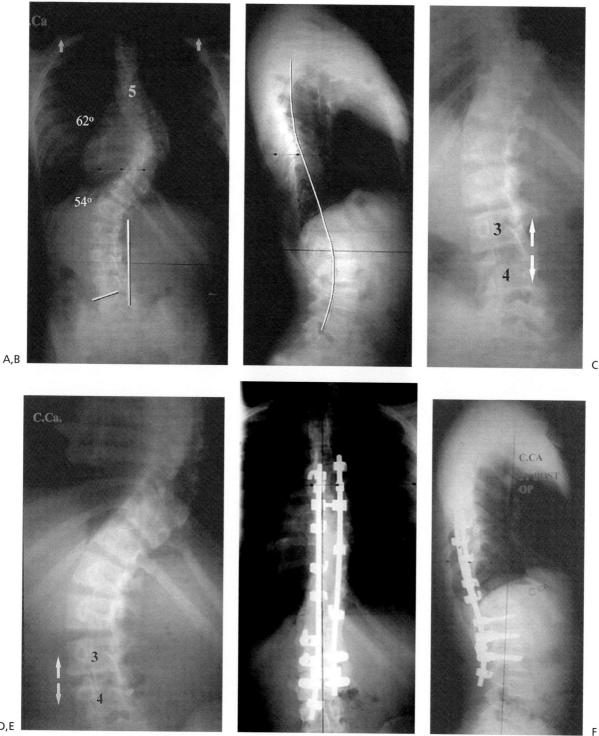

A,B

C

D,E

F

FIGURE 10. A–J: This boy, aged 12 years 7 months, had a type IIB curve that is fused to L3, which is the mobile vertebra on side-bending radiographs, whereas the lumbar end vertebra is L4. The mobile vertebra is the most cephalad lumbar vertebra, and its distal end plate would overcorrect or at least be parallel to the proximal end plate of the adjacent caudal vertebra on side-bending radiographs (**C, D**). Final follow-up shows good correction and appropriate balance. *(Figure continues.)*

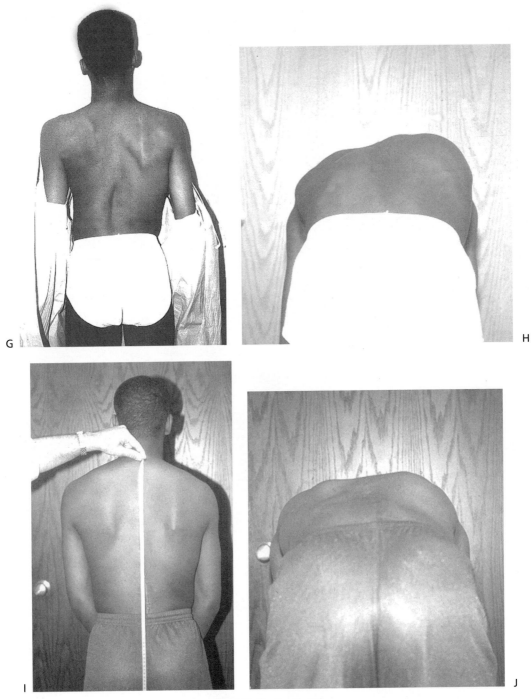

FIGURE 10. *Continued.*

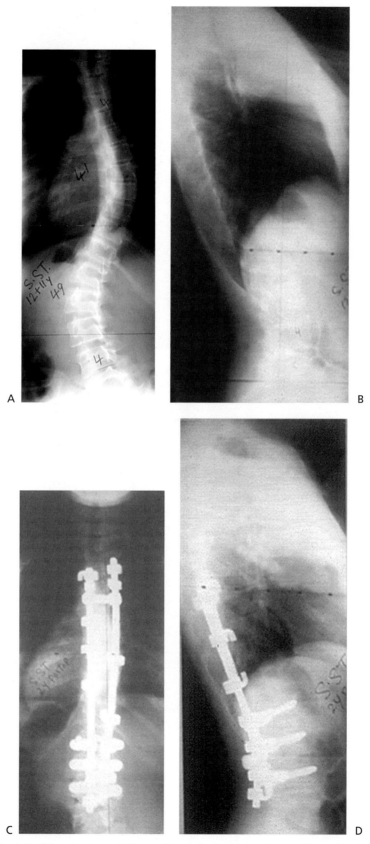

FIGURE 11. A–D: This patient, aged 12 years 11 months, had a type I curve. The end lumbar vertebra is L4, but with the pedicle screws, the fusion ended at L3 (which is the mobile vertebra on the side-bending radiographs), with excellent correction and coronal and sagittal balance.

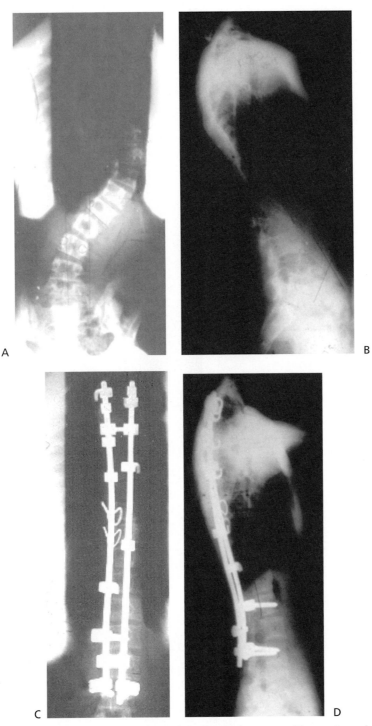

FIGURE 12. **A–D:** This girl, aged 12 years 1 month, had an 80-degree type IV curve. It was fused to the mobile vertebra, which is L3, with excellent outcome. The residual curve is 17 degrees.

rigid fixation to avoid pseudarthrosis and loss of correction, and to avoid unnecessary proximal extension of instrumentation into the upper lumbar levels. Pedicle screws satisfy these goals. They are the only possible fixation because hooks are not feasible when the posterior arch is loose or was removed for decompression (Fig. 13,[85]).

Absence of Posterior Arch

Pedicle screws are the only bone anchor in the absence of a posterior arch, such as in patients with myelomeningocele (Fig. 14), and in the management of spinal tumor or in decompression in spinal stenosis, such as in patients with achondroplasia (1,70).

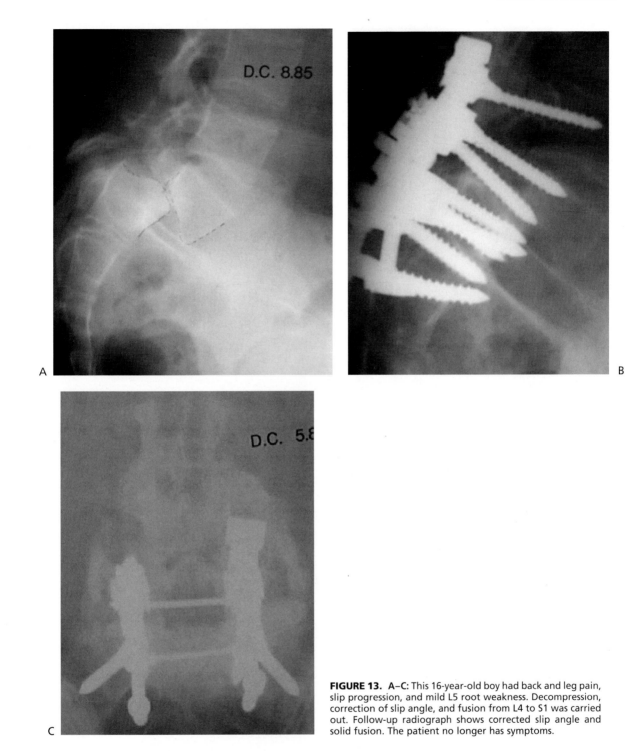

FIGURE 13. A–C: This 16-year-old boy had back and leg pain, slip progression, and mild L5 root weakness. Decompression, correction of slip angle, and fusion from L4 to S1 was carried out. Follow-up radiograph shows corrected slip angle and solid fusion. The patient no longer has symptoms.

Excision of Congenital Lumbar Hemivertebra

The growth of lumbar hemivertebra would cause congenital scoliosis and significant coronal imbalance. Excision of the hemivertebra restores the balance, corrects the scoliosis, and halts the progression. Fixation with pedicle screws accomplishes rigid fixation with short fusion, which is of utmost importance in the lumbar spine to preserve as many mobile segments possible (Figs. 15, 16).

Paralytic Scoliosis in Cerebral Palsy Patients

Patients with cerebral palsy, especially those with spastic athetoid, have significant trunk imbalance, spasticity, and abnormal body movements. Therefore, coronal and sagittal balance and

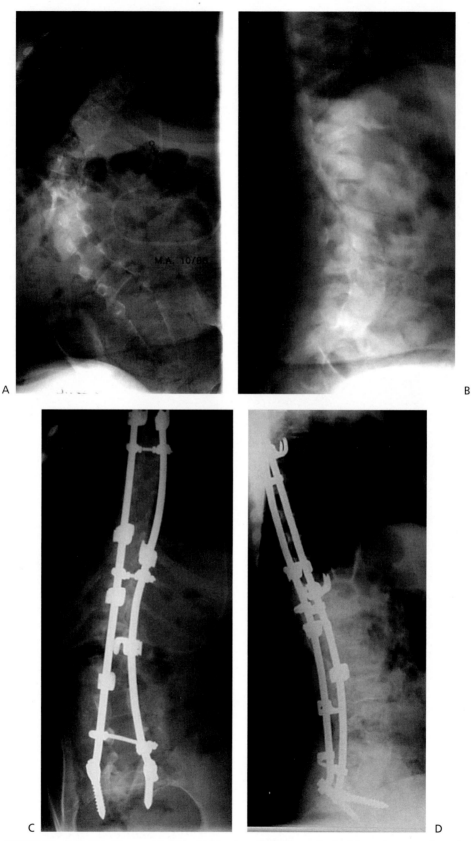

FIGURE 14. A–D: This 11-year-old girl had L4-level myelomeningocele. Pedicle screws were the only possible fixation for the caudad end of the construct, where the laminae are missing. At follow-up, she had a balanced spine with strong fixation.

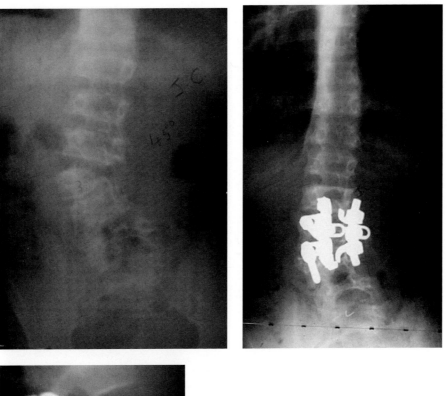

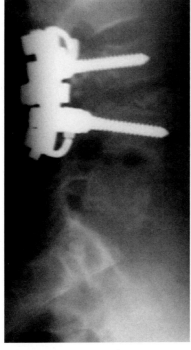

FIGURE 15. **A–C:** This boy, aged 12 years 7 months, had progressive congenital scoliosis because of L3 hemivertebra, which was excised from a posterior approach (modified eggshell operation). The L1 to L4 curve was 46 degrees before surgery and 8 degrees on follow-up after it was fused from L2 to L4 with pedicle screws.

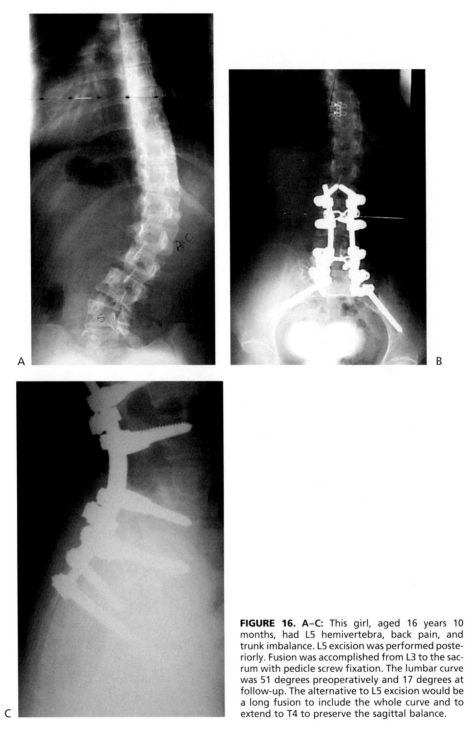

FIGURE 16. A–C: This girl, aged 16 years 10 months, had L5 hemivertebra, back pain, and trunk imbalance. L5 excision was performed posteriorly. Fusion was accomplished from L3 to the sacrum with pedicle screw fixation. The lumbar curve was 51 degrees preoperatively and 17 degrees at follow-up. The alternative to L5 excision would be a long fusion to include the whole curve and to extend to T4 to preserve the sagittal balance.

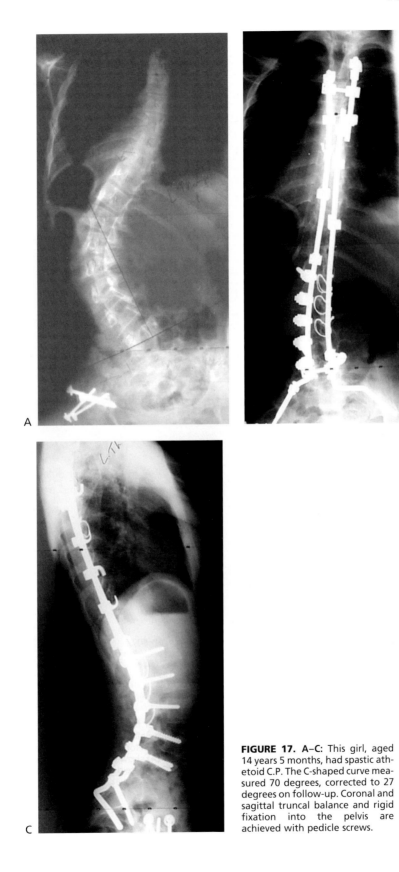

FIGURE 17. A–C: This girl, aged 14 years 5 months, had spastic athetoid C.P. The C-shaped curve measured 70 degrees, corrected to 27 degrees on follow-up. Coronal and sagittal truncal balance and rigid fixation into the pelvis are achieved with pedicle screws.

tween frontal balance, hook configuration and fusion levels. *Orthop Trans* 15(1).

39. Ibrahim K, Bueche M (1996): *The effect of using lumbar pedicle screws on fusion extension, curve correction and spinal balance in adolescent idiopathic scoliosis instrumentation.* Annual Meeting of the Scoliosis Research Society, Ottawa, Ontario, Canada, September.

40. Ibrahim K, Bueche M (1997): The effect of using lumbar pedicle screws on fusion extension, curve correction and spinal balance in adolescent idiopathic scoliosis instrumentation. *Orthop Trans* 21(327).

41. Ibrahim K, Goldberg BJ (1989): Cotrel-Dubousset instrumentation for right thoracic curves: relationship between results and distal fusion level. *Orthop Trans* 13(3):606–607.

42. Ibrahim K, Sofiyan M, Liao Y, et al. (1998; 1999): *Spinal balance in adolescent idiopathic scoliosis (AIS): type II curves after instrumentation with CD and Isola system.* Presented at the Annual Meeting of the North American Spine Society. San Francisco, California, October 1998; at the Annual Meeting of the Pediatric Orthopedic Society of North America, Orlando, Florida, May 1999; and at the Annual Meeting of the American Orthopaedic Association, Sun Valley, Idaho, June 1999.

43. Jacobs RR, Schlaepfer F, Mathys R, et al. (1984): A locking hook spinal rod system for stabilization of fracture-dislocations and correction of deformities of the dorsolumbar spine: a biomechanical evaluation. *Clin Orthop* 189:168–177.

44. Kahanovitz N, Arnoczky SP, Levine DB, et al. (1984): The effects of internal fixation on the articular cartilage of unfused canine facet joint cartilage. *Spine* 9:268.

45. King AG, Tahmoush KM, Thomas KA (1997): *Biomechanical testing of pedicle screw versus laminar hooks as distal anchors for scoliosis instrumentation.* Presented at the Annual Meeting of the Scoliosis Research Society, St Louis, MO, September.

46. King HA, Moe JH, Bradford DS, et al. (1983): The selection of fusion levels in thoracic idiopathic scoliosis. *J Bone Joint Surg Am* 65:1302–1313.

47. Knapp DR, Price CT, Jones ET, et al. (1992): Choosing fusion levels in progressive thoracic idiopathic scoliosis. *Spine* 17:1159–1165.

48. Krag MH (1988): Lumbosacral fixation with the Vermont spinal fixator. In: Lin PM, Gill K, eds. *Lumbar interbody fusion: principles and techniques of spine surgery.* Rockville, MD: Aspen.

49. Krag MH, Beynnon BD, Pope MH, et al. (1986): An internal fixator for posterior application to short segments of the thoracic, lumbar, or lumbosacral spine: design and testing. *Clin Orthop* 203:75–98.

50. Krag MH, Weaver DL, Beynnon BD, et al. (1988): Morphometry of the thoracic and lumbar spine related to transpedicular screw placement for surgical spinal fixation. *Spine* 13:27–32.

51. Lenke LG, Bridwell KH, Baldus C, et al. (1992): Cotrel-Dubousset instrumentation for adolescent idiopathic scoliosis. *J Bone Joint Surg Am* 74:1056–1067.

52. Leong JC, Lu WW, Zheng Y, et al. (1998): Comparison of the strengths of lumbosacral fixation achieved with techniques using one and two triangulated Scarl screws. *Spine* 23(21):2289–2294.

53. Liljenqvist UR, Halm HF, Link TM (1997): Pedicle screw instrumentation of the thoracic spine in idiopathic scoliosis. *Spine* 22(19):2239–2245.

54. Luque ER (1982): Anatomic basis and development of segmental spinal instrumentation. *Spine* 7:256–259.

55. Marchesi D, Scheider E, Glauser P, et al. (1988): Morphometric analysis of the thoracolumbar and lumbar pedicles, anatomo-radiologic study. *Surg Radiol Anat* 10:317–322.

56. Mazda K, Khairouni A, Pennecot GF, et al. (1998): The ideal position of sacral transpedicular endplate screws in Jackson's intrasacral fixation: an anatomical study of 50 sacral specimens. *Spine* 23(19):2123–2126.

57. Mirkovic S, Abitol JJ, Steinman J, et al. (1991): Anatomic considerations for sacral screw placement. *Spine* 16:289–294.

58. Molitor CJ, Wiltse LL, DiMartino PP, et al. (1991): Vascular and neurological anatomy of the lumbosacral spine as it relates to injury by pedicle screw placement (Abstract). *Proc North Am Spine Soc.*

59. Nasca RJ, Johnson LP (1988): Harrington-Bobechko instrumentation in the treatment of scoliosis: a preliminary report. *Spine* 13:246–249.

60. Olsewski JM, Simmons EH, Kallen FC, et al. (1990): Morphometry of the lumbar spine: anatomical perspectives related to transpedicular fixation. *J Bone Joint Surg Am* 72:541–549.

61. Pashman RS, Hu SS, Schenel MJ, et al. (1993): Sacral screw loads in lumbosacral fixation for spinal deformity. *Spine* 18(16):2465–2470.

62. Peek RD, Thomas JC, Weinstein J, et al. (1988): Lumbar spine fusion with pedicle screws and rods. *Proc Int Soc Study Lumbar Spine.*

63. Pfaundler S, Ebeling U, Reulen HJ (1989): Pedicle origin and intervertebral compartment in the lumbar and upper sacral spine. *Acta Neurchir* (Wein) 97:158–165.

64. Phillips WA, Hensinger RN (1988): Wisconsin and other instrumentation for posterior spinal fusion. *Clin Orthop* 229:44–51.

65. Porter RW, Pavitt D (1987): The vertebral canal. 1. Nutrition and development, an archaeological study. *Spine* 12:901–906.

66. Puno RM, Bechtold JE, Byrd JE, et al. (1987): Biomechanical analysis of five techniques of fixation for the lumbosacral junction. *Proc Orthop Res Soc.*

67. Purcell GA, Markoff KL, et al. (1981): Twelfth thoracic-first lumbar vertebral mechanical stability of fractures after Harrington rod instrumentation. *J Bone Joint Surg Am* 63:71.

68. Puschel J, Zielke K (1984): Transpedicular vertebral instrumentation using VDS instruments in ankylosing spondylitis. *Proc Scoliosis Res Soc.*

69. Resina J, Alves AV (1977): Technique of correction and internal fixation for scoliosis. *J Bone Joint Surg Br* 59:159–165.

70. Rogers WB, Williams MS, Schwend RM, et al. (1997): Spinal deformity in myelodysplasia: correction with posterior pedicle screw instrumentation. *Spine* 22(20):2435–2443.

71. Rossier AB, Cochran TP (1984): The treatment of spinal fractures with Harrington compression rods and segmental sublaminar wiring: a dangerous combination. *Spine* 9:796–799.

72. Roy-Camille R, Saillant G, Bertreaux D, et al. (1976): Osteosynthesis of thoraco-lumbar spine fractures with metal plates screwed through the vertebral pedicles. *Reconstr Surg Traumatol* 15:2–16.

73. Ruland CM, McAfee PC, Warden KE, et al. (1991): Triangulation of pedicular instrumentation: a biomechanical analysis. *Spine* 16:S270–S276.

74. Saillant G (1976): Etude anatomique despedicules vertebraex: application chirurgcale. *Rev Chir Orthop* 62:151–160.

75. Sato S, Asher MA (1996): *Comparison of laminar hook to pedicle screw anchors for the correction of double structural adolescent idiopathic scoliosis.* Presented at the Annual Meeting of the Scoliosis Research Society. Ottawa, Ontario, Canada, September.

76. Schlicke L, Schulak J (1980): The simultaneous use of Harrington compression and distraction rods in a thoracolumbar fracture dislocation. *J Trauma* 20:177–179.

77. Schreiber A, Suezawa Y, Jacob HAC (1986): Preliminary report of 40 patients: dorsal spinal fusion with a transpedicular distraction and compression system. *Orthop Rev* 15:93–96.

78. Scoles PV, Linton AE, Latimer B, et al. (1988): Vertebral body and posterior element morphology: the normal spine in middle life. *Spine* 13:1082–1086.

79. Simmons EH, Capicotta WN (1988): Posterior transpedicular Zielke instrumentation of the lumbar spine. *Clin Orthop* 236:180–191.

80. Smith SA, Abitol JJ, Carlson GD, et al. (1993): The effects of depth of penetration, screw orientation, and bone density on sacral screw fixation. *Spine* 18(8):1006–1010.

81. Steffee AD, Biscup RS, Sitkowski DJ (1986): Segmental spine plates with pedicle screw fixation: a new internal fixation device for disorders of lumbar and thoracolumbar spine. *Clin Orthop* 203:45–53.

82. Stovall DO Jr, Goodrich JA, Lundy D, et al. (1997): Sacral fixation technique in lumbosacral fusion. *Spine* 22(1):32–37.

83. Suk SI, Lee CK, Min HJ, et al. (1994): Comparison of Cotrel-Dubousset pedicle screws and hooks in the treatment of idiopathic scoliosis. *Int Orthop* 18(6):341–346.

84. Suk SI, Lee CK, Kim WJ, et al. (1995): Segmental pedicle screw fixation in the treatment of thoracic idiopathic scoliosis. *Spine* 20(12):1399–1405.

85. Suk SI, Lee CK, Kim WJ, et al. (1997): Adding posterior lumbar interbody fusion to pedicle screw fixation and posterolateral fusion

after decompression in spondylolytic spondylolisthesis. *Spine* 22(2): 210–219.

86. Thomas JC, Haye W, Wiltse LL, et al. (1988): Review of deep wound infection complicating pedicle screw fixation of the lumbar spine. *Proc Int Soc Study Lumbar Spine.*

87. Urban JP, Holm S, Maroudas A, et al. (1982): Nutrition of the intervertebral disc: effect of fluid flow on solute transport. *Clin Orthop* 170: 296.

88. Wenger D, Miller S, Wilkerson J (1981): Evaluation of fixation sites for segmental instrumentation of the human vertebra (Abstract). *Proc Scoliosis Res Soc.*

89. Xu R, Ebraheim NA, Yeasting RA, et al. (1995): Morphometric evaluation of the first sacral vertebra and the projection of its pedicle on the posterior aspect of the sacrum. *Spine* 20(8):936–940.

90. Zielke K, Strempel AV (1986): Posterior lateral distraction spondylodesis using the twofold sacral bar. *Clin Orthop* 203:151–158.

91. Zindrick MR, Knight GW, Carnevale T, et al. (1992): Pedicle morphology of the immature spine (Abstract). *Proc Assoc Bone Jt Surg* 44: 53.

92. Zindrick MR, Knight GW, Carnevale T, et al. (1992): Pedicle morphology of the immature spine (Abstract). *Proc Scoliosis Res Soc* 26.

93. Zindrick MR, Wiltse LL, Doornik A, et al. (1987): Analysis of the morphometric characteristics of the thoracic and lumbar pedicles. *Spine* 12:160–166.

94. Zindrick MR, Wiltse LL, Widell EH, et al. (1986): A biomechanical study of intrapeduncular screw fixation in the lumbosacral spine. *Clin Orthop* 203:99–112.

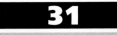

THEORIES AND MECHANISMS
OF ANTERIOR DEROTATIONAL
SPINAL SYSTEMS

THOMAS G. LOWE

Scoliosis represents both a coronal and a sagittal plane deformity with torsion. The goals of treatment with any instrumentation system should be directed at correction of all three components of the deformity, balancing the spine over the pelvis, and providing adequate long-term stability to promote an arthrodesis of the instrumented segments of the spine. The last and equally important goal of treatment is to preserve as many motion segments as possible, thereby minimizing the risk for back pain later in life related to degenerative disc disease (10). Anterior derotation instrumentation systems have been shown to provide coronal correction similar to posterior systems, better sagittal control and rotational correction than posterior systems, and usually, a reduced number of instrumented segments than posterior instrumentation systems. The success rate of fusion is equal to that of posterior instrumentation systems.

There have been a number of reported complications related to the present generation of posterior multisegmented hook systems (20). Associated hypokyphosis of the thoracic spine has proved difficult to correct with all of the available posterior instrumentation systems, primarily related to biomechanical limitations of posterior instrumentation (2). Thoracolumbar kyphosis and coronal decompensation of the uninstrumented curve have both been frequent complications of posterior instrumentation systems (20), primarily related to lack of anterior column support and the derotation maneuver, respectively (2–4). Likewise, better correction of rotation can be achieved because corrective forces are applied directly to each vertebral body, the part of the spine that is the most rotated. Crankshaft phenomenon can develop in skeletally immature patients (Risser 0, open triradiate cartilage) who undergo posterior instrumentation and fusion for scoliosis. Also, in slender patients, prominent posterior instrumentation is not an uncommon sequela after posterior surgery for scoliosis (2,7). Anterior instrumentation and fusion for scoliosis avoids the extensive paraspinous muscle dissection associated with the use of posterior instrumentation systems, which appears to significantly affect postoperative rehabilitation.

Finally, from a biomechanical standpoint, an anterior fusion is loaded in compression, which biologically favors a successful arthrodesis.

HISTORICAL REVIEW OF ANTERIOR DEROTATION SYSTEMS FOR SCOLIOSIS

Dwyer and Schafer (1974) developed the first anterior system designed for the treatment of scoliosis (8). The system was designed for lumbar and thoracolumbar curves and consisted of a cable and screw design. This system provided only compression but gave excellent coronal correction. It proved to be very kyphogenic because there was no mechanism for dealing with the sagittal (or rotational) component of the deformity, and breakage was common because of its unconstrained cable and screw design (19,22). Pseudarthrosis was a common sequela (22).

In the late 1970s, Zielke and colleagues reported on the use of an anterior instrumentation system (VDS) that consisted of a 3.2-mm threaded rod-screw design (29). These investigators emphasized the need for a derotational maneuver, which was incorporated into this system. Zielke began applying its use to thoracic as well as lumbar and thoracolumbar curves as long as the curve was flexible (12). Several investigators have reported good results with this system (22–26). Zielke demonstrated that frequently one or more distal levels could be saved with this system and that associated hypokyphosis of the thoracic spine could be improved. Use of the system demonstrated less instrumentation kyphosis in the thoracolumbar and lumbar spine because of the use of the "derotator," but maintenance of lordosis was difficult because of the flexible rod, and rod breakage was common (6). This system is still being used frequently for thoracolumbar and lumbar curves. The use of anterior structural support in the lumbar spine has decreased the incidence of rod breakage greatly with Zielke instrumentation.

In the late 1980s, Harms improved on the Zielke system by providing a stronger threaded rod system with a better locking mechanism for the screw (Moss system) (2,16). He emphasized the importance of avoiding a derotational maneuver in the thoracic spine and further promoted the treatment of thoracic curves by anterior instrumentation, relying entirely on compression for

T. G. Lowe: Woodridge Orthopaedic and Spine Center, P.C., Wheat Ridge, CO 80033.

coronal correction and correction of hypokyphosis. In 1992, a multicenter anterior spine study group was organized to analyze prospectively the results of anterior instrumentation compared with posterior instrumentation for thoracic adolescent idiopathic scoliosis (2). Results have confirmed that anterior instrumentation is comparable to posterior instrumentation as far as coronal correction is concerned but that anterior instrumentation is superior to posterior instrumentation for the correction of hypokyphosis. Results also indicated that thoracic curves could be fused shorter when anterior instrumentation was used. A 4% pseudarthrosis rate was noted, which was similar to that reported with posterior systems. There were also some negative results gleaned from the study. There was a high rod breakage rate (11.5%), and hyperkyphosis was noted to occur in patients with a normal preoperative kyphosis related to the flexible rod and inability to provide structural grafting in the thoracic spine.

Because of these complications, semirigid, smooth rods (4 and 5 mm) have been developed for thoracic curves. Early results have demonstrated a marked reduction in rod breakage as well as thoracic hyperkyphosis. Obviously, longer follow-up will be necessary to document the success of these implant modifications.

Turi and colleagues in 1993 were the first to report on the use of smooth, rigid (6 and 7 mm TSRH) anterior instrumentation for thoracolumbar and lumbar adolescent idiopathic scoliosis (28). Curve correction is based on precontouring the rod to the sagittal contour of the segments to be instrumented. After the rod is inserted, it is rotated to the sagittal plane, and compression is applied. This methodology of anterior scoliosis correction was a major step in the use of anterior implants for correction of thoracolumbar and lumbar curves. Several other smooth, rigid rod systems using this technique of curve reduction have emerged and are discussed in subsequent chapters. Because of some loss of sagittal contour secondary to lack of interbody support, the use of structural grafts or cages with these rigid systems has resulted in even better maintenance of sagittal profile (2,16).

In 1991, Kaneda published some early results with his double-rod system, which provides segmental vertebral body purchase by means of a two screws and a plate at each level (17). Curve correction is achieved by rod rotation followed by compression. Structural grafting is used to maintain the physiologic sagittal profile. The Kaneda system is the most rigid of the systems available.

Thus, from the rather unsophisticated screw-cable concept devised by Dwyer has evolved several biomechanically sound methods of dealing with single adolescent idiopathic scoliosis curves of the thoracic, thoracolumbar, and lumbar spine.

SEGMENTAL SAGITTAL PLANE CONSIDERATIONS

Because anterior derotational spine systems are all potentially kyphogenic and because the correction of adolescent idiopathic scoliosis curves by anterior instrumentation involves conversion of the coronal plane deformity into a physiologic sagittal profile by rod rotation maneuvers and interbody structural grafting, a

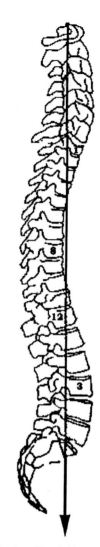

FIGURE 1. Normal sagittal profile of spine. Lumbar lordosis is normally 30 degrees greater than thoracic kyphosis. The transitional zone (T10 to L2) is normally slightly lordotic or "neutral," and the sagittal vertical axis passes through the body of T1 and is within 1 cm of the sacral promontory.

brief description of the normal sagittal profile of the spine is included. Figure 1 depicts the normal sagittal contour of the spine. The thoracic and lumbar spines are "balanced" when the "plumb line" from the center of the vertebral body of T1 passes within 1 cm of the sacral promontory on a 36-inch standing lateral radiograph of the spine. The arms should be elevated no more than 45 degrees above the vertical to preserve the normal sagittal contour and balance of the spine.

The normal thoracic kyphotic curve from T1 to T12 should measure between 20 and 45 degrees. The normal lumbar lordotic sagittal curve between L1 and S1 is normally 20 to 30 degrees larger than the thoracic kyphosis and ranges between 40 and 65 degrees. The thoracolumbar junction, T10 to L2, is a transitional zone between the two curves and normally ranges between neutral and 10 degrees of lordosis. T8 constitutes the apex of the thoracic kyphosis and should be horizontally oriented. L3 constitutes the apex of the lumbar lordosis and should also be horizontally oriented. These ranges of measurements constitute the normal physiologic sagittal profile of the adolescent spine (1). Maintaining or restoring physiologic sagittal curves and balance is equal in importance to establishing coronal curve correction and balance when using anterior derotational instrumentation systems. Restoration of a physiologic sagittal profile provides the best opportunity for minimizing low back pain in later adult life secondary to degenerative disc disease in the uninstrumented segments.

INDICATIONS FOR ANTERIOR DEROTATIONAL SYSTEMS FOR ADOLESCENT IDIOPATHIC SCOLIOSIS

Thoracolumbar and Lumbar Curves

Most adolescent idiopathic thoracolumbar (King IV) and lumbar (King I) curves are well suited for anterior instrumentation and fusion (22,27). Usually, one or more distal levels can be saved when compared with posterior instrumentation systems (15). Curves greater than 75 degrees, especially if very structural, would be better managed by a combined anterior and posterior approach with posterior instrumentation. Curves with a lower end vertebra, below L4, are not candidates for anterior instrumentation systems because of anatomic difficulties, such as iliac crest, iliac vessels, and so forth. If there is a thoracic hyperkyphosis or a structural thoracic curve that requires surgical treatment, anterior instrumentation and fusion is contraindicated.

When anterior derotational systems are used in the thoracolumbar or lumbar spine, structural interbody support should always be provided. Figure 2 illustrates the ability to save a distal level and the use of anterior structural support in King IV curves.

Thoracic Curves

The most suitable thoracic curves for anterior instrumentation and fusion are those associated with hypokyphosis (2,16). Usually, several proximal and distal levels can be saved when compared with posterior instrumentation systems. Because of the inability to use structural grafts or cages above T10 related to small discs and limited mobility, anterior instrumentation systems are "kyphogenic." The systems using smaller, flexible rods create more kyphosis than do the larger, more rigid rod systems. Thoracic curves with a normal kyphosis are best managed with the larger rod systems, which, when contoured carefully, preserve the sagittal profile of the thoracic spine. Thoracic curves associated with hyperkyphosis should always be managed with posterior instrumentation systems.

In double major curves (King II), when the lumbar curve is less than 40 degrees and corrects beyond 20 degrees on side bending, a selective thoracic fusion can be considered a good option, avoiding a long fusion of both curves (18). In that situation, it is important to leave a small residual curve in the instrumented segments to accommodate the uninstrumented lumbar curve. Figure 3 illustrates the principle of selective thoracic curve instrumentation and fusion in a King II curve pattern. Likewise,

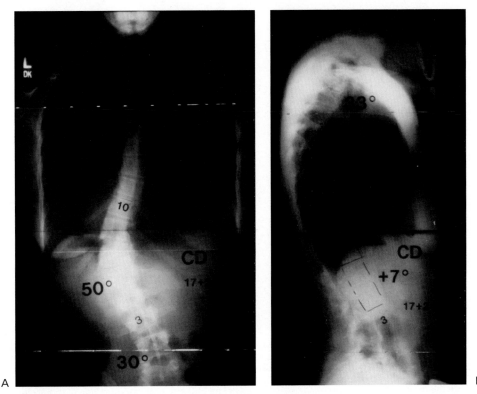

FIGURE 2. A and B: Preoperative radiographs of a girl aged 13 years, 9 months with a progressive thoracolumbar (King IV) scoliosis despite brace treatment. The patient had a Cobb angle of 50 degrees, a normal sagittal profile, and thoracolumbar kyphosis. *(Figure continues.)*

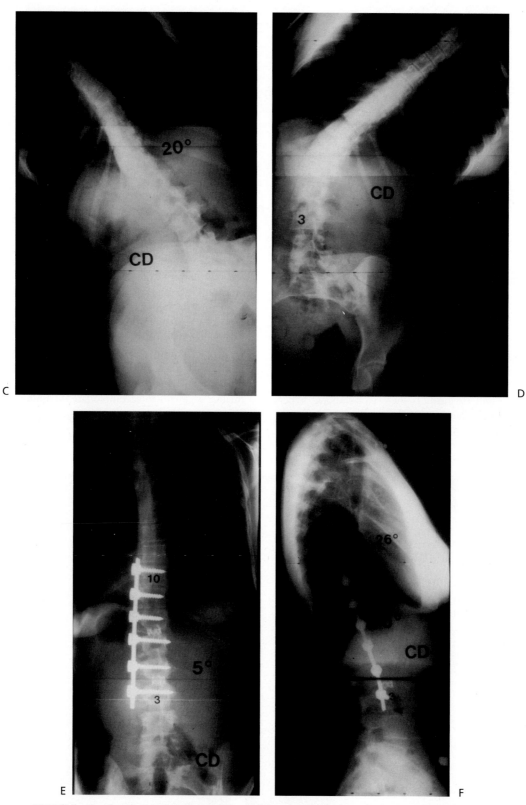

FIGURE 2. *Continued.* **C and D:** Preoperative radiographs of a girl aged 13 years 9 months with a progressive thoracolumbar (King IV) scoliosis despite brace treatment. The patient had a Cobb angle of 50 degrees, a normal sagittal profile, and thoracolumbar kyphosis. **E and F:** Postoperative radiographs of the same patient 1 year after anterior fusion and instrumentation of levels within the Cobb angle. Note the structural support (mesh cages) at all levels below T12. Also note the correction of thoracolumbar kyphosis and the coronal deformity.

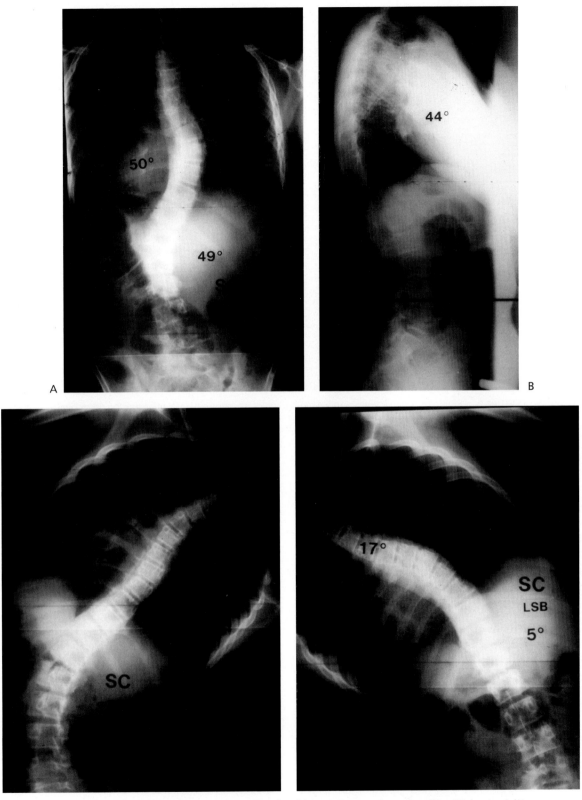

FIGURE 3. A to D: Preoperative radiographs of a girl aged 12 years, 9 months with a 50-degree right thoracic and 49-degree lumbar scoliosis. Note the normal sagittal profile of the thoracic spine and flexibility of the lumbar curve. *(Figure continues.)*

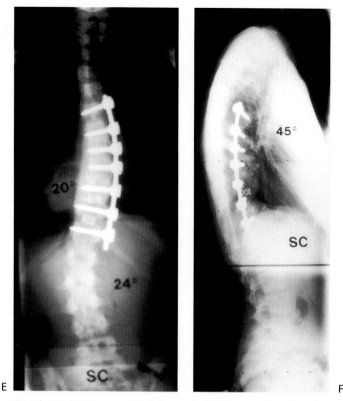

FIGURE 3. *Continued.* **E and F:** Postoperative radiograph of the same patient demonstrating correction of the thoracic curve to 20 degrees with spontaneous correction of the lumbar curve to 24 degrees. Note that no increase in thoracic kyphosis occurred because of structural grafting at the thoracolumbar junction and use of a rigid rod system.

in double thoracic curves in which the upper thoracic curve is less than 40 degrees and corrects to 20 degrees or less on the bending anteroposterior radiograph and the shoulder tilt is less than 10 degrees, a selective anterior instrumented fusion of the primary thoracic curve is a good option. Again, a small residual curve in the instrumented segments should be left to accommodate the uninstrumented curve to avoid increased shoulder tilt. If hyperkyphosis is present in either of the thoracic curves, anterior instrumentation and fusion are contraindicated. Thoracic curves greater than 75 degrees are best managed by posterior instrumentation systems (21). Obviously, a patient who would not tolerate a thoracotomy for any reason should not be considered for anterior instrumentation and fusion.

DETERMINATION OF INSTRUMENTATION LEVELS

Thoracolumbar and Lumbar Curves

Two methods of determining instrumentation levels for thoracolumbar and lumbar curves have evolved, and each method has been used successfully.

The most commonly used method is to include all levels within the Cobb end vertebrae on the erect posteroanterior radiograph (22–25). The end vertebrae are the most angled verte-

brae of the curve, as shown in Figure 4A. When using this method, the distal end vertebra should be horizontal on the reverse side-bending anteroposterior radiograph. If it is not horizontal, the instrumentation should be extended distally to the first level that is horizontal.

Another method that is commonly used for flexible thoracolumbar or lumbar curves is called the *short-segment method,* which was developed by John Hall (13,14). Levels to be instrumented are determined by the erect posteroanterior radiograph. First, the most horizontal element at the apex of the curve is noted. If this is a disc, it is necessary to instrument two vertebrae above and below the apical disc, giving a three-disc, four–vertebral body fusion area. If the most horizontal element is a vertebral body, it is necessary to instrument one vertebral body above and below the apical body, resulting in a two-disc, three–vertebral body fusion area, as shown in Figure 4B. Rotation does not appear to be a factor in selection of levels to be fused.

Thoracic Curves

The determination of fusion levels in the thoracic spine is based on measurements from the erect posteroanterior and side-bending radiographs. All of the levels within the Cobb angle are included, as shown in Figure 4A. In addition, if the end plates of the next distal vertebra, either proximally or distally, are parallel, and there is less than 10 degrees of motion between those end

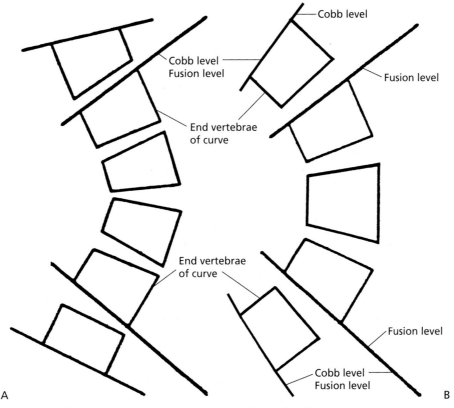

FIGURE 4. A: The end vertebrae of the Cobb angle are the standard fusion levels for thoracic, thoracolumbar, or lumbar curves. **B:** The short-segment (Hall) method of anterior fusion levels for thoracolumbar curves. Note that the apex is vertebra T7. The fusion levels would be T6 to T8 even though the Cobb angle levels are T5 to T9.

plates on the side-bending radiographs, the fusion level should include that next vertebra. In addition, if there is a junctional kyphosis greater than 10 degrees distally, that level should be included as well as provided with interbody support. A junctional kyphosis above the curve would necessitate a posterior instrumented fusion. Again, rotation does not appear to affect fusion level selection.

BIOMECHANICAL CONSIDERATIONS

The more flexible rod or cable and screw systems are primarily compression systems and have little potential for correction of torsion (13,22,23,25,28). Coronal correction is based on the flexibility achieved by the discectomies. They are extremely kyphogenic by themselves, which can be used to advantage in the thoracic spine when hypokyphosis is present, as shown in Figure 5. In the thoracolumbar and lumbar spine, structural interbody support should always be provided to maintain the sagittal contour and provide sharing to avoid excessive rod breakage and pseudarthrosis. Figure 6 demonstrates the use of a flexible rod system in the thoracolumbar spine. The newer larger diameter smooth rod-screw systems, such as Moss-Miami, C-D Horizon, Isola, and TSRH, all use several forces for scoliosis correction, including cantilever bending, rod rotation, and compression

(2,27). First, the rod is prebent into the physiologic sagittal contour of the segments to be instrumented. Next, the rod is inserted into the screws at one end of the curve and delivered into the screws at the opposite end by cantilever bending. The rod is then rotated into the sagittal profile of the instrumented segments, and finally, compression is applied to the apex of the curve, completing the correction maneuvers. Figures 7 and 8 demonstrate the correction of scoliosis in the thoracic and thoracolumbar spine using a rigid rod system. These systems are more successful in controlling torsion than the posterior multisegmental systems because of the anterior release provided by the discectomies and segmental purchase of screws in the vertebral body, the most rotated element of the spine. These systems are less kyphogenic because of their stiffness and rotational capability. In the thoracolumbar and lumbar spine, interbody structural support should always be provided, as with the more flexible rod-screw systems. The Kaneda double-rod system is the most rigid of all the systems available (17).

All these systems have staples for the screws that increase purchase strength when screws are placed centrally in the vertebral body. Screws must always be bicortical to achieve adequate bone purchase. It is important not to apply excessive compression between screws because this may result in some plowing of the screw in the vertebral body, weakening fixation of the spine.

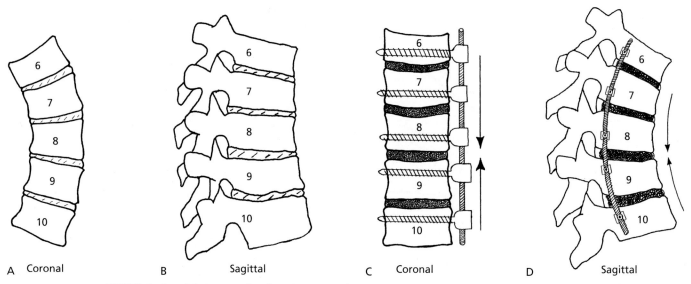

A   Coronal   B   Sagittal   C   Coronal   D   Sagittal

FIGURE 5. A and B: Preoperative thoracic curve and sagittal contour. **C and D:** Postoperative curve correction using flexible rod system and morselized bone graft. Correction is by compression only. Note the increased thoracic kyphosis after instrumentation, which is unavoidable with flexible rod systems.

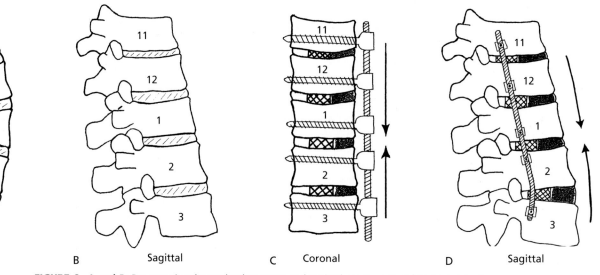

A   Coronal   B   Sagittal   C   Coronal   D   Sagittal

FIGURE 6. A and B: Preoperative thoracolumbar curve and sagittal contour. **C and D:** Postoperative curve correction using flexible rod system and structural grafts to preserve lordosis. Correction was by compression only, but structural grafts maintain lordosis.

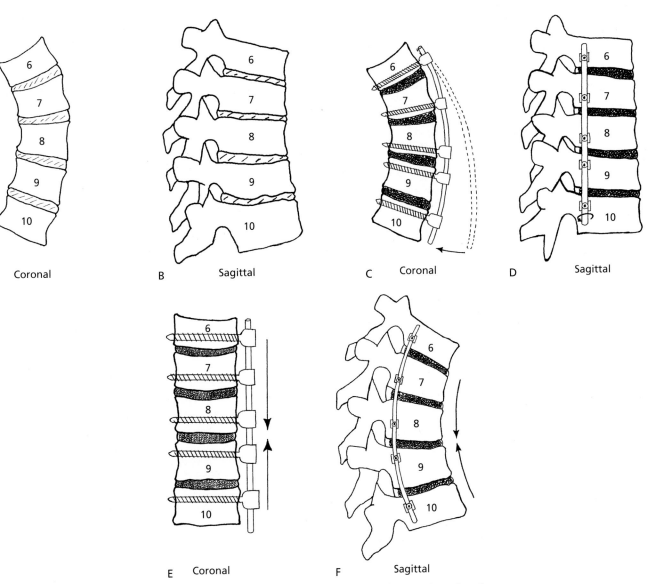

A   Coronal

B   Sagittal

C   Coronal

D   Sagittal

E   Coronal

F   Sagittal

FIGURE 7. A and B: Preoperative thoracic curve and sagittal contour. **C and D:** After discectomy, morselized graft is packed between the vertebral bodies. Initial correction is achieved with a rigid rod system by contouring the rod to the sagittal profile of the spine. The rod is attached to screws proximally and delivered to lower screws by cantilever bending. **E and F:** The rod is rotated to the sagittal plane (kyphosis), and segmental compression is then applied, completing the corrective maneuvers.

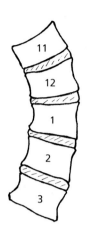

A   Coronal

B   Sagittal

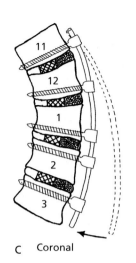

C   Coronal

D   Sagittal

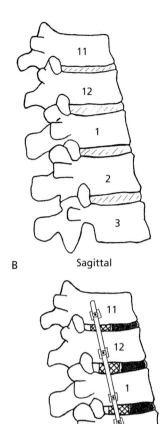

E   Coronal

F   Sagittal

FIGURE 8. A and B: Preoperative thoracolumbar curve and sagittal contour. **C and D:** After discectomy, structural support is achieved, and morselized graft is inserted between vertebral bodies to maintain the normal sagittal contour. A rigid rod is contoured to the sagittal profile. The rod is then attached to proximal screws and delivered to lower screws by cantilever bending. **E and F:** The rod is rotated to the sagittal contour of spine (lordosis), and segmental compression is applied to the construct as a final step.

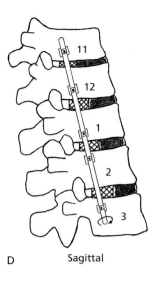

TECHNICAL CONSIDERATIONS

Interbody Fusion

In the thoracic spine (above T10), the discs are small and relatively immobile. In rigid, large-magnitude curves, it is helpful to remove first the rib head, which overlies the posterior quarter of the disc. After the rib head is removed and the posterior disc and annulus are removed, an appreciable amount of mobility is obtained. In curves of less than 60 degrees, which are flexible on the side-bending radiographs, it is usually not necessary to remove the rib heads to remove the posterior portion of the disc and annulus. Lamina spreaders are essential to clean out the disc space thoroughly. Above T10, morselized rib graft is tightly packed into each disc space.

In the thoracolumbar and lumbar spine, after discectomies are complete, it is important to insert either titanium mesh cages or structural allografts to provide anterior column support. Without structural grafting, kyphosis inevitably develops within instrumented segments. Along with the structural support, morselized autograft is packed tightly into each interbody space.

Screw Placement

Screws should always have bicortical purchase. They are usually placed horizontally in the midbody position with a staple and

should be angled slightly anteriorly to avoid the neural canal. Either the surgeon or an assistant should place his or her index finger around the front of the spine to the opposite side of the vertebral body to help determine the exact trajectory of the screw. Screws can also be placed adjacent to the end plate without a staple and without loss of bone purchase. When using the "juxta" end plate position, the screw should be placed adjacent to the inferior end plate above the apex of the curve and adjacent to the superior end plate below the apex for maximal strength. This technique allows for preservation of the segmental vessels.

Rod Contouring

When the small, flexible, threaded rods are used (e.g., Zielke and Moss instrumentation), no contouring is needed. The rod is merely pushed into the screws, and compression is applied.

When the larger, smooth rods are used, proper contouring is important because the rod will hold the spine in the profile of the contoured rod after it has been inserted and rotated into the sagittal plane. For most flexible curves, the rod is contoured to match the physiologic sagittal profile of the spine over the segments to be instrumented. No in situ bending should be done after the construct has been completed because of the likelihood of screw pullout or loosening.

In large-magnitude, rigid curves, a residual curve should be left in the rod based on the side-bending anteroposterior radiographs. Likewise, in patients with double structural curves (King II and V), in whom a selective single curve fusion is being considered, a residual curve should be left in the rod to accommodate the structural portion of the uninstrumented curve; otherwise, coronal decompensation of the spine will occur.

Need for Thoracoplasty

Most adolescent idiopathic scoliosis thoracic curves with angular rib prominences should be considered for thoracoplasty unless preoperative pulmonary function studies indicate significant restrictive lung disease (4). It is usually necessary to remove portions of the periapical four or five ribs of the thoracic curve. The transthoracic operative approach lends itself nicely to internal thoracoplasty. If the rib heads are going to be removed to facilitate exposure of the posterior disc, the rib head and an additional 2 cm of rib are removed. If the rib heads are not going to be removed, a 2- to 3-cm section is removed lateral to the rib head. Gelfoam strips are placed in the resected rib beds, and the pleura is closed. A chest tube is always required after internal thoracoplasty.

SELECTION OF FLEXIBLE VERSUS STIFF ROD SYSTEMS

Flexible Rod Systems

The major advantage of the flexible rod anterior systems is ease of insertion. No contouring of the 3.2-mm rod and little of

the 4-mm rod system is needed. The major disadvantage is the difficulty in maintaining the physiologic sagittal profile in the thoracic spine in patients with a normal kyphosis as demonstrated in Figure 9. In the thoracolumbar and lumbar spine, structural support can be used, but in the thoracic spine, only morselized autograft can be used, which when combined with a flexible rod, always results in some degree of increased kyphosis.

The primary indication for the use of the flexible rod systems would be a stiff, high-magnitude thoracic curve with associated hypokyphosis, as demonstrated in Figure 10, or a thoracic curve in a very small patient. These systems can also be used in the thoracolumbar or lumbar spine with structural interbody support, but patients should be braced for 3 months after surgery with a thoracolumbar standing orthosis (TLSO) brace because of increased risk for rod breakage.

Rigid Rod Systems

For thoracic curves, the larger rod anterior systems have the advantage of providing better control of the sagittal profile and are less kyphogenic. Figure 11 demonstrates the use of a rigid rod system for a thoracic curve. The disadvantage is that they are less forgiving; hence, contouring must be precise, and the rod rotation maneuver may exert large torsional forces at the bone-screw interface, especially in very structural curves. The larger rod systems should be used primarily for flexible thoracic curves with a normal sagittal profile or hypokyphosis.

The larger rod anterior systems should be used for most thoracolumbar and lumbar curves for better control of the sagittal

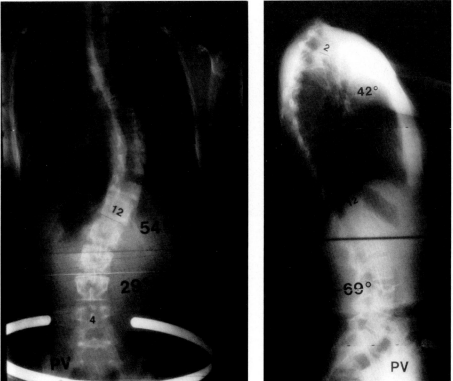

FIGURE 9. A and B: Preoperative radiographs of a girl aged 13 years, 6 months with a 54-degree thoracic curve and thoracic kyphosis of 42 degrees. *(Figure continues.)*

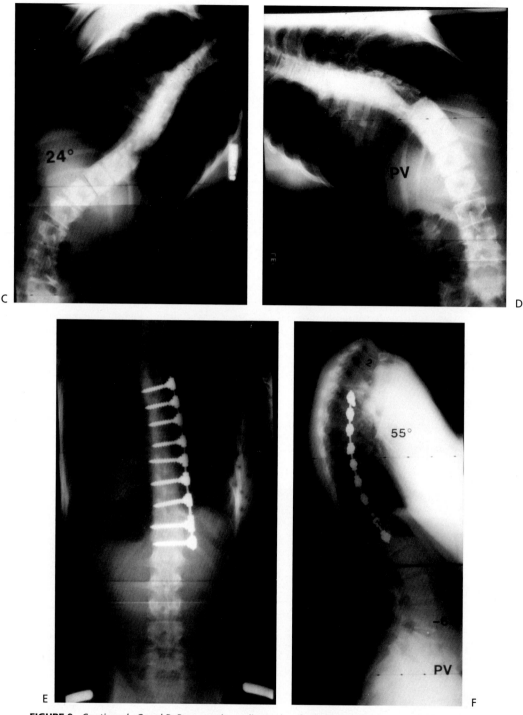

FIGURE 9. *Continued.* *C and D:* Preoperative radiographs of a girl aged 13 years, 6 months with a 54-degree thoracic curve and thoracic kyphosis of 42 degrees. **E and F:** Postoperative radiographs of the same patient after anterior fusion with flexible rod instrumented from T4 to T12. Morselized rib graft was packed at each level; however, hyperkyphosis of 55 degrees developed. The use of a rigid rod system probably would have prevented the hyperkyphosis.

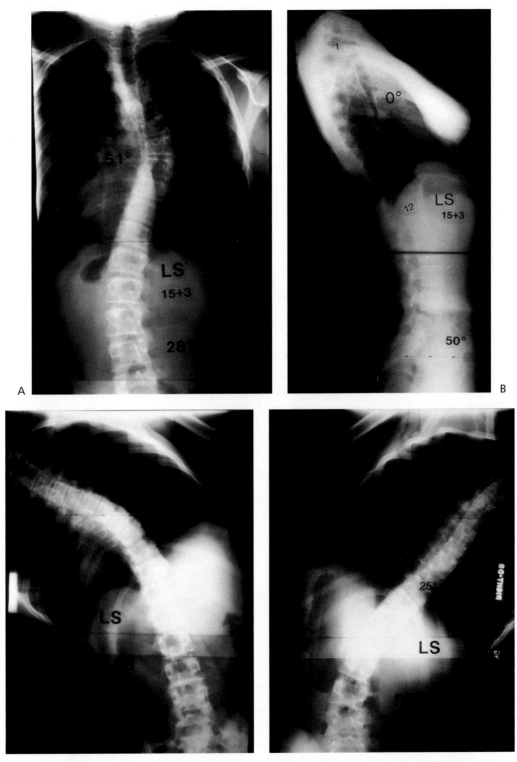

FIGURE 10. A to D: Preoperative standing posteroanterior and lateral radiographs of a girl aged 15 years, 3 months with a progressive right thoracic scoliosis associated with hypokyphosis. *(Figure continues.)*

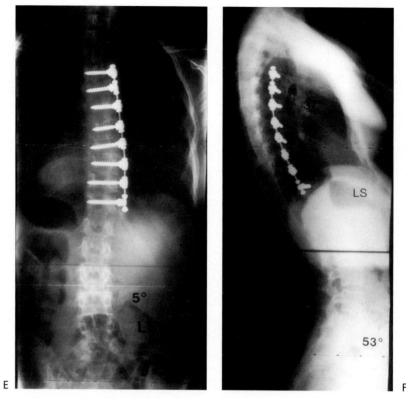

FIGURE 10. *Continued.* **E and F:** Postoperative radiographs of the same patient 1 year after anterior fusion and instrumentation from T5 to T12 within the Cobb angle, with correction of scoliosis as well as hypokyphosis.

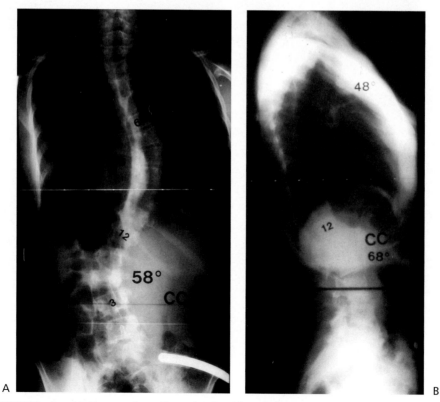

FIGURE 11. **A and B:** Preoperative radiographs of a girl aged 14 years, 2 months with a double major King II curve pattern. Note flexibility of the lumbar curve. *(Figure continues.)*

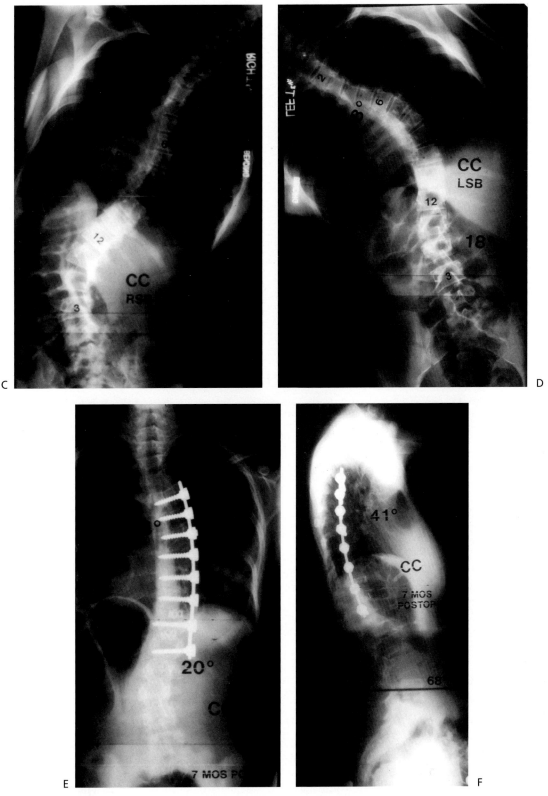

FIGURE 11. **C and D:** Preoperative radiographs of a girl aged 14 years, 2 months with a double major King II curve pattern. Note flexibility of the lumbar curve. **E and F:** A selective anterior fusion of only the thoracic curve was done with resultant spontaneous correction of the lumbar curve over the following 15 months. No increase in thoracic kyphosis occurred because of rigid rod and anterior column support at the thoracolumbar junction. Residual curve was left in the instrumentation to accommodate the uninstrumented curve and to avoid decompensation. *(Figure continues.)*

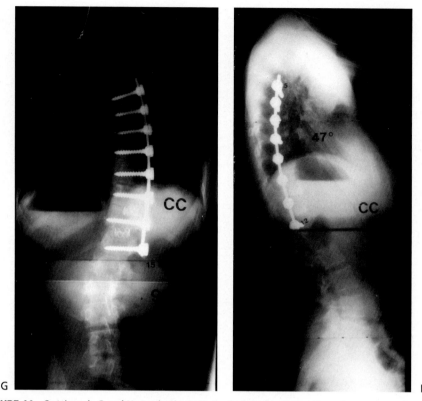

FIGURE 11. *Continued.* **G and H:** A selective anterior fusion of only the thoracic curve was done with resultant spontaneous correction of the lumbar curve over the following 15 months. No increase in thoracic kyphosis occurred because of rigid rod and anterior column support at the thoracolumbar junction. Residual curve was left in the instrumentation to accommodate the uninstrumented curve and to avoid decompensation.

profile and to decrease the risk for breakage. Structural interbody support should always be provided. In the thoracic spine, these systems are ideally suited for flexible curves associated with either normal or hypokyphosis. Because of their larger diameter, they are better able to control the sagittal contour of the thoracic spine even though true structural support is not provided. If they are used for stiff curves, only a minimal rotational maneuver should be performed because of the likelihood of screw pullout or loosening.

COMPLICATIONS RELATED TO ANTERIOR SPINAL SYSTEMS FOR SCOLIOSIS

Inadequate Exposure

The patient should always be placed in a straight lateral position preoperatively to ensure that appropriate exposure is obtained. In thoracic curves in which the upper level to be instrumented is above T10, an endotracheal tube (Uni-Vent), which allows collapse of the ipsilateral lung, should be used during the procedure. The level of the thoracotomy is determined by the upper level to be instrumented. If more than six levels are to be instrumented, a double thoracotomy is usually required, but this can always be performed through a single thoracotomy incision. Options include rib removal or working between ribs, which is

somewhat more difficult but preserves the contour of the chest wall (2).

Screw Loosening and Pullout

All screws should be bicortical to avoid pullout. Screws that do not adequately purchase the opposite cortex lose about 40% of their pullout strength, which almost always results in loss of fixation, especially at the upper levels where pullout forces are the greatest. Screw loosening can also occur during the cantilever maneuver, rod rotation, or final compression. Excessive force should be avoided when performing these maneuvers.

Hyperkyphosis

All the anterior derotation systems are kyphogenic. The smaller threaded-rod systems are more kyphogenic than the larger-diameter rod systems. It is important to use structural grafts or cages in the thoracolumbar and lumbar spines to prevent loss of lordosis. Figure 12 illustrates postoperative loss of lumbar lordosis because anterior structural support was not provided; this case required revision surgery. When anterior instrumentation systems are being used for thoracic curves, some increase in thoracic kyphosis is likely to occur related to the fact that structural interbody grafts or cages usually cannot be used because of the small disc

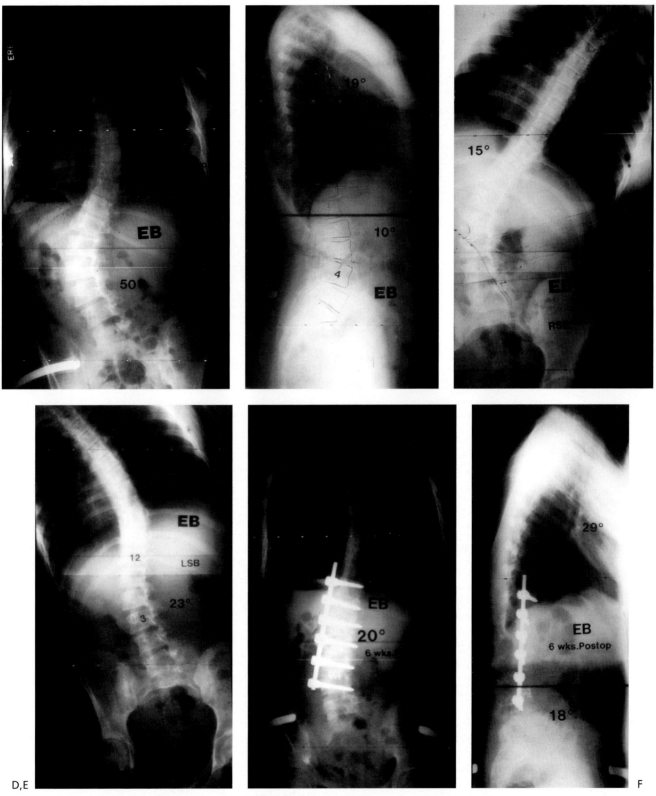

A,B

C

D,E

F

FIGURE 12. A to D: Preoperative radiographs of girl aged 15 years, 6 months with a progressive left thoracolumbar (King II) curve of 50 degrees. Note the normal sagittal profile preoperatively. **E and F:** Postoperative radiographs of the same patient taken 6 weeks after surgery show marked loss of lumbar lordosis despite rigid rod fixation because structural support was provided only at L3 to L4. *(Figure continues.)*

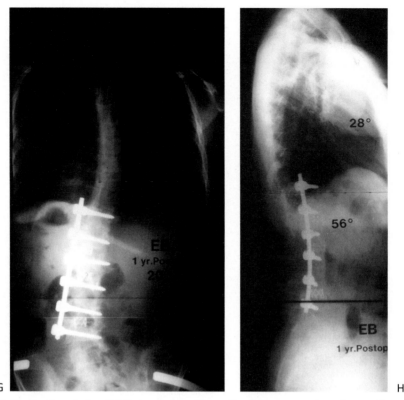

FIGURE 12. *Continued.* **G and H:** Postoperative radiographs of the same patient after revision surgery with insertion of structural support and reinstrumentation at all levels with restoration of normal sagittal profile.

spaces. The increase in kyphosis can be minimized by tightly packing disc spaces and using the more rigid systems (2,16).

Decompensation of Uninstrumented Curve

Uninstrumented curve decompensation may occur in two ways. The first cause of decompensation is failure to select the appropriate levels to be instrumented. When either fusing too long or too short, decompensation in the coronal plane almost always occurs. The levels to be instrumented should include all levels between the upper and lower Cobb levels. A level should be added distally if the lower Cobb vertebra and the vertebra below it have parallel end plates and there is less than 10 degrees motion between the two vertebrae on side-bending anteroposterior radiographs.

The second cause of decompensation is overcorrection of the primary curve when there is more than one structural curve (King II and V). If not enough residual curve is left in the instrumented curve to accommodate the structural component of the uninstrumented curve, decompensation usually results.

Pulmonary

On occasion, adolescent patients undergoing thoracotomy and thoracoplasty develop postoperative pulmonary complications, including atelectasis, pneumonitis, and pneumothorax. In the

near future, many of these curves will be approached thoracoscopically, which should lower the incidence of these complications. The use of an incentive spirometer at the bedside and in the early postoperative period has been helpful. A group of 40 adolescent patients are being followed with preoperative and postoperative pulmonary function tests, and although an initial decrease in pulmonary function occurs, it appears to return to its preoperative level by the 2-year follow-up (11).

Pseudarthrosis

Although rod breakage was noted to occur with a high incidence (10.5%), pseudarthrosis has not been more frequent with the posterior multisegmented hook systems (4%) (2,16). Theoretically, the incidence of pseudarthrosis should be low because the fusion is loaded in compression and the interbody space has an excellent blood supply. Longer follow-up studies are needed to evaluate the true incidence of pseudarthrosis.

Neurologic

No neurologic complications related to the use of anterior derotational spinal systems have been reported in the peer-reviewed literature thus far. Anterior instrumentation avoids distractive forces known to be associated with neurologic complications. Most of these systems are in their infancy, with relatively small numbers of cases spread out over several centers. Only as more data is collected over time will the true incidence of neurologic complications be defined.

SUMMARY

The anterior derotational spinal systems for adolescent idiopathic scoliosis appear to be equal to the posterior systems as far as coronal correction is concerned; however, correction in both the sagittal and horizontal planes appears to be superior. Furthermore, one or more distal segments can usually be saved when compared with fusion levels instrumented posteriorly, which allows for greater flexibility and a lessened incidence of low back pain related to degenerative disc disease. When only a single curve requires surgical management in the adolescent idiopathic scoliosis patient, anterior instrumentation and fusion provide a reasonable alternative to the more conventional posterior instrumentation systems. Certainly, anterior instrumentation systems are widely accepted for thoracolumbar and lumbar curves. The only major disadvantages of anterior instrumentation systems is that they can be used only for correction of a single curve, and they cannot be used for thoracic curves if there is an associated hyperkyphosis. Longer follow-up results are needed before the definitive role of anterior instrumentation for thoracic curves can be established.

REFERENCES

1. Bernhardt M, Bridwell K (1989): Segmental analysis of the sagittal plane alignment of the normal thoracic and lumbar spine and the thoracolumbar junction. *Spine* 14:17.
2. Betz R, Harms J, Clements D III, et al. (1999): Comparison of anterior and posterior instrumentation for correction of adolescent thoracic idiopathic scoliosis. *Spine* 24(3) 225.
3. Bridwell KH, McAllister JW, Betz RR, et al. (1991): Coronal decompensation produced by Cotrel-Dubousset "derotation" maneuver for idiopathic right thoracic scoliosis. *Spine* 16:769–777.
4. Bridwell KH (1994): Surgical treatment of adolescent idiopathic scoliosis: the basics and the controversies. *Spine* 19:1095.
5. Chapman M, Bridwell KH, Lenke LG, et al. (1995): *Assignment of risk factors for transition syndrome: an analysis of patients who have broken down above or below a solid fusion.* Presented at the 30th annual meeting of the Scoliosis Research Society, Asheville, NC, September 13–17, 1995.
6. Chapman MP, Hamill CL, Bridwell KH (1996): *Can we lordose the spine with Zielke instrumentation anteriorly?* Exhibit at the 31st annual meeting of the Scoliosis Research Society, Ottawa, Ontario, Canada, September 25–28, 1996.
7. Dubousset J, Herring JA, Shufflebarger HL (1989): The crankshaft phenomenon. *J Pediatr Orthop* 9(5):541.
8. Dwyer AF, Schafer MF (1974): Anterior approach to scoliosis: results of treatment in fifty-one cases. *J Bone Joint Surg Br* 56:218–224.
9. Ecker ML, Betz RR, Trent PS (1989): Computer tomography evalua-

10. Ginsburg HH, Goldstein L, Haake PW: *Longitudinal study of back pain in postoperative idiopathic scoliosis: long-term follow-up.* Presented at the 30th annual meeting of the Scoliosis Research Society, Asheville, NC, September 13–17, 1995.
11. Graham E, Lenke L, Lowe T, et al. (1999): *Prospective pulmonary function evaluation following open thoracotomy for anterior thoracic spinal fusion in adolescent idiopathic scoliosis.* Presented at the 34th annual meeting of the Scoliosis Research Society [oral presentation]. San Diego, CA, September 1999.
12. Grehl J, Zielke K (1997): Anterior Zielke instrumentation in thoracolumbar and lumbar curves. In: Bridwell KH, Dewald R, eds. *The textbook of spinal surgery.* Philadelphia: Lippincott-Raven, pp. 627–640.
13. Hall JE, Millis MB, Snyder BD (1997): Short segment anterior instrumentation for thoracolumbar scoliosis. In: Bridwell KH, Dewald R, eds. *The textbook of spinal surgery.* Philadelphia: Lippincott-Raven, pp. 665–674.
14. Hall JE (1981): Current concepts review: Dwyer instrumentation in anterior fusion of the spine. *J Bone Joint Surg Am* 63:1188–1190.
15. Hamill CL, Lenke LG, Bridwell KH (1996): The use of pedicle screw fixation to improve correction in the lumbar spine of patients with idiopathic scoliosis: is it warranted? *Spine* 21:1241–1249.
16. Harms J, Jeszensky D, Beele B: Ventral correction of thoracic scoliosis. In: Bridwell KH, Dewald R, eds. *The textbook of spinal surgery.* Philadelphia: Lippincott-Raven, pp. 611–626.
17. Kaneda K, Shono Y, Satoh S (1996): New anterior instrumentation for the management of thoracolumbar and lumbar scoliosis. *Spine* 21: 1250–1262.
18. King HA, Moe JH, Bradford DS, et al. (1983): The selection of fusion levels in thoracic idiopathic scoliosis. *J Bone Joint Surg Am* 65:1302.
19. Kohler R, Galland O, Mechin H (1990): The Dwyer procedure in the treatment of idiopathic scoliosis: A 10-year follow-up review of 21 patients. *Spine* 15:75–80.
20. Lenke LG, Bridwell KH, Baldus C (1992): Cotrel-Dubousset instrumentation for adolescent idiopathic scoliosis. *J Bone Joint Surg Am* 1992;74:1056–1067.
21. Lowe TG: Combined anterior-posterior surgery for scoliosis. In: Whitecloud TS III, Harms J, eds. *Anterior spinal column reconstruction.* In Press.
22. Lowe TG, Peters JD (1993): Anterior spinal fusion with Zielke instrumentation for idiopathic scoliosis: a frontal and sagittal curve analysis in 36 patients. *Spine* 18:423–426.
23. Luk KD, Leong JC, Reyes L, et al. (1989): The comparative results of treatment of idiopathic thoracolumbar and lumbar scoliosis using Harrington, Dwyer, and Zielke instrumentation. *Spine* 14:275–280.
24. Moe JH, Purcell GA, Bradford DS (1983): Zielke instrumentation (VDS) for the correction of spinal curvature. *Clin Orthop* 180: 133–153.
25. Ogiela DM, Chan DPK (1986): Ventral derotation spondylodesis: a review of 22 cases. *Spine* 11:18–22.
26. Puno RM, Johnson JR, Osterman PA, et al. (1989): Analysis of the primary and compensatory curvatures following Zielke instrumentation for idiopathic scoliosis. *Spine* 14:738–743.
27. Thompson JP, Transfeldt EE, Bradford DS, et al. (1990): Decompensation after Cotrel-Dubousset instrumentation of idiopathic scoliosis. *Spine* 15(9):927.
28. Turi M, Johnston CE II, Richards BS (1993): Anterior correction of idiopathic scoliosis using TSRH instrumentation. *Spine* 18:417–422.
29. Zielke K, Stunkat R, Beaujean F (1976): Ventral derotation spondylodesis. *Arch Orthop Unfalchi* 85:257–260.

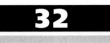

ANTERIOR INSTRUMENTATION: TECHNIQUES

RANDAL R. BETZ

THORACIC SCOLIOSIS

Indications

The advantages of using anterior instrumentation for correction of thoracic scoliosis include the potential to save two or more distal fusion levels (Figs. 1, 2) and ability to correct hypokyphosis (less than 20 degrees of kyphosis). In addition, in skeletally immature patients, anterior release and fusion may be indicated, and insertion of anterior instrumentation potentially involves less surgery than a combined anterior and posterior procedure (1).

In most cases in which two or more distal levels can be saved, the curves are classified as King II, III, or IV or as type IA,B,C or IIIC by the Lenke classification (18), where there is a risk of the patient being unbalanced after posterior instrumentation of the thoracic curve alone. The number of fusion levels to be saved needs to be predicted. The lower instrumented vertebra (LIV), using anterior thoracic instrumentation, is the end vertebral body of the Cobb measurement; otherwise, if there are two parallel vertebrae, the more distal vertebrae is used. This can then be compared with the predicted posterior LIV either by the stable vertebrae or the Cotrel-Dubousset method (3,30). In the Cotrel-Dubousset method, the disc below the proposed LIV on a bending radiograph must reverse 5 degrees and the LIV have less than 20% rotation in the mature patient or be neutral in the immature patient. In cases in which there is evidence of a thoracolumbar kyphosis on the preoperative radiographs and in which posterior instrumentation would need to be longer, anterior instrumentation may save fusion levels (29).

Residual hypokyphosis has been reported to occur in up to 60% of cases after posterior multisegmented hook-rod systems (1,19,29), and anterior instrumentation can consistently correct hypokyphosis and thoracic lordosis.

Surgical Technique

Approach

The usual approach to the thoracic spine involves a double thoracotomy (1,12). Generally for predicted anterior instrumenta-

tions of seven or fewer levels, a single incision through the interspace may be all that is required. For more than seven levels, a double thoracotomy is usually necessary to provide adequate exposure for disc clean-out, anterior support, and instrumentation.

Open Technique

The patient is intubated with a double lumen tube for one-lung ventilation so that at the site of the thoracotomy, the lung can be kept deflated for most of the procedure to facilitate exposure of the anterior spine, similar to that which is done for thoracoscopy.

The patient is then placed in a lateral decubitus position and prepped and draped in the standard fashion. A single skin incision is made, approximately paralleling the eighth rib as is standard for thoracotomy. The serratus anterior muscle is then mobilized and detached anteriorly. An incision is then made in the intercostal space (at about T4–5 for instrumentation of T5). A second incision is then made between the intercostal space of about three to four ribs distally (at T8–9 for instrumentation of T12). These intercostal space incisions can be adjusted proximally or distally, depending on the levels of the spine to be instrumented. For a short anterior instrumentation (seven or fewer levels), a single incision of the intercostal space may be all that is required. The most proximal level instrumented to date has been T3 (Fig. 3).

If the preoperative analysis of the patient suggests that a thoracoplasty is indicated for cosmesis, it is easiest to perform it at this stage. Small pieces of rib are resected as posteriorly as possible in the intervening ribs between the two intercostal space entrances and above and below. For example, in the previous example, pieces of the ribs of T5, T6, T7, T8, and T9 about 2 cm in length would be removed. If there is a long rib deformity, additional pieces of ribs can be removed, such as from T4 or T10. It is best to do this at this stage because the instrumentation will have minimal effect on correcting the rib deformity, and the rib resections will then facilitate mobilization of the chest wall to make the discectomies and instrumentation easier to perform. The pieces of rib are used for bone grafting.

After thoracoplasty, the use of a large chest spreader extending from the T4–5 interspace down to the T9 rib spread wide ex-

R. R. Betz: Shriners Hospitals for Children, Philadelphia PA 19140.

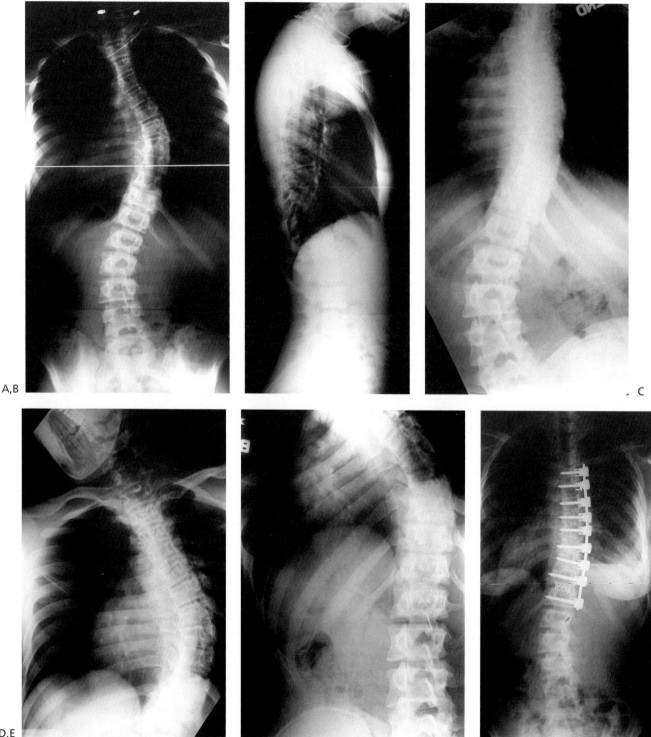

A,B

C

D,E

F

FIGURE 1. A: This is a 15-year-old girl with a 53-degree right thoracic curve, a 35-degree compensatory lumbar curve, and a 20-degree upper thoracic curve. **B:** Lateral radiograph showing a hypokyphotic spine of 10 degrees as measured from T5 to T12. **C:** The right supine-bending film of the right thoracic curve shows the curve to reduce to 25 degrees. **D:** The left upper thoracic supine-bending film shows the curve reducing to 13 degrees. **E:** The left lumbar supine bend shows the lumbar spine to reduce to 5 degrees. The first disc to show 5 degrees of reversal is L3 on L4. However, it remains significantly rotated on both supine bend and erect anteroposterior radiograph; therefore, posterior instrumentation would need to go to L4. This curve would be classified as a King 2½ or a type 1B negative curve by the Lenke classification. **F:** The thoracic curve was instrumented along the Cobb curve from T5 to T12, plus T4 to afford better purchase because of the cantilever effect. Four distal fusion levels were saved. In addition, the patient had a partial rib resection from T5 to T11. The thoracic curve was reduced to 13 degrees, with the lumbar curve measuring 19 degrees. *(Figure continues.)*

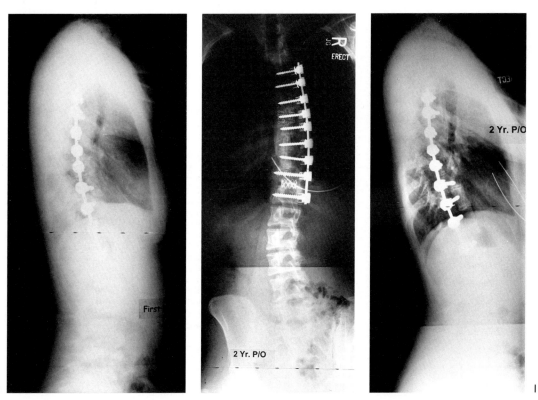

G,H   I

FIGURE 1. *Continued.* **G:** The lateral radiograph shows correction of the sagittal alignment to a more normal profile of 24 degrees. **H:** Two-year follow-up radiograph shows maintenance of correction. The thoracic curve has maintained its correction at 13 degrees, and the lumbar curve has decreased from 19 degrees to 15 degrees. **I:** The sagittal profile is maintaining at 25 degrees.

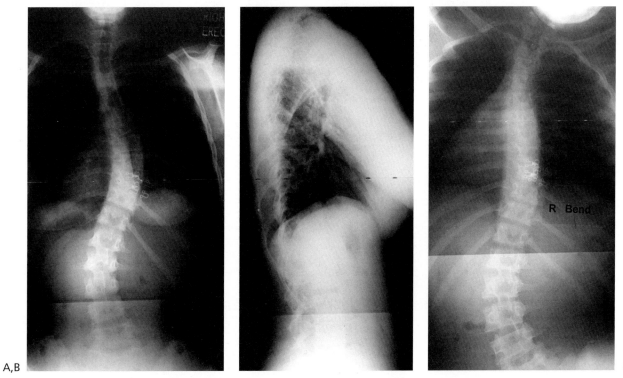

A,B   C

FIGURE 2. **A:** This is a 15-year-old girl with a 42-degree right thoracic curve, a 21-degree upper thoracic curve, and a 37-degree lumbar curve. She has a large rib prominence. **B:** Sagittal profile shows 18 degrees of kyphosis from T5 to T12. **C:** The right thoracic supine-bending film shows the thoracic curve to have reduced to 22 degrees. *(Figure continues.)*

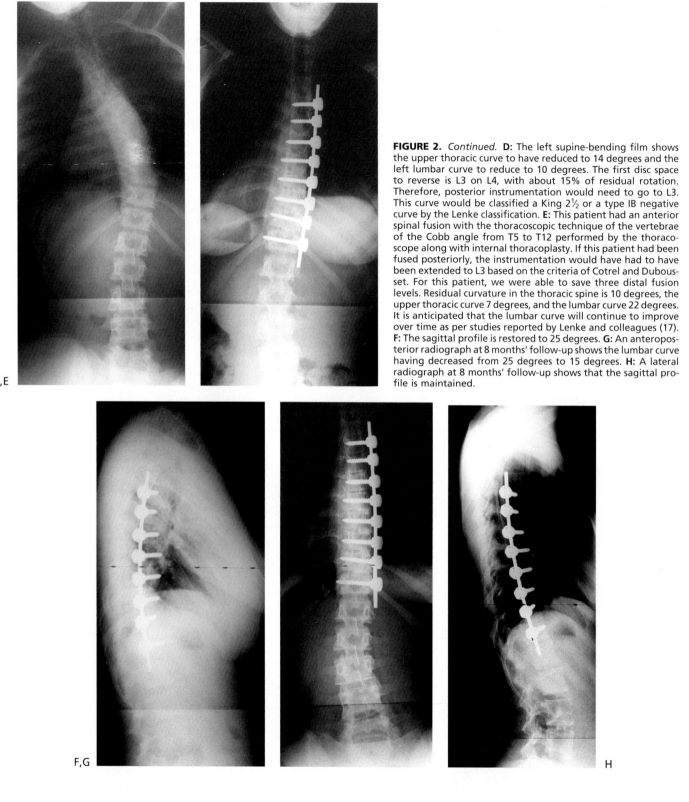

D,E

F,G

H

FIGURE 2. *Continued.* **D:** The left supine-bending film shows the upper thoracic curve to have reduced to 14 degrees and the left lumbar curve to reduce to 10 degrees. The first disc space to reverse is L3 on L4, with about 15% of residual rotation. Therefore, posterior instrumentation would need to go to L3. This curve would be classified a King 2½ or a type IB negative curve by the Lenke classification. **E:** This patient had an anterior spinal fusion with the thoracoscopic technique of the vertebrae of the Cobb angle from T5 to T12 performed by the thoracoscope along with internal thoracoplasty. If this patient had been fused posteriorly, the instrumentation would have had to have been extended to L3 based on the criteria of Cotrel and Dubousset. For this patient, we were able to save three distal fusion levels. Residual curvature in the thoracic spine is 10 degrees, the upper thoracic curve 7 degrees, and the lumbar curve 22 degrees. It is anticipated that the lumbar curve will continue to improve over time as per studies reported by Lenke and colleagues (17). **F:** The sagittal profile is restored to 25 degrees. **G:** An anteroposterior radiograph at 8 months' follow-up shows the lumbar curve having decreased from 25 degrees to 15 degrees. **H:** A lateral radiograph at 8 months' follow-up shows that the sagittal profile is maintained.

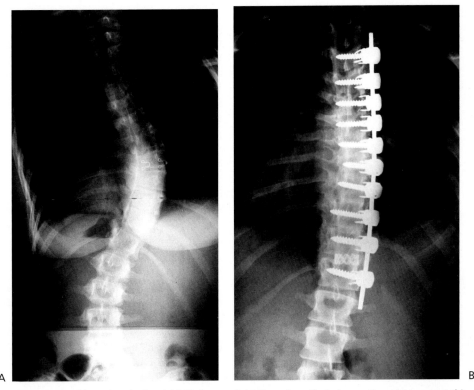

FIGURE 3. **A:** This patient had a rigid 65-degree right thoracic scoliosis. In an attempt to correct this by means of cantilever effect, proximal instrumentation was extended to T3 when T4 and T5 were found intraoperatively to have weak bone structure. **B:** One year after surgery, showing continued maintenance of curve correction with instrumentation from T3 to T12.

poses most of the spine. Then, using a Buckholder retractor, the segment of intervening ribs (T5 to T8) can be pulled either proximally or distally, depending on which aspect of the spine the surgeon is working on.

A radiograph should be obtained with a large needle in a disc space to confirm the anatomic levels. Because only selected fusion levels are performed using anterior instrumentation, it is absolutely critical to be correct in the levels.

Next, the segmental vessels are ligated over each of the vertebral bodies to be instrumented. Some surgeons do not ligate the vessels but mobilize them and plan on slightly eccentric placement of the screw and staple or use no staple at all (personal communication with Dr. Thomas Lowe, Harms Study Group meeting, Toronto, July 1996).

Staples are then inserted into the vertebral bodies. These are aligned so that they are in about the same anatomic position in each vertebral body, being as far posterior as possible while ensuring no possibility of penetration of the spinal canal with the staple prongs. An awl is then used to make the hole, and the screws are inserted.

Proximal screw stability is an issue with all anterior thoracic instrumentation (Fig. 4). If the upper level of the fused Cobb angle is T5, consider going to T4 so that two vertebrae instead of one are now holding the upper end of the curve. In the most proximal vertebrae (e.g., T4), the most proximal screw is inserted eccentrically into the vertebral body. It is placed in the superior one third, but in the same position posteriorly as the other screws. This appears to add increased strength by butting the screw threads up against the superior end plate of the vertebral body. A slightly longer proximal screw is necessary so that the screw extends a bit out of the staple in order to align the rod with the other screws. I use one or two washers to take up this space, and the screw must be at least 5 mm through the far cortex. If the screw measurement was 25 and one would normally put in a 30 to allow the threads to stick out 5 mm, a 35-mm screw with two washers is used. I have noted no instances of proximal screw pullout using this technique. All screw tips should be palpated on the concave side of the vertebral body. Using some form of string or the electrocautery cord, the appropriate length of rod can then be measured from proximal to distal screw. The rod should be cut the exact length of the measurement, allowing about $\frac{1}{8}$ inch extra on each end. The rod is then prebent to parallel the normal kyphosis of the area of the spine to be instrumented.

Before rod insertion, bone grafting must be performed. Small pieces of rib can be used from the rib resection performed earlier if a thoracoplasty was done. If not, or if additional rib graft is necessary, it can be obtained by subperiosteally exposing the superior surface of exposed ribs in both thoracotomy incisions, taking the superior longitudinal half of each of those ribs (e.g., T5 and T9 in the previous example). These ribs can then be left in large pieces for support-type grafts or cut into smaller pieces to accommodate grafting at the apex.

Beginning distally, the disc spaces are wedged open and the

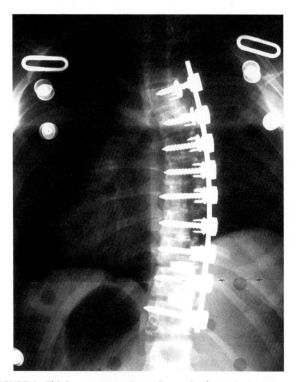

FIGURE 4. This is a postoperative radiograph of anterior instrumentation inserted through an open thoracotomy. Note that the proximal screw appears to have backed out of the proximal vertebral body. Methods to correct this are noted in the text, but the preferred method would be to include two washers and add extra length to the screw, making sure it has at least 5 mm protrusion on the far concave side.

interspaces packed. It is important to pack the inferior discs between T11 and L2 firmly with bone graft to full anatomic height. Structural types of anterior support, either autogenous or synthetic (e.g., titanium cage) should be used to help ensure maintenance of the sagittal profile. When grafting the apical vertebrae, the original sagittal contour must be considered. If the starting sagittal profile is lordotic or very hypokyphotic, only a small amount of graft can be inserted in the disc on the concave anterior portion at the apex of the curve to allow the kyphosis to occur during compression with instrumentation. If, however, the patient starts with normal kyphosis (greater than or equal to 20 degrees), the apical disc space should be wedged open to a normal height and bone graft applied solidly on the concave half of the disc space to a normal anatomic position had the disc been left intact. This still allows the convex side of the disc to compress. It is critical that the sagittal profile be controlled by the amount of bone graft because the rod will be applied only in compression.

After the bone grafting has been completed, the rod is inserted such that the sagittal alignment is established and the first two proximal nuts tightened. It is important to remember to straighten out the operating table if it has been bent to facilitate the thoracotomy and disc exposure. In addition, it helps to have the anesthesiologist remove the axillary roll and to pull on the lower arm at the axillary level to help facilitate correction of the curvature. With the rod inserted, a cantilever force is applied proximally, and the remaining nuts are inserted.

At this point, the surgeon must decide on the anticipated coronal correction that needs to be obtained. If there is a structural upper thoracic curve, only modest correction can be obtained in the main thoracic curve equal to the correction seen on bending radiographs of the upper thoracic curve. If there is no residual structural proximal thoracic compensatory curve, an almost complete reduction of the coronal main curve can be obtained. Correction is obtained using a compressor and compressing each screw toward the apex. All the correction should not be obtained in the first pass; the compression should be done slowly and sequentially. The surgeon should be careful, especially with the end vertebrae, because torquing of the screw could translate it out of the vertebral body. Therefore, it is recommended that the surgeon use the antitorque device that goes over the rod and provides countertorque while the "innies and outies" (Moss-Miami system) are finally tightened.

Neurologic function should be assessed, with either a wake-up test or spinal cord monitoring, and the surgeon should then adequately visualize the appearance of the spine, possibly by radiograph, for correction. Additional bone grafting can then be undertaken.

The parietal pleura is subsequently reapproximated. A chest tube is inserted, and the chest thoracotomy incision is closed in the standard fashion. Double thoracotomy and thoracoplasty appear to present no problem to chest stability. Provided there is no loosening of screws and there is a stable construct, I do not use postoperative immobilization. A case example using this technique is illustrated in Figure 1.

Variations of Thoracic Instrumentation
Flexible The Zielke 3.2-mm rod and the Harms-Moss 3.2-mm and 4-mm threaded rods have been used for correction of anterior scoliosis (1,11). Harms has reported that the flexible rod works well for control of correction of the thoracic hypokyphosis and for more controlled correction when there is a severe deformity of the thoracic spine. These flexible rods correct by controlled compression, in contrast to the single solid rods, most of which correct by cantilever. The flexible rods in the rigid curves have less chance of screw pullout than the solid rods, which risk screw pullout with cantilever effect (12). The major problem with flexible rods is rod breakage, reported to be 31% in one series (1) and 11% in another (12), although most patients are symptom free with no loss of correction and no pain.

Solid Solid rod systems known to work in the thoracic spine include the 4- and 5-mm Moss-Miami, the M-8 system, and Isola. Some of the systems are made of titanium and some of stainless steel. In my experience with the Harms' Study Group, there have been more broken 5-mm than 4-mm Moss-Miami stainless-steel rods. It is theorized that there is settling of bone graft and that the 4-mm rod may allow the spine to collapse slightly and then go on to heal, and that the 5-mm rod may be too stiff and prevents the spine from getting contact when the bone resorbs. The spine then develops pseudarthrosis, and the rod breaks.

Longer-term results with titanium regarding optimal rod diameter and stiffness are not yet available.

Thoracoscopic Technique

After it has been decided that an anterior approach may be of benefit, a minimally invasive option for the approach may be considered. Thoracoscopic and minimally invasive techniques have advanced considerably over the last decade (6,16,21,28). Dickman and colleagues (5) compared costs of open to thoracoscopic surgery and found that the length of stay in the intensive care unit with open procedures was one third that of the thoracoscopic procedure, hospital stay was half as long, and the need for narcotic medication was half as frequent, but this study looked at one-level discectomy or corpectomy procedures only. Newton and associates (25) compared open anterior release and fusion to the thoracoscopic procedure for deformity and showed no difference in length of hospital stay but higher costs with the thoracoscopic procedure. Most surgeons still believe that the advantages of the thoracoscopic procedure include muscle sparing and improved cosmesis, but these are yet to be proved.

A question that arises in using the thoracoscopic approach for anterior release and fusion is whether adequate spine flexibility can be obtained. Wall and coauthors (33) looked at biomechanical flexibility obtained after thoracoscopic and open discectomy in swine and found it to be comparable, and similar results were obtained in a goat model by Newton and colleagues (24). The only clinical study comparing thoracoscopic release and open release was done by Newton and associates (25) in a small series of ten patients in each group. This study showed no statis-

tically significant difference in the amount of correction obtained using posterior instrumentation when the anterior release was done either as an open procedure or thoracoscopically.

The next question that arises is whether adequate disc annulus and end plate can be removed to create a good bed for fusion with thoracoscopic techniques. Huntington and coworkers (13) compared open and thoracoscopic discectomies in a sheep model and found no statistically significant difference between the two approaches. In addition, they found no statistical difference in the number of discs that had half of their end plate resected. Bunnell (2) reported that more than half of the disc end plate had to be resected to obtain an adequate anterior spinal fusion (ASF).

Several variations of thoracoscopic instrument insertion have been developed. The technique used by myself and Dr. David Clements includes making three portals anterolaterally to perform annular release, disc removal, end plate obliteration, fusion, and thoracoplasty (if needed). Additional portals are subsequently made in the posteroaxillary line perpendicular to the vertebral bodies for placement of vertebral body screws. These screws are bicortical and are visualized on the undersurface, facilitated by the use of the anterior portals. No intraoperative fluoroscopy or cannulated guide pins are needed. The rod is inserted, followed by the remainder of the 4-mm Moss-Miami system of innies and outies, correction is obtained by cantilever, the rod is rotated for sagittal plane alignment, and the spine is com-

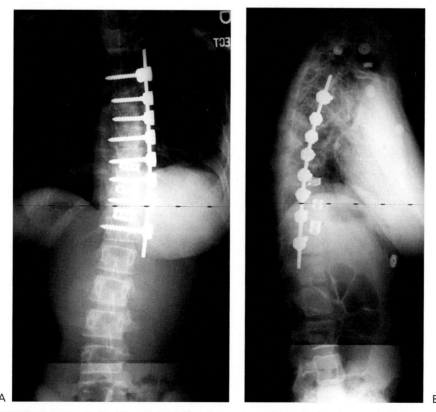

FIGURE 5. Anteroposterior **(A)** and lateral **(B)** postoperative radiographs showing anterior instrumentation inserted thoracoscopically, including intervertebral spacers.

pressed with a specially designed compression device. This is illustrated in Figures 2 and 5. The average operating room time for endoscopic instrumented cases is 6 to 7 hours, most of which is needed for meticulous discectomy, grafting, and thoracoplasty. The actual instrumentation takes $1\frac{1}{2}$ to 2 hours.

In contrast, another method being developed for thoracoscopic technique is that of Picetti and coworkers (27), who use posterolateral portals only for the discectomy approach and the insertion of the instrumentation. They also use a cannulated pin and intraoperative radiographic imaging.

Dual Rod Systems

Other authors have reported on use of anterior instrumentation for thoracic scoliosis. Most recently, Kaneda and colleagues (14) reported excellent coronal and sagittal correction with their dual-rod system. In addition, they obtained only 15% axial correction before rib head resection and 58% after rib head resection.

Results and Complications

Harms and colleagues (12) reported the results of 101 patients who underwent ventral instrumentation using the Harms-Moss system between 1988 and 1994. Average correction was 73% (range, 32% to 100%), and the sagittal plane improved from an average of 10.9 degrees of hypokyphosis to a normal kyphosis averaging 27.9 degrees postoperatively. Spontaneous correction of the lumbar curve averaged 14.7 degrees (range, 0 to 47 degrees), and spontaneous correction of the upper thoracic curve averaged 16.2 degrees (range, 0 to 47 degrees). The rod fractured in 11 cases (11%), with 4 of the 11 being associated with pseudarthrosis and 3 of the 4 requiring revision surgery. The authors also reported a 22% incidence of proximal screw pullout.

Clinical Results

Betz and coworkers (1) reported the results of a comparison study of 78 patients with ASF with Harms instrumentation and 100 patients with posterior multisegmented hook-rod systems. Average coronal correction of the main thoracic curve was 58% in the anterior group and 59% in the posterior group ($P = .92$). Analysis of sagittal contour showed that the posterior systems failed to correct a preoperative hypokyphosis (sagittal T5 to T12 less than 20 degrees) in 60% of cases, whereas 81% were normal postoperatively in the anterior group. However, hyperkyphosis (sagittal T5 to T12 greater than 40 degrees) occurred postoperatively in 40% of the anterior group when the preoperative kyphosis was greater than 20 degrees. Postoperative coronal balance was equal in both groups. An average of 2.5 (range, 0 to 6) distal fusion levels were saved using the anterior spinal instrumentation, with variation depending on criteria used for determining posterior fusion levels. Selective fusion of the thoracic curve was performed in 76 of 78 patients (97%) of the anterior group and in only 18 of 100 (18%) of the posterior

group (Fig. 6). Although these results were supportive of the anterior instrumentation, there were problems with the 3.2-mm flexible rod used. Surgically confirmed pseudarthrosis occurred in four of 78 (5%) patients in the anterior group. Loss of correction greater than 10 degrees occurred in 18 of 78 (23%) patients in the anterior group. Rod breakage occurred in 24 (31%) of the anterior group. Most patients with rod breakage did not have symptoms. The author now uses a 4-mm Moss-Miami solid rod system.

Spontaneous Correction of the Lumbar Curve

Commonly asked questions concerning selected fusion of the thoracic curve with anterior instrumentation is whether the spontaneous correction of the lumbar curve will continue to hold up over time and whether it any better than selected posterior instrumentation. In a study by Lenke and colleagues (17), not only did the lumbar curve spontaneously reduce predictably, but also this correction either stayed improved or, on occasion, continued to improve over a 2-year follow-up. Although a similar pattern occurred in the posterior (control) group, the amount of correction obtained in comparing anterior to posterior was dramatically different. Overall, for thoracic curvatures instrumented selectively with ASF, these patients obtained a 58% correction, and the lumbar curve spontaneously corrected 56% at 2-year follow-up. In the posterior group, only 38% correction was obtained in the thoracic curve and, likewise, spontaneous correction of the lumbar curve was only 37%. This was found to be even more significant in the King II curves, in which the mean thoracic curves were 65 degrees in the anterior group and 67 degrees in the posterior group. The mean residual curve in the anterior group was 27 degrees and in the posterior group 49 degrees, with 59% and 27% correction, respectively. Similarly, the residual curves at 2 years' follow-up in the lumbar region were only 21 degrees in the anterior group and 37 degrees in the posterior group (50% and 30% correction, respectively).

Although skeletal immaturity was originally thought to be an indication for anterior instrumentation to prevent crankshaft, the Harms Study Group noted a large degree of hyperkyphosis in these immature patients at 2-year follow-up, with more than 70% of the patients having sagittal curvatures greater than 40 degrees from T5 to T12. D'Andrea and colleagues (4) reported the possible phenomenon of progressive sagittal kyphosis after ASF in an immature patient. They showed that in Risser 0 patients who underwent ASF, 60% developed kyphosis greater than 40 degrees, as compared with only 27% of Risser 1 to 4 patients. The curves that progressed after the ASF did so an average of 15 degrees. Therefore, when performing ASF on immature patients, several members of the Harms Study Group are reducing the amount of residual kyphosis at the time of surgery through use of structural interbody grafts, anticipating a 15-degree progression of sagittal deformity as the patient matures. The exact cause of this progressive sagittal kyphosis is unclear. D'Andrea and colleagues (4) speculate that it may be due to overgrowth of the posterior elements with a solid ASF.

Pulmonary Function

In a study by Graham and associates (9), 44 patients with thoracic adolescent idiopathic scoliosis, with an average age of 15

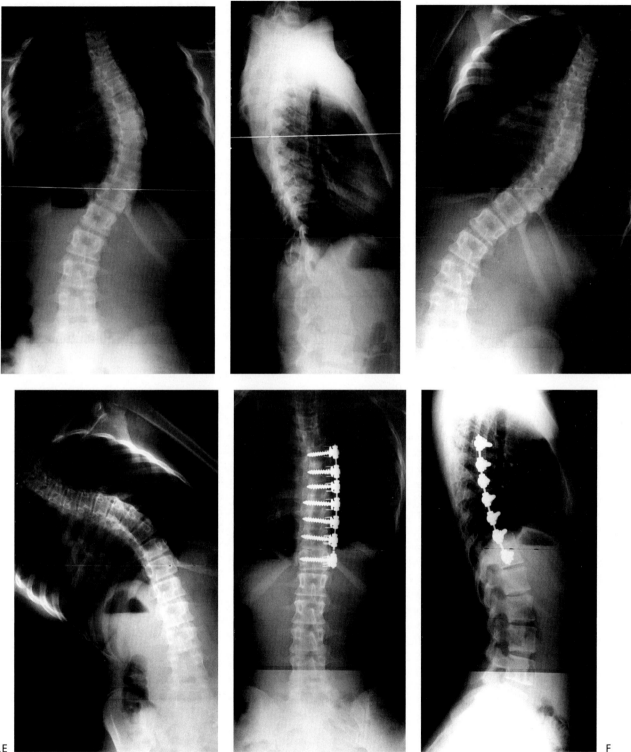

A,B

C

D,E

F

FIGURE 6. A: This patient has a 55-degree right thoracic scoliosis, an 18-degree upper thoracic compensatory curve, and a 38-degree lumbar compensatory curve. **B:** The sagittal profile shows 12 degrees of thoracic kyphosis. **C:** The right thoracic side-bending radiograph shows the curve to reduce only to 40 degrees. **D:** The left side-bending film shows the first disc space to reduce is L2–3. It is neutral back on the erect film (see part **A**). This curve would be classified as a King 3 or a type IA negative curve by the Lenke classification. Proposed posterior fusion levels would be to L2 by both the stable vertebrae and by the Cotrel-Dubousset method. **E and F:** The patient had an anterior spinal fusion from T6 to T12. Eight-year follow-up shows maintenance of the coronal and sagittal alignment of 23 degrees.

years, 2 months (range, 10 to 20 years) had pulmonary function tests consisting of volume (FVC) and flow (FEV_1) parameters and total lung capacity (TLC). The results showed a significant temporary decline in pulmonary function absolute values of 27% FVC, 15% FEV_1, and 11% TLC at 3 months' follow-up, with continued improvement and eventually showed no statistical difference between preoperative and 2-year postoperative values. There was no significant effect when comparing single to double thoracotomies in those patients with or without an internal thoracoplasty, or in patients younger than 15 years of age (n = 22) versus those 15 years of age or older (n = 22).

Thoracoscopic Approach Versus Open Thoracotomy

In a study by Betz and colleagues (unpublished), 19 patients had anterior instrumentation inserted thoracoscopically. The average age at surgery was 14 years, and the average preoperative curve was 50 degrees. Follow-up ranged from 1 to 30 months. These patients were randomly matched with 19 patients having open thoracotomy for insertion of anterior instrumentation by age, curve degree, and curve types according to Lenke and colleagues (18). In this study, the average age at surgery was 14 years, and the average preoperative curve was 48 degrees. Follow-up ranged from 11 to 26 months. Both thoracoscopic and open techniques included partial rib resection for thoracoplasty with autogenous rib grafting in all patients. The 4-mm Moss-Miami single rod was used. In the thoracoscopic versus open groups, results were as follows: coronal correction rates were 67% ± 6% and 54% ± 8%, respectively; no patient's plumb line was out of balance (more than 2 cm) in either group; one patient in each group had more than 10 degrees of shoulder asymmetry; the sagittal measurements at T5 to T12 were 24 degrees preoperatively to 22 degrees postoperatively and 21 degrees preoperatively to 33 degrees postoperatively, respectively; rates of normal postoperative sagittal profile (20 to 40 degrees at T5 to T12) were 63% and 67%, respectively; residual hypokyphosis (less than 20 degrees) rates were 31% and 12%, respectively; hyperkyphosis (more than 40 degrees) rates were 6% and 21%, respectively; estimated blood loss measurements were 1.028 ± 363 mL and 484 ± 170 mL, respectively; and average operating room times were 7 hours and 4.5 hours, respectively. One patient in the thoracoscopic group had residual pleural effusion, and two patients in the open group had recurrent pneumothorax after the chest tube was discontinued. Two patients in the thoracoscopic group had a delayed peroneal palsy that did not present until 24 hours after surgery and completely resolved within 4 weeks. This was thought to be secondary to the prolonged operative time with the weight of the upper leg on the lower leg, which sustained the peroneal palsy. It was encouraging in this preliminary study to see that the thoracoscopic technique of insertion of anterior instrumentation was producing similar results radiographically to the open technique. Although the operating room time is prolonged (with subsequent increase in blood loss) and there were two peroneal nerve injuries secondary to the prolonged procedure, these instances should decrease as skill and technology improve.

THORACOLUMBAR AND LUMBAR SCOLIOSIS

Indications

For idiopathic scoliosis, it has been reported that the indications include saving one or more distal fusion levels and immaturity (22,26). Saving the distal fusion levels can be done by predicting the lower instrumented vertebral level anteriorly as that vertebra having less than 15-degree tilt to the pelvis on bending films and less than 20% rotation (23). This lower instrumented vertebral level can then be compared with a predicted level for posterior. Another technique, pioneered by Hall and colleagues (10), provides overcorrection of the instrumented apical segment of thoracolumbar and lumbar curves and is performed to stop fusion at either L1 or L2, further saving additional fusion levels.

Anterior instrumentation may be indicated in myelodysplasia because of the absent posterior elements and the difficulty in posterior instrumentation. It can be extremely helpful when there is a marked pelvic obliquity because of the derotation of the thoracolumbar and lumbar spine segments that can be performed with the anterior instrumentation.

Approach

Thoracolumbar and lumbar approaches are well described in other chapters in this text. Generally, one needs to enter the retroperitoneal space or the thorax through an interspace above the proposed upper instrumented level. Some surgeons prefer to take the rib; however, upon closure, especially after the convexity has been corrected and straight, this leaves a defect in the chest wall. Harms (personal communication) has promoted going through the intercostal space, which leaves less of a chest wall deformity. If one needs to harvest bone graft of the rib, the surgeon can take a longitudinal half of the rib (both above and below) and still leave the chest wall intact.

One can shorten the length of the incision and extend the exposure by using a puncture approach to place in the proximal or distal screw. This involves making a small incision in the interspace above to get the proper angulation for screw insertion. Angled screwdrivers are available; however, sometimes, there is not enough room between the rib and the vertebral body for it to work appropriately, and the puncture technique is helpful. It is strongly recommended that an intraoperative radiograph be obtained. Although the ribs and their attachment to the spine can be a guideline, one can be misled and off a level because of the deformity that sometimes exists. If one is too distal, the opportunity for saving a fusion level is lost. If one is too proximal, there is a high risk for decompensation. Controversy still exists about whether to remove the segmental vessels. Most surgeons ligate the vessels, and in a large series reported by Winter and colleagues (34) of more than 1,000 cases, there were no instances of intraoperative paralysis secondary to vessel ligation.

Creation of a periosteal sleeve is still controversial. It has been proposed by Dubousset (personal communication) to be important in obtaining fusion, especially with flexible anterior instrumentation. The disadvantages of this include more blood loss and the tedious exposure required. A thorough discectomy is essential for anterior instrumentation alone to hold in the thoracolumbar and lumbar spine. It is essential to use a device (disc spreader) to spread the disc such that end plate and posterior annulus can be removed all the way back to the posterior longitudinal ligament, maximizing the area of exposure for bone grafting.

Variations of Thoracolumbar and Lumbar Instrumentation

Flexible

Flexible systems available include the Zielke, Dwyer, and Harms-Moss systems of 3.2- and 4-mm rods (7,8,15,20,22,31). The derotation maneuver for derotating the lumbar spine and maintaining lordosis was popularized by Zielke and reported in the English literature by Ogiela and Chan (26) and Moe and colleagues (22). The biggest problem with flexible rods has been the development of an average of 13- to 20- degree kyphosis in the instrumented segment (20). Prevention of this problem has been promoted by the use of solid, rigid rods (32) and through the use of structural grafts for interbody spacers to provide anterior support (12).

Solid

Solid rods include the use of TSRH as reported by Turi and colleagues (32); CD-Horizon, Moss-Miami, Synergy, and Isola. Anterior structural support as repoted by Harnes and colleagues appears to be most important with use of single solid rods for maintaining kyphosis and obtaining bone healing, although published reports of long-term studies are pending. Hall and coauthors (10) reported on a short-segment overcorrection technique using solid rods and overcorrection of the apical segment, fusing three or four segments. If the apex of the curve is a vertebral body, Hall and coauthors fuse three segments, one body above and one below the apex. If the apex is a disc, they fuse two vertebral bodies above and two below, for a four-segment construct. A solid dual-rod system (Kaneda Anterior Spinal System, or KASS) has been reported to provide excellent coronal and sagittal results. The dual-rod system requires two screws in each vertebral body (14).

Results and Complications

Since 1983, Hall and coauthors (10) have performed either three- or four-segment anterior instrumentation on patients with thoracolumbar and lumbar scoliosis. They have reported on 26 patients with either Dwyer or VDS instrumentation and on 18 patients with TSRH instrumentation, with coronal correction rates averaging 100% and 108%, respectively. Development of kyphosis in the instrumented segment averaged 10 degrees in the Dwyer-VDS group and 9.9 degrees in the TSRH group. To date, no patient in Hall's series has required extension of the fusion because of increased deformity distal to the lower instrumented vertebrae, nor have any patients had pain in an oblique segment below the fusion. Longer follow-up is required to deter-

mine whether the oblique segment below the instrumentation becomes a clinical concern.

REFERENCES

1. Betz RR, Harms J, Clements DH III, et al. (1999): Comparison of anterior and posterior instrumentation for correction of adolescent thoracic idiopathic scoliosis. *Spine* 24:225–239.
2. Bunnell WP (1982): Anterior spinal fusion: experimental evaluation of technique. *J Pediatr Orthop* 2:469–477.
3. Chopin D, Morin C (1991): Cotrel-Dubousset instrumentation for adolescent idiopathic scoliosis. In: Bridwell KH, DeWald RD, eds. *The textbook of spinal surgery*. Philadelphia: JB Lippincott, p. 198.
4. D'Andrea LP, Betz RR, Lenke LG, et al. (2000): The effect of continued spinal growth on sagittal contour in patients treated by anterior instrumentation for adolescent idiopathic scoliosis. *Spine* 25:813–818.
5. Dickman CA, Mican C (1996): Thoracoscopic approaches for the treatment of anterior thoracic spinal pathology. *BNI Quarterly* 12:14–19.
6. Dubois F, Icard P, Berthelot G, et al. (1990): Coelioscopic cholecystectomy: preliminary report of 36 cases. *Ann Surg* 211:60–62.
7. Dwyer AF, Newton NC, Sherwood AA (1969): Anterior approach to scoliosis: a preliminary report. *Clin Orthop* 62:192–202.
8. Dwyer AF, Schafer MF (1971): Anterior approach to scoliosis: results of treatment in fifty-one cases. *J Bone Joint Surg Br* 56:218–224.
9. Graham EJ, Lenke LG, Lowe TG, et al. (1999): *Prospective pulmonary function evaluation following open thoracotomy for anterior thoracic spinal fusion in adolescent idiopathic scoliosis.* Presented at the Scoliosis Research Society annual meeting, San Diego, September 1999.
10. Hall JE, Millis MB, Snyder BD (1997): Short segment anterior instrumentation for thoracolumbar scoliosis. In: Bridwell KH, DeWald RL, eds. *The textbook of spinal surgery*. Philadelphia: Lippincott-Raven Publishers, pp. 665–674.
11. Hammerberg KW, Zielke K (1985): *VDS instrumentation for idiopathic thoracic curvatures.* Presented at the American Academy of Orthopaedic Surgeons annual meeting, Las Vegas, January 1985.
12. Harms J, Jeszenszky D, Beele B (1997): Ventral correction of thoracic scoliosis. In: Bridwell KH, DeWald RL, eds. *The textbook of spinal surgery*. Philadelphia: Lippincott-Raven, pp. 611–626.
13. Huntington CF, Murrell WD, Betz RR, et al. (1998): Comparison of thoracoscopic and open thoracic discectomy in a live ovine model for anterior spinal fusion. *Spine* 23:1699–1701.
14. Kaneda K, Shono Y, Satoh S, et al. (1997): Anterior correction of thoracic scoliosis with Kaneda anterior spinal system: a preliminary report. *Spine* 22:1358–1368.
15. Kostuik JP, Carl A, Ferron S (1989): Anterior Zielke instrumentation for spinal deformity in adults. *J Bone Joint Surg Am* 71:898–912.
16. Landreneau RJ, Mack MJ, Hazelrigg SR, et al. (1992): Video-assisted thoracic surgery: basic technical concepts and intercostal approach strategies. *Ann Thorac Surg* 54:800–807.
17. Lenke LG, Betz R, Harms J, et al. (1999): Spontaneous lumbar curve correction following selective anterior or posterior thoracic fusion in adolescent idiopathic scoliosis. *Spine* 24:1663–1671. Presented at the North American Spine Society annual meeting, New York City, October 1997.
18. Lenke LG, Betz RR, Harms J, et al.: A new and comprehensive classification system of adolescent idiopathic scoliosis. *Spine*. In press.
19. Lenke LG, Bridwell KH, Baldus C, et al. (1992): Cotrel-Dubousset instrumentation for adolescent idiopathic scoliosis. *J Bone Joint Surg Am* 74:1056–1067.
20. Lowe TG, Peters JD (1993): Anterior spinal fusion with Zielke instrumentation for idiopathic scoliosis: a frontal and sagittal curve analysis in 36 patients. *Spine* 18:423–426.
21. Mack MJ, Regan JJ, Bobechko WP, et al. (1993): Application of thoracoscopy for diseases of the spine. *Ann Thorac Surg* 56:736–738.

22. Moe JH, Purcell GA, Bradford DS (1983): Zielke instrumentation (VDS) for the correction of spinal curvature. *Clin Orthop* 180: 133–153.

23. Nash CL Jr, Moe JH (1969): A study of vertebral rotation. *J Bone Joint Surg Am* 51:223–229.

24. Newton PO, Cardelia JM, Farnsworth CL, et al. (1998): A biomechanical comparison of open and thoracoscopic anterior spinal release in a goat model. *Spine* 23:530–535.

25. Newton PO, Wenger DR, Mubarak SJ, et al. (1997): Anterior release and fusion in pediatric spinal deformity: a comparison of early outcome and cost of thoracoscopic and open thoracotomy approaches. *Spine* 22:1398–1406.

26. Ogiela DM, Chan DPK (1986): Ventral derotation spondylodesis: a review of 22 cases. *Spine* 11:18–22.

27. Picetti GD III, Blackman RG, O'Neal K, et al. (1998): Anterior endoscopic correction and fusion of scoliosis. *Orthopedics* 21:1285–1287.

28. Regan JJ, Mack MJ, Picetti GD (1994): A technical report on video-assisted thoracoscopy in thoracic spinal surgery: preliminary description. *Spine* 19:1087–1091.

29. Richards BS, Birch JG, Herring JA, et al. (1989): Frontal plane and sagittal plane balance following Cotrel-Dubousset instrumentation for idiopathic scoliosis. *Spine* 14:733–737.

30. Shufflebarger HL (1994): Theory and mechanisms of posterior derotation spinal systems. In: Weinstein SL, ed. *The pediatric spine: principles and practice*. New York: Raven, p. 1518.

31. Swank SM, Brown JC, Williams L, et al. (1982): Spinal fusion using Zielke instrumentation. *Orthopedics* 5:1172–1182.

32. Turi M, Johnston CE, Richards BS (1993): Anterior correction of idiopathic scoliosis using TSRH instrumentation. *Spine* 18:417–422.

33. Wall E, Bylski-Austrow D, Shelton F, et al. (1996): *Spine flexibility after open versus endoscopic discectomy*. Presented at the Pediatric Orthopaedic Society of North America annual meeting, Phoenix, May 1996.

34. Winter RB, Lonstein JE, Denis F, et al. (1996): Paraplegia resulting from vessel ligation. *Spine* 21:1232–1233.

LUMBOSACRAL INSTRUMENTATION

GUY A. LEE
BRYAN W. CUNNINGHAM
PAUL C. MCAFEE

Improved treatment of spinal deformities is increasingly dependent on improved fixation at the bone-metal interface. Spinal instrumentation has revolutionized the surgical treatment and management of pediatric spinal disorders. Previous techniques using Harrington distraction required excessive dissection and resulted in loss of lumbar lordosis. Pedicle screw fixation has become increasingly widespread, and instrumented reductions of spondylolistheses are rapidly becoming a more accepted technique (27).

Disorders of the lumbosacral junction in children parallel many of the deformities observed in adults. However, the morphologic differences in the pediatric spine require difficult techniques for spinal fixation and fusion. The pediatric spine possesses the potential for future growth, which can lead to the onset of adult deformities (51). In addition, fixation is many times limited because of the smaller, often dysplastic anatomic structures of the pediatric spine. This can be easily managed with instrumentation specifically designed for the pediatric population. Pediatric tissue has a thicker, more biologically active periosteum, which has not achieved its optimal bone mineral density. Therefore, it deforms at a lower peak pressure and absorbs more energy to ultimate failure (34).

POSTERIOR LUMBOSACRAL INSTRUMENTATION AND FIXATION

Lumbosacroiliac Spinal Kinematics

The anatomic considerations and complex biomechanical properties of the lumbosacral and sacroiliac junctions collectively pose a formidable challenge to the surgical application and outcome performance of spinal instrumentation. From a kinematic standpoint, the lumbosacral junction presents itself as the most active transition zone in the spine. Based on flexion-extension radiographs, the motion characteristics in the normal lumbar spine of young adults demonstrates that maximal lumbar translation

and rotation occur at the L5 and L4 vertebral levels, respectively (59). In vitro and in vivo studies have demonstrated the L5 to S1 joint to exhibit sagittal and coronal plane range of motions as high as 17 and 12 degrees, respectively, under normal physiologic loads (40,47,48). Moreover, the magnitude of these displacements has been shown to exhibit twofold increases after L5 to S1 posterior element excision (40). Coupled with these kinematic properties, experimental studies have demonstrated the lumbosacral junction to carry and transfer compressive forces up to eleven times the superincumbent body weight (43). In a classic series of investigations conducted by Nachemson and colleagues, the loads on the lower lumbar discs have been shown to range from 700 Newton standing to as high as 3,400 Newtons (760 lb) in a flexural posture while holding weight (42,44,45).

In contrast to the motions exhibited at the lumbosacral junction, the sacroiliac articulations present a transition zone where the highly mobile lower lumbar segments join the rather immobile sacroiliac region. The immobilization properties can be attributed to a number of factors, including the wedge-shaped keystone configuration of the sacroiliac junction, strong anterior and posterior sacral articular capsule, and surrounding ligaments. In fact, the collective tensioning properties of the posterior sacroiliac and interosseous ligaments on the sacrum, combined with the syndesmotic nature of the sacroiliac joint, actually results in the sacroiliac articulation becoming more stable under increasing loads (41,57). The combination of high loads and large ranges of motion at the lower lumbar levels juxtaposed to a nearly immobile sacral region poses a formidable biomechanical challenge to the spinal instrumentation and surgical techniques used to reconstruct the lumbosacral spine (57).

The treatment of spondylolysis and spondylolisthesis in children requires a basic understanding of lumbosacral kinematics. Most children respond to conservative treatment and never need to have surgery (15). The goals of surgery for spondylolysis and spondylolisthesis are reduction of back and radicular pain, prevention of further slip, stabilization of L5 to S1, restoration of posture and gait, and improved appearance (3). Lumbosacral fusion with instrumentation has many advantages over uninstrumented in situ fusion. Internal fixation should eliminate the approximately one third risk for slip progression even with a successful in situ arthrodesis (3,15,26). With instrumentation, a more complete L5 nerve root decompression can be performed

G. A. Lee: Orthopaedic Specialty Center, Willow Grove, Pennsylvania 19090.

B. W. Cunningham: Department of Orthopaedic Surgery, Union Memorial Hospital, Baltimore, Maryland 21218.

P. C. McAfee: The Johns Hopkins Hospital, Scoliosis and Spine Center, Towson, Maryland 21204.

without the potential for further instability or slippage. Spinal stabilization results in higher fusion rates, preservation of lordosis, and better correction of deformity (17).

Basic Instrumentation Concepts

Much of the scientific basis for the design of instrumentation to stabilize the lumbosacral junction has been obtained through investigations using animal tissue, human cadaveric tissue, or synthetic surrogate models. The following provides a systematic approach to the concepts of lumbosacral spinal instrumentation. Purchase of the vertebral bodies in the lumbosacral spine can be achieved with pedicle screws, laminar hooks and sublaminar wires. From a vertebral attachment standpoint, transpedicular fixation offers several advantages to hook- and wire-based systems. It affords immediate, three-column stabilization to the operative levels, which is biomechanically superior to correction of deformities through single-column fixation. In vitro testing has demonstrated that pedicle screw–based systems maximally reduce intersegmental three-dimensional motion and enhance the strength of fixation compared with laminar hook and wire systems (1,4,49). However, in osteopenic conditions, laminar hooks have proved to be significantly more resistant to failure from posteriorly directed forces than spinous process wires or transpedicular fixation (11). This increased resistance to failure from posteriorly directed forces and independence from decreased bone mineral density may indicate that laminar hooks are superior to spinous process wiring and transpedicular fixation in patients with decreased bone mineral density (11).

Recent work by Zdeblick (60) justified rigid internal fixation with pedicle screws. The increased apparent fusion rate also received clinical success in lumbar or lumbosacral fusions compared with semirigid devices or uninstrumented fusions. Intuitively, instrumentation becomes more beneficial for multilevel fusions because the fusion rate is significantly lower than for single-level fusions. Posterolateral arthrodeses involving the outer portions of the facet joints, transverse processes, and intertransverse space are biomechanically superior to a Hibbs posterior fusion (57).

Fixation to the Sacrum

For short fusions, L4 or L5 to the sacrum, pedicle screw fixation to the sacrum should provide enough stability for a solid fusion (18). There a several anatomic considerations with regard to transpedicular screw placement, including depth of penetration and screw orientation. In the lower lumbar levels, medial angulation and transfixation of lumbar pedicle screw fixation have been shown to improve the stabilizing properties in multilevel reconstructions (10). Moreover, screw triangulation permits oblique screw orientation, thereby posing less interference with the proximal adjacent facets (31); improves the length of screw purchase (5); and enhances fixation, particularly in the osteoporotic case (39,49). Purchase of the anterior cortex, although mechanically favorable (5,61), is not clinically ideal. Satisfactory purchase can be achieved with fixation extending into the anterior half of the vertebral body, with pullout strengths decreased by only 20% compared with anterior cortex purchase (5).

Bicortical sacral screw fixation has proved to increase the strength of fixation (54,61); however, screw orientation in the sacrum has offered different results based on the direction of applied load (9,54,61). Bending moments in the S1 screws are highest under anterior flexural loading conditions because of the large cantilever effect of the distal anchorage sites (46). Although physiologic load application is multidirectional on the first sacral screw, the predominant force is perpendicular to the screw axis and is directed in flexion. In pursuance to this loading mode, Carlson and colleagues (9) and Smith and coauthors (54) determined that anteromedial screw positioning in S1 resulted in the greatest load to failure and least amount of screw rotation compared with anterolateral positioning. Moreover, the regional bone density in the centrum of the first sacral body was greater than that in the lateral alar region, thereby enhancing screw fixation (54). An anatomic study conducted by Asher and Strippgen suggested that anteromedial orientation increases the available screw purchase surface area compared with anterolateral orientation (5). Coupled with the risk for neurovascular injury, medial angulation is the preferred technique, assuming accurate purchase of the anterior sacral cortex (Fig. 1). The anterior safe zone is larger than the lateral safe zone and easier to visualize fluoroscopically and intraoperatively. At the S2 pedicle level, 45-degree anterolaterally directed screws provide better fixation than medially directed screws; however, the potential risk for neurovascular injury must be considered (61). S1 laminar hook and sublaminar wire fixation alone are of questionable effectiveness based on a high incidence of clinical complications (2,38) and minimal fixation strength (24,39) (63% incidence of wire or hook cutout) and are probably not indicated without adjunctive S1 pedicle screw fixation (56).

Biomechanics of Lumbosacral Fixation

Considering the volume of articles published on the lumbosacral spine, there exists a paucity of information investigating the comparative biomechanical properties of different reconstruction techniques (23,24,30,39). McCord and colleagues (39) undertook a comprehensive investigation comparing the stabilizing properties of 11 different lumbosacral fixation constructs and their abilities to resist destructive flexural moments around the lumbosacral junction. The findings introduce the biomechanical concept of a lumbosacral pivot point located at the intersection of the middle osteoligamentous column and L5 to S1 intervertebral disc (Fig. 2). As reported by McCord and colleagues, those techniques employing S1 fixation alone—hooks, wires, and screws—afforded the least resistance to counteract effectively the flexural moment around the pivot point and failed precipitously by means of device cutout. Adjunctive S2 screw fixation was found to increase significantly the stabilizing effect of the construct, whereas S2 hooks, although they improved fixation, were highly dependent on applied preload.

As reported by Stovall and coworkers, however, the placement of a down-going hook in the S1 neuroforamina effectively distracted against the S1 pedicle screw offered the dual biomechanical advantage of increasing stiffness and preventing S1 screw pullout (56). Fixation using an iliosacral screw, which employs screw purchase of the ilium and S1 obtained in a linear

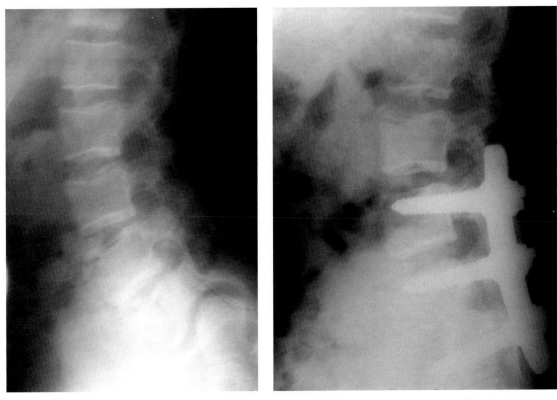

FIGURE 1. **A:** Preoperative lateral radiograph of a 10-year-old female with a grade 4 spondylolisthesis. **B:** Postoperative radiograph showing reduction of the slip and restoration of sagittal alignment. Note bicortical purchase in the sacrum.

fashion, offered no significant improvement in the fixation strength over S1 fixation alone. The theoretical advantage of iliosacral fixation between the ilium and sacrum permits the correction and stabilization forces to be distributed between two points rather than concentrated at a single point. The iliosacral

point of fixation has the additional advantage of lateral placement to the long axis of the spine, providing a longer moment arm and thereby reducing the force required for correction of a given spine deformity.

As reported by McCord and colleagues, the two lumbosacral

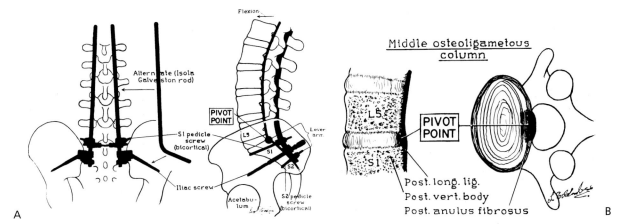

FIGURE 2. **A:** Crossing the sacroiliac joint is biomechanically justified only by fixation that extends anterior to the pivot point. Note the significant anterior extent of the iliac purchase compared to the bicortical S1 or S2 screws. **B:** Lumbosacral pivot point at the intersection point of the middle osteoligamentous column and L5 to S1 intervertebral disc. (**A and B,** from McCord DH, Cunningham BW, Shono Y, et al. [1992]: Biomechanical analysis of lumbosacral fixation. *Spine* 17:S235–S243, with permission.)

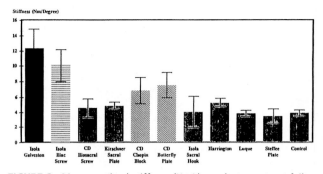

FIGURE 3. Mean maximal stiffness (Nm/degree) at construct failure. (From McCord DH, Cunningham BW, Shono Y, et al. [1992]: Biomechanical analysis of lumbosacral fixation. *Spine* 17:S235–S243, with permission.)

constructs that offered the greatest resistance to the flexural moment around the pivot point entailed S1 medial pedicle screws and iliac purchase using a Galveston-type technique (39) (Fig. 3). Importantly, however, it was concluded that crossing the sacroiliac joint using rods or screws is biomechanically justified only when fixation extends anterior to the projected image of the middle osteoligamentous column on the lateral radiograph. Despite the increased fixation, Wood and associates, using strain-gauged pelvises, concluded that instrumentation of the lumbosacroiliac joint may lead to a device-related osteopenic condition, predisposing patients to late insufficiency—type pelvic fractures as activity levels increase (58).

ILIUM AND ILIOSACRAL FIXATION

Longer posterior spinal fusions usually require enhanced fixation using the sacrum, pelvis, or both. The Galveston technique 2 of iliac wing purchase has become one of the more common methods of fixation. (Fig. 4). Using this technique, iliac fixation ends anteriorly to the axis of rotation in flexion-extension, supplying a more stable buttress to the flexion forces across the lumbosacral junction. A 90-degree bend is made in the rod lateral to S1 and then placed in the thick column of bone between the cortical tables of the posterosuperior iliac spine just above the sciatic notch. The Galveston technique may be combined with a S1 pedicle screw to add further to the stability to this construct. A more acute bend in the rod is occasionally necessary to gain entry into the pelvis. A modification of the Galveston technique requires the use of iliac screws. Iliac screws are generally 7 to 8 mm in diameter and placed in the ilium similar to the Galveston rod. The screws are technically easier to place but require connection to the lumbar construct.

As discussed previously, the use of iliosacral screws is another option to obtain purchase, using both the sacrum and the ilium for fixation, when pelvic obliquity or sacroiliac joint disruption is present. The advantage of the iliosacral screw is its increased resistance to pullout because of purchase in multiple cortices. In addition to the inner and outer iliac table, the posterior sacral cortex, the subchondral bone, and the S1 superior end plate are also engaged, providing a minimum of four sites of cortical

purchase (19). The screws are usually at least 7 mm in diameter and fully threaded. They are inserted over a K wire placed from the iliac wing to the anterior aspect of the sacral promontory at the end plate of S1. The screw is placed through a connector located in the sacroiliac junction. The connector is then used as an anchor for lumbar rod attachment. In a review of 28 patients with this type of fixation, Farcy and associates (20) concluded that the most important intraoperative observation was radiographic confirmation of screw position and reported a 95% fusion rate at 2-year follow-up.

Jackson Technique

Despite the increased fixation strength afforded by deep purchase of the ilium, when crossing or bridging the sacroiliac joint, rod breakage and loosening in the ilium are occasionally observed (7,50). Moreover, these techniques are difficult, demanding, and potentially dangerous. As an alternative to indirect purchase of the ilia by means of the sacroiliac joint, Jackson and McManus (28) proposed a technique of insertion of the rods into the lateral sacral mass, creating a "sacroiliac buttress" of the rods. The rods and screws interlock in the sacrum, protecting the sacral screws from cantilever pullout under anterior flexural loads. Using this technique, the implants can be "buttressed" posteriorly and laterally without crossing the sacroiliac joint (28) and have demonstrated improved stability under flexural and rotational loading modes compared with the Galveston technique (23). The overall concept of lumbosacral fixation using the iliosacral buttress is that anterior placement of the rods and other implants in the pelvis—nearer the instantaneous axis of rotation—offers advantages in reducing moment arms acting on the implants (25,39). Sacral screws with closed oblique canals and strong ductile rods are used. The rod is introduced through the oblique canal sacral screw and then driven into the sacrum. The rods can then be contoured, which aids in reduction of a slip (Fig. 5).

Anterior Constructs

The efficacy of anterior lumbar interbody fusion (ALIF) compared with posterior lumbar interbody fusion (PLIF) remains controversial (35). PLIFs can be technically demanding and carry a higher risk for neurologic injury. However, posterior pedicle screw fixation can be combined with anterior fixation through the same incision. ALIFs require a separate larger anterior exposure incurring a greater risk to vascular structures and require a separate incision for posterior fixation. With the anterior approach, there is less risk for root injury, and the disc can be completely excised. With the advances in video-assisted spine surgery, the risk and morbidity associated with open anterior surgery should be reduced (13,37).

In consideration of the fact that 80% of the spinal load is transmitted across the intact intervertebral disc (8), anterior interbody reconstruction provides a mechanically favorable alternative to enhance further the rigidity of posterior segmental fixation and to maximize deformity correction. In attempts to quantify anterior column loads when using posterior segmental fixation, Duffield and coauthors demonstrated that in a correctly

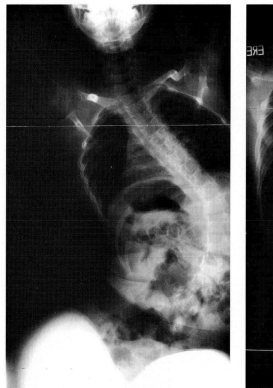

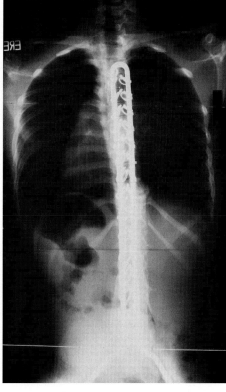

A

B

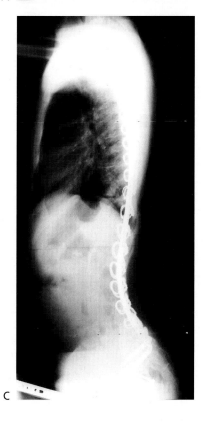

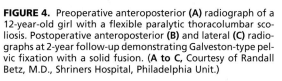

C

FIGURE 4. Preoperative anteroposterior **(A)** radiograph of a 12-year-old girl with a flexible paralytic thoracolumbar scoliosis. Postoperative anteroposterior **(B)** and lateral **(C)** radiographs at 2-year follow-up demonstrating Galveston-type pelvic fixation with a solid fusion. (**A to C,** Courtesy of Randall Betz, M.D., Shriners Hospital, Philadelphia Unit.)

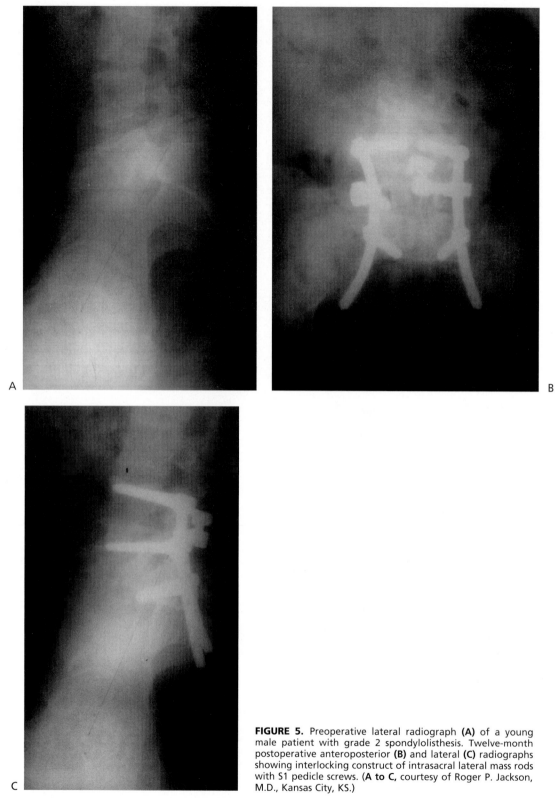

FIGURE 5. Preoperative lateral radiograph **(A)** of a young male patient with grade 2 spondylolisthesis. Twelve-month postoperative anteroposterior **(B)** and lateral **(C)** radiographs showing interlocking construct of intrasacral lateral mass rods with S1 pedicle screws. (**A to C,** courtesy of Roger P. Jackson, M.D., Kansas City, KS.)

instrumented two–motion-segment construct, 75% of the normal physiologic axial load is still predicted to pass through the vertebral bodies (16). Moreover, excessive preloading of the instrumentation through distraction or improper longitudinal element contouring may predispose the instrumentation to increased stress and possible cantilever fatigue failure of the screws. In addition, using a "worst-case scenario corpectomy loading configuration," Cunningham and colleagues concluded that pedicle screw spinal implant systems exhibit bending strengths below the normal load distribution through the anterior column, and in the absence of adequate anterior column support, normal physiologic loads exceed the strengths of all systems (14).

Interbody Fusion

Patients with smaller-grade spondylolistheses (grade I or II) are reasonable candidates for interbody fusion. An ALIF provides a viable option for patients presenting with back pain only and no history of leg pain (29). If there is a history of leg discomfort, a PLIF should be considered so that the nerve roots can be adequately explored and decompressed. Placement of an interbody graft within the disc space places it in a position to experience a compressive load, whereas a posterolateral graft experiences compression only by the overlying muscle. The increased vascularity of the disc space, as well as a favorable biomechanical environment, has resulted in increased fusion rates over standard posterior lateral fusions (33). The interbody bone grafts available include both allograft and autograft. Allograft may be in the form of femoral rings or the newer threaded cortical dowels. More rigid interbody devices (BAK, Sulzer SpineTech, Minneapolis) and Ray TFC (Surgical Dynamics, Inc., Norwalk, CT) were developed with the emphasis on providing a more rigid distraction-fixation device in combination with the bone-healing properties of autograft (29).

Anterior interbody reconstruction using cylindrical cages and femoral ring allografts has shown to decrease S1 screw strain (46) and at the same time to increase construct stiffness (23,30,32). Moreover, Kostuik and associates recommended the use of anterior L5 to S1 fixation in long constructs, particularly scoliosis surgery requiring instrumentation of the lumbosacral junction (30). Based on the work of Shirado and colleagues, transpedicular screw fixation augmented with posterior interbody arthrodesis for spondylolisthesis has been shown to improve rigidity significantly at the lumbosacral junction (52).

The placement of interbody cages anteriorly or posteriorly has been described elsewhere; however, special consideration should be given to their placement. The cages should be placed in a distracted disc space to maximize annular tension, allowing for compression of the cage when the distraction is released (6). With anterior cage placement, attention must be paid to the midline so that the cages are not positioned too far lateral, compromising the neuroforamen and compressing the exiting rather than transversing nerve root. Generally, after performing a complete discectomy, the channel is tapped long and the cage countersunk so that cancellous autograft bone can be placed anterior and lateral to the cage. On follow-up lateral radiographs, trabecular bridging bone anterior to the cage can easily be visualized, providing a "sentinel sign" of successful arthrodesis (36) (Fig. 6). Use of cancellous autograft within the cages is recommended

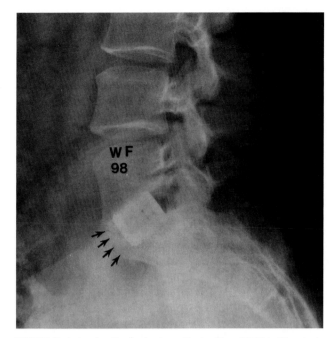

FIGURE 6. Lateral radiograph of a patient with solid L5 to S1 anterior BAK fusion with anterior bridging bone ("sentinel sign").

because of the higher rates of pseudarthroses with allograft and local bone (36).

TRANSVERTEBRAL FIXATION

Spondylolisthesis presents one of the most biomechanically challenging deformity conditions to the stabilizing effectiveness of posterior instrumentation. Although fixation at an increasing distance from the axis of rotation affords greater leverage and resistance to motion around the instantaneous axis of rotation (57), inadequate anterior column support leads to a potentially unstable mechanism (21) and an "instrumentation load-bearing" configuration. To augment segmental posterior fixation in such cases, both anterior and posterior lumbar interbody arthrodeses present viable options. Moreover, Speed was among the first to report the use of anterior transsacral (L5 to S1) fibular dowel fixation in the surgical management of medium- to high-grade spondylolisthesis (55). Cunningham and colleagues documented that an anterior L5 to S1 transsacral fibular dowel exhibits stiffness levels equivalent to a threaded fusion cage alone and posterior transpedicular fixation alone (12). Moreover, the combination of posterior screw fixation from L4 to S1 combined with transsacral L5 to S1 fixation provided significantly more stability than either reconstruction alone (Fig. 7).

The similar levels of functional unit stability when comparing transsacral techniques to pedicle screws may be attributable to the L5 to S1 axis of rotation. Transsacral fixation crosses the axis of rotation—posterior third of the lumbosacral junction (22)—whereas transpedicular fixation provides cantilever support to the axis. The clinical importance of these findings may relate to the surgical management of medium- to high-grade (grade III to IV) spondylolisthesis. In cases of high-grade slips

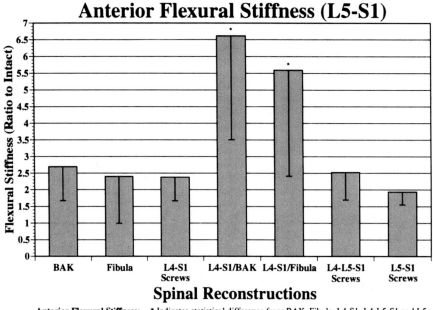

Anterior Flexural Stiffness (L5-S1)

Anterior Flexural Stiffness: - * Indicates statistical difference from BAK, Fibula, L4-S1, L4-L5-S1 and L5-S1 reconstructions (Repeated Measures ANOVA F=9.63, p<0.001). Significance is indicated at p<0.05 and error bars equal one standard deviation.

FIGURE 7. Flexion-extension stiffness in kN/M.

or other conditions in which transpedicular purchase of L5 is compromised, posterior L4 to S1 screws, combined with transsacral fixation, obviates the need for an L5 screw, and at the same time improves stability of the lumbosacral junction. The transsacral graft can be place from either anterior or posterior position. Because of excessive traction on the sacral nerve roots in order to pass the graft, this procedure usually requires

a two-stage approach. Placement of the graft is performed through an anterior approach, followed by supplemental posterior arthrodesis.

In a series by Smith and Bohlman (53), all of 11 patients achieved a solid arthrodesis after a one-stage posterior decompression with posterolateral fusion and transvertebral fibular fixation (Fig. 8).

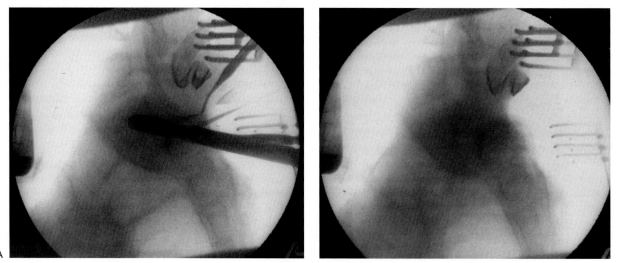

FIGURE 8. A 13-year-old girl with a high-grade type 1 (dysplastic) spondylolisthesis. She had experienced progression and failure of symptom relief from a previous L4 to sacrum in situ fusion. She had evidence of a severe L5 radiculopathy, including numbness in the L5 nerve distribution and a weak extensor hallucis longus (EHL). Straight-leg lifting was possible to only 2 inches off the examination table. Gait was waddling with a short stride length. Bowel and bladder control was normal. **A:** The 10-mm cannulated drill in place. **B:** The fibular bone graft in place in the operating room. *(Figure continues.)*

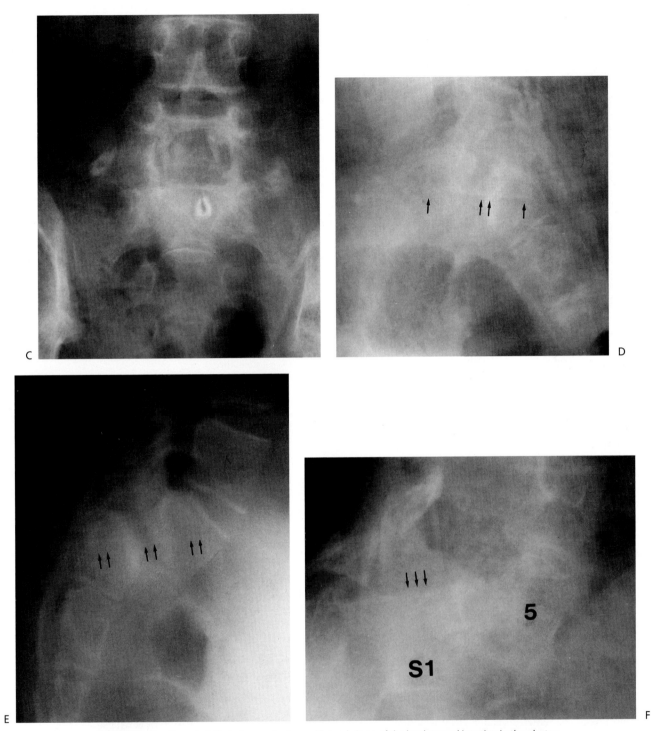

FIGURE 8. *Continued.* **C, D:** Anteroposterior and lateral views of the lumbosacral junction in the plaster pantaloon 1 week after surgery. The patient was managed postoperatively in a pantaloon spica for 6 months. **E and F:** Lateral and oblique views 6 months after surgery show good graft incorporation. The radiculopathy resolved completely, and the patient could perform the straight-leg raise to 90 degrees. (Case courtesy of Stuart L. Weinstein, M.D., University of Iowa. Reprinted with permission from Lovell W., Winter R., eds. [2000]: *Atlas of Pediatric Orthopedic Surgery,* 3rd ed. Philadelphia: Lippincott Williams & Wilkins.)

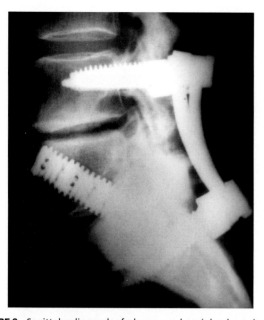

FIGURE 9. Sagittal radiograph of a human cadaveric lumbar spine with L5 to S1 anterior threaded transvertebral fusion cage and supplemental L4 to S1 pedicle screw fixation. (Case courtesy of Stuart Weinstein, M.D., University of Iowa. Reprinted with permission from Lovell W., Winter R., eds. [2000]: *Atlas of Pediatric Orthopedic Surgery,* 3rd ed. Philadelphia: Lippincott Williams & Wilkins.)

Because of the morbidity associated with harvesting a fibular graft, the use of a long, threaded cage packed with cancellous autograft can be an alternative. As discussed previously, this configuration is biomechanically equivalent to fibular autograft or posterior pedicle screw fixation (Fig. 9).

SUMMARY

From a clinical standpoint, the lumbosacral junction presents itself as the most challenging region of the spine to obtain a successful spinal arthrodesis. These motions and loads collectively contribute to the high incidence of lumbar spine pathology at the L5 to S1 level. The reason for this, in part, can be attributed to the tremendous loads encumbered by body weight coupled with the large ranges of motion and activities involving powerful muscle forces. In addition, this region of the spine serves as a transition zone, where the highly mobile lower lumbar segments adjoin the rather immobile sacral region.

REFERENCES

1. Abumi K, Punjabi M, Duranceau J (1989): Biomechanical evaluation of spinal fixation devices. Part III. Stability provided by six spinal fixation devices and interbody graft. *Spine* 14:1249.
2. Allen BL Jr, Ferguson RL (1984): The Galveston technique of pelvic fixation with L-rod instrumentation of the spine. *Spine* 9:388–94.
3. Amundson G, Edwards C, Garfin S (1998): Spondylolisthesis. In: Rothman R, Simeone F, eds. *The spine.* Philadelphia: WB Saunders, pp. 835–886.
4. Asazuma T, Stokes IA, Moreland MS, et al. (1990): Intersegmental

spinal flexibility with lumbosacral instrumentation: an in vitro biomechanical investigation. *Spine* 15:1153–1158.
5. Asher MA, Strippgen WE (1986): Anthropometric studies of the human sacrum relating to dorsal transsacral implant designs. *Clin Orthop* 203:58–62.
6. Bagby G (1988): Arthrodesis by the distraction-compression method using a stainless steel implant. *Orthopaedics* 11:931–934.
7. Boachie-Adjei O, Dendrinos GK, Ogilvie JW, et al. (1991): Management of adult spinal deformity with combined anterior-posterior arthrodesis and Luque-Galveston instrumentation. *J Spinal Disord* 4: 131–141.
8. Brown M (1980): Lumbar spine fusion. In: BE Finneson, ed. *Low back pain.* Philadelphia: JB Lippincott.
9. Carlson GD, Abitbol JJ, Anderson DR, et al. (1992): Screw fixation in the human sacrum: an in vitro study of the biomechanics of fixation. *Spine* 17:S196–S203.
10. Carson WL, Duffield RC, Arendt M, et al. (1990): Internal forces and moments in transpedicular spine instrumentation: the effect of pedicle screw angle and transfixation—the 4R-4bar linkage concept. *Spine* 15: 893–901.
11. Coe JD, Warden KE, Herzig MA, et al. (1990): Influence of bone mineral density on the fixation of thoracolumbar implants: a comparative study of transpedicular screws, laminar hooks, and spinous process wires. *Spine* 15:902–907.
12. Cunningham B, Haggerty C, Oda I, et al. (1999): *Trans-sacral fixation using the BAK threaded fusion cage: an in vitro biomechanical analysis.* Presented at the Scoliosis Research Society; September 25, 1999; San Diego, California.
13. Cunningham B, Kotani Y, Mcnulty P, et al. (1998): Video-assisted thoracoscopic surgery versus open thoracotomy for anterior thoracic spinal fusion. *Spine* 23:1333–1340.
14. Cunningham BW, Sefter JC, Shono Y, et al. (1993): Static and cyclical biomechanical analysis of pedicle screw spinal constructs. *Spine* 18: 1677–1688.
15. Dandy D, Shannon M (1971): Lumbosacral subluxation: group 1 spondylolisthesis. *J Bone Joint Surg Br* 53:578–595.
16. Duffield RC, Carson WL, Chen LY, et al. (1993): Longitudinal element size effect on load sharing, internal loads, and fatigue life of trilevel spinal implant constructs. *Spine* 18:1695–1703.
17. Emery S (1999): In situ decompression and fusion techniques for spondylolisthesis. *Semin Spine Surg* 11:34–47.
18. Esses SI, Doherty BJ, Crawford MJ, et al. (1996): Kinematic evaluation of lumbar fusion techniques. *Spine* 21:676–684.
19. Farcy J, Margulies J (1996): Iliosacral screw fixation. In: Marqulies JY, Floman Y, Farcy JPC, et al., eds. Lumbosacral and spinopelvic Fixation. Philadelphia: Lippincott-Raven, pp. 601–610.
20. Farcy JP, Rawlins BA, Glassman SD (1992): Technique and results of fixation to the sacrum with iliosacral screws. *Spine* 17:S190–S195.
21. Gaines RW Jr, Carson WL, Satterlee CC, et al. (1991): Experimental evaluation of seven different spinal fracture internal fixation devices using nonfailure stability testing: the load-sharing and unstable-mechanism concepts. *Spine* 16:902–909.
22. Gertzbein SD, Holtby R, Tile M, et al. (1984): Determination of a locus of instantaneous centers of rotation of the lumbar disc by moire fringes: a new technique. *Spine* 9:409–413.
23. Glazer PA, Colliou O, Lotz JC, et al. (1996): Biomechanical analysis of lumbosacral fixation. *Spine* 21:1211–1222.
24. Guyer DW, Yuan HA, Werner FW, et al (1987): Biomechanical comparison of seven internal fixation devices for the lumbosacral junction. *Spine* 12:569–573.
25. Haher TR, Bergman M, O'Brien M, et al. (1991): The effect of the three columns of the spine on the instantaneous axis of rotation in flexion and extension. *Spine* 16:S312–S318.
26. Harris I, Weinstein S (1987): Long-term follow-up of patients with grade III and IV spondylolisthesis. *J Bone Joint Surg Am* 63:960–969.
27. Hu S, Deckey J (1999): Reduction techniques for spondylolisthesis. *Semin Spine Surg* 11:48–55.
28. Jackson R, McManus A (1993): The iliac buttress: a computed tomographic study of sacral anatomy. *Spine* 18:1318–1328.

29. Jenis L, An H (1999): Posterior lumbar interbody fusion for spondylolisthesis. *Semin Spine Surg* 11:56–65.
30. Kostuik JP, Valdevit A, Chang HG, et al. (1998): Biomechanical testing of the lumbosacral spine. *Spine* 23:1721–1728.
31. Krag M (1990): Biomechanics of transpedicle spinal fixation. In: Weinstein JN, Wiesel S, eds. *The lumbar spine.* Philadelphia: WB Saunders, p. 916.
32. Lee CK, Langrana NA (1984): Lumbosacral spinal fusion: a biomechanical study. *Spine* 9:574–581.
33. Lin P, Cautilli R, Joyce M (1983): Posterior lumbar interbody fusion. *Clin Orthop* 180:154–167.
34. Mardjetko S, Lubicky J (1996): Disorders of the spinopelvic junction: indications for fixation and fusion—pediatric aspects. In: Margulies JY, Floman Y, Farcy JPC, et al., eds. *Lumbosacral and spinopelvic fixation.* Philadelphia: Lippincott-Raven, pp. 129–142.
35. Margulies J, Armour E, Kohler-Ekstrand C, et al. (1999): Revision of fusion from the spine to the sacropelvis: considerations. In: Margulies JY, Abei M, Farcy JPC, eds. *Revision spine surgery.* Philadelphia: CV Mosby, pp. 623–630.
36. McAfee P, Cunningham B, Lee G, et al. (1999): Revision strategies for salvaging or improving failed cylindrical cages. *Spine* 24:2147–2153.
37. McAfee P, Regan J, Geis P, et al. (1998): Minimally invasive anterior retroperitoneal approach to the lumbar spine: emphasis on the lateral BAK. *Spine* 23:1476–1483.
38. McAfee PC, Bohlman HH (1985): Complications following Harrington instrumentation for fractures of the thoracolumbar spine. *J Bone Joint Surg Am* 67:672–686.
39. McCord DH, Cunningham BW, Shono Y, et al. (1992): Biomechanical analysis of lumbosacral fixation. *Spine* 17:S235–S243.
40. McGlashen KM, Miller JA, Schultz AB, et al. (1987): Load displacement behavior of the human lumbo-sacral joint. *J Orthop Res* 5:488–496.
41. Miller J, Schultz A, Anderson G (1987): Load-displacement behavior of sacroiliac joints. *J Orthop Res* 5:92.
42. Nachemson A (1966): The load on lumbar disks in different positions of the body. *Clin Orthop* 45:107–122.
43. Nachemson A, Elfstrom G (1970): Intravital dynamic pressure measurements in lumbar discs: a study of common movements, maneuvers and exercises. *Scand J Rehabil Med Suppl* 1:1–40.
44. Nachemson A, Morris J (1964): In vivo measurements of intradiscal pressure. *J Bone Joint Surg Am* 46:1077–1092.
45. Nachemson AL, Schultz AB, Berkson MH (1979): Mechanical properties of human lumbar spine motion segments: influence of age, sex, disc level, and degeneration. *Spine* 4:1–8.
46. Pashman RS, Hu SS, Schendel MJ, et al. (1993): Sacral screw loads in lumbosacral fixation for spinal deformity. *Spine* 18:2465–2470.
47. Pearcy M, Portek I, Shepherd J (1984): Three-dimensional x-ray analysis of normal movement in the lumbar spine. *Spine* 9:294–297.
48. Pearcy MJ, Tibrewal SB (1984): Axial rotation and lateral bending in the normal lumbar spine measured by three-dimensional radiography. *Spine* 9:582–587.
49. Ruland CM, McAfee PC, Warden KE, et al. (1991): Triangulation of pedicular instrumentation. A biomechanical analysis. *Spine* 16: S270–S276.
50. Saer EHD, Winter RB, Lonstein JE (1990): Long scoliosis fusion to the sacrum in adults with nonparalytic scoliosis: an improved method. *Spine* 15:650–653.
51. Schufflebarger H (1991): Prevention of the crankshaft phenomenon. *Spine* 16:409.
52. Shirado O, Zdeblick TA, McAfee PC, et al. (1991): Biomechanical evaluation of methods of posterior stabilization of the spine and posterior lumbar interbody arthrodesis for lumbosacral isthmic spondylolisthesis: a calf-spine model. *J Bone Joint Surg Am* 73:518–526.
53. Smith M, Bohlman H (1990): Spondylolisthesis treated by a single-stage operation combining decompression with in situ posterolateral and anterior fusion. *J Bone Joint Surg Am* 72:415–421.
54. Smith SA, Abitbol JJ, Carlson GD, et al. (1993): The effects of depth of penetration, screw orientation, and bone density on sacral screw fixation. *Spine* 18:1006–1010.
55. Speed K (1938): Spondylolisthesis: treatment by anterior bone graft. *Arch Surg* 37:175–189.
56. Stovall DO Jr, Goodrich JA, Lundy D, et al (1997): Sacral fixation technique in lumbosacral fusion. *Spine* 22:32–37.
57. White A, Punjabi M (1990): *Clinical biomechanics of the spine.* Philadelphia: JB Lippincott.
58. Wood K, Schendel M, Ogilvie J, et al. (1996): Effect of sacral and iliac instrumentation on strains in the pelvis. *Spine* 21:1185–1191.
59. Yoshioka T, Tsuji H, Hirano N, et al. (1990): Motion characteristic of the normal lumbar spine in young adults: instantaneous axis of rotation and vertebral center motion analyses. *J Spinal Disord* 3: 103–113.
60. Zdeblick TA (1993): A prospective randomized study of lumbar fusion. *Spine* 18:1673.
61. Zindrick MR, Wiltse LL, Widell EH, et al. A biomechanical study of intrapedicular screw fixation in the lumbosacral spine. *Clin Orthop* 203:99–112.

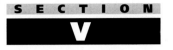

SECTION
V

COMPLICATIONS OF SURGERY

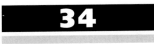

COMPLICATIONS OF SPINAL SURGERY

STEPHEN J. TREDWELL
CHRISTOPHER W. REILLY

Complications of a medical treatment are usually considered in relation to a specific operation or disease entity, such as complications of spondylolisthesis surgery or complications of anterior spinal approaches. This chapter draws complications together under various headings that relate to the nature of the patient's difficulty rather than to the individual's gross anatomical defect or the surgical procedure used. Two factors not normally considered complications—pain and blood loss—are discussed to emphasize their importance to the patient's overall well-being. This chapter also deals with the concepts of materials failure in two areas. One section details complications arising from biologic failures, such as pseudarthrosis, and the other deals with problems arising from implant or mechanical failure. In each section of this chapter, the groups at risk are identified, suggestions for avoiding complications made, and treatment procedures for these complications outlined.

PAIN

As for all surgical patients, pain control for children undergoing spinal surgery begins long before the initial anesthetic is administered. To treat these children effectively, surgeons must reassess and improve their understanding of acute physiologic pain.

The classic perception that painful stimuli act on small-caliber unmyelinated nerve fibers in the periphery, which in turn connect with second-order neurons in the dorsal horn and then through the spinal thalamic tracts to the thalamic areas of the brain, is inaccurate. As the vast proliferation of journals and texts on pain attests, what a patient perceives to be a painful stimulus and how that patient responds to that stimulus is a complex and incompletely understood physiologic process.

Woolf separates pain into two groups based on the intensity of and response to the noxious stimuli (115). Acute physiologic pain, that is, pain produced by high-intensity stimuli that have the potential to damage normal tissue, is transmitted by primary afferent neurons that have a relatively high threshold, and the result, reflex or avoidance, is aimed at protecting the body from injury. Acute pathologic pain, on the other hand, results from abnormal activation of the afferent system and produces a hyperalgesic state.

Postoperatively, patients experience pain as a result of peripheral tissue damage and the associated inflammatory response. These stimuli serve to lower the threshold of the afferent system and also to change the central neural reaction to the normal input. Consequently, stimuli not normally considered noxious begin to produce pain, whereas those that are normally painful produce an exaggerated and prolonged response.

Acute pathologic pain depends on afferent input. The light level of general anesthetic techniques currently in use does not prevent this flood of afferent stimuli.

The surgical patient's acute pain threshold can be altered by providing a peripheral local anesthetic blockade before noxious stimuli, by administration of a preoperative narcotic, and/or by administration of an antiinflammatory medication before and after stimulus (98). If the noxious stimuli normally transmitted under general anesthetic are prevented from reaching the spinal cord by adjunctive local block, sensitization and resulting hyperalgesia can be prevented or reduced. McQuay et al. showed that preoperative morphine administration can successfully decrease postoperative pain in the first 5 hours after surgery, presumably by suppressing the spinal cord's ability to reach a hyperexcitable state (67). Anti-inflammatory drugs act peripherally as cyclooxygenase inhibitors, reducing the synthesis of prostaglandins that act directly on the peripheral receptors to lower their threshold of stimuli. Because these three strategies act at different levels in pain perception and transmission, they are probably best used in concert rather than individually.

Administration of epidural morphine has been advocated by Amaranth et al. (4) to reduce the total narcotic requirements in the early postoperative period, but use of epidural morphine presents a slight risk of respiratory depression. Respiratory function of patients receiving this type of analgesic regimen must be closely monitored.

A combination of epidural morphine and bupivacaine has also proven to be an effective pain regimen. The adverse effects of this treatment include pruritis, nausea, and urinary retention.

S. J. Tredwell and C. W. Reilly: Department of Orthopedic Surgery, British Columbia's Children's Hospital, Vancouver, British Columbia, Canada V6H 3V4.

A review of 71 patients by Shaw et al. continued epidural control of pain with a combination of morphine bupivacaine for the first 3 days after surgery (94). Shaw reported 90% with satisfactory control of postoperative pain using the technique.

The emotional state of the patient, both pre- and postoperatively, is as important as the pharmacologic methods used for pain prevention. A relaxed preoperative patient often experiences less postoperative pain. Access to a sufficient dose and frequency of analgesia postoperatively can preserve this emotional stability and therefore decrease pain. Patient-controlled analgesia or continuous opioid infusion provides better pain control than bolus intramuscular (IM) or intravenous (IV) narcotics administered by an intermediary.

The review of Beaulieu et al. involving 100 adolescent patients supports this thesis (6). This study reported improved pain control along with excellent control of side effects, which included nausea and vomiting in 45% and pruritis in 15% of the patients. Respiratory depression can occur in patient-controlled analgesia with higher boluses in the range of 25 mg/kg.

Children undergoing spinal surgery should receive preoperative medication, including an opioid. Postoperative narcotics should be administered in adequate dosages and should be patient-controlled. Injection of local anesthetic to the initial incision mutes the resulting afferent barrage and therefore is an integral part of an overall pain prevention strategy. Although postoperative pain is an inevitable consequence of spinal surgery, planning and sensitivity to the plight of patients can lessen their discomfort.

PULMONARY DYSFUNCTION

Pulmonary difficulties represent the most common perioperative cause of increased morbidity after spinal surgery. Preoperative assessment should be tailored to the patient's baseline pulmonary function and risk factors. Patients can be classified into two easily recognizable groups: those with preexisting pulmonary compromise and those without. Healthy patients with normal underlying pulmonary function should be evaluated with a careful history and physical examination. Vedantam and Crawford established little correlation between preoperative pulmonary function results and postoperative complication rates; therefore, routine pulmonary function tests are not indicated for patients with healthy pulmonary function (107). Patients with preoperative pulmonary compromise who require careful preoperative assessment include those with muscle diseases, cerebral palsy, infantile or juvenile-onset idiopathic scoliosis, and severe congenital scoliosis.

Careful preoperative evaluation and management of high-risk patients can allow pulmonary management problems to be anticipated and thereby minimized. If possible, the patient should be scheduled at a time of maximum pulmonary health, avoiding periods of high community viral pulmonary infection rates; smoking should be eliminated in the patient's environment; and reversible reactive airway disease should be aggressively managed.

Pulmonary function studies are a key component of the pre-

operative workup in the high-risk group. The interpretation of these results is complex, and the degree of pulmonary compromise may be overestimated. Patient effort can be variable, especially that of patients with cognitive impairment or patients younger than 5 years. Some neuromuscular patients cannot achieve an efficient seal despite mouthpiece modification. The scoliotic spinal deformity itself clearly leads to a progressive deterioration in pulmonary function once it exceeds 70 degrees, characterized by a restrictive breathing pattern and reduced vital capacity. With careful pulmonary management, patients with vital capacities of 30% can be successfully treated. Problems with alveolar gas exchange are a late-developing component of pulmonary deterioration in progressive scoliosis. Rarely, pediatric patients with severe curves will present with an elevated CO_2 identified on arterial blood gas measurement. This group may have a primary hypoxic drive; therefore, careful postoperative care requires ventilation.

Patients with muscular dystrophy require careful pulmonary planning before surgery. The classic patient with Duchenne muscular dystrophy shows a predictable decrease in pulmonary function secondary to the disease itself, the progressive scoliosis, and the associated cardiomyopathy. This condition, together with the general weakness of the skeletal muscles due to this disease, makes the postoperative period hazardous. The combination of decreased pulmonary function and gradual increase in scoliosis allows a surgical window of opportunity in patients who are wheelchair-bound, whose spinal curve is between 30 degrees and 50 degrees, and whose pulmonary functions show vital capacity greater than 40%. During this optimum surgical period, simple posterior instrumentation achieves a virtually straight spine and allows ease of positioning during the late stages of the muscular dystrophy.

Pulmonary problems during the optimum surgical period are significant but not overwhelming. Preoperative physiotherapy is essential. Surgical instrumentation with a posterior segmental system allows early postoperative mobilization (102). Planned anesthetic and intensive care unit consultation permits the patient to remain intubated in an intensive care unit during the first 12 to 24 hours after surgery. Postoperative intubation produces a good respiratory toilet, provides for gradual weaning from the respirator, and lessens the effort required for the patient to breathe (26).

As the muscular dystrophy progresses and respiratory function becomes poorer, the scoliotic curve becomes larger and more rigid. Therefore, at some point operative intervention poses an equal or a greater hazard than the natural history of the disease. Patients with severe cardiomyopathy and severe respiratory compromise are often best treated with a palliative program and by being provided with a molded insert in their chair to make them as comfortable as possible. Tilt-in-space capability on the patient's power wheelchair leads to improved patient comfort and endurance as well as minimization of the effect of gravity on curve progression. Surgical intervention in such severe cases carries a high risk of significant perioperative morbidity and mortality for little practical gain. Vital capacity deterioration below 30% of predicted is a major concern in this patient group. It is an indicator of poor tissue quality in addition to severe pulmonary compromise. At this stage in the disease, the patient's muscles, including paraspinal muscles, have been largely replaced by fibrofatty tissue. This increases the risk of infection in a patient group that will not tolerate multiple surgical debridements.

Patients with spinal muscular atrophy do not have the associated cardiomyopathy of those in the dystrophy group. Many patients with Werdnig-Hoffmann or Kugelberg-Welander disease develop a curve before age 10 years. Bracing allows an additional two or three years of growth before surgery is indicated. Again, segmental posterior instrumentation to allow early postoperative mobilization is important, as is maintenance of an endotracheal tube for the first day or two following surgery (17).

Patients with cerebral palsy have three potential problems that may affect respiratory function. The first problem stems from the general weakness and lack of coordination of these patients. They are primarily diaphragm breathers and have a poor cough mechanism. A respiratory physiotherapist should be involved in their treatment both before and after surgery.

The second problem involves patients with severe quadriplegic involvement. Patients with large curves often have gastrointestinal problems, typically gastric reflux with aspiration. Preoperative assessment by a gastroenterology team often identifies this problem, and appropriate medical/surgical management can prevent postoperative problems.

The third problem involves central control of respiration. Some severely affected patients with spastic quadriparesis have died suddenly in the postoperative period with no better explanation than a broad diagnosis of respiratory failure with no obvious pulmonary disease. These patients may have experienced central respiratory death. Although this may not be preventable, preoperative family counseling should include this cause of sudden death as a risk.

Patients with severe congenital scoliosis, particularly those who undergo surgery in late childhood or early adolescence, may actually have a greater decrease in functioning lung volume than predicted values. The basic anatomy and physiology of the lung shows a standard number of alveoli present at birth, but these alveoli are not fully developed. Complete development and inflation of the alveolar buds occurs by approximately 8 years of age. In patients with severe scoliosis in the first years of life and secondary restriction of the size of the thoracic cage, complete development and inflation of the alveolar buds may not occur. These patients and those with severe infantile idiopathic scoliosis should undergo thorough pulmonary function testing before surgery (Fig. 1).

Pehrsson et al. (79) studied 115 patients with untreated idiopathic scoliosis with onset in the infant and juvenile period. Of the 54 deaths from natural causes in this group, 21 were caused by respiratory failure and 17 resulted from cardiovascular disease. Increased mortality was also noted in patients with congenital scoliosis and other scolioses when onset occurred in infancy or early childhood, but this study could not demonstrate early mortality in any form of adolescence-onset scoliosis.

Intraoperative pulmonary difficulty can occur with combined anterior and posterior spinal procedures. Chest tube placement is routine after anterior transthoracic approaches; however, in sequential front and back procedures, the chest tube can become blocked when the patient is moved to the prone position. Positive-pressure ventilation can rapidly lead to a tension pneumothorax. In isolated posterior procedures, severe chest wall deformity can allow the pleural cavity to be easily opened inadvertently. A pneumothorax should be considered if ventilatory pressures increase or if the patient's general condition deteriorates.

Air embolism can lead to rapid cardiorespiratory collapse (63). Patients undergoing kyphectomy are at risk for air embolism. The apex of the kyphos is elevated significantly with the patient prone. As the lordotic portion of the curve above the apex is dissected out, massive bleeding can be encountered, which usually stems from foraminal vessels and the epidural veins running along the posterior longitudinal ligament. If the patient's intravascular volume is low, the venous pressure will drop during mechanical expiration and air may be entrained. The Trendelenburg position, used to reduce epidural venous pressure and reduce bleeding, can actually increase the risk of air embolism.

Postoperative management of high-risk patients requires a team approach. Early mobilization, incentive spirometry, and chest physiotherapy are key tools for minimizing pulmonary complications. Good pain management also plays a critical role in allowing patients to mobilize and to cooperate with their therapy. Combined anterior and posterior spinal fusion patients are at greatest risk for atelectasis. Interestingly, in 30 sequential anterior and posterior spinal surgery patients at Children's Hospital in Vancouver, British Columbia, the dependent or downside lung was more frequently and more severely involved (Fig. 2). At the completion of the anterior and posterior procedures, the lung is routinely reinflated prior to extubation. Physiotherapy should be directed to both lung fields.

Postoperative fluid management should be carefully monitored. Advances in surgical techniques continue to lead to reductions in intraoperative blood loss. Most patients are euvolemic or hypervolemic at the completion of the surgery. Postoperative fluid loss needs to be followed more closely after anterior surgery because large, unrecognized losses after posterior procedures are unusual. Antidiuretic hormone (ADH) secretion has been recognized in scoliosis patients as leading to low urine output despite euvolemia. Crystalloid boluses will not improve urine output in this setting and will lead to deterioration in pulmonary status. Neuromuscular scoliosis patients are at particular risk. Abnormalities of peripheral vasomotor tone may lead to hypotension in the postoperative period despite adequate central venous pressure. Repetitive fluid boluses will increase the patient's pulmonary complication rate; he or she may be better treated with judicious use of vasopressors.

A pneumothorax can occur after posterior surgery. A lung air leak can be produced because of surgical penetration of the chest or can occur spontaneously due to an underlying lung bleb. Thoracoplasty increases the risk of pneumothorax, and insertion of a chest tube may be required. Revision anterior surgery can produce significant air leaks due to intrapleural scarring that must be taken down during the surgical approach. Prolonged chest tube drainage may be required, and intraopera-

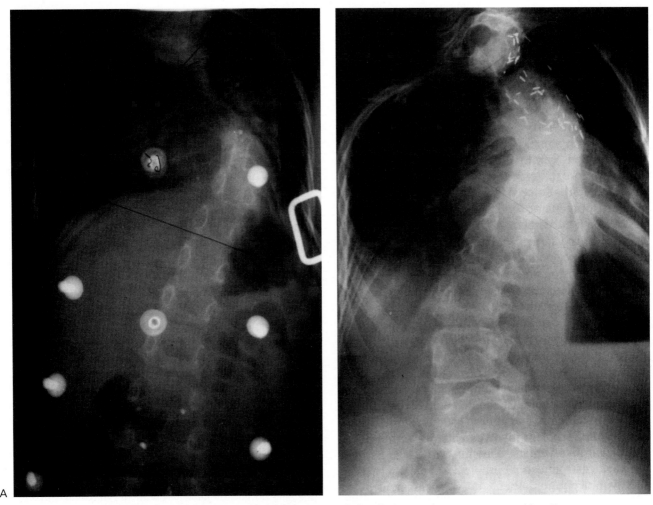

FIGURE 1. A: A 4-year-old girl with 65-degree congenital scoliosis secondary to unsegmented bar. **B:** Same patient at age 16 after multiple anterior and posterior procedures to stabilize the curvature, with rib deformity and small chest cavity apparent. Vital capacity is 25% of normal. The patient has dyspnea on exertion.

tive thoracic surgical consultation should be considered in cases involving recognized high-flow air leaks.

Significant hemothoraces should be recognized on the postoperative chest radiographs. The bleeding is commonly due to an intercostal vessel and may be seen after rib resection. After anterior surgery, prolonged bloody chest tube output may also be due to a segmental vessel injury. The vessels laceration may occur during chest closure, especially if sutures are used around the ribs to approximate the chest wall. In both anterior and posterior cases, prolonged blood loss should be managed with thoracotomy and ligation of the vessel.

Intraoperative thoracic duct injury can lead to a chylothorax and should be repaired if recognized. Postoperative management includes maintenance of chest tube drainage and reduction of fat intake, which in difficult cases may require prolonged total parenteral nutrition. Thoracic duct injuries are difficult to repair, and the distal duct may be difficult to identify and ligate after

previous anterior surgery. This complication can be difficult to manage.

Pulmonary function is not significantly improved postoperatively in idiopathic scoliosis patients. If a thoracoplasty is completed at the time of surgery, there is a reduction in postoperative function that takes 2 years to return to preoperative levels. In adult scoliosis, there may be a permanent reduction in pulmonary function after thoracoplasty (57).

Pulmonary function has been noted to decrease slightly or remain the same after combined anterior and posterior procedures, with some loss in anterior and posterior fusions for Scheuermann disease (47). Patients with the lordotic curves associated with Marfan syndrome have shown decreased postoperative respiratory function, perhaps potentiated by the pectus excavatum deformity of the chest. Segmental instrumentation in neuromuscular curves with early postoperative mobilization causes little decrease in lung function.

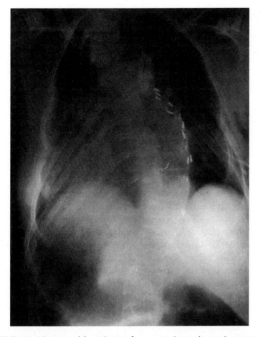

FIGURE 2. A 12-year-old patient after anterior release in preparation for posterior instrumentation as second stage. Postoperative atelectatic change evident on the nonoperated side responded to simple physiotherapy.

NEUROLOGIC COMPLICATIONS

The most devastating complication of spinal surgery is postoperative neurologic damage. Postoperative neurologic problems were rare before the advent of implantable spinal instrumentation. With today's increasing ability to correct and control spinal deformity, more stress is placed on the contents of the spinal canal.

Spinal deformity correction impacts on the spinal cord in two ways: coincidental and direct. Coincidental damage occurs through distraction of the neural elements themselves or through interference with the blood supply to the spinal cord. Direct injury to the cord arises from improper placement of a hook or sublaminar wire or from an inadvertent fracture of the lamina and impingement of the contents during surgical exposure.

Most cases of Brown-Séquard syndrome can be traced to direct intraoperative cord contusion. Anterior spinal artery damage manifests as a predominance of motor over sensory loss, with the greatest preservation of posterior column function. Because most case reports classify neurologic damage as complete or incomplete, a true determination of the percentage of vascular as compared with pure distraction of neural elements is not possible.

With a complication as catastrophic as paraparesis or paraplegia, the major emphasis must be prevention; therefore, the first step requires recognition of high-risk cases. Patients with greatest risk are those with short-arc kyphosis (congenital kyphosis, neurofibromatosis, and skeletal dysplasia) and those with postinfection kyphosis (59). In such patients, the risk is proportional to the size of the kyphosis and the rigidity of the curve. Winter et al. detailed the risk of spinal cord and/or anterior spinal artery damage from preoperative traction in this group (113).

A second factor increasing operative risk is intraspinal anomaly. This occurs primarily in congenital scoliosis patients. McMaster reported 18% occult anomalies in 251 cases of congenital scoliosis cases (66). In a urodynamics study of children with congenital spinal anomalies, Goldberg et al. reported abnormal results in 40% (41). In McMaster's series, the most common anomaly evident on myelogram was diastematomyelia; cysts, teratoma, tethering of the cord, lipoma, and lipofibroma were also noted. The highest incidence of anomaly was evident in the unilateral unsegmented bar with a contralateral hemivertebra. In congenital deformities (kyphotic or scoliotic), preoperative traction is contraindicated, and preoperative myelography or magnetic resonance imaging (MRI) is mandatory (Fig. 3).

Also to be considered for MRI are younger children with rapidly progressive curvatures. Although not as ominous as first reported in the literature, left thoracic curves still deserve detailed neurologic examination. Zadeh reported on 12 children with persistent absent superficial abdominal reflexes, 10 of whom showed syringomyelia on MRI (119). Yngve screened 65 normal adolescents and young adults for the presence of superficial abdominal reflexes (116). His results showed that 15% of the study group had an absence of abdominal reflexes in all quadrants. However, no subjects showed presence of the reflex on one side and absence on the other. Difficulties in preoperative evaluation lead some investigators to examine the use of routine MRI of neurologically normal idiopathic scoliotic patients. Shen in 1996 and Winter in 1997 reported on a combined total of 212 clinically normal adolescent idiopathic scoliotic patients who underwent preoperative MRI (95,112). Neither study supported the validity of MRI as a preoperative tool for otherwise normal adolescent idiopathic scoliotic patients.

Less specific risk factors include the rigidity and size of the curve. In scoliotic deformities, a large, rigid curve represents a high-risk situation both in correction of the curve and in instrumentation systems that demand insertion of hooks or wires into the rigid apex (103). These are the curves that are at risk of intraoperative laminar fracture and spinal cord damage.

Even with adequate preoperative assessment, intraoperative monitoring is important. In 1973, Vauzelle et al. reported functional monitoring of the spinal cord during spinal surgery (106). They described the wake-up test, which gained rapid acceptance in the 1970s and early 1980s. Patients with preexisting neurologic problems, such as myelomeningocele, cerebral palsy, and spinal muscular atrophy, or patients with mental retardation are poor candidates for this test. This technique carries a risk of extubation and makes it difficult for the anesthesiologist to use halothane or to modify the patient's blood pressure. In addition, the intraoperative wake-up test relies on motion of toes and feet only, and therefore can miss subtle lesions.

Hoppenfeld et al. reported a different form of clinical examination following surgery (49). They observed that a transient ankle clonus is normal and expected in patients recovering from general anesthetic and that absence of transient ankle clonus during arousal from anesthetic is indicative of neurologic defect. This observation was made on 1,006 patients who underwent spinal surgery. Nine patients failed to show ankle clonus on

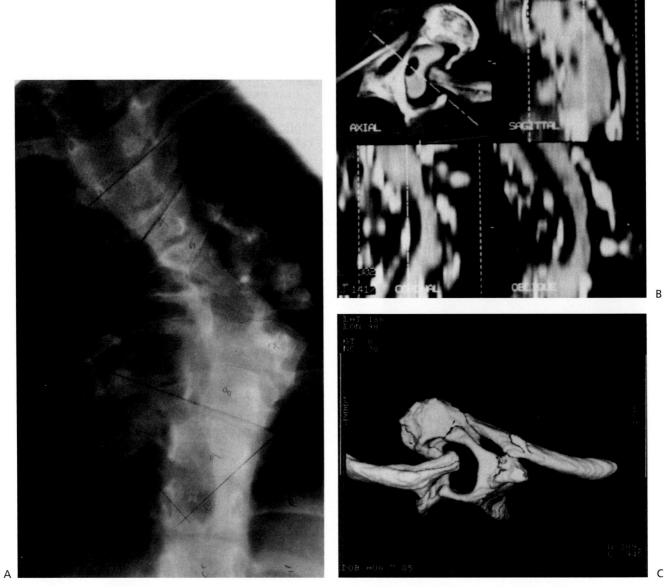

FIGURE 3. The value of preoperative myelography. **A:** Anteroposterior (AP) spine of an 8-year-old girl with a severe focal midthoracic scoliosis initially believed to be of congenital etiology. Neurologic examination was entirely normal. The curve had progressed 20 degrees in the previous year. **B:** Computed tomography myelograms showing rib dislocation into the canal with compression of the dural sac. **C:** Three-dimensional reconstruction of the involved apical area showing rib intrusion into the canal. Further work-up demonstrated the etiology of the curve to be neurofibromatosis.

emerging from general anesthetic; six of the nine had a neurologic deficit. There were no false-negative results in this series; however, there were three false positives, indicating that the presence of ankle clonus portends an intact spinal cord.

Another useful technique for monitoring of spinal cord function is either by evoking somatosensory evoked potential (SEP) or motor evoked potential (MEP) (111). However, these methods also pose problems. Technical difficulties arise from the choice of anesthetic agents, such as halothane, and the use of depressants, such as droperidol. Use of intrathecal opioids for

pain control does not mask monitoring; therefore, it has no noticeable effect on SEP/MEP latency or amplitude (42). In addition, a decrease in core temperature increases SEP latency and decreases its amplitude. Unfortunately, neither SEP nor MEP monitors the entire spinal cord.

When SEP monitoring is used, York et al. recommend that a latency change of 15% or an amplitude change of 50% be considered an indication for major concern (118). Edgar et al., reporting on use of epidural leads as compared with the leads of York et al., use an amplitude change of 40% as the upper limit (35). Despite intraoperative monitoring, delayed lesions of the spinal cord can still occur, appearing in the early postoperative period (40).

Certain diagnostic groups are more difficult to monitor than others. A combination of SEPs and MEPs reported by Ecker showed that 31 of 34 cerebral palsy patients could be monitored (34). Cortical SEPs are more affected by anesthetics when recorded from patients with neuromuscular disease than with routine idiopathic scoliosis.

The total incidence of spinal cord damage during corrective surgery for scoliosis has become increasingly hard to document because of the proliferation of new instruments and the varying degree to which intraoperative monitoring is performed. In 1975, McEwen et al. reported an incidence of 1.17% in a review of 9,680 cases submitted by members of the Scoliosis Research Society (65). In 1983, part of that same society reported an incidence of 0.72%. The difference between these two studies is probably not significant. The reports from the Society showed that incomplete spinal cord lesions outnumbered complete lesions by 3:2. As the monitoring systems became more sophisticated, the reporting levels changed to include transient changes in evoked potentials. In 1984, Wilbur et al. published one of the first reports detailing changes in SEPs during spinal instrumentation (111). Their report of a 4% incidence rate of patients showing change reflects an increased sensitivity of this type of monitoring rather than an absolute increase in pathology.

In 1998, Bridwell reported on a retrospective study of 1,090 patients undergoing corrective spine surgery (16). Among these patients, he found four major neurologic defects (0.39%). Three of the four were vascular and one had a mechanical component. All four resulted from complex surgeries that included ligation of the convex segmental vessels.

Although most neurologic complications secondary to vascular compromise occur during surgery, there are at least five cases reported since 1995 of the compromise delayed to the postoperative period.

The important issue is not the incidence of complications but rather the fact that complications do exist and that no spinal reconstructive service can avoid the problem completely. When complications are diagnosed intraoperatively, either by wake-up test or spinal cord monitoring, the universal recommendation is to modify or remove the internal fixation device. However, guidelines for management of a case that appears in the early postoperative period are not as clear. Although the initial response may be to remove the equipment as an emergency procedure, existing data do not support this action. This is especially true of an incomplete lesion. McEwen et al. reported no difference in the course of incomplete lesions whether the rods were left in or removed (65). The possible morbidity associated with a second surgical procedure must be considered, especially with implants that involve sublaminar wires.

In the event of a neurologic complication during surgery, first ensure that the patient's blood pressure has returned to normal and that the circulating volume is physiologic. Intraoperative myelography may be performed if mechanical compromise is suspected. Intraoperative steroid administration should be started immediately according to spinal injury protocols. If the spine has been elongated, the implant should be removed.

Preoperative steroid prophylaxis is indicated for the cord in high-risk patients. Research on animal models demonstrated that early intervention with steroids produced significant benefit. These studies showed that the experimental group receiving steroid treatment before trauma fared better than groups receiving steroid treatment post trauma. Sensible prophylaxis now appears to indicate the use of preoperative steroids in patients who have a preexisting neurologic lesion or in rigid kyphotic patients undergoing anterior decompression and strut grafting.

Use of intraoperative hypotension to reduce blood loss is attractive. Using a dog model, Kling et al. demonstrated that with classic hypotensive techniques spinal cord blood flow decreases with hypotension (52). The dog model shows evidence of an autoregulation phenomenon with a return to normal blood flow approximately 35 minutes after onset of hypotension. Intraoperative maintenance of fluid volumes is important; if intraoperative hypotension is used, a latency period that allows for return of normal blood flow should be observed. Because this latency in humans is unknown, it is advisable that distraction not be carried out until hypotension has persisted for at least 30 minutes. The instrumentation implanted during scoliosis correction can also cause delayed neurologic problems (41). Kornberg et al. and Hale et al. report radicular problems related to the lower hook in Harrington instrumentation systems (55,44). All of Hale's patients had been instrumented at L5 and had migration of the hook through the lamina and into the canal. This complication typifies two problems: first, the inability to contour the Harrington system to the normal lordosis results in a force directed onto the lamina so that penetration into the canal can occur, and second, instrumenting down to the fifth lumbar vertebra should be avoided.

Surgery for spondylolisthesis in children and adolescents also carries a risk of neurologic problems. Bradford and Boachie-Adjei reported that the natural history of severe spondylolisthesis includes deficits in nerve root and/or bladder (14). Schonecker et al. reported 12 patients in whom simple posterolateral fusion for severe spondylolisthesis resulted in cauda equina syndrome (91). Decompression in this situation involves removal of the posterior superior ridge of the body of the S1 vertebra, usually through a posterior approach. This suggests that preoperative evaluation of severe spondylolisthesis patients by myelography or MRI may identify cases of severe impingement of the dorsal superior ridge of S1. In these cases, decompression may be performed electively as part of the initial procedure.

In procedures that involve reduction of the severe spondylolisthesis, neurologic complications have also been reported. Three of the 22 patients with grade IV and V spondylolisthesis reported by Bradford and Gotfried sustained postoperative neurologic problems (11).

Neurologic complications are an unavoidable consequence of any reconstructive spinal surgery. Through identification of high-risk patients, careful planning, intraoperative monitoring, and meticulous technique, the devastating effects of these neurologic complications can be minimized.

BLOOD LOSS

Control of blood loss during spinal surgery is an important objective. Two goals are paramount: first, reducing the actual amount of blood lost; and second, minimizing use of homologous blood when transfusion is required.

Some disorders place the patient at greater risk of blood loss than others. For example, neuromuscular scoliosis with its combination of osteoporosis and hypotonia can lead to increased blood loss and decreased ability of the body to compensate for the blood lost. Patients with neurofibromatosis may have abnormal vascular anatomy that exacerbates the problems of blood loss.

Blood loss can be reduced by various techniques. First, the patient should be positioned so that the abdomen lies free and compression of the inferior vena cava is avoided. The frame popularized by Relton and Hall accomplishes this, as do some specially designed spinal tables.

Second, surgical technique can be modified to minimize blood loss. Moe suggested injecting the incision line with dilute epinephrine solution (71). The use of electrocautery minimizes blood loss during dissection. Intraoperative hypotension has been commonly used, but potential risks do exist relating to spinal cord blood flow and renal dysfunction. Rylance et al. reported 43 patients whose blood loss averaged 725 mL when systolic blood pressure was held between 60 and 70 mm Hg (87). They noted no abnormalities in renal function and no significant changes in spinal cord monitoring. However, in a well-controlled study, Lennon et al. showed that hypotension did not add to blood conservation (58).

There may be special places for the use of hypotensive anesthesia. Fox used a hypotensive anesthetic technique that maintained systolic blood pressure between 75 and 85 mm Hg to examine 19 patients with Duchenne muscular dystrophy. He reported a significant reduction in blood loss using a posterior fixation system with sublaminar wiring.

Preoperative desmopressin has been recommended by Kobrinsky et al. (54), but this agent has a possible complicating effect because it is an antidiuretic and may compound the normal postoperative oliguric state. Guay et al. and Theroux et al. were unable to demonstrate a beneficial effect of desmopressin in a prospective, randomized, double-blind study (43).

Preoperative use of erythropoietin has a theoretical advantage in scoliosis surgery. Vitale et al. examined a series of 178 pediatric patients, 44% of whom received preoperative erythropoietin (108). This retrospective review found that the idiopathic subgroup within the main group showed a reduction in the need for blood transfusion. Of the erythropoietin-treated group, 3.9% required blood by transfusion compared with 23% of the non-treated idiopathic scoliosis group.

Tredwell and Sawatzky reported on a study of 33 patients undergoing corrective surgery for adolescent idiopathic scoliosis where intraoperative fibrin sealant was used to control blood loss (105). When applied to denuded cancellous bone during surgery, the application of fibrin sealant resulted in a significant reduction in blood loss: from an average of 894 mL (or 88 mL per level fused) to 672 mL (or 67 mL per level fused). Coincidentally, this study also noted a significant reduction in blood loss, when the randomized controls were compared with a historical control group. This observation underscores the principle that all studies of blood loss should be prospective and, as far as possible, single- or double-blinded. Comparison of a new treatment with a historical control will always have two significant variables, making the results invalid.

Blood lost may be replaced with either whole blood or blood components. The use of large volumes of packed red blood cells to replace lost blood carries with it a risk of increased coagulability. Murray et al. reported on a group of adolescent patients who lost more than 50% of their blood volume during posterior spinal surgery (76). Crystalloid plus packed red cell replacement resulted in 17 of 32 patients developing increased surgical bleeding as a result of decreased clot formation and increased clotting time. This was probably due to a dilution-related coagulopathy.

Use of autologous, predonated blood is the least hazardous method of replacing blood lost during surgery. Autologous blood can be harvested up to 5 weeks before surgery, stored, and returned to the patient. Moran et al. (72) in a series of 116 pediatric patients reported that 89% of the spinal surgeries were successfully completed using only predonated autologous blood. In a subset of 79 individuals with adolescent idiopathic scoliosis, only two required homologous blood transfusions. These results have been supported by Murray et al., who reported 135 of 144 adolescent idiopathic scoliosis surgeries completed using only predonated autologous blood, thus avoiding homologous blood transfusions (75).

Although screening of donated blood has become more accurate, there are still risks associated with homologous blood transfusion. These include coagulation disorders, febrile reactions, isoimmunization, citrate toxicity, and viral contamination. Of these complications, viral contamination remains the most difficult to control. While recent attention has been directed to the human immunodeficiency virus (HIV), hepatitis acquired through transfusion is a more common complication.

Extensive posterior spinal surgery often requires postoperative wound drainage. McCall and Bilderback reported that the administration of premarin, 1 mm/kg IV, immediately postoperatively resulted in a 37% decrease in postoperative drainage (62).

Reduction of blood loss is critical to the well-being of all surgical patients. Positioning of the patient as well as the use of specific surgical techniques can reduce the amount of blood lost during surgery. In addition, a comprehensive program of autologous blood donation can minimize or eliminate the need for homologous blood transfusion. With implementation of an effective blood loss control program, the risk to patients from transfusion reactions and/or blood-borne diseases can be reduced dramatically.

FLUID AND ELECTROLYTE BALANCE

Control of fluid balance in scoliosis patients begins in the operating room and is linked to control of blood loss. In most patients, monitoring should continue for the first 2 or 3 days of recovery until postoperative ileus is alleviated and the patient is able to take fluids by mouth. During this monitoring period, problems related to hypovolemia and inappropriate secretion of ADH can be confused.

Urine output is commonly used as the monitor of fluid balance. In patients aged 2 to 5 years, acceptable urine output is 2 mL/kg per hour; from age 5, 0.5 to 1 mL/kg per hour is acceptable. A decrease in urinary output during the first 12 hours after spinal surgery is common. The hypovolemic patient typically produces urine with high osmolality and low sodium; the patient's serum also shows high osmolality but normal sodium. The indicated treatment in such cases is volume replacement.

The opposite problem involves ADH release after surgery, which is a normal part of the body's stress reaction (24). The increase in ADH causes retention of free water, resulting in hypertonic urine that is high in sodium and serum that is hypoosmolar with reduced sodium. The indicated treatment is fluid restriction; if fluid is to be given, it should be isotonic.

The syndrome of inappropriate ADH secretion is defined by serum sodium less than 130, serum osmolality less than 275 mOsm/L, and urine sodium greater than 50 mEq/L. To avoid an incorrect diagnosis, test results should also include central venous pressure greater than 5 cm H_2O, absence of azotemia, and normal adrenal function.

In the immediate postoperative period, crystalloid replacement should be with isotonic solutions. In a series of 20 patients receiving hypotonic solution in the immediate postoperative period, Burrows et al. reported that 14 developed oliguria and 5 showed symptoms sufficient to suggest inappropriate ADH secretion (19). Burrows further recognized the need for use of isotonic rather than hypotonic solutions. McPhee reports that this concept was beneficial when applied to the patient before and during surgery as well as postoperatively. McPhee was able to significantly suppress inappropriate ADH secretion by using isotonic saline pre- and intraoperatively.

Patients with extreme inappropriate ADH secretion show clinical signs of restlessness and agitation that can progress to coma. Oliguria secondary to inappropriate ADH secretion can result in fluid overload and pulmonary interstitial edema if improperly diagnosed and if large volumes of crystalloid are given. As long as the patient's sodium level is greater than 130, a bolus of normal saline may be used. If the patient fails to respond, serum osmolality, urine sodium, and urine osmolality should be checked before a repeat challenge is used. Diuretics are not indicated in the initial treatment of patients with inappropriate ADH secretion; most respond to fluid restriction. The results of the study of Burrows et al. suggest that some cases of inappropriate ADH secretion can be prevented by use of isotonic fluids only during the postoperative period.

Fluid and electrolyte balance of spinal surgery patients must be monitored during the recovery period. Because symptoms can indicate conflicting complications, care must be taken to ensure that the diagnosis is accurate and that the patient receives the appropriate treatment.

GENITOURINARY COMPLICATIONS

Genitourinary complications after spinal surgery in children are common. The incidence of infection varies between subject groups. In at-risk patients, preoperative urinalysis and urine culture is indicated together with aggressive management of preoperative infections. At special risk are children with paraplegia, both traumatic and that secondary to meningomyelocele. In this patient subgroup, abnormal urodynamics and preexisting pathology in the kidney and bladder are often present and need to be well described prior to surgery. By lengthening the trunk and introducing rigidity into a collapsing deformity, self-catheterization may also become more difficult.

In the postoperative period, an overly distended bladder is predisposed to infection; thus, postoperative regimens that produce bladder distention should be avoided. When patients are treated with postoperative IV morphine, extra care should be taken because one side effect of this narcotic is decreased efficiency of bladder emptying. In high-risk patient groups, an indwelling catheter should be used to monitor fluid and electrolyte balance in the early postoperative period. This catheter may be removed after the morphine dosage is reduced. Use of indwelling catheters avoids the need for intermittent catheterization, which poses a risk of infection if the bladder becomes overly distended and hypotonic between catheterizations.

Urine culture and sensitivity determination should be performed in all spinal patients for whom intermittent catheterization is contemplated. An accurate record of the patient's awareness of the catheter being passed should also be kept. Because decreased ability to void may be one of the only signs of neurologic problems, early detection by sensory examination is important. The highest risk patients for this occult presentation of neurologic problem are severe spondylolisthesis patients who may develop a cauda equina syndrome.

Anterior spinal procedures can cause damage to the kidney itself or to the collecting system. Direct injury to the ureter has been reported as has blunt injury to the kidney (97). The latter can cause bleeding, which may result in early obstruction from a clot. Late obstruction secondary to scar tissue surrounding the ureter has also been reported. Any patient whose urine output alters in the first week postoperatively must be investigated thoroughly.

Chan and Chow (21) and Cleveland et al. (22), in three and one case, respectively, reported retroperitoneal fibrosis with urethral obstruction to be a long-term problem related to the anterior approach spinal procedures.

Sexual complications secondary to anterior approaches have received widespread attention. In 1984, Flynn and Price reported an incidence of retrograde ejaculation of 0.42% and impotence of 0.44% (36). One quarter of patients with retrograde ejaculation improved spontaneously. Flynn and Price concluded that the approach was not related to the complication. However, many surgeons have subsequently switched to retroperitoneal rather than transperitoneal dissection for anterior approaches in the region of the presacral plexus.

Although genitourinary complications after spinal surgery are common in children, the incidence of infection varies between subject groups. The groups at highest risk are patients with meningomyelocele and paraplegia. All children in the paralytic group undergoing corrective spinal surgery should undergo preoperative urinalysis and urine culture. When necessary, preexisting infections must be controlled before surgery rather than managed afterward.

GASTROINTESTINAL COMPLICATIONS

Postoperative ileus is common to most spinal surgical procedures. Posterior approaches that distract the spine may also distract the innervation of the posterior peritoneum, causing reactive ileus. During anterior procedures with extraperitoneal approaches, mere handling of the peritoneum can induce paralytic ileus. This intestinal obstruction is usually short-lived (approximately 36 to 48 hours), but it can be prolonged by injudicious use of early oral fluids or by electrolyte imbalance.

A more serious problem occurs when the superior mesenteric artery obstructs the duodenum. Superior mesenteric or cast syndrome has been reported with hyper lordosis of the lumbar spine secondary to cast immobilization as well as in situations of prolonged bed rest with weight loss (73). The mechanism of obstruction appears to be the same in all cases. The mesentery is dragged down, reducing the angle created by the superior mesenteric artery and the aorta in such a way that the duodenum is obstructed. This is also believed to be the mechanism of obstruction that occurs after correction of scoliosis in which the upper lumbar spine may be placed in distraction.

Delayed onset is a common characteristic of superior mesenteric artery syndrome, usually appearing from the second to fifth day after surgery. The first sign of the problem is often intermittent vomiting every 8 to 12 hours. If ignored, this syndrome can lead to profound electrolyte imbalance.

Once suspected, the diagnosis can be confirmed radiographically. A plain radiograph shows a deleted gastric shadow, and a water-soluble contrast study shows the obstruction. If the water-soluble study is chosen as part of the patient's medical evaluation, the radiology staff should position the patient in both left and right lateral positions to observe gastric emptying. Often it is the right lateral position that facilitates emptying. After this study, the patient can be positioned in optimum alignment. Once diagnosed, the currently recommended treatment includes maintenance of IV fluids and electrolyte balance as well as insertion of a double-lumen gastric tube to facilitate gastric emptying and jejunal alimentation. Aggressive early treatment usually solves the problem, but some cases can be prolonged (74).

Patients at risk are those with neuromuscular curves, especially severely involved spastic quadriparetic patients. For this group, active prophylaxis is recommended. Children should be admitted at least 2 weeks before surgery to a center that can monitor gastric hyperalimentation. A nasogastric tube should be passed, and hyperalimentation should be given until the child's weight gain is between 2 and 5 kg.

Although gastrointestinal complications are common in spinal surgery patients, few are serious and the effects of most are short-lived. More serious problems may have late onset in patients with hyperlordosis of the lumbar spine coupled with prolonged cast immobilization. In such cases, care must be taken to ensure an accurate timely diagnosis and appropriate treatment.

INFECTION

As with any surgical procedure, spinal operations in children create the risks of superficial and/or deep infection. Superficial infection involves the skin and the subcutaneous area, but neither reaches into the lower planes of the surgical dissection or compromises the implant. Superficial infections are best managed aggressively with local debridement, frequent dressing changes, and antibiotics in cases that become systemic or show evidence of extensive involvement.

Deep infections reach beyond the subcutaneous areas to involve the implant and the bony skeleton as well as the surrounding tissues. These infections are much more serious and may result in loss of fixation and/or chronic bone infection. As with all complications, certain patients are at greater risk than others. Kretzler and Renshaw (56), Stevens and Beard (100), and Gersoff and Renshaw (39) all reported increases in infection rates in neuromuscular curves with special risk for meningomyelocele patients. Meningomyelocele accounted for an infection rate of 11% in Kretzler's and Renshaw's series and 8% in Banta's (7). Although idiopathic scoliosis operations generally produce an infection rate of 1% or less, the infection rate in scoliosis surgery for neuromuscular curves ranges from 4% to 14% depending on the series reported (17).

Meningomyelocele patients present an added risk for infection. These patients have three areas where infection prevention requires special attention. The first results from preexisting genitourinary tract infection; therefore, adequate urologic screening is an essential part of the preoperative workup. A chronic bladder infection is important in younger children, and in older males prostatitis may also present as a chronic reservoir of infection. The preoperative urine culture in this group should be retained for reference.

The second area of difficulty in meningomyelocele patients deals with peroneal hygiene. This problem also arises with other groups of patients with significant physical handicaps, especially those confined to wheelchairs. As these children enter their teenage years, toileting can become progressively more difficult. If the child assumes this responsibility, as is common at this age, resulting incomplete peroneal hygiene leads to colonization of the natal cleft. This is especially true in obese patients as well as in patients with limited upper extremity function. The colonized cleft can easily spread contaminates to wounds that involve the lower part of the lumbar spine. Good practice mandates that preparation for surgery include culture of this area as well as thorough skin preparation.

A third area of skin colonization can be a concern in all patients who are on chronic antibiotics as well as in meningomyelocele patients. The natural flora of the skin can change with the chronic use of antibiotics. This is one of the possible avenues for the emergence of methacycline-resistant *Staphylococcus aureus* strains.

Another problem area in the meningomyelocele patient has to do with skin closure. Because of the earlier closure of the meningomyelocele defect, many of these children present with a relatively immobile scars; therefore, skin coverage following surgery can be a problem. Preoperative assessment by the plastic surgical service and perhaps even securing a plastic surgeon's involvement in the surgical closure may alleviate this problem. Tissue expanders can be a valuable preoperative adjunct to spinal surgery in meningomyelocele patients.

Early diagnosis is critical in the management of deep infection. Superficial cultures and a subfascial aspiration with the needle entry point away from the midline can be performed on the hospital ward. However, if a clinical suspicion is high, the patient should be taken to the operating room and undergo wound exploration.

The technique for management of an established deep infection remains controversial. Primary wound closure over suction irrigation systems, following radical surgical débridement, and appropriate antibiotic coverage has been successful in some cases, but the recurrence rate with this procedure may be unacceptably high. A more radical method of wound debridement, antibiotic coverage, packing, and allowing the wound to heal by secondary intent coupled with programmed and meticulous dressing changes was reported by Kretzler and Renshaw with good results in 19 cases. Unfortunately, healing by secondary intent requires prolonged hospitalization, produces significant scarring, and may be impractical in some patients whose wounds lack paraspinal muscles, such as the spina bifida group.

A third method midway between the previous two initiates the wound care with repeated debridement and packing of the wound opening with bactericidal dressings such as providine-soaked gauze. Following repeated débridement and primary control of the infection, the wound is closed over antibiotic-impregnated beads. The antibiotic in the beads must be targeted as specifically as possible to the infecting organism. Used appropriately, this is an efficient and highly efficacious technique.

In cases of established infection, removal of the hardware is seldom indicated as an initial event, although in the face of chronic longstanding infection removal may be indicated.

In all cases of spinal surgery in children, prevention of infection involves meticulous examination of the skin for distant areas of infection. In patients with adolescent idiopathic scoliosis, excessive acne over the back is a relative indication to postpone surgery. Judicious use of antibiotics and isotretinoin may be indicated; however, enlisting the assistance of a dermatologist can be important and worthwhile under these circumstances.

In the operating room, unnecessary traffic should be restricted, wound preparation should be augmented with iodoform-impregnated polyethylene adhesive sheeting, and antibiotic coverage should begin at induction of anesthesia and continue for the first 24 hours postoperatively.

Current research indicates that allograft bone used in cases of neuromuscular scoliosis has no higher infection rate than autograft bone. McCarthy and Peek reported an infection rate of 9.3% in 32 patients with neuromuscular curves treated with bone from a bone bank (64).

The nutritional status of the patient before and after surgery may also bear on the individual's susceptibility to infection (50). One third of adult patients undergoing elective surgery are malnourished. Simple laboratory tests, such as serum transferrin, albumin, and total lymphocyte count, have shown that 70% of patients in the adult population in whom complications develop had abnormalities in one or more tests. Rainey-Macdonald et al. developed a nutritional index to identify malnourished patients: the index is calculated as 1.2 times serum albumin plus 0.013 times transferrin minus 6.43 (81). A negative index indicates a malnourished state; a positive index indicates a nutrition-

ally sound condition. The index correlates positively with risk of postoperative infection.

Although the risk of infection is common to all surgical procedures, certain patient groups of children undergoing spinal surgery are at greater risk. In most reviews, patients with neuromuscular curves and those with meningomyelocele reported the highest rates of infection. Careful monitoring of such patients during the postoperative period should minimize the effects of these complications.

SURGICAL FAILURE

One of the goals of spinal surgery in children is to correct and stabilize the deformity, a process that often includes use of an implant and/or a bony arthrodesis. Failure to achieve this goal can result from either biologic or instrument failure.

Biologic Failure

This section addresses problems of biologic stability after initial correction of spine deformity.

The major biologic problem in spinal surgery is pseudarthrosis or failure of fusion. Difficulties in obtaining fusion are affected by four factors: the site of the attempted fusion in the spine, the immobilization method used at the point of fusion, the tensile or compression forces acting on the graft, and the ability of the body to incorporate the graft.

The problems associated with fusion in spondylolisthesis are typical of biologically caused pseudarthroses. Because the common fusion area in spondylolisthesis is posterior, the geometry of the slip places the fusion mass in tension, which inhibits osteogenesis. Neutralization of this tension can be achieved with external immobilization by hip spica or with posterior compressive instrumentation (i.e., pedicle screw and rod constructs) or anterior strut grafting, but only if placement of the graft is truly in such alignment that it acts as a neutralizing force. Neutralization can also be accomplished by anterior support with grafts or cages. Reconstruction stabilization of the anterior column gains its greatest efficiency when it also reestablishes a normal sagittal contour.

Surgical alternatives for preventing pseudarthrosis or significant progression in spondylolisthesis need to be balanced against what is considered a satisfactory fusion rate for a particular patient, that is, the degree of surgical intrusion must be weighed against the chances that fusion will be successful. Stanton et al. reviewed 20 cases of simple posterolateral fusion stabilized with a pantaloon hip spica (99). One of the 20 patients developed a delayed neurologic complication, one developed pseudarthrosis, and two increased their slip significantly before progressing to fusion. Of these four patients, two required further surgery. This constitutes a biologic failure rate of 10%, divided equally between pseudarthrosis and slip progression. Pizzutillo et al. reviewed 40 patients with posterolateral fusion and spica immobilization of whom 23 were grade 3 or greater (80). Two patients had postoperative progression of their slip—a biologic failure rate of 5%. All patients eventually healed. Bradford reported on

22 patients, with loss of correction requiring anterior fusion in two patients, a biologic failure rate of 9%.(15)

These studies compose a group of 82 patients that can provide comparison for other stabilization methods. The expected biologic failure rate is 5% to 10%. This includes both pseudarthrosis and progression of slip during the healing period, and it is split equally between progression of slip greater than 10%, most of which eventually progress to union, and true pseudarthrosis requiring another operation.

A less efficient procedure fuses the vertebrae in situ and omits the hip spica cast. Seitsalo et al., in a review of 93 children with simple in situ fusion for slips of 50% or greater, reported an initial reoperation rate for nonunion or progression of 19% (92). Seitsalo also reported the natural history of slips of 30% or less in 149 children; minor slips followed a moderately benign course (93). In this latter series, 77 patients were treated by fusion and 72 were treated without surgery. No statistical difference in slip progression between the two groups was observed in an average follow-up period of 13 years.

This suggests that in slips greater than 50% the optimum course is in situ fusion and hip spica (37). The added effort needed for the hip spica appears to be balanced by a reduction of almost 50% in the biologic failure rate as compared with the rate of the groups without external stabilization.

More elaborate two-stage stabilization has been proposed by DeWald et al. (29). They studied posterior instrumentation from L1 to the sacrum and fusion from L4 to the sacrum, also posterior, followed by anterior fusion for slips greater than 50%. In this group, one of the 14 patients showed loss of correction, a biologic failure rate of 7%. Bradford and Gotfried reported a small group of slips greater than 75% (11). Among 16 patients, 6 had delayed union and 1 had pseudarthrosis, a biologic failure rate of 43%. Bradford and Boachie-Adjei (14) reported 22 patients with slips greater than 50% in which anterior and posterior procedures produced a biologic failure rate of 19%. These staged procedures may be indicated in a subgroup of patients with slips greater than 50%, but a prudent course of treatment based on the least invasive surgical technique does not support use of a more elaborate procedure as initial treatment for slip progression or pseudarthrosis.

This analysis ignores the possible long-term biologic failure that can be induced by retention of the lumbosacral kyphosis produced with in situ fusion. This abnormal kyphosis may induce premature degeneration in the levels above. Harris and Weinstein reviewed the natural history of severe spondylolisthesis (grades 3 and 4) treated nonsurgically in 11 patients; however, only one patient had significant symptoms, even though half the group had used a back brace at some time (45). This suggests that combined anterior-posterior approaches should be reserved for cases in which late mechanical problems arise, as in severe symptomatic spondyloptosis, or when posterior procedures have failed. The benefit of fusing slips less than 30% without significant follow-up before fusion apparently is slight.

Fusion for scoliosis also runs the risk of biologic failure. Because of the length of the fusion in most procedures and because most posterior procedures are not combined with anterior fusions, some pseudarthrosis is expected. The highest risk lies in attempts to fuse to the sacrum (10,47). Each instrumentation system available approaches fusion to the sacrum differently. This multiplicity of devices results from the difficulty of achieving fusion at this level where the fusion is expected to continue up into the spine. The long lever arm of the proximal fusion creates stress at the lumbosacral level and thus increases the pseudarthrosis rate. Although certain screw positions and screw plates address this problem, the lack of solid bone in the sacrum makes fixation difficult. Currently, the transiliac Luque rod, popularized by the Galveston group, gives satisfactory results, especially in neuromuscular curves (3). Boachie-Adjei et al., in 46 neuromuscular cases, showed that Galveston alignment augmented by anterior fusion resulted in a pseudarthrosis rate of 6% and a rod fracture rate of 9% (10). The technique described by Roger Jackson involving pedicle screw fixation of S1 and extension of the rod into the sacrum and ilium lateral to the midline has reported favorable results.

Pure posterior fusion has the disadvantage of bridging vertebral segments leaving the anterior disc intact. The presence of the intact anterior disc potentially allows for micromotion across the disc space. Except in cases requiring fusion to the sacrum, one can neutralize the micromotion at the disc level with posterior instrumentation coupled with a posterior fusion technique that removes the facet joints and incorporates an autologous bone graft. This procedure can reduce the pseudarthrosis rate to 2% to 5% (30).

Dodd et al. noted no difference between use of allografts and autografts (31). This is noteworthy for treatment of patients with neuromuscular scoliosis in whom availability of autografts is limited.

Special circumstances do exist in the scoliosis group. The subgroups of scoliosis secondary to neurofibromatosis and Marfan syndrome in which dysplastic changes of bone occur have high pseudarthrosis rates. Savini et al. recommended anterior and posterior procedures for both the Marfan dystrophic curve and the neurofibromatosis curve (89,90). Risebourough also recommended a combined anterior and posterior procedure in cases with a radiated spine secondary to tumor (84), and Banta recommended its use in the meningomyelocele group in which the posterior elements are poor (7).

Generally, combined anterior and posterior procedures are recommended in nonidiopathic curvatures in which the bone is dysplastic or the posterior elements are suboptimal. In the Marfan and neurofibromatosis subgroups, curves of less than 50 degrees that do not show dystrophic change can be handled with posterior instrumentation, but adjunctive anterior fusion should be considered for larger curves.

Neuromuscular curves caused by cerebral palsy or polio benefit from an anterior and posterior approach. Boachie-Adjei et al. reported a 6% pseudarthrosis rate and improved correction of pelvic balance with the combined approach (10). O'Brien et al. reported similar findings in polio patients (78).

Kyphosis of any cause presents the difficulty of placing tension on a posterior bone graft. Neutralization with some form of posterior compression to counteract the distraction force or anterior strut is of benefit in achieving a high fusion rate.

The kyphoses can be grouped into two major structural curves: large arc and small arc. The large-arc curves are represented by the Scheuermann and paralytic groups. The short-arc curves include the congenital curves, as well as the dystrophic curves of neurofibromatosis, Marfan's syndrome, and posterior element deficiency (e.g., meningomyelocele or iatrogenic post laminectomy). The short-arc curves as a group demand both anterior and posterior fusion. The anterior procedure consists of a neutralizing strut so that the posterior fusion no longer is placed under tension stress and can form a solid arthrodesis. The exception to this general rule is a small congenital kyphosis of less than 50 degrees for which an initial posterior fusion may be attempted (114).

Anterior strut grafting serves two mechanical/biologic purposes: mechanical support and neutralization of posterior stresses, and establishment of anterior fusion. These two goals tend to be mutually exclusive. Streitz et al. reported anterior fibular strut grafting in a series of 20 patients; 15% of whom showed a pseudarthrosis (101). Bradford et al. reported 48 anterior strut grafts using both the fibula and the iliac crest as donor sites (12). Strut graft fracture occurred in five patients, each with an apical vertebra 4 cm or more distant from the strut. This suggests that gradual weakening of the graft before incorporation and revascularization were the cause of this biologic failure.

The addition of a vascularized rib strut graft has been proposed. McBride and Bradford reported six patients in whom this technique was used; all achieved solid fusion with rapid incorporation of the bone graft (61). J. A. Koos, speaking to a Canadian orthopaedic group in 1991, reported a similar technique used in the grossly osteoporotic spines of tuberculous patients in South Africa. Koos's results also demonstrated rapid incorporation and stabilization using a vascularized graft. Although addition of a vascularized rib strut involves a more invasive procedure, it should be considered when high-risk factors exist. These high-risk factors include, but are not limited to, a large kyphosis in which the bridging strut will be placed anteriorly more than 4 cm away or in patients with exceedingly porotic bone in whom the anterior strut may not be stable. The recent introduction of structurally strong cages that incorporate bone graft material while retaining stability provides another option that is probably less invasive and less technically demanding.

Biologic failures other than pseudarthroses can also occur in scoliosis. The stress risers produced by the rigid posterior fusion can induce failure above or below the fused segment. Friedman and Micheli, and Blasier and Monson reported patients who acquired spondylolisthesis after fusion (9,38). In the former, spondylolisthesis occurred below the fusion in the lumbar spine, and in the latter, it occurred above a posterior lumbar fusion. These complications are rare but should be included in the differential diagnosis of pain outside the fused area.

Failure of the spine above or below the fused area can also be secondary to growth or failure of the mechanical strength of the spinal column. This group of complications is best exemplified by the kyphotic falloff above the rod observed in some patients with a growing rod (instrumented curve without fusion to allow further spinal growth), especially those associated with axial osteoporosis, such as the arthrogrypotic spine, or associated with Marfan syndrome as reported by Amis and Herring (5). Failure to include structural curves in the fused segment or extending the correction too far into the compensatory segment can upset the balance of the spinal column and result in a pro-gression of the curve in the sagittal plane as well as in the coronal plane (Fig. 4).

Broom et al. reported a tendency for cephalad progression of deformity when fusion or instrumentation ends at or below the fourth thoracic vertebra (17). This reemphasizes the importance of sagittal contours and of ending instrumentation in high-risk groups of neuromuscular scoliosis patients higher in the thoracic spine. Bradford et al., reviewing a series of patients with Scheuermann kyphosis, noted caudal falloff of correction when the posterior arthrodesis did not extend past the transition area in the thoracolumbar spine (13).

Finally, the so-called crankshaft phenomenon involves continued anterior growth of a posterior tether (Fig. 5). This phenomenon was first described by Dubousset et al. (32). In all of their patients the spine had fused posteriorly at Risser 0–1 and had continued anterior vertebral growth, which expressed as a spiral deformation rotating around the posterior tether formed by the fusion and instruments. A variation of the crankshaft phenomenon was described by Rodgers et al. as an increase in the occipital cervical lordosis in young children following occipital cervical fusion (86). Previously, this particular complication was often misdiagnosed as a pseudarthrosis or bending of the graft (108). Dubousset et al. (32) recommended recognition of the potential problem and its prevention with adjunctive anterior fusion to stop the growth in that direction. The extent of prophylactic anterior fusion required is still undefined.

Avoidance of the crankshaft phenomenon has been the focus of several publications. Sanders followed 43 patients who were Risser 0 at the time of posterior spinal fusion (88). He concluded that in patients with an open triradiate cartilage surgery performed before or during peak trunk growth velocity had a high likelihood of displaying crankshaft phenomenon postoperatively. Therefore, surgical planning in the immature patient should include an assessment of skeletal maturity. If the opportunity exists to study growth over time, peak growth velocities can be determined. If time is restricted, patients who are Risser 0 Tanner 1 with open triradiate cartilages and a bone age of 11 years or less are often at high risk. In these patients, the addition of an anterior procedure should be considered.

Diagnosis of biologic failure can be difficult. Serial radiographic examination shows curve progression and decompensation only if radiographic position is standardized. Because the plane of deformity of the crankshaft phenomenon is rotatory, it may not be as easily identified on routine radiographs as it is clinically.

The diagnosis of pseudarthrosis is perhaps the most difficult. Clinical indicators are pain and/or progression of curvature. Plain radiographs are not usually helpful. Use of bone scanning, especially of the more sophisticated programs that allow tomography, can be useful. Radiographic polytomograms are often difficult to interpret but may also display occult pseudarthrosis. Dawson et al. report a correlation of almost 96% with the use of tomography (27).

If no instrumentation has been used, as in cases of spondylolisthesis with posterolateral fusion or congenital scoliosis, CT with three-dimensional reconstruction can prove valuable in localizing fusion defects (Fig. 6).

Treatment of biologic failure involves extension of the fusion

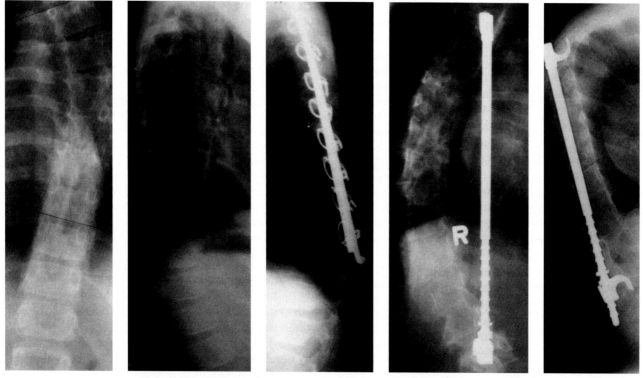

A,B,C   D,E

FIGURE 4. A: Anteroposterior (AP) and lateral radiographs of a 10-year-old patient with neurofibromatosis; the curvature is progressive in the AP projection, and focal thoracolumbar kyphosis is apparent. **B:** Lateral radiograph taken 9 months postoperatively shows failure to address the thoracolumbar kyphosis and the tendency to further progression. Extending the instrumentation and fusion into the upper lumbar spine would have avoided this complication. **C:** An 11-year-old patient with growing rod for connective tissue disorder. **D:** The upper hook ended at T5 with resulting kyphotic falloff. Placement at T1 or T2 may have avoided this complication.

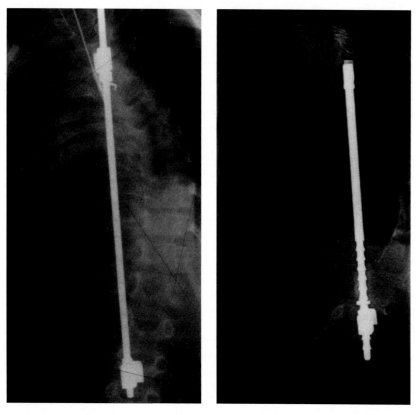

A,B

FIGURE 5. A: A 6-year-old girl with infantile idiopathic scoliosis and growing rod. **B:** Same patient at age 12 years with the final growing rod in place. Significant increase in rotation about the posterior tether of the rod is evident even though the spine was unfused.

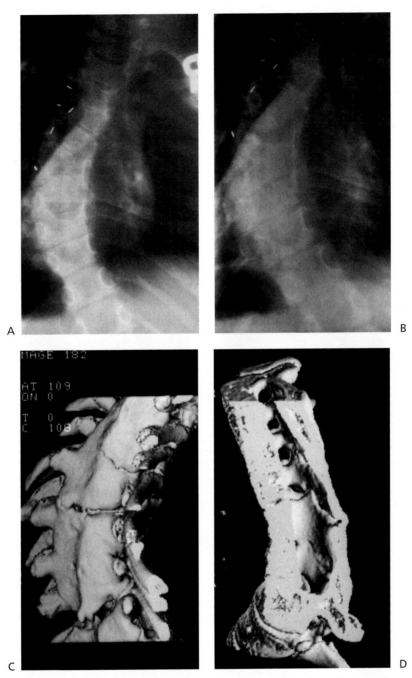

FIGURE 6. **A:** A 9-year-old patient with in situ anterior and posterior fusion for neurofibromatosis scoliosis performed at age 6. **B:** Same patient at age 11 years with progression of curvature. **C:** Three-dimensional reconstruction of computed tomography scan of spine suggests apical pseudarthrosis. **D:** Cut-away reconstruction shows pseudarthrosis.

for curves that have become imbalanced. This may entail osteotomy and/or anterior support and is especially important in kyphotic curvature.

Patients who exhibit the crankshaft phenomenon should be studied for the degree of maturity of their spine. Children with more than 12 to 18 months of spinal growth remaining and who demonstrate the rotatory changes associated with the crankshaft phenomenon should be considered for anterior fusion. If the

patient is nearing the end of growth, accepting the increase in deformity may be the prudent course of action because the deformity will not progress once growth is completed. Nachemson's findings should be considered when assessing patients nearing the end of their growth. The author reviewed 63 patients who were Risser 0 at the time of surgery and noted that despite the fact that the crankshaft phenomenon occurred in the majority of patients, the resulting increase of Cobb and rotational deformity was mild to moderate. This suggests that the addition of an anterior procedure be reserved for the immature patient at the greatest risk.

Analysis of the cause of the lack of fusion should precede pseudarthrosis repair. For fusion masses that heal under tension, compressive instrumentation across the pseudarthrosis with bone grafting as necessary may be indicated. For anterior fusions with pseudarthrosis of the strut and mechanical fatigue, addition of vascularized rib strut may be considered. Anterior augmentation of a posterior pseudarthrosis repair may also be added.

In children, laminectomy over long distances produces a biologically unstable condition with falloff into kyphosis; this is often evident after surgical procedures for tumors (51). Prevention of this complication is largely a matter of education. In high-risk situations (a younger child with a laminectomy in the cervical or high thoracic spine), addition of a simple posterior fusion after a laminectomy is often indicated though rarely implemented. Once the kyphosis starts, posterior fusion is unlikely to be successful. Therefore, the treatment strategy is to realign the spine before stabilizing it—a procedure that does not necessarily require open surgery (Fig. 7). In younger children, if the complication is detected early in the healing process, cervical kyphosis can occasionally be treated with halo traction to realign the spine followed by immobilization in a halo thoracic brace. This accomplishes two goals: first, it realigns and reestablishes normal spinal contours; and second, it removes the posterior tension load and allows spontaneous posterior fusion. If such treatment is unsuccessful and posterior elements are deficient, an anterior fusion is usually indicated.

Pseudarthrosis is a common complication in all reconstructive spinal surgery. Four factors affect the body's ability to obtain fusion: the site of the attempted fusion in the spine, the immobilization method used at the point of fusion, the tensile or compression forces acting on the graft, and the ability of the spine to incorporate the graft. Although high-risk procedures exist, one must plan surgical correction keeping the biologic limitations in mind to ensure the best possible chance of successful fusion.

Biologic complications resulting in a failure of fusion constitute only a portion of the total picture of surgical failure. As spinal implants and instruments become more sophisticated, failure of these mechanical devices becomes an increasing factor.

Instrument Failure

The use of surgical implants to obtain and maintain surgical correction in spinal reconstructive surgery was popularized by Paul Harrington with the development of the distraction compression system that bears his name. Since the introduction of the Harrington system, implants have continued to be modified and redesigned. Although these systems provide obvious benefit to patients, their use involves risks and concerns.

An implant system can fail in three major ways: inadequate mechanical strength built into the implant system can cause fracture of a rod or wire; mechanical connectors can loosen or disengage; and the implant system simply may not accomplish its physical objective.

Material failure is commonly linked to pseudarthrosis. Failure of fusion will produce a stress riser at that level, and the micromotion of the pseudarthrosis will lead to stress failure of the metal implant. Therefore, fractured rods are often a radiographic sign indicating the need for further investigation of pseudarthrosis.

Herndon et al. reported early experiences with Luque's segmental system (47). They had a rod failure of 19% and noted an increase in failures with the smaller diameter rods and with rods that extended to the pelvis. They recommended external support for cases in which the smaller rods were used. The newer devices designed by Cotrel, Dubousset, and TSRH have double upright constructs connected with rigid cross-links to form a rectangular construct. These groups have not reported early mechanical failures, but the construct has not been in use long enough to report 15- to 20-year failure rates.

Patients at risk for mechanical failure include those with high-risk pseudarthrosis, such as neurologic curves, those with a long fusion mass, especially those extending down to the pelvis, and those in whom a small-diameter implant must be used (47).

If the patients at risk can be identified preoperatively, addition of anterior fusion will not only decrease the pseudarthrosis rate but will also reduce the stress on the rods. External support in paralytic scoliosis cases will decrease stress on the rod system during the first 6 to 8 months. The strength of the rod itself can be augmented by constructs that allow the rods to be rigidly joined. It is important not to equate the strength of the construct with the stiffness of the rod. The latter physical characteristic does not necessarily strengthen the system. What it may do is add increased segmental stress, causing laminar fracture in cases in which rod contouring is not exact.

The second form of material failure is an early complication related to hook displacement. In the posterior systems, this is best prevented by accurate preoperative assessment of the site, appropriate choice of hooks, and compulsive preparation of hook sites intraoperatively.

Curves that are instrumented without fusion to allow further spinal growth to occur (the growing rod) create special conditions for materials failure. The indications for the growing rod are usually confined to curves in patients aged 4 to 7 years in whom bracing has failed and in whom increased spinal growth is desirable. Of necessity, these systems are fixed only at the cephalad and caudad ends of the curve, and because of the size of the child, small-scale hooks and rods are used. Dislodgement in this flexible system is quite common, often despite careful hook site preparation and postoperative protection. Complications can be minimized by creating hook sites top and bottom and by fusing the two vertebrae adjacent to each hook site. Sublaminar mercelene tapes may also be used to anchor the rod more firmly at either end. The complication rates in the growing rod group are high, but attempts to adapt the Luque system to the growing rod approach have not been successful (33,83).

In the commonly used multiple-hook systems (Cotrel-Dubousset, TSRH, Isola), the hook site at risk is the most distal hook on the convexity of the major curve. When this hook must be placed cephalad, alignment of the shoe with the lamina becomes critical. In the upper lumbar spine, the laminae are not parallel with the final alignment of the rod but instead slope anteriorly from caudad to cephalad. If the shoe of the hook is

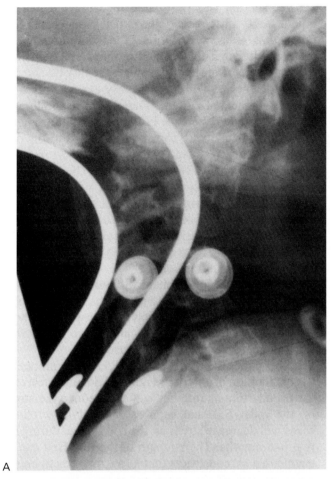

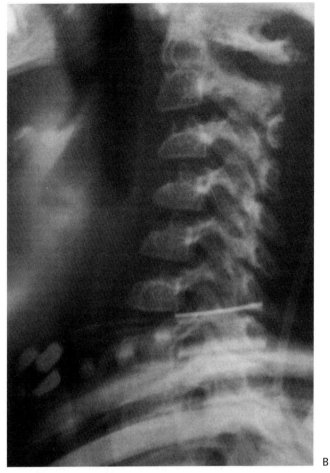

A

B

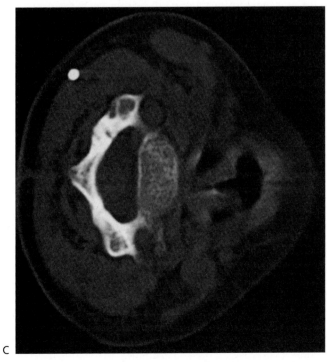

C

FIGURE 7. **A:** A 4-year-old child with significant cervical kyphosis after posterior craniotomy and removal of the arch of C1 plus laminoplasty of C2–C4 for benign tumor. **B:** Same patient after halo-femoral traction and halo brace wear for 3 months. **C:** Computed tomography scan of C3 shows healing of the laminoplasty.

not aligned parallel with the lamina, it can easily pull out. This problem can be avoided by properly placing the hook and by contouring the distal rod in a slight lordotic tilt to allow parallel alignment of the shoe of the hook with the lamina and by adding a caudad-facing hook at the level above.

In the multiple-hook systems, dislodgement of one hook is not necessarily an indication for operative reexploration. If no correction is lost, external support with a cast or brace may be used until bony fusion occurs. Reexploration then allows either reseating or removing the hook without unduly jeopardizing the long-term result.

With a small-diameter threaded rod, it is essential not to lock the rod to the screw with nuts on either side of the screw head. The nuts should be placed only on the side where tightening will move the screw toward the center of the curve, causing compression. Sublaminar wires are an integral part of both the Luque and the Isola systems. Mastering the technique for passing these wires is critical because improper technique can create focal stress. Generally, a double wire is stronger than a single wire with a thicker diameter. Wire twisting with the wires at 45 degrees is less likely to produce focal stress risers than tying [8], but excessive twisting will cause fatigue failure. In most cases, a technique that pushes the rod to the lamina is preferable to a situation in which the wire pulls the vertebra to the rod. The latter situation may cause the wire to cut through softer bone or may result in longer wire loops in other situations that are more vulnerable to fatigue. As in the multiple-hook system, the existence of a fractured wire is not necessarily an indication for its removal [8].

Currently, the most controversial aspect of instrument failure is imbalance [104]. Spinal deformity in scoliosis has three possible planes of deformity: frontal, sagittal, and axial. Each vertebra that is acted on during the correction process has six possible variables in correction. Three of these are in the planes of displacement: the anteroposterior plane, the vertical plane, or the medial-lateral plane. The other three are in the planes of rotation: around the vertical axis, tilt in the sagittal plane, and tilt in the frontal plane. These variables may occur in combination with each other. Unfortunately, the displacement resulting from these six variables is not well understood.

The Harrington system aimed at correction of deformity in one plane only: its distraction compression mode corrected in the coronal plane. The major corrective force was distraction. Compensatory movements occurred in the sagittal plane and minimally in rotation. The effect of the single-plane corrective force was to create imbalance with respect to a decrease in thoracic kyphosis and a decrease in lumbar lordosis [1,20,69]. Coronal plane imbalance with the Harrington system occurred but was rare. With addition of the Luque sublaminar wires, deliberate correction in two planes became possible [70]; the spine could now be recontoured so that thoracic kyphosis was preserved and lumbar lordosis was not diminished.

The anterior instrumentation systems are also capable of correcting in two planes: coronal and rotatory. Sagittal plane imbalance remains difficult to address [71]. All of these systems tend to apply a kyphotic force [53]. Use of anterior interbody bone grafts or cages in an attempt to prevent this has been partially successful, but the tendency to kyphosis remains. Anterior systems should not be used in isolation in patients with a preexisting kyphosis; anterior release and posterior instrumentation works better in these areas. When anterior and posterior instrumentation systems are combined, as in neurologic curves, ending the anterior instrumentation at L2 or L3 and extending the posterior instrumentation further down allows shaping in a more physiologic sagittal contour.

The multihook system popularized by Cotrel added the theoretical possibility of rotational correction. Intraoperative stereophotogammetry has demonstrated that each individually instrumented vertebra shows unique movement along or about an axis that has x, y, and z components. The resulting correction improves both the sagittal and the coronal deformity. Correction also moves the plane of maximum deformity back toward the neutral or sagittal plane.

Guidelines for the posterior instrumentation systems that have the potential for three-dimensional correction are difficult to delineate. The King classification of scoliotic deformity was derived from the results of Harrington's uniplanar posterior instrumentation. These King guidelines stress analysis of the flexibility of the curve and fusion to the neutrally rotated vertebra [104]. The guidelines for Cotrel and Dubousset emphasize analysis of the neutral end vertebrae as determined by side bending to note both rotation and correction of disc wedging. Cotrel and Dubousset also stress analysis of lateral radiographs to ensure that the upper part of instrumentation extends above the lordotic or hypokyphotic segment of the curve in the upper thoracic spine and that the lower end of the instrumentation encompasses the thoracolumbar kyphosis when it exists.

Given the significant difference in correction mechanisms between the pure distraction and the multihook systems, using the guidelines for one group on the other may result in trunk imbalance or focal kyphotic deformity.

Distal extension of the fusion and instrumentation into the lumbar spine has mechanical and biologic implications [1,70]. True distraction equipment will produce flat-back syndrome if the instrumentation is carried to L4 or below. Flat-back syndrome produces imbalance in the sagittal plane and may require corrective osteotomy. According to Casey et al., regardless of whether the rod was contoured or a square-ended rod and hook was used, the lumbar lordosis was decreased with Harrington instrumentation [20]. They noted that lumbar lordosis was decreased above L4 and increased below, suggesting that there was increased stress on the unfused areas. Hayes et al. reviewed a series of cases involving Harrington instrumentation with an average follow-up of 11 years [46]. They noted an increase in low back pain in patients fused to L4, and those fused to L3 or L4 had significantly more translational motion in the intact disc spaces. They also noted a retrolisthesis in 80% of patients fused to L4 and in 40% of those fused to L3. This complication did not occur in patients fused to a higher level, suggesting that the long-term outcome of sagittal imbalance in the lumbar spine may be increased degeneration [23]. Michel and Lalain noted morphologic change in unfused lumbar vertebrae followed for more than 10 years [69]. They noted that unfused vertebral bodies tended to become more elongated and more trapezoidal, which tended to reconstitute the lumbar lordosis and to correct sagittal plane imbalance to a degree.

With currently available segmental systems, the flat back may be avoided; however, even with accurate sagittal contours, if instrumentation is carried to L4 or below, the number of free-motion segments in the lumbar spine is drastically reduced, setting the stage for subsequent biologic failure.

The effect of spinal alignment produced by the instrumentation is of special importance in the function of patients with neuromuscular curvatures. Patients who are primarily dependent on wheelchairs must be warned that their center of gravity after surgery will be higher than it was preoperatively, making balancing in the wheelchair more difficult. The shoulders also will be raised farther from the ground and the arms will not reach as far down on the wheel, resulting in decreased ability of the patient to power the chair. Although balance can be relearned, some functional loss may be permanent. Brown et al. reviewed 84 patients with spinal muscular atrophy who had been operated on for scoliosis, noting that the ability to perform activities such as drinking, self-feeding, and self-hygiene decreased in the early postoperative period but had improved 5 years later (18). They also noted that many surgical patients did not regain their preoperative skill level despite this improvement. Mazur et al., in a review of 49 patients with meningomyelocele who had undergone spinal surgery, noted that although the ability to walk decreased, sitting balance and function improved (60).

As advances are made in spinal implants and corrective surgery, the risk of complications from instrument failure increases. An implant system usually fails for one of three major reasons. First, inadequate mechanical strength of the implant system may cause a rod or wire to fracture. Second, the mechanical connectors may loosen or disengage. Third, the implant system may not achieve the physical objective that it was intended to accomplish. Although complete elimination of instrument failure may be impossible, such failure must be considered in the planning and management of children's spinal surgery to ensure better outcome of the reconstructive procedure.

SPECIAL CIRCUMSTANCES

Uncommon diagnoses that lead to spinal surgery in children present unique situations that must be evaluated on their own merits to limit risks to the patient. Although positioning during surgery is a concern for all patients, patients with restricted joint motion have a special risk, that is, patients with arthrogryposis or some of the skeletal dysplasias, such as metatropic dwarfism or diastrophic dwarfism. These children must be positioned to ensure that no harm comes to shoulders or elbows because of their stiffness (25). Patients with excessive motion must be positioned in a way that protects their upper cervical alignment, that is, patients with syndromes involving upper cervical spine instability, such as Down syndrome, Morquio syndrome, and other dysplasias that involve the axial skeleton (117). After patients with excessive motion have been positioned, a lateral radiograph should be taken to ensure that the cervical spine is aligned in a way that will not cause harm.

Surgeons should also be cognizant of pressure over the axilla and brachial plexus. Ulnar nerve electrodes and early intraoperative monitoring or assessment will help in this area as well. Other possible pressure points include the anterior superior iliac spine, where prolonged pressure can result in meralgia paresthetica (103).

All bony prominences should be inspected before the patient is positioned, appropriately padded during the surgery, and charted after the procedure. Pressure sores resulting from improper positioning have been reported, and at least one case of pressure to the eyes causing loss of vision has been documented (110).

Unique diagnoses present unique sets of problems. Prader-Willi syndrome is marked by hypogonadism, early childhood obesity, variable mental deficiency, and behavior disorders that include hyperphagia. This genetic disorder also has a high incidence of scoliosis. In a literature review, Rees et al. reported an incidence of 5% to 85% (82). In their own series, there was an incidence of five cases of scoliosis in seven patients.

Management of Prader-Willi patients can be complicated by their behavior disorder. When necessary, bracing should be a thoracolumbosacral orthosis. This type of high-profile brace is the safest for patients with moderate retardation and combative personality.

Scoliosis surgery in a Prader-Willi patient is difficult because of the patient's size and because of the lack of postoperative cooperation. Segmental instrumentation is preferable in this group of patients because of its capability of spreading out the corrective force. Progression of the curve greatly exceeding 45 to 50 degrees should be an indication for surgery, and these patients should not be allowed to progress to a degree of curvature for which both anterior and posterior interventions are needed (77).

In a review on Prader-Willi patients, Dearlove and Dobson noted that in the early stages of the condition those at or below the 50th percentile of weight present no specific problems (28). However, this study reported that children who are heavier than the 97th percentile have a combination of difficulties, including difficult intravenous access and sleep apnea.

Behavior disorders also complicate the treatment of familial dysautonomia patients. Although it is usually tried, bracing has only variable success in this group. Brace pressure sores can be a major problem, and compliance is difficult to regulate. Surgical intervention also poses special problems. Albenese and Bobechko reported at least one complication in each of their surgically treated patients (2). Again, because of the degree of difficulty in postoperative management, early surgical intervention with segmental fixation and long-term monitoring of patients is indicated. Even with this treatment, late hook displacement and pseudarthroses can occur (85). Both Kaplan and Rubery noted the rigidity of these curves and the difficulty in obtaining significant correction. Therefore, surgical strategies have been aimed at early intervention and stabilization of the curve. These two studies also reported an increase in overall complications and especially in pulmonary compromise.

Patients with arthrogryposis present to the spinal clinic for both exaggerated lordosis and exaggerated scoliosis. Soft-tissue contracture makes bracing difficult, and the combination of contracture and mild osteoporosis complicate surgical correction (25). A segmented instrumentation system is more successful in osteoporotic bone. This group of patients must have adequate sagittal balance at completion of surgery. Curves that are not fused high enough into the thoracic spine tend to progress into kyphosis above, and curves not fused below the transition between the thoracic and lumbar spine may develop focal thoracolumbar kyphosis below.

Surgical correction of patients with the connective tissue disorder known as Marfan syndrome is associated with specific hazards. Preoperative assessment of the cardiothoracic status of such patients is essential. At least one incident of tracheal compression occurred after correction in Marfan syndrome (68), and the tracheal malacia that these children have may cause respiratory problems. One anecdotal report of C1–2 instability in unrecognized Marfan syndrome produced quadriplegia owing to improper positioning of the patient during surgery.

The Ehler-Danlos group also may be a increased risk. Vogel and Lubicky reported three patients with Ehler-Danlos syndrome who developed neurologic complications postoperatively, suggesting that in either of these groups meticulous intraoperative monitoring and more modest surgical goals are indicated (109).

Certain uncommon situations lead to particular complications that require special attention. The uniqueness of these patients belies all attempts to find general courses of treatment and/or widely accepted rules for their management. Each anomaly, and often each patient in an anomalous group, requires individual evaluation with regard to the best preoperative preparation, surgical plan, and postoperative management regimen to achieve the desired outcomes.

CONCLUSION

This chapter discusses the complications of spinal surgery in children. By taking an anatomical approach rather than a procedural or disease approach, complications are treated as systemic malfunctions instead of isolated notations on the patient's chart. Areas central to a child's well-being, such as pain and blood loss, are discussed as they relate to the patient's recovery and the overall success of the surgical procedure. Finally, this chapter identifies and outlines treatments for at-risk groups in each area of complication.

ACKNOWLEDGMENT

The author gratefully acknowledges the editorial assistance provided by Lawrence A. Davis, M.A.

REFERENCES

1. Aaro S, Ohlen G (1983): The effect of Harrington instrumentation on the sagittal configuration and mobility of the spine in scoliosis. *Spine* 8:570–575.
2. Albanese SA, Bobechko WP (1987): Spine deformity in familial dysautonomia (Riley-Day syndrome). *J Pediatr Orthop* 7:179–183.
3. Allen BL Jr, Ferguson RL (1986): Neurologic injuries with the Galveston technique of L-rod instrumentation for scoliosis. *Spine* 11:14–17.
4. Amaranath L, Andrish JT, Gurd AR, et al. (1989): Efficacy of intermittent epidural morphine following posterior spinal fusion in children and adolescents. *Clin Orthop* 249:223–226.
5. Amis J, Herring JA (1984): Iatrogenic kyphosis: a complication of Harrington instrumentation in Marfan's syndrome. A case report. *J Bone Joint Surg Am* 66:460–464.
6. Beaulieu P, Cyrenne L, Matthews S, et al. (1996): Patient-controlled analgesia after spinal fusion for idiopathic scoliosis. *Int Orthop* 20(5):295–299.
7. Banta JV (1990): Combined anterior and posterior fusion for spinal deformity in myelomeningocele. *Spine* 15:946–952.
8. Bernard TN Jr, Johnston CE II, Roberts JML, et al. (1983): Late complications due to wire breakage in segmental spinal instrumentation. Report of two cases. *J Bone Joint Surg Am* 65:1339–1345.
9. Blasier RD, Monson RC (1987): Acquired spondylolysis after posterolateral spinal fusion. *J Pediatr Orthop* 7:215–227.
10. Boachie-Adjei O, Lonstein JE, Winter RB, et al. (1990): Management of neuromuscular spinal deformities with Luque's segmental instrumentation. *J Bone Joint Surg Am* 71:548–562.
11. Bradford DS, Gotfried Y (1987): Staged salvage reconstruction of grade IV and V spondylolisthesis. *J Bone Joint Surg Am* 69:191–202.
12. Bradford DS, Ganjavian S, Antonious D, et al. (1982): Anterior strut-grafting for the treatment of kyphosis. Review of experience with forty-eight patients. *J Bone Joint Surg Am* 64:680–690.
13. Bradford DS, Ahmed KB, Moe JH, et al. (1980): The surgical management of patients with Scheuermann's disease: a review of twenty-four cases managed by combined anterior and posterior spine fusion. *J Bone Joint Surg Am* 62:705–712.
14. Bradford DS, Boachie-Adjei O (1990): Treatment of severe spondylolisthesis by anterior and posterior reduction and stabilization. A long-term follow-up study. *J Bone Joint Surg Am* 72:1060–1066.
15. Bradford DS (1988): Closed reduction of spondylolisthesis. An experience in 22 patients. *Spine* 13:580–587.
16. Bridwell KH, Lenke LG, Baldus C, et al. (1988): Major intraoperative neurologic deficits in pediatric and adult spinal deformity patients. Incidence and etiology at one institution. *Spine* 23(3):324–331.
17. Broom MJ, Banta JV, Renshaw TS (1989): Spinal fusion augmented by Luque-rod segmental instrumentation for neuromuscular scoliosis. *J Bone Joint Surg Am* 71:32–44.
18. Brown JC, Zeller JL, Swank SM, et al. (1989): Surgical and functional results of spine fusion in spinal muscular atrophy. *Spine* 14:763–770.
19. Burrows FA, Shutack JG, Crone RK (1983): Inappropriate secretion of antidiuretic hormone in a postsurgical pediatric population. *Crit Care Med* 11:527–531.
20. Casey MP, Asher MA, Jacobs RR, et al. (1987): The effect of Harrington rod contouring on lumbar lordosis. *Spine* 12:750–753.
21. Chan FL, Chow SP (1983): Retroperitoneal fibrosis after anterior spinal fusion. *Clin Radiol* 34:331–335.
22. Cleveland RH, Gilsanz V, Lebowitz RL, et al. (1978): Hypernephrosis from retroperitoneal fibrosis after anterior spinal fusion: a case report. *J Bone Joint Surg Am* 60:996–997.
23. Cochran T, Irstam L, Nachemson A (1983): Long-term anatomic and functional changes in patients with adolescent idiopathic scoliosis treated by Harrington rod fusion. *Spine* 8:576–584.
24. Cowley DM, Pabari M, Sinton TJ, et al. (1988): Pathogenesis of postoperative hyponatraemia following correction of scoliosis in children. *Aust N Z J Surg* 58:485–489.
25. Daher YH, Lonstein JE, Winter RB, et al. (1985): Spinal deformities in patients with arthrogryposis. A review of 16 patients. *Spine* 10:609–613.
26. Daher YH, Lonstein JE, Winter RB, et al. (1985): Spinal deformities in patients with muscular dystrophy other than Duchenne. A review of 11 patients having surgical treatment. *Spine* 10:614–617.
27. Dawson EG, Clader TJ, Bassett LW (1985): A comparison of different methods used to diagnose pseudarthrosis following posterior spinal fusion for scoliosis. *J Bone Joint Surg Am* 67:1153–1159.
28. Dearlove OR, Dobson A: *Anaesthesia and Prader-Willi syndrome.* Department of Paediatric Anaesthesia, Royal Manchester Children's Hospital, Pendlebury, UK.
29. DeWald RL, Faut MM, Taddonio RF, et al. (1981): Severe lumbosa-

cral spondylolisthesis in adolescents and children. Reduction and staged circumferential fusion. *J Bone Joint Surg Am* 63:619–626.

30. Dickson JH, Erwin WD, Rossi D (1990): Harrington instrumentation and arthrodesis for idiopathic scoliosis. A twenty-one year follow-up. *J Bone Joint Surg Am* 72:678–683.

31. Dodd CA, Fergusson CM, Freedman L, et al. (1988): Allograft versus autograft bone in scoliosis surgery. *J Bone Joint Surg Br* 70:431–434.

32. Dubousset J, Herring JA, Shufflebarger H (1989): The crankshaft phenomenon. *J Pediatr Orthop* 9:541–550.

33. Eberle CF (1988): Failure of fixation after segmental spinal instrumentation without arthrodesis in the management of paralytic scoliosis. *J Bone Joint Surg Am* 70:696–703.

34. Ecker ML, Dormans JP, Schwartz DM, et al. (1996): Efficacy of spinal cord monitoring in scoliosis surgery in patients with cerebral palsy. *J Spinal Disord* 9(2):159–164.

35. Edgar MA, Waller C, Patterson M, et al. (1987): A checklist for spinal cord monitoring: is it true- or false-positive change? *J Bone Joint Surg Br* 69:854.

36. Flynn JC, Price CT (1984): Sexual complications of anterior fusion of the lumbar spine. *Spine* 9:489–492.

37. Freeman BL III, Donati NL (1989): Spinal arthrodesis for severe spondylolisthesis in children and adolescents. A long-term follow-up study. *J Bone Joint Surg Am* 71:594–598.

38. Friedman RJ, Micheli LJ (1984): Acquired spondylolisthesis following scoliosis surgery. A case report. *Clin Orthop* 190:132–134.

39. Gersoff WK, Renshaw TS (1988): The treatment of scoliosis in cerebral palsy by posterior spinal fusion with Luque-rod segmental instrumentation. *J Bone Joint Surg Am* 70:41–44.

40. Ginsburg HH, Shetter AG, Raudzens PA (1985): Postoperative paraplegia with preserved intraoperative somatosensory evoked potentials. Case report. *J Neurosurg* 63:296–300.

41. Goldberg C, Dowling FE, Fogarty J (1989): Occult neuro-dysfunction in congenital spinal deformity. In: *Proceedings of the combined meeting of the Scoliosis Research Society and the European Spinal Deformity Society,* Amsterdam.

42. Goodarzi M, Shier NH, Grogan DP (1996): Effect of intrathecal opioids on somatosensory-evoked potentials during spinal fusion in children. *Spine* 21(13):1565–1568.

43. Guay J, Reinberg C, Rivard GE, et al. (1990): DDAVP does not reduce bleeding during spinal fusion for idiopathic scoliosis. *Can J Anaesthesiol* 37:S14.

44. Hale DD, Dawson EG, Delamarter R (1989): Late neurological complications of Harrington rod instrumentation. *J Bone Joint Surg Am* 71:1053–1057.

45. Harris IE, Weinstein SL (1987): Long term follow up of patients with grade II and IV spondylolisthesis. *J Bone Joint Surg Am* 69:960–969.

46. Hayes MA, Tompkins SF, Herndon WA, et al. (1988): Clinical and radiological evaluation of lumbosacral motion below fusion levels in idiopathic scoliosis. *Spine* 13:1161–1167.

47. Herndon WA, Sullivan JA, Yngve DA, et al. (1987): Segmental spinal instrumentation with sublaminar wires. A critical appraisal. *J Bone Joint Surg Am* 69:851–859.

48. Herndon WA, Emans JB, Micheli LJ, et al. (1981): Combined anterior and posterior fusion for Scheuermann's kyphosis. *Spine* 6:125–130.

49. Hoppenfeld S, Gross A, Andres C, et al. (1997): The ankle clonus test for assessment of the integrity of the spinal cord during operations for scoliosis. *J Bone Joint Surg Am* 79(2):208–212.

50. Jensen JE, Jensen TG, Smith TK, et al. (1982): Nutrition in orthopedic surgery. *J Bone Joint Surg Am* 64:1263–1272.

51. Johnston CE II (1986): Post laminectomy kyphoscoliosis following surgical treatment for spinal cord astrocytoma. *Orthopedics* 9:587–594.

52. Kling TF, Fergusson NV, Leach AB, et al. (1985): The influence of induced hypotension and spine distraction on canine spinal cord blood flow. *Spine* 10:878–883.

53. Kohler R, Galland O, Mechin H, et al. (1990): The Dwyer procedure in the treatment of idiopathic scoliosis. A ten year follow-up review of 21 patients. *Spine* 15:75–80.

54. Kobranisky NL, Letts RM, Patel LR, et al. (1987): 1-Desamino-8-D-arginine vasopressin (Desmopressin) decreases blood loss in patients having Harrington rod spinal fusion surgery. *Ann Intern Med* 107:446–450.

55. Kornberg M, Herndon WA, Rechtine GR (1985): Lumbar nerve root compression at the site of hook insertion. *Spine* 10:853–855.

56. Kretzler JE, Renshaw TS (1991): Wound infections following spinal fusion surgery. In: *Proceedings of the Annual Meeting of the Pediatric Orthopaedic Society of North America,* Dallas, Texas.

57. Lenke LG, Bridwell KH, Blanke K, et al. (1995): Analysis of pulmonary function and chest cage dimension changes after thoracoplasty in idiopathic scoliosis. *Spine* 20(12):1343–50

58. Lennon RL, Hosking MP, Gray JR, et al. (1987): The effect of intraoperative blood salvage and induced hyoptension on transfusion requirements during surgical procedures. *Mayo Clin Proc* 62:1090–1094.

59. Lonstein JE, Winter RB, Moe JH, et al. (1980): Neurologic deficits secondary to spinal deformity. A review of the literature and report of 43 cases. *Spine* 5:331–355.

60. Mazur J, Menelaus MB, Dickens DR, et al. (1986): Efficacy of surgical management of scoliosis in myelomeningocele: correction of deformity and alteration of functional status. *J Pediatr Orthop* 6:568–575.

61. McBride GG, Bradford DS (1983): Vertebral body replacement with femoral neck allograft and vascularized rib strut graft. A technique for treating post-traumatic kyphosis with neurological defect. *Spine* 8:406–415.

62. McCall RE, Bilderback KK (1997): Use of intravenous Premarin to decrease postoperative blood loss after pediatric scoliosis surgery. *Spine* 22(12):1394–1397.

63. McCarthy RE, Lonstein JE, Mertz JD, et al. (1990): Air embolism in spine surgery. *J Spinal Disord* 3(1):1–5.

64. McCarthy RE, Peek RD, Morrissy RT, et al. (1986): Allograft bone in spinal fusion for paralytic scoliosis. *J Bone Joint Surg Am* 68:370–375.

65. McEwen DG, Bunnell WP, Sriram K (1975): Acute neurological complications in the treatment of scoliosis. *J Bone Joint Surg Am* 57:404.

66. McMaster MJ (1984): Occult interspinal anomalies and congenital scoliosis. *J Bone Joint Surg Am* 66:588–601.

67. McQuay HJ, Carroll D, Moore RA (1988): Postoperative orthopedic pain—the effect of opiate premedication and local anaesthetic blocks. *Pain* 33:291–295.

68. Mesrobian RB, Epps JL (1986): Midtracheal obstruction after Harrington rod placement in a patient with Marfan's syndrome. *Anesth Analg* 65:411–413.

69. Michel CR, Lalain JJ (1985): Late results of Harrington's operation. Long-term evolution of the lumbar spine below the fused segments. *Spine* 10:414–420.

70. Mielke CH, Lonstein JE, Denis F, et al. (1989): Surgical treatment of adolescent idiopathic scoliosis. A comparative analysis. *J Bone Joint Surg Am* 71:1170–1177.

71. Moe JH, Purcell GA, Bradford DS (1983): Zielke instrumentation (VDS) for the correction of spinal curvature. Analysis of results in 66 patients. *Clin Orthop* 180:133–153.

72. Moran MM, Kroon D, Tredwell SJ, et al. (1992): The role of autologous blood transfusions in adolescents undergoing spinal surgery. In: Proceedings of the Canadian Orthopaedics Meeting, June 1992, Toronto, Canada.

73. Moskovich R, Cheong-Leen P (1986): Vascular compression of the duodenum. *J R Soc Med* 79:465–467.

74. Munns SW, Morrissy RT, Golladay ES, et al. (1984): Hyperalimentation for superior mesenteric-artery (cast) syndrome following correction of spinal deformity. *J Bone Joint Surg Am* 66:1175–1177.

75. Murray DJ, Forbes RB, Titone MB, et al. (1997): Transfusion management in pediatric and adolescent scoliosis surgery. Efficacy of autologous blood. *Spine* 22(23):2735–2740.

76. Murray DJ, Pennell BJ, Weinstein SL, et al. (1995): Packed red cells in acute blood loss: dilutional coagulopathy as a cause of surgical bleeding [see comments]. *Anesth Analg* 80(2):336–342; comments in *Anesth Analg* 80(2):215–216.

77. Nelson CL, Poskarich CL (1990): Nutritional status and outcome

in orthopedic patients. In: Esterhai JL, Gristina AC, Poss R, eds. *Musculoskeletal infection.* American Academy of Orthopedic Surgery.

78. O'Brien JP, Yau AC, Gertzbin S, et al. (1975): Combined staged anterior and posterior correction and fusion of the spine in scoliosis following poliomyelitis. *Clin Orthop* 110:81–89.

79. Pehrsson K, Larsson S, Nachemson A, et al. (1991): Mortality and causes of death in patients with untreated scoliosis. In: *Proceedings of the 25th Annual Meeting of the Scoliosis Research Society,* September.

80. Pizzutillo PD, Mirenda W, MacEwen GD (1986): Posterolateral fusion for spondylolisthesis in adolescence. *J Pediatr Orthop* 6:311–316.

81. Rainey-Macdonald CG, Holliday RL, Wells GA, et al. (1983): Validity of a two-variable nutritional index for use in selecting candidates for nutritional support. *J Parent Ent Nutr* 7:15–20.

82. Rees D, Jones MW, Owen R, et al. (1989): Scoliosis surgery in the Prader-Willi syndrome. *J Bone Joint Surg Br* 71:685–688.

83. Rinsky LA, Gamble JG, Bleck EE (1985): Segmental instrumentation without fusion in children with progressive scoliosis. *J Pediatr Orthop* 5:687–690.

84. Riseborough EJ (1977): Irradiation induced kyphosis. *Clin Orthop* 128:101–106.

85. Robin GC (1984): Scoliosis in familial dysautonomia. *Bull Hosp Joint Dis Orthop Inst* 44:16–26.

86. Rodgers WB, Coran DL, Kharrazi FD, et al. (1997): Increasing lordosis of the occipitocervical junction after arthrodesis in young children: the occipitocervical crankshaft phenomenon. *J Pediatr Orthop* 17(6):762–765.

87. Rylance PB, Carli F, McArthur SE, et al. (1988): The effect of induced hypotension and tissue trauma on renal function in scoliosis surgery. *J Bone Joint Surg Br* 70:127–129.

88. Sanders JO, Little DG, Richards BS (1997): Prediction of the crankshaft phenomenon by peak height velocity. *Spine* 22(12):1352–1356; discussion 1356–1357.

89. Savini R, Cervellati S, Beroaldo E (1980): Spinal deformities in Marfan's syndrome. *Ital J Orthop Traumatol* 6:19–40.

90. Savini R, Parisini P, Cervellati S, et al. (1983): Surgical treatment of vertebral deformities in neurofibromatosis. *Ital J Orthop Traumatol* 9:13–24.

91. Schoenecker PL, Cole HO, Herring JA, et al. (1990): Cauda equina syndrome after in situ arthrodesis for severe spondylolisthesis at the lumbosacral junction. *J Bone Joint Surg Am* 72:369–377.

92. Seitsalo S, Osterman K, Hyvarinen H, et al. (1990): Severe spondylolisthesis in children and adolescents. A long-term review of fusion in situ. *J Bone Joint Surg Br* 72:259–265.

93. Seitsalo S (1990): Operative and conservative treatment of moderate spondylolisthesis in young patients. *J Bone Joint Surg Br* 72:908–913.

94. Shaw BA, Watson TC, Merzel DI, et al. (1996): The safety of continuous epidural infusion for postoperative analgesia in pediatric spine surgery. *J Pediatr Orthop* 16(3):374–377.

95. Shen WJ, McDowell GS, Burke SW, et al. (1996): Routine preoperative MRI and SEP studies in adolescent idiopathic scoliosis. *J Pediatr Orthop* 16(3):350–353.

96. Siller TA, Dickson JH, Erwin WD (1996): Efficacy and cost considerations of intraoperative autologous tranfusion in spinal fusion for idiopathic scoliosis with predeposited blood. *Spine* 21(7):848–852.

97. Slawski DP, Bridwell KH, Manley CB (1990): Acute renal obstruction after combined anterior and posterior arthrodeses on the convex side of the spine. A case report. *J Bone Joint Surg Am* 72:1259–1261.

98. Stanley TH, Ashbern MA, Fine PG (1991): *Anaesthesiology in pain management.* Dordrecht: Kluwer Academic Publishers.

99. Stanton RP, Meehan P, Lovell WW (1985): Surgical fusion in childhood spondylolisthesis. *J Pediatr Orthop* 5:411–415.

100. Stevens DB, Beard C (1989): Segmental spinal instrumentation for neuromuscular spinal deformity. *Clin Orthop* 242:164–168.

101. Streitz W, Brown JC, Bonnet CA (1977): Anterior fibula strut grafting in the treatment of kyphosis. *Clin Orthop* 128:140–148.

102. Taddonio RF (1982): Segmental spinal instrumentation in the management of neuromuscular spinal deformity. *Spine* 7:305–311.

103. Thompson GH, Wilber RG, Shaffer JW, et al. (1985): Segmental spinal instrumentation in idiopathic scoliosis. A preliminary report. *Spine* 10:623–630.

104. Thompson JP, Transfeldt EE, Bradford DS, et al. (1990): Decompensation after Cotrel-Dubousset instrumentation of idiopathic scoliosis. *Spine* 15:927–931.

105. Tredwell SJ, Sawatzky B (1990): The use of fibrin sealant to reduce blood loss during Cotrel-Dubousset instrumentation for idiopathic scoliosis. *Spine* 15:913–915.

106. Vauzelle C, Stagnara P, Jouvinroux P (1973): Functional monitoring of spinal cord activity during spinal surgery. *Clin Orthop* 93:173–178.

107. Vedantam R, Crawford AH (1997): The role of preoperative pulmonary function tests in patients with adolescent idiopathic scoliosis undergoing posterior spinal fusion. *Spine* 22(23):2731–2734.

108. Vitale MG, Stazzone EJ, Gelijns AC, et al. (1998): The effectiveness of preoperative erythropoietin in averting allogenic blood transfusion among children undergoing scoliosis surgery. *J Pediatr Orthop B* 7(3):203–209.

109. Vogel LC, Lubicky JP (1996): Neurologic and vascular complications of scoliosis surgery in patients with Ehlers-Danlos syndrome. A case report. *Spine* 21(21)2508–2514.

110. West J, Askin G, Clarke M, et al. (1990): Loss of vision in one eye following scoliosis surgery. *Br J Ophthalmol* 74:243–244.

111. Wilber RG, Rhompson GH, Shaffer JW, et al. (1984): Postoperative neurological deficits in segmental spinal instrumentation. A study using spinal cord monitoring. *J Bone Joint Surg Am* 66:1178–1187.

112. Winter RB, Lonstein JE, Heithoff KB, et al. (1997): Magnetic resonance imaging evaluation of the adolescent patient with idiopathic scoliosis before spinal instrumentation and fusion. A prospective, double-blinded study of 140 patients. *Spine* 22(8):855–888.

113. Winter RB, Moe JH, Lonstein JE (1984): Posterior spinal arthrodesis for congenital scoliosis. An analysis of the cases of two hundred and ninety patients, five to nineteen years old. *J Bone Joint Surg Am* 66:1188–1197.

114. Winter RB, Moe JH, Lonstein JE (1985): The surgical treatment of congenital kyphosis. A review of 94 patients age 5 years or older, with 2 years of more follow-up in 77 patients. *Spine* 10:224–231.

115. Woolf CJ (1983): Evidence for a central component on post-injury pain hypersensitivity. *Nature* 306:686–688.

116. Yngve D (1997): Abdominal reflexes. *J Pediatr Orthop* 17(1):105–108.

117. Yong-Hing K, Kalamchi A, MacEwen GD (1979): Cervical spine abnormalities in neurofibromatosis. *J Bone Joint Surg Am* 61:695–699.

118. York DH, Chabot RJ, Gaines RW (1987): Response variability of somatosensory evoked potentials during scoliosis surgery. *Spine* 12:864–875.

119. Zadeh HG, Sakka SA, Powell MP, et al. (1995): Absent superficial abdominal reflexes in children with scoliosis. An early indicator of syringomyelia. *J Bone Joint Surg Br* 77(5):762–767.

INDEX

Page references for figures are followed by an f, and page references for tables are followed by a t.